Arsenic Pollution

T0185658

RGS-IBG Book Series

Published

Forthcoming

Arsenic Pollution

A Global Synthesis

Peter Ravenscroft, Hugh Brammer
and Keith Richards

WILEY-BLACKWELL

A John Wiley & Sons, Ltd., Publication

This edition first published 2009
© 2009 Peter Ravenscroft, Hugh Brammer and Keith Richards

Blackwell Publishing was acquired by John Wiley & Sons in February 2007. Blackwell's publishing program has been merged with Wiley's global Scientific, Technical, and Medical business to form Wiley-Blackwell.

Registered Office
John Wiley & Sons Ltd, The Atrium, Southern Gate, Chichester, West Sussex, PO19 8SQ, United Kingdom

Editorial Offices
350 Main Street, Malden, MA 02148-5020, USA
9600 Garsington Road, Oxford, OX4 2DQ, UK
The Atrium, Southern Gate, Chichester, West Sussex, PO19 8SQ, UK

For details of our global editorial offices, for customer services, and for information about how to apply for permission to reuse the copyright material in this book please see our website at www.wiley.com/wiley-blackwell.

The right of Peter Ravenscroft, Hugh Brammer and Keith Richards to be identified as the authors of this work has been asserted in accordance with the Copyright, Designs and Patents Act 1988.

All rights reserved. No part of this publication may be reproduced, stored in a retrieval system, or transmitted, in any form or by any means, electronic, mechanical, photocopying, recording or otherwise, except as permitted by the UK Copyright, Designs and Patents Act 1988, without the prior permission of the publisher.

Wiley also publishes its books in a variety of electronic formats. Some content that appears in print may not be available in electronic books.

Designations used by companies to distinguish their products are often claimed as trademarks. All brand names and product names used in this book are trade names, service marks, trademarks or registered trademarks of their respective owners. The publisher is not associated with any product or vendor mentioned in this book. This publication is designed to provide accurate and authoritative information in regard to the subject matter covered. It is sold on the understanding that the publisher is not engaged in rendering professional services. If professional advice or other expert assistance is required, the services of a competent professional should be sought.

Library of Congress Cataloging-in-Publication Data

Ravenscroft, Peter.
  Arsenic pollution : a global synthesis / Peter Ravenscroft, Hugh Brammer, and Keith Richards.
    p. cm.
  Includes bibliographical references and index.
  ISBN 978-1-4051-8602-5 (hardcover : alk. paper)—ISBN 978-1-4051-8601-8 (pbk. : alk. paper) 1. Arsenic compounds—Environmental aspects. 2. Arsenic wastes—Environmental aspects. I. Brammer, H. II. Richards, K. S. III. Title.
  TD196.A77R38 2009
  363.738′49–dc22

                                                            2008013330

A catalogue record for this book is available from the British Library.

Set in 10/12pt Plantin by SPi Publisher Services, Pondicherry, India

1   2009

Contents

Figures

Tables

Series Editors' Preface

The RGS-IBG Book Series only publishes work of the highest international standing. Its emphasis is on distinctive new developments in human and physical geography, although it is also open to contributions from cognate disciplines whose interests overlap with those of geographers. The Series places strong emphasis on theoretically-informed and empirically-strong texts. Reflecting the vibrant and diverse theoretical and empirical agendas that characterize the contemporary discipline, contributions are expected to inform, challenge and stimulate the reader. Overall, the RGS-IBG Book Series seeks to promote scholarly publications that leave an intellectual mark and change the way readers think about particular issues, methods or theories.

For details on how to submit a proposal please visit:
www.rgsbookseries.com

Kevin Ward
University of Manchester, UK

Joanna Bullard
Loughborough University, UK

RGS-IBG Book Series Editors

Acknowledgements

Many persons have assisted in the preparation of this book through discussions and the supply of information, and are listed in alphabetical order below: Bill Adams (Department of Geography, Cambridge) for discussion, support and encouragement; Feroze Ahmed (Bangladesh University of Engineering and Technology) for reviewing Chapter 7; Kazi Matin Ahmed (Dhaka University) for discussions regarding Bangladesh, and reviewing Chapter 8; David Banks of Holymoor Consultancy for clarifications regarding arsenic in Norway; Bob Bredberg regarding the geology of Madoc, Ontario; Robert Brinkman (ex-FAO) for discussion of many subjects, especially regarding soils and agriculture; Dipankar Chakraborti, Amir Hossain and Bashkar Das (Jadavpur University, Kolkata) for hospitality, discussions and guiding one of the authors on a tour of the Technology Park Project; Chris Daughney of GNS Science for information on groundwater quality monitoring in New Zealand; Wole Gbadebo (University of Agriculture, Abeokuta) and Othniel Habila (UNICEF) for access to information on arsenic testing in Nigeria; Meera Hira-Smith (University of California, Berkeley) for arranging a visit to Project Well in West Bengal and discussions regarding dug wells; Guy Howard (DFID) for access to information and discussion concerning the RAAMO study in Bangladesh; Richard Johnston (UNICEF) for access to information concerning arsenic in Burkina Faso; K. Kestutis (Geological Survey of Lithuania) for providing data on As concentrations in Lithuania; Craig Meisner (Cornell University), G. Pannaulah (CIMMYT) and Richard Loeppert (Texas A&M University) for discussions regarding agriculture in Bangladesh and photographs of diseased rice plants; I.T. Mbotake (University of Buea) regarding arsenic in Cameroon; John McArthur (University College London) for many valuable discussions, especially regarding geochemistry, Bangladesh and West Bengal, and reviewing chapters 2 and 3; the NGO Forum for Water Supply (Bangladesh), especially M.A. Hasnat, for arsenic education materials; Ross Nickson (UNICEF) for information on arsenic in India, many helpful discussions, and for reviewing Chapter 6; Kirk Nordstrom (US Geological Survey) for information regarding Fairbanks, Alaska and other discussions; Ryuji Ogata (JICA) for data on deep wells in Bangladesh; Roberto Oyarzun (Madrid University) for information on river and sediment chemistry in Chile; Stanislav Rapant (Geological Survey, Bratislava) regarding arsenic pollution in Slovakia; V.K. Saxena (National Geophysical research Institute) for information on geothermal waters in India; Arup Sengupta (Lehigh University) and S. Sarkar, D. Ghosh and Samir Bag (Bengal Engineering College, Kolkata) for assistance in visiting arsenic removal plants in West Bengal; Allan Smith (University of California, Berkeley) for helpful comments regarding the health effects of arsenic; Ondra Sracek, for many valuable discussions and reviewing sections on South and Central America; Philip Stickler and Ian Agnew (Department of Geography, Cambridge) for their diligence in drafting the figures; Rafaella Vivona (IRSA) from providing information regarding arsenic in Italy; Rob Ward (Environment Agency) for information on arsenic in England and Wales; Richard Wilson (Harvard University) or helpful discussions; Scott Wilkinson (University of Canterbury) for access to his thesis on arsenic in New Zealand; Severn-Trent Services Ltd for photographs of arsenic removal plants in the UK; and any others we have overlooked.

The authors organised an international interdisciplinary meeting on *Arsenic: the Geography of a Global Problem,* on 29 August 2007 during the Annual Conference of the Royal Geographical Society/Institute of British Geographers at the RGS in London. Presentations at the conference are at: http://www.geog.cam.ac.uk/research/projects/arsenic/symposium/. Contributors came from several affected countries and concerned research groups, and included: George Adamson, K Matin Ahmed, Feroze Ahmed, Nupur Bose, William Burgess, Johanna Buschmann, Vicenta Devesa, Ashok Ghosh, M. Manzurul Hassan, Meera M Hira-Smith, Mohammad Hoque, Guy Howard, Jiin-Shuh Jean, John M. McArthur, Andrew Meharg, Debapriya Mondal, Bibhash Nath, Ross Nickson, David Polya, Mahmuder Rahman, Sudhanshu Sinha, Allan H. Smith, Ondra Sracek, Farhana Sultana, Richard Wilson and Yan Zheng. We are grateful for their involvement in an event designed to heighten interest in and concern for the arsenic contamination problem, and to Clarissa Brocklehurst, Ross Nickson and Oluwafemi Odediran for arranging a UNICEF meeting at the RGS on 30th August to follow up issues raised during the conference. Presentations and discussion over these two days contributed significantly to our thinking about the content of the book.

Finally, we are especially grateful to Downing College, Cambridge, and particularly to Dr Susan Lintott, for supporting this whole project and making possible the financial arrangements for its successful prosecution and conclusion.

Preface

Readers may be surprised to learn that the most severe effect of human impact on environmental systems is *not* climate change. But that is what this book sets out to show.

One similarity between global warming and the arsenic crisis is that in both, human actions accentuate risks associated with otherwise natural phenomena. Another is that the consequences affect the global poor most severely. Indeed, this dimension is already obvious from the history of the arsenic crisis. Nearly 50 million people in south and east Asia have, for some decades, drunk water contaminated with arsenic at levels above the *old* WHO standard of 50 ppb. Many already have clinical symptoms of arsenicosis, leading to this being referred to as history's largest mass poisoning. By contrast, the USA has diverse sources and types of arsenic contamination in water supplies, but little evidence that this has a significant effect, because of better water treatment and better general health in the population.

What is less widely understood is the latency of the effects of chronic arsenic poisoning. Even if a solution to the problem of water supply quality is found soon, many who have been drinking contaminated water will still suffer cancer in spite of switching to clean water. Furthermore, arsenic ingestion is often estimated from water intake alone, although it is increasingly apparent that an additional loading arises from arsenic in food, especially from paddy rice grown with contaminated irrigation water. Soils thus irrigated may accumulate arsenic to phytotoxic levels, creating a problem of latent effects on crop yields.

That we find ourselves in this position reflects badly on both environmental science and the development process. Water becomes naturally contaminated by arsenic in several ways, and we must understand how this arises under different geological, geomorphological and geographical circumstances. The environmental sciences have not always successfully anticipated this sensitivity to specific circumstances, and one consequence of emphasis on climate change is a global focus that tends to avoid the issue of such sensitivity, and its potential meaning for regionally vulnerable populations. Questions that transcend disciplinary boundaries also still offer challenges; the reductive dissolution of arsenic might have been understood sooner had groundwater chemists talked at an earlier stage to marine geochemists. These shortcomings meant that science was unprepared for the consequences when development agencies sought to solve the problem of enteric disease caused by polluted surface water supplies, by providing shallow tube wells. These wells tapped aquifers in which precisely that process of reductive dissolution had elevated the dissolved arsenic concentrations to unhealthy levels.

Since these events, and the belated recognition of the consequential mass poisoning, research in the field has burgeoned, and it is now timely to synthesise the knowledge gained. In doing so, we examine the geochemistry of arsenic and its mobilisation, and the geomorphologies and geologies that define the geography of these processes. We suggest simple tools to identify areas where high levels of arsenic in groundwater might be expected, but have yet to be identified. We assess the risks for crop production and food contamination, and review the health and social effects, observed and potential. We then consider mitigation options, through water-supply substitution and point-of-use treatment; and their additional risks (e.g., drawdown of arsenic into overexploited deeper aquifers, and disposal of arsenic wastes generated by treatment procedures). And we examine these issues not only in general, but also as geographies, characterised by spatial diversity and multiple knowledge bases.

One of us, Hugh Brammer, not only contributed to the book, but also supported the research and the linked conference (see Acknowledgements, p. xxi) financially. His desire to do so arose from his experience in Bangladesh working on soils, agriculture and disaster preparedness, and his belief in the capacity of geography to facilitate better understanding of both the mobilisation of arsenic, and the cultural context of the management of its effects and their mitigation.

We hope this book will be valued as a synthesis of current knowledge about arsenic contamination and the crisis it has caused, and about what needs to be done to accelerate mitigation. We hope it will help to disseminate information and spread realisation of the nature and scale of the problem to a wider range of professionals and publics so that pressure to act on these issues will grow. We also offer it as an example of the practical value of geography in helping to tackle environmental and development problems with multidisciplinary dimensions and regionally differentiated consequences.

Keith Richards
Vice-President (Research), RGS-IBG (2004-2007)
18 August 2008
Department of Geography, University of Cambridge

Abbreviations

AA	activated alumina
AD	alkali desorption
AAS	atomic absorption spectrometry; with variants, the generally preferred analytical method for analysis of arsenic in water.
ADI	average daily intake
AMD	acid mine drainage
ARP	arsenic removal plant
As(III)	trivalent arsenic, normally referring to the arsenite ion in solution
As(V)	pentavalent arsenic, normally referring to the arsenate ion in solution
a.s.l	above sea level
ASM	arsenical skin manifestation
ASV	anodic stripping voltammetry; an analytical technique for measuring ions in solution
BFD	Blackfoot Disease; a serious peripheral vascular disease common in Taiwan
b.g.l.	below ground level
BGS	British Geological Survey
BMI	body mass index
BP	before present (years); used in radiometric dating to mean years before 1950.
BV	bed volumes; normally referring to the volume treatment medium in arsenic removal plants.
CI	confidence interval (normally 95% or 99%)
CLD	chronic lung disease
CVD	cardiovascular disease
DALY	disability adjusted life years
DCH	Dhaka Community Hospital

DMA^{III}	dimethylarsinous acid
DMA^V	dimethylarsinic acid
DO	dissolved oxygen
DOC	dissolved organic carbon
DOM	dissolved organic matter (similar to DOC)
DPHE	Department of Public Health Engineering (Bangladesh)
DTW	deep tubewell. This term has different meanings for irrigation and water supply. In irrigation in Bangladesh and India it is a high-capacity (50–60 L/s) motorised well equipped with a vertical-turbine or submersible pump. For water supply, however, it does refer to the depth of the well
DWS	drinking water standard
EC	electrical or electrolytic conductivity; a simple and reliable measure of the TDS content of water
Eh	a measure (normally in millivolts) of the oxidising (positive values) or reducing (negative values) potential of a water
FAO	Food and Agriculture Organization (of the United Nations)
GAC	granulated activated carbon
GF-AAS	graphite furnace atomic absorption spectrometry
GV	(WHO) guideline value (for drinking water)
ha	hectare
HACRE	*Hidroarsenicismo Cronico Regional Endemico* (chronic endemic regional hydroarsenicism). This term is applied to the characteristic symptoms of arsenic poisoning in Cordoba Province of Argentina.
HH	household
ICP	inductively coupled plasma (spectrometry). An analytical method suitable for analysis of arsenic and a broad spectrum of other elements
IHD	ischaemic heart disease, related to poor heart circulation
IRP	iron-removal plant
K$_d$	distribution coefficient; a measure of partitioning of contaminants between the solid and liquid phases
LGM	Last Glacial Maximum; the peak of the final Pleistocene glaciation between 18,000 and 30,000 years ago, when sea level fell to about 120–130 m below its present level
MDI	maximum daily intake
MIT	Massachusetts Institute of Technology
MMA^{III}	monomethylarsonous acid
MMA^V	monomethylarsonic acid
MCL	maximum contaminant/concentration level
MRL	minimal risk level
NCPF	non-cirrhotic portal fibrosis (a liver disease)

NOAEL	no observed adverse effect level
NOM	natural organic matter
OR	odds ratio. Statistical term used by epidemiologists, similar to the 'prevalence odds ratio' and 'risk ratio'. OR is used in case-control studies; it is the ratio of the odds of exposure in the affected group to the odds of exposure in the control group. An odds ratio of 2 means that people in the studied group are twice as likely to be afflicted as in the control group.
PAHO	Pan American Health Organisation
PHED	Public Health Engineering Directorate (West Bengal, India)
POU	point of use (treatment system).
ppb	parts per billion; a unit of concentration equivalent to μg/L in dilute solutions.
ppm	parts per million; a unit of concentration equivalent to mg/L in dilute solutions.
PSF	pond sand filter
QFR	quartz:feldspar:rock fragments ratio; normally describing sand composition
RD	reductive dissolution
R_f	retardation factor; a measure of how much the movement of a contaminant is retarded compared with the water in which it is dissolved
RSSCT	rapid small scale column testing (in water treatment studies)
RWH	rainwater harvesting
SMR	standardised mortality ratio. SMR is calculated after adjusting the age distribution of the group studied to fit that of an international standard age-distribution to ensure unbiased comparisons between different regions of the world
SO	sulphide oxidation
SOES	School of Environmental Studies, at Jadavpur University in Kolkata
SSAAB	South and Southeast Asian Arsenic Belt
SSF	slow sand filter
STW	shallow tubewell. The term is used in Bangladesh and India to describe a medium capacity (10–15 L/s) motorised irrigation wells equipped with a surface-mounted centrifugal pump.
TCLP	toxicity characteristic leaching procedure; a US Environmental Protection Agency test for assessing the pollution of waste prior to disposal
TDS	total dissolved solids (in water)
TTC	thermo-tolerant coliforms
UP	Uttar Pradesh (India)
WHO	World Health Organization

Glossary

Arsenicosis	A term describing the characteristic clinical effects of chronic arsenic poisoning
Arteriosclerosis	Medical term referring to hardening and/or narrowing of the arteries
Authigenic	A mineral or crystal formed in a sediment after its deposition
Block	This term has special meaning in West Bengal, an administrative unit equivalent to the Bangladeshi term upazila
Bowen's disease	A pre-cancerous form of skin lesion
Framboidal	Adjective derived from the French word for raspberry, usually applied to describe a form of authigenic pyrite
Hepatic	Concerning the liver
Hyperpigmentation	Darkening of the skin
Hypopigmentation	Lightening of the skin
Ischaemia	Restriction in blood supply with resultant damage of tissue
Keratosis	Skin disease producing painful corn-like growths or nodules
Melanosis	Darkening of the skin (opp. Leucomelanosis)
Myocardial infarction	Heart attack
Palaeosol	An ancient, normally buried, soil horizon
Raynaud's syndrome	A debilitating condition that causes periods of severely restricted blood flow to the fingers and toes, and sometimes the nose or ears
Renal	Concerning the kidneys
Transmissivity	The result of multiplying the permeability of an aquifer by its thickness – its water transmitting capacity
Upazila	An administrative unit in Bangladesh, a subdivision of a district, and roughly equivalent to a county

Chapter One

Introduction

1.1 Background

Arsenic, a notorious poison, is now recognised to be one of the world's greatest environmental hazards, threatening the lives of several hundred million people. Andrew Meharg (2005), in his book *Venomous Earth*, presents fascinating accounts of the use of arsenic for murder, medicine and wallpaper[1]. Sometimes known as the King of Poisons, arsenic has been known to humankind for thousands of years, being used to harden bronze in the Middle East around 3000 BC, and prized as a dye by the Egyptians, Greeks and Romans. In the fifth century BC, Hippocrates suggested using arsenic compounds as an ulcer treatment, while in the first and second centuries AD, the Roman Emperor Nero and Mithridates, King of Pontus, both used arsenic to murder their enemies. However, we will not describe the human use and abuse of arsenic further, because that is not the purpose of this book. Here, we are concerned with the insidious, creeping effects of naturally occurring arsenic in rocks and soils, which finds its way into underground water and streams, or is drawn into the roots of plants. This arsenic, withdrawn from the ground by wells and used for drinking, does not kill suddenly, but in the past 20 or 30 years has surely accounted for many more deaths than all the arsenical poisonings in history.

Long-term exposure to low levels of arsenic in food and water produces a broad array of effects on human health that are often described by the catch-all term arsenicosis. Early symptoms are non-specific effects such as muscular weakness, lassitude and mild psychological effects. These are followed by characteristic skin ailments such as changes in skin pigmentation and progressively painful skin lesions, known as keratosis. At the same time, arsenic causes a wide range of other effects on health, including diseases of the liver and kidney, cardio-vascular and peripheral vascular diseases, neurological effects, diabetes and chronic and acute lung disease. Continued exposure to arsenic can lead to gangrene, cancers of the skin, lung, liver, kidney and bladder, and thereby to death.

Because the effects of arsenic depend on cumulative exposure, the symptoms are most commonly seen in adults and, because of lifestyle, in men more than in women. As symptoms develop, a person's ability to live a normal life is reduced. Sufferers may become unable to work, severely affecting the welfare of their families. Meanwhile, so long as exposure continues, the patient's condition will continue to deteriorate, while their ability to cope with the illness is reduced. The stigma of arsenic poisoning revealed in the symptoms of arsenicosis, and even of simply owning a polluted well, gives rise to social impacts such as ostracism and social and economic exclusion, with the burden falling disproportionately on women.

Naturally occurring arsenic in groundwater used for drinking and cooking is a catastrophe of global proportions. The World Health Organization (WHO) described the situation in Bangladesh as 'the largest poisoning of a population in history' (Smith et al., 2000). It is estimated that in 1998–99 around 27 million people were drinking water containing more than the national standard of 50 parts per billion (ppb) of arsenic. To this total should be added another 6 million people in the adjoining area of West Bengal in India. Worse, the WHO and many countries now consider 50 ppb unsafe, and recommend a limit of only 10 ppb. At this level, around 50 million people in Bangladesh, about 40% of the total population, and about 12 million people in West Bengal, are consuming dangerous concentrations of arsenic. If the statistics were not dire enough, these countries, striving to reduce the burden of poverty, are desperately ill-equipped to cope with the additional disease burden of arsenicosis. Moreover, suffering falls disproportionately on the poor, who are malnourished, drink more well-water, eat more arsenic in their diet and are less able to resist the toxic effects of arsenic than their better-off counterparts. Indeed, there is evidence that, within affected regions, the poor are most likely to show clinical symptoms of arsenicosis.

1.2   The Nature of Arsenic Pollution

Some of the features that made arsenic such an attractive poison – that it is colourless, tasteless and odourless – also contributed to its late discovery as an environmental contaminant. Further, when exposure is continuous over a period of years, arsenic is toxic at very low concentrations. In the past, it was no simple task to measure arsenic concentrations in water, and so, because it was not recognised as a problem, it was not routinely tested for. Unfortunately, in many parts of the world, arsenic is naturally present in groundwater that is easily accessible and otherwise fit for drinking. Because it is in water used for drinking and cooking, and sometimes in staple foods as well, arsenic may be consumed in large quantities and for long periods. However, arsenic is almost never found in natural waters at concentrations that are acutely poisonous[2]. Chronic poisoning involves a long latent period before clinical symptoms develop. When water containing tens to a few hundreds of ppb is consumed continuously, symptoms of arsenicosis typically become apparent after periods of 2–10 years.

Natural arsenic pollution occurs in diverse geological and climatic conditions. It occurs most commonly in sands deposited by large rivers, and most of the worst cases are found in the tropical river basins of Asia. However, arsenic-contaminated groundwater is found in unconsolidated sediments and sedimentary, igneous and metamorphic rocks ranging in age from a few thousand to more than a billion years old. Arsenic pollution is found in climates ranging from the hot and humid tropics, to Arctic Alaska and hyperarid deserts. Despite this diversity, in any given location, contamination usually has a well-defined relationship to particular strata, or to particular depths of wells.

In many areas where groundwater contains high levels of arsenic, so too do the soils. Although the quantities vary greatly, most plants take up arsenic through their roots and into the edible parts. Where arsenic-rich groundwater is used for irrigation, the arsenic content of soils gradually builds up, and leads to more arsenic being taken up by plants. Thus, the effects of arsenic in food and water are both additive and cumulative. The worst conditions occur in the subsistence rice economies of Asia, where rice is irrigated with arsenic-contaminated water. The diet of the rural poor typically comprises locally grown rice with little fruit, vegetables or meat, and so a deficiency of vitamins, minerals and protein reduces their ability to resist the toxic effects of arsenic. If their food is cooked in, and washed down with, polluted well-water, the daily intake of arsenic can be ten times the recommended maximum. Thus, poverty and environmental hazards combine to exacerbate the suffering of poor, rural populations.

1.3 History of Natural Arsenic Contamination

1.3.1 Early discoveries

Although almost unknown 25 years ago, natural arsenic contamination affects more than 70 countries in the world (Figure 1.1). Unlike arsenic in minerals, such as orpiment and realgar, the occurrence of arsenic in natural waters has been known for barely 100 years. The earliest measurement of arsenic in natural water was by the famous German chemist Fresenius

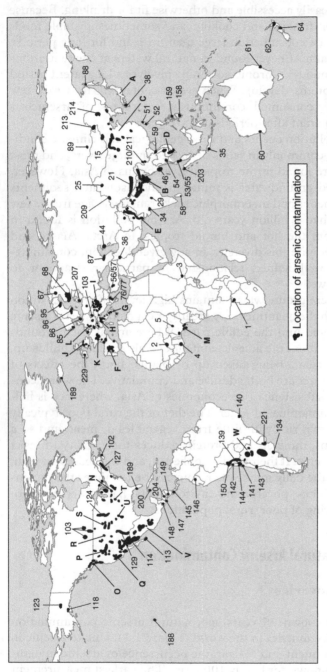

Figure 1.1 Global distribution of arsenic contamination. Note that the size of each affected area should not be confused with either the intensity and severity of pollution, or the numbers of people affected, which are elaborated in Chapters 8–10. The map numbers are detailed in Table 1.2. Where the numbered locations are too close to show on the map, groups of affected regions are identified by letter. Asia: A, 37, 39–41 & 43; B, 10, 11, 31–33, 154–157 and 205; C, 13, 14, 16–20, 22–24, 26; D, 12, 58, 201 and 202; E, 9, 28, 30, 47, 48 and 49 (see Fig. 8.1). Europe: F, 92, 93, 96 and 200; G, 80, 82, 83, 191 and 198; H, 79, 81, 166, 194, 195 and 215; I, 65, 78, 90, 91, 151, 161, 223; J, 97, 98, 216–220; K, 69–72, 152, 164; L, 73–75, 84, 165, 192 (see Fig. 9.17). Africa: M, 6–8, 190 (see Fig. 10.6). North America: N, 100, 101, 123, 133; O, 99, 104, 131, 132 and 187; P, 121, 170–174, 182; Q, 116, 117, 130, 175, 177, 188, 193; R, 126, 169, 176, 183, 186; S, 107, 119, 168, 184; T, 122, 178, 179, 181, 185; U, 128, 167; V, 106, 110–112, 115 (see Fig. 9.1). South America: W, 135–138 (see Fig 10.1).

at Wiesbaden Spa in 1885 (Schwenzer et al., 2001). Although historically interesting, this water was not consumed in sufficient quantities to cause illness. The earliest report of arsenic poisoning from well-water, which apparently caused skin cancer, was from Poland in 1898 (Mandal and Suzuki, 2002), although ironically there are no later reports from Poland. The first major case of endemic disease caused by arsenic in drinking water was reported in the 1920s in Cordoba Province of Argentina (Bado, 1939), where it is associated with a type of skin cancer known as Bel Ville disease. Although this affected thousands, perhaps tens of thousands, of people, it was little known outside Argentina until the end of the 20th century.

1.3.2 The mid-twentieth century

From the 1930s to the 1970s, there were few discoveries of natural arsenic contamination, although minor occurrences were noted in Canada (Wyllie, 1937) and New Zealand (Grimmett and McIntosh, 1939). In the 1960s, arsenic poisoning from well-water became well known in Taiwan, which has a special place in the history of epidemiological studies of arsenic. In Taiwan, arsenic caused a range of severe illnesses, including Blackfoot Disease, which is almost unique to southwest Taiwan. However, there were no international publications concerning the science of its occurrence, and the Taiwan case was largely unknown amongst water scientists[3]. Arsenic contamination is not only an issue in the developing world. The USA is, in fact, one of the most widely affected countries in the world, although the health impacts are quite small. The USA has been curiously slow to recognise and respond to the extent of contamination. A classic paper on the geochemistry of arsenic by Onishi and Sandell (1955) only recorded arsenic in hot springs and volcanic exhalations. A 1969 survey of 1000 water supplies reported that only 0.5% exceeded 10 ppb and 0.2% exceeded 50 ppb, and stated that arsenic represented 'no current threat to public health in the US' (Ferguson and Gavis, 1972). However, later surveys of water supplies reported that 1% exceeded 50 ppb and 8% exceeded 10 ppb (Ryker, 2003). In the 1970s, arsenic contamination was identified in Nova Scotia in Canada, where 25% of people drinking water with >50 ppb showed mild clinical symptoms (Grantham and Jones, 1977). Around the same time, almost the whole population of Antofagasta in northern Chile was exposed to 800 ppb As between 1958 and 1971, resulting in widespread and severe illness. However, the death toll attributed to arsenic-induced cancer, lung and heart disease in the decades following commissioning of a municipal treatment plant was about four times higher than during the period of peak exposure (Yuan et al., 2007).

1.3.3   The late twentieth century

Until the 1980s, the picture that emerges is one of isolated problems that did not attract international attention. The reasons are unclear, but there are probably three main explanations. First, arsenic was not routinely tested for in many countries, and second, there was a relatively poor knowledge of the health effects of low levels of arsenic. The third reason is cultural. The two major problems at the time (Argentina and Taiwan) were poorly known in Europe and North America and did not resonate with public health officials. Also, because arsenic was not perceived to be a problem in the home territories of the former colonial powers of Europe, they did not 'export' arsenic-testing protocols to their former colonies.

With hindsight, the 1980s may be seen as the period when the extent of pollution began to be recognised. Arsenic poisoning related to well-water was discovered in West Bengal (India) in 1983[4], although it took the rest of the decade for the size of the affected area to be appreciated. At about the same time, arsenic pollution was recognised in Hungary (Varsányi et al., 1991) and Xinjiang Province in China (Sun, 2004). However, in the political climate of the Cold War, there was apparently little awareness of the two latter problems in the west. Meanwhile, there was growing recognition of arsenic pollution in North America, with investigations of glacial aquifers in the mid-west by Matisoff et al. (1982), and a landmark publication by Welch et al. (1988) that documented 28 occurrences of groundwater arsenic in the southwest USA. While investigations in India and China had been triggered by medical diagnoses, the occurrences in the USA were not associated with clinical symptoms of arsenic poisoning.

In tropical Asia, drinking water was traditionally drawn from surface water or very shallow dug wells, and bacterial pollution of these water sources gave rise to epidemics of diarrhoeal diseases such as cholera and dysentery. Although the use of groundwater supplies began in the 1930s, it accelerated particularly after 1970 and into the 1990s, partly as a result of a deliberate policy promoted by UNICEF to reduce child mortality associated with enteric diseases. Tens of millions of cheap, shallow tubewells were drilled to obtain microbiologically safe drinking water. The major aim was to avoid polluted surface water sources that had caused widespread diarrhoeal disease. To this end, there was considerable success: in Bangladesh, between 1960 and 1996, child mortality dropped from 151 to 83 per thousand (Meharg, 2005). However, the switch from surface water did not occur without cost. For while the policy was largely successful in reducing enteric disease, and millions of deaths from this cause were prevented, in some areas the shallow tubewells that were substituted tapped arsenic-polluted groundwater, leading to chronic poisoning on a massive scale.

In the 1990s, arsenic pollution of groundwater burst from obscurity to receive the attention of the international press (e.g. Bearak, 1998), and radio and television networks such as CNN and the BBC. This transformation essentially took place in India and Bangladesh between 1994 and 1998, thanks particularly to the efforts of Dipankar Chakraborti and his colleagues at the School of Environmental Studies (SOES) at Jadavpur University in Kolkata, who described arsenic pollution in six districts of West Bengal as 'the biggest arsenic calamity in the world' (Das et al., 1994). For 10 years this was effectively unknown, even in neighbouring Bangladesh, except to a handful of individuals who chose to ignore or suppress the information. The tipping point was an international conference organised by Chakraborti in Kolkata in 1995. Almost overnight, the plight of millions of people in West Bengal was brought to the attention of the world's scientists, aid agencies and international media. The message was carried to Bangladesh, where geologists knew that the contamination must extend across the border, although none anticipated it would cover more than half of the country. Unlike its gradual revelation in West Bengal, Bangladesh progressed from discovery to comprehensive national mapping in two and a half years, and doctors soon began to recognise the symptoms of arsenic poisoning. From indifference in 1995, by the end of 1997, United Nations agencies, the World Bank and five bilateral donors were ready to commit millions of dollars to assist the Bangladesh Government implement a mitigation programme.

A second landmark conference took place in Dhaka in February 1998, organised by SOES and the Dhaka Community Hospital (DCH), which reiterated the magnitude of the problem in West Bengal, and revealed the even greater scale of contamination in Bangladesh. For the first time, the current scientific explanation of the pollution in Bengal was presented (Ahmed et al., 1998), showing that the cause was geological, and not anthropogenic, and acted as a stimulus for testing in surrounding countries. Over the next few years, extensive pollution was discovered in the river basins of Nepal, Myanmar, Cambodia, Vietnam and Pakistan (e.g. Jain and Ali, 2000; Nordstrom, 2002). Ironically, it was not until later that arsenic pollution was identified upstream from West Bengal in the Indian States of Bihar, Uttar Pradesh and Assam on the Ganges and Brahmaputra floodplains. Meanwhile, expanding studies in China discovered severe arsenic pollution in Inner Mongolia and Shanxi Provinces.

1.3.4 The twenty-first century

Since 2000, arsenic contamination has been found in other parts of the world, and new discoveries are regularly reported. In many parts of the world, especially Africa and South America, there is still a grave shortage of information, and it seems inevitable that more cases will be found in the future. However, new discoveries have also been driven by the lowering of drinking water standards in many countries. From the middle of the 20th century, most countries specified a standard of 50 ppb, but in 1993, the WHO reduced its guideline value for drinking water to 10 ppb. Beginning with Germany in 1996, many countries have adopted the new guideline as a legal standard, leading to major testing programmes, so that countries that previously did not have an arsenic problem suddenly acquired one, and were obliged to retrofit arsenic treatment to many existing public supplies. However, the countries that face the most severe problems, mostly poor and in Asia, have retained 50 ppb as the standard for drinking water.

Where arsenic contamination has been discovered recently, one of the puzzles is to know how long the poisoning has been going on. Is it a new phenomenon, or has it always been present, and why was it not recognised before? In most cases, there are no clear answers to these questions, yet it is widely perceived that extensive arsenicosis is a recent phenomenon, and this has led many people to assume an anthropogenic cause. While this is generally incorrect, and arsenic has been present in groundwater for thousands of years, there is a human connection because of the deliberate shift towards groundwater supply in the 20th century.

1.3.5 The growth of knowledge

Knowledge of arsenic contamination has expanded enormously in the past two to three decades. Commenting on the first diagnosis of arsenic poisoning due to well-water in India, Datta and Kaul (1976) noted that the only equivalent reports of arsenical skin lesions were from Chile and Taiwan. While overlooking Argentina, they were correct in principle. Likewise, Fowler (1977), summarising the conclusions of an international conference intended to 'assess the current level of scientific knowledge about arsenic as an environmental toxicant and to identify areas of needed research', observed that the most important sources of arsenic exposure were non-ferrous smelting and burning of arsenic-rich coal. He 'suggested' that steel smelters, burning of impregnated wood, and abandoned mines should be studied. Finally, he noted that 'natural sources of environmental arsenic release such as volcanoes and hotsprings were also recognised as important.' The occurrence of non-geothermal arsenic in aquifers or soils received no mention.

The subsequent growth of knowledge is reflected in the literature consulted during the preparation of this book. Although far from comprehensive, a database of 1100 publications explicitly concerning arsenic was compiled, for the period up to the end of 2006. Classified by decade (Table 1.1), over 90% of all publications were produced after 1990. The database included 789 geographically related publications, of which the largest group, 444

Table 1.1 Publications concerning arsenic by decade

Period	Publications Number	%
1931–40	3	0.3
1941–50	1	0.1
1951–60	1	0.1
1961–70	5	0.5
1971–80	26	2.4
1981–90	47	4.3
1991–2000	208	18.9
2001–2006	810	73.6

Source: Authors' database

publications, concerned arsenic in Asia, of which 83% had been published since the year 2000.

Because of the history of arsenic as a poison, the occurrence of accidental industrial poisonings, and its use as a medicine, medical investigators were reasonably well prepared to anticipate the symptoms of chronic arsenic poisoning. Earth and environmental scientists, however, were ill-prepared to respond to the discoveries of the 1980s and 1990s. The causes of the few known natural cases of arsenic pollution in Argentina, Chile, India and Taiwan were not seriously investigated until at least the late 1980s. It is hardly surprising, therefore, that the initial discoveries in other countries were met with confusion and uncertainty and, in some cases, denial. Until recently (Hiscock, 2005), the general texts on groundwater chemistry (e.g. Appelo and Postma, 1996; Langmuir, 1997) and hydrogeology included negligible descriptions of natural arsenic contamination[5].

1.4 Arsenic Pollution

The environmental literature makes diverse use of the terms contamination and pollution. Some authors use the term pollution when the cause is anthropogenic, while others use it as a measure of severity. In discussing arsenic in groundwater, an anthropogenic distinction is not particularly helpful. In many cases, the background levels are harmful, and in others, naturally elevated concentrations of arsenic have been modified by human action. Here we follow Chapman (2007) in using contamination to refer to the presence of a substance where it would not normally occur, or at concentrations above the natural background, whereas pollution is contamination that results in actual or potential adverse biological effects.

However, arsenic in drinking water has no well-defined threshold for adverse health effects, so we apply this distinction loosely, preferring the term contamination where health effects are not apparent, or less likely.

1.4.1   Unnatural pollution by arsenic

Humans have often polluted their environment with arsenic, usually in the processing of geological materials such as coal and metaliferous ores (Han et al., 2003). In mining, pollution may occur from improper disposal of wastes from sulphide-rich ores (Abrahams and Thornton, 1987; Williams, 2001). Exposed to air and rainwater, sulphides are oxidised to produce sulphate-rich, acid mine drainage (AMD) that often contains high arsenic concentrations. Arsenic-rich spoil heaps, such as from the Cornish tin-mines, have left a legacy of contaminated soil that prevents their use for food crops more than a 100 years after the mines were abandoned. Arsenic pollutes the air through the smelting of sulphide ores. Airborne arsenic may be inhaled, but also accumulates as fallout on soils, from where it may be taken up by crops or enter streams in runoff. Globally, the burning of coal has been the major anthropogenic input of arsenic to the surface environment (Han et al., 2003). Some coals contain high concentrations of arsenic, the worst case being in Guizhou Province of China, where power stations cause extensive air pollution, and even worse health effects result from burning coal inside households (Ding et al., 2001). Although now largely abandoned, arsenical pesticides were widely applied to orchards and cotton and rice fields in the USA, resulting in serious soil contamination (Peryea, 2002; Renshaw et al., 2006). In addition, chromated copper arsenate compounds have been widely used as wood preservatives, although this practice is now being discouraged (Hingston et al., 2001). Arsenic is also mobilised by other polluting activities such as landfill (Hounslow, 1980) and oil spills (Burgess and Pinto, 2005).

Important sources of knowledge about chronic arsenic poisoning were tragic industrial accidents such as the Manchester Beer Incident (which provided part of the basis for the original 50 ppb standard for arsenic in water), and the contamination of milk powder and soy sauce in Japan (Pershagen, 1983; Dakeishi et al., 2006). Historically, arsenic has been used as a medicine, and is still used in some cancer treatments, where the side-effects may be tolerated. Arsenical medicines were particularly popular in the 19th century until their association with keratosis and skin cancer was recognised. Some were simply quack medicines, but others such as Fowler's Solution were still in use in the 1970s (Meharg, 2005). Fowler's *Liquor Arsenicalis* was a 1% solution of potassium arsenite, taken internally, and was promoted as a cure for ague, fever and headache. One of the more bizarre cases of arsenic poisoning is that of the Styrian arsenic eaters in 19th century Austria (Meharg, 2005). The Styrian peasants believed that arsenic conferred plumpness to the figure and improved the complexion as well as aiding digestion and having aphrodisiac properties. These people consumed arsenic trioxide with food, at gradually increasing doses, eventually consuming doses that would normally be considered fatal. This latter observation suggests that the human body can develop a degree of tolerance to arsenic[6] (Przygoda et al., 2001).

1.4.2   Natural arsenic pollution

Arsenic in the natural environment

Arsenic is not a rare element in the Earth's crust, but it is unusual to find high concentrations in water. Although arsenic is found in some silicate minerals, such as biotite, the most important accumulations are found in two distinct mineral associations, sulphides and oxides, which themselves reflect how dissolved arsenic may be removed from groundwater. Arsenic can form sulphide minerals such as orpiment, realgar and arsenopyrite, and it also substitutes for sulphur, to be trapped in more common minerals such as pyrite (iron sulphide), chalcopyrite (copper sulphide), galena (lead sulphide) and sphalerite (zinc sulphide). These minerals commonly form in areas of hydrothermal activity, and are often associated with metal ores. However, pyrite, the most abundant of these minerals, also forms in swamps, peat basins, beneath the beds of lakes and seas, and in some aquifers. The important point is that they are stable when there are no sources of oxygen, but they are easily broken down by oxidation. Oxide minerals do not take arsenic into their structure, but have a great capacity to adsorb arsenic onto their surface. Iron oxides are the most important minerals in controlling the occurrence of arsenic in groundwater. In contrast to sulphides, oxides are formed in environments where there are ready sources of oxygen, and conversely break down and dissolve in anaerobic environments. Thus, there are two competing means of trapping arsenic in minerals, under oxidising and reducing conditions, and so arsenic contamination occurs where, for reasons described later, neither sulphides nor oxides can remove arsenic from solution.

The causes of natural arsenic pollution of groundwater

In natural waters, arsenic is usually found in one of four chemical associations, which occur in more-or-less predictable geological and climatic settings, and each of which is associated with a characteristic cause, or mobilisation mechanism. The water types and mobilisation mechanisms are themes that recur throughout the book because they determine not only where arsenic is found, but also how it may be avoided, how it affects agriculture, and how it may best be treated. The four mechanisms are described below in order of decreasing importance:

1 **Reductive dissolution** occurs when iron oxides, onto which arsenic is adsorbed, break down under the influence of decaying organic matter (which consumes oxygen sources) and dissolve, thereby releasing arsenic in the process. The groundwater produced by these processes is always strongly reducing, with high concentrations of iron and bicarbonate, while nitrate and sulphate are absent.
2 **Alkali desorption** occurs at high pH (≥8.0) and in the presence of dissolved oxygen, nitrate or sulphate, producing waters which can be termed 'alkali-oxic', and which have low concentrations of iron and manganese.
3 **Sulphide oxidation** occurs where sulphide minerals such as pyrite or arsenopyrite are exposed to oxygen, often at the water table, to produce waters that are typically both acid (pH 1–6) and sulphate-rich, but not necessarily high in iron.
4 **Geothermal** waters from deep, sometime volcanic, sources leach arsenic from the country rocks. The waters are distinguished primarily by elevated temperature, and usually also by a correlation of arsenic with chloride.

Soils, irrigation and agriculture

Combined exposure from food and water can significantly increase the disease burden from arsenic. In many affected areas, moderately high levels of arsenic are found in natural soils. Arsenic may be taken up through the roots of plants to accumulate in the edible parts. Where soil is the only source of arsenic, uptake by plants declines over time. However, greater problems may develop where arsenic in irrigation water accumulates in the soil and leads to increasing uptake by plants. In general, as a proportion of dry mass, leafy vegetables and some spices may take up the most arsenic, but when adjusted for dietary intake, grains such as rice make the largest contribution to human exposure. In some Asian countries this can be a larger source of exposure than drinking water. High concentrations of arsenic in soil can be toxic to rice, and can dramatically reduce yields. This worrying phenomenon has recently been recognised in South Asia (e.g. Duxbury and Panaullah, 2007), but as Reed and Sturgis (1936) noted 'arsenic toxicity in soils is no new problem'.

Extent of natural arsenic contamination

Known sites of natural arsenic contamination of surface and groundwater are listed in Table 1.2 and their locations shown in Figure 1.1[7]. The reader should take care not to confuse geographical extent with significance. The quality of mapping varies between sources; contamination is not necessarily

Table 1.2 Locations of natural arsenic contamination of surface and groundwaters. See Chapters 8 to 10 for details of individual occurrences. Locations marked as "Unspecified" are assigned a nominal location in the centre of the country, and Map ID refers to location numbers on Figure 1.1

Map ID	Name/location	Maximum As (ppb)	Map ID	Name/location	Maximum As (ppb)
Asia			211	Yunnan (S)	200
Afghanistan			26	Zhongmou, Zhengzhou	186
9	Logar and Ghazni		*India*		
Bangladesh			27	Assam	657
10	Chittagong coastal plain		28	Chandigarh	545
11	Bengal Basin	4000	29	Chattisgarh	1930
Cambodia			30	Himachal Pradesh	
12	Cambodia	1700	31	Nagaland	278
China			32	Thoubal (Manipur)	986
13	Datong Basin	1530	33	Tripura	444
14	Houshayu, near Beijing	91	34	Vapi (Gujarat)	
15	Inner Mongolia, Huhhot	1480	153	Chennai	146
212-2	Inner Mongolia		157	Uttar Pradesh and Bihar	
16	Jilin Province	360	205	Son River, Garwha District	1654
17	Jinchuan, Sichuan	287	*Indonesia*		
18	Liaoning Province		35	Citarum River	279
19	Linbei, Wuhe, Anhui	500	203	Aceh	
20	Ningxia Province		*Iran*		
21	Qinghai–Tibet Plateau	126,000	36	Kurdistan	104
22	Shanxi	2783	*Japan*		
23	Tongxiang, Zhejiang	70	37	Fukui	50
24	Weichang, Hebei	48	38	Fukuoka–Kumamoto	370
25	Xinjiang Province	880	39	Niigata Plain	10
209	W. Xinjiang–Tarim		40	Osaka	11
210	Yunnan (N)	200	41	Sendai	

(cont'd)

Table 1.2 (cont'd)

Map ID	Name/location	Maximum As (ppb)
Japan (cont'd)		
42	Shinji Plain	114
43	Takatsuki	60
Kazakhstan		
44	South Mangyshlak	1500
Lao PDR		
201	Inchampasak and Sarava	54
202	Attapeu Province	112
Malaysia		
45	Kampong Sekolah	
Mongolia		
232	Dornod Steppe	
233	Gobi Altai–Hovd	
234	Arkhangai	
Myanmar		
46	Irrawaddy Delta	
Nepal		
154	Terai (W)	2620
155	Terai (E)	
156	Kathmandu Valley	
Pakistan		
47	Indus Valley, Punjab	972
48	Kalalanwala, Punjab	1900
49	Indus Valley, Sindh	906
Philippines		
158	Mount Apo	
159	Greater Tongonan	

Map ID	Name/location	Maximum As (ppb)
Finland		
	SW Finland	2230
France		
68	Aquitaine	49
69	Massif Central	100
70	Pyrenees	
71	Vosges Mts	
152	Centre	49
164	W–C France	49
Germany		
73	Bavaria	150
74	Paderborn	38
75	Wiesbaden	100
Greece		
76	E. Thessaly	125
77	Thessaloniki	
Hungary		
78	Tisza interfluve	4000
151	SW Hungary	4000
160	Danube valley	
161–2	W. Hungary	
Ireland		
229	Unspecified*	32
Italy		
79	Anzasca Valley, Piedmont	
80	Etna	6390
81	Siena	14

Country	No.	Location	
Russia	88	Sakhalin	10,000
Saudi Arabia	231	Jubail	
Sri Lanka	50	Near Colombo	
Taiwan	51	NE Taiwan	3000
	52	SW Taiwan	1410
Thailand	53	Hat Yai	1000
	54	Nakorn Chaisi	100
	55	Ron Phibun tin belt	5000
Turkey	56	Afyon, Heybeli Spa	1240
	57	Emet–Hisarcik	700
Vietnam	58	Mekong River	500
	59	Red River	3050
Europe			
Belgium	192	Neogene, Flanders	60
Croatia	65	Eastern Croatia	612
Czech Republic	163	Celina–Mokrsko	1500
Denmark	66	Fensmark	30
Finland	67	Finnish Lapland	35
Italy	82	Stromboli, Vulcano	130
	83	Vesuvius	92
	166	Po Basin	
	191	Tiber Valley	52
	194	Emilia–Romagna	1300
	195	Lombardia	>400
	196	Veneto	480
	197	Toscana	14
	198	Lazio	52
	199	Ischia	460
Lithuania	207	Unspecified*	33
Netherlands	82	Gouda	15
	165	Brabant	44
Norway	85	Unspecified*	19
Poland	230	Sudetes Mts	140
Romania	86	Unspecified*	176
Russia	87	East Caucasus foothills	1500
	89	Trans-Baikal	700
Slovakia	90	W. Slovakia	39
	221	E. Slovakia	
Slovenia	91	Radovijica	559
Spain	92	Castellon–Valencia	14

(cont'd)

Table 1.2 (cont'd)

Map ID	Name/location	Maximum As (ppb)	Map ID	Name/location	Maximum As (ppb)
Spain (cont'd)			170	Washington	
93	Duero Basin	290	171–2	Oregon	
94	Madrid Basin	91	173–4	Nevada	
206	Salamanca	52	175	Carson Desert, Nevada	1000
Sweden			176	Yellowstone	1000
95	S. Sweden	200	177	Arizona	1000
96	Uppsala	300	178	Ohio	
Switzerland			179	Indiana	
215	Malcantone watershed	300	180	Florida	
UK			181	Arkansas	
97	Bridgwater		182	Idaho	
98	West Midlands	30	183–4	Montana	
220	Carlisle Basin	233	185	Kentucky	
219	Vale of York	39	186	Utah	
218	Manchester–E. Cheshire	57	187	Washington	
217	Liverpool–Rufford	355	188	San Joaquin valley	2600
216	North Humberside	63	193	Owens Lake	163,000
			228	Newark Basin, Pennsylvania	70
North America			South America		
Canada			Argentina		
99	Bowen Island	580	134	Bahia Blanco	500
100	Cobalt, Ontario		135	Tucuman	1000
101	Madoc, Ontario	3780	136	Cordoba	3810
102	Nova Scotia	1050	137	San Antonio de los Cobres	220
103	Saskatchewan	117	138	Santiago del Estero	14,969
104	Sunshine Coast/Powell Is.	>1000			

No.	Region	Location	Value
Mexico			
106	North central Mexico		
110	Durango		624
111	Guanajuato–Salamanca		
112	Rio Verde river basin		54
113	San Antonio, Baja California		410
114	Sonora		305
115	Zimapán		1100
USA			
107	Grass Mt, S. Dakota		117
116	California		1000
117	Sierra Nevada		110
118	Cook Inlet basin		
119	Dakota		
120	Fairbanks, Alaska		1370
121	Idaho		
122	Illinois		266
123	Michigan		220
124	Minnesota, Iowa		145
125	N. Idaho		
126	Nebraska		
127	New England		408
128	Oklahoma		232
129	Rio Grande		264
130	Southwest USA		1300
131	Washington State		33,000
132	Willamette Basin, Oregon		2150
133	Wisconsin		12,000
167	Kansas		
168	Nebraska		
169	Colorado		

No.	Region	Location	Value
Bolivia			
139		Altiplano	1000
Brazil			
140		Iron Quadrangle	250
Chile			
141		Antofagasta	870
142		Rio Camarones	1252
143		Rio Elqui	110
144		Rio Loa	2000
Costa Rica			
145		Unspecified*	
Cuba			
200		Isle of Youth	
Ecuador			
146		Rio Tambo	5080
El Salvador			
147		Lake Ilopango	770
Guatemala			
148		Unspecified*	
Honduras			
204		Unspecified*	
Nicaragua			
149		Sebaco–Matagalpa	1320
Peru			
150		Lake Aricota	500
221		Uruguay — SW Uruguay	58
Africa			
1		Okavango Delta	117
Burkina Faso			
2		Yatenga	1630

(cont'd)

Table 1.2 (cont'd)

Map ID	Name/location	Maximum As (ppb)
Cameroon		
190	Ekondo Titi	2000
Ethiopia		
3	Rift Valley	96
Ghana		
4	Obuasi	557
Nigeria		
7	Rivers State	
5	Kaduna	220
6	Ogun State	
8	Wari – Port Harcourt	780
Australasia		
Australia		
60	Perth	800

Map ID	Name/location	Maximum As (ppb)
61	Stuarts Point, NSW	337
New Zealand		
62	Waikato River	1320
63	Waiotapu valley	260
64	Wairu Plain	50
237	N. Hawkes Bay	
238	Bay of Plenty	
Ocean Basins		
Guam		
208	Tumon Bay	1
Iceland		
189	Iceland	48
USA		
188	Hawaii	70

*Locations marked as 'unspecified' are assigned a nominal location in the centre of the country in Figure 1.1.

continuous within the map areas, and both arsenic concentrations and population densities vary enormously between and within areas. Arsenic contamination is very unevenly distributed between the continents. In terms of the exposed population, by far the worst pollution is found in Asia, especially in a band running from Pakistan, along the southern margins of the Himalayan and Indo-Burman ranges, to Taiwan, which we refer to as the South and Southeast Asian Arsenic Belt (SSAAB). In this area, groundwater in shallow alluvial aquifers is both the main source of drinking water and an important source of irrigation water. In India, Bangladesh and Taiwan, exposure has resulted in widespread clinical effects, ranging from skin lesions to cancer and death, yet in Nepal, Cambodia and Vietnam there have been few diagnoses of arsenicosis to date. Elsewhere, pollution of alluvial aquifers has resulted in severe arsenicosis in at least three provinces of China.

In North America, the USA is affected by extremely widespread and diverse cases of arsenic contamination, but the concentrations are typically lower than in Asia and diagnosed cases of arsenicosis are almost unknown. Europe has one severe case of arsenic pollution in Hungary, and many low-level occurrences that, as in the USA, were probably detected because of more intensive testing of water sources. South America contains two areas of severe arsenic pollution (the Pampean Plains of Argentina and the Pacific Plains of Chile) that have both resulted in extensive arsenicosis and many deaths due to cancer, heart and lung disease. Elsewhere in South and Central America, arsenic contamination occurs along the volcanic mountains of the Pacific Rim.

In Africa, there are few reported occurrences of arsenic contamination. The only extensive, and reasonably well documented, case of arsenic pollution in Africa is in southwest Ghana, which is partly anthropogenic, and has been known for more than about 10 years. It appears that, in large areas of Africa, groundwater has simply not been tested. In Australasia, New Zealand is quite widely affected, but in Australia only two minor occurrences have been reported. There is very little information from the ocean basins, although arsenic has been reported from geothermal sources on Hawaii and Iceland.

1.5　Risk, Perception and Social Impacts

The promotion of shallow tubewells to reduce the incidence of enteric disease had the unintended consequence of creating a new risk of mass chronic poisoning. This is an example of the self-generated risks with unmanageable outcomes that characterise Ulrich Beck's 'risk society' (Beck, 1992). In the risk society, the social production of risk involves hazards that are produced by society itself, and that undermine the established safety systems of the state's existing risk assessments (Beck, 1996). Furthermore, responsibility for the risk is indeterminate because the chain of decision-making is so convoluted and institutionalised that the attribution of blame is often impossible. Beck (1999) describes this as the 'travesty of the hazard technocracy', and it is exemplified by the unsuccessful outcome of the class action brought by 400 Bangladeshi villagers against the British Geological Survey (BGS) for failing to test for arsenic (Annexe 8.1). The BGS was deemed to be insufficiently 'proximate' to be directly responsible, although this lack of proximity reflects the complex structure of corporate, institutional and individual decision-making that typifies the risk society, and protects against legal liability even where it can be argued there was a failure to exercise a duty of care.

These issues must, however, also be judged in the light of the evolving understanding of the effects of exposure to arsenic contamination, which demonstrates the transition from ignorance of an environmental problem to a quantifiable risk (Wynne, 1980, 1994). To make the statements about risk (of health consequences of ingesting arsenic) that are quoted in Chapter 5 requires an ability to quantify the associated odds. However, these risks may have wide margins for error because, for example, of the very large sample sizes required to estimate probabilities at low doses. Uncertainty, however, is a lower-order problem than both ignorance and indeterminacy. In the case of uncertainty, the parameter is known, but its value is subject to error. Ignorance, on the other hand, implies a complete lack of knowledge about the existence of a parameter (the 'unknown unknowns' of Donald Rumsfeld, 12 February 2003). Equally, indeterminacy represents an open-ended state in which it may be known that a problem exists, but there are multiple, unknown and non-linear ways in which it can manifest itself. Quantifiable risk requires extensive data to remove the layers of ignorance, indeterminacy and uncertainty that surround environmental problems, and in some circumstances the sampling intensity required to achieve confidence in risk estimation is prohibitively expensive. This may indeed be true of arsenic mobilisation in alluvial sediments, where local variability in the stratigraphy is high, and closely separated wells may differ greatly in arsenic concentration.

A third set of issues arises in the estimation of the medical risks associated with arsenic ingestion, and how these are translated into regulatory standards for arsenic in water and food (section 5.4.3). It is evident that chronic poisoning depends on cumulative ingestion, which implies that a precautionary approach would specify a low standard. However, dose-response curves at low dose may be non-linear, and because it is difficult to extrapolate reliably to these concentrations, the future cancer burden is highly uncertain given the latency periods for such diseases. These estimates are further complicated when food is an important source of exposure. Epidemiological data also have to allow for subpopulations having distinctive susceptibilities, and failing to recognise this may underestimate the risks to the most vulnerable populations. The severe health impacts of drinking water with more than 100 ppb As are not disputed, but the consequences of drinking water containing arsenic in the range of 10–50 ppb (i.e. the difference between the present and previous WHO guideline values) has received much discussion. Some have suggested that developing countries should delay adopting a lower standard in order to prioritise the worst affected groups, and optimise use of limited financial resources. However, an alternative, morally defensible position would be to adopt the lower standard, and implement it through a phased but time-limited programme.

1.6   Water-supply Mitigation

Historically, most water supplies were originally developed from local surface water sources and subsequently, due to the pressures of population growth and pollution, the source of supply has shifted to either groundwater or surface water transported from a remote source. There are three approaches to mitigating arsenic polluted water supplies: treat the contaminated water; resink the well at some distance away or at different depth; or develop a surface-water supply. There is no single best solution. Treating groundwater always involves significant cost and effort in operation and maintenance, and methods must be matched to the water quality, the size of installation, and the skills of the operators. Developing deeper groundwater is popular, but involves risks of contamination over time. Surface water, drawn from ponds or streams, must be treated to remove microbial contamination, and requires a higher level of management, or else acute bacterial infections may be substituted for chronic arsenic poisoning.

Approaches to mitigating contaminated water supplies have varied greatly between countries, reflecting the extent and rate of discovery of the problem, and their economic condition. In the USA, where the extent of contamination emerged slowly, public authorities took responsibility, abandoning the most polluted sources, installing treatment at others, and occasionally importing surface water. In Taiwan, public authorities constructed a reservoir and piped water to the affected villages. In Chile, a municipal treatment plant was built to supply the whole city of Antofagasta. In Hungary, state utilities installed treatment plants at some wells, and piped in uncontaminated groundwater to replace others. In all these examples, arsenic exposure has been greatly reduced. In South Asia, there is still massive exposure of the rural population. To date, the main response has focused on surveying private wells and raising awareness to encourage arsenic avoidance. In West Bengal, government has played a leading role, initially installing thousands of small treatment plants, and later piping supplies from high-capacity deep tubewells and surface-water treatment plants to groups of villages. In Bangladesh, guided by donors, the government has promoted a demand-led approach, which has resulted in installing thousands of deep hand-pumped tubewells. In other states of India and in Nepal, Cambodia and Vietnam, mitigation is less advanced, although Vietnam and Nepal have promoted domestic and small community arsenic removal plants (ARPs).

Currently, tens of millions of people continue to depend on arsenic-polluted groundwater as a source of drinking water and for irrigation. Greatly increased mitigation efforts are needed to reduce, and eventually eliminate, exposure to arsenic, and thus to begin to reduce the current and growing burden of disease.

1.7   Structure and Scope of the Book

1.7.1   Objectives

The primary purpose of this book is to satisfy the need for an up-to-date, interdisciplinary and global perspective on arsenic pollution for researchers, both established and just entering the field, and for practitioners in arsenic mitigation, government officials, aid and development administrators and workers in non-government organisations. The recent recognition of the scale of natural arsenic pollution means that such a book could not have been written earlier. Further, as indicated above, anything written more than about five years ago will have overlooked three-quarters of the published material. Although there is a risk that this work could quickly become obsolete, we doubt that it will, because we believe that the past 10 years have been a special period in the history of arsenic research, and new ideas, as opposed to new data, will not be produced as quickly in the next 10 years. Most existing knowledge is scattered amongst hundreds of journal articles, conference proceedings and reports, which we attempt to synthesise. We anticipate that most readers will approach this book with knowledge of one or more of the technical areas covered, and hope that, after reading this book, they will feel comfortable to discuss and work with specialists in all subject areas. We also hope that the reader will gain a truly global perspective of arsenic pollution.

The book is divided into two main parts, each with a distinct focus. Chapters 2–7 approach arsenic pollution from the technical–disciplinary approaches of geochemistry, hydrology, health and water supply. In Chapters 8–10 we address arsenic pollution from a geographical perspective, seeking to present an integrated account of the characteristics, impacts and activities in each region. As far as practicable, the technical and geographical chapters are cross-referenced to minimise duplication, but the reader seeking more information on a specific subject should refer first to the corresponding technical or geographical chapter. Finally in Chapter 11, we summarise and synthesise the major findings and conclusions, and try to predict future trends of discovery, occurrence and impact.

1.7.2 Terminology

Inevitably, the literature uses different units. However, so far as it is sensible to do so, we have used consistent units and tried to help the reader by using forms that are specific to each medium. For concentrations of arsenic in water, we use parts per billion (ppb) as standard, which is equivalent to micrograms per litre (μg/L)[8]. Occasionally, we quote arsenic concentrations in water in units of parts per million (ppm), but only when referring to extreme concentrations. For other solutes in water, we use either ppb or ppm, equivalent to milligrams per litre (mg/L), as appropriate to make the concentrations easily comprehensible. For arsenic concentrations in soil, we use milligrams per kilogram (mg/kg) as standard, since it helps in differentiating solid and liquid concentrations in complex sections of text. Where referring to arsenic concentrations in plant materials and foodstuffs, we express these in units of micrograms per kilogram (μg/kg), to differentiate the different media (i.e. water, soil and food) within the text; this also makes the quantities of arsenic in food numerically comparable to those in water (in ppb or μg/L).

The most severely affected area of the world is the delta of the Ganges, Brahmaputra and Meghna rivers, which form a large part of Bangladesh and the adjoining Indian state of West Bengal. Geologically, these areas form a continuum, known as the Bengal Basin, and have demographic and cultural similarities. The areas face very similar problems, and where we refer to matters of common concern, we use the term Bengal Basin, or simply Bengal where there is no geological significance.

NOTES

1 It has been suggested that arsenical dyes in wallpaper were responsible for the accidental poisoning of Napoleon Bonaparte during his imprisonment on St Helena.
2 Acute poisoning follows from the ingestion of a few grams of arsenic over a short space of time, and results in life-threatening illness. Chronic poisoning results from months or years of low-level arsenic exposure, and causes no immediate suffering.

3   As judged by the absence of references in standards texts in water engineering, hydrogeology or geochemistry.
4   An earlier discovery in northern India by Datta and Kaul (1976) was largely ignored.
5   The reasons for this are not clear. Although the most affected areas were remote from the authors, contamination was widespread in the USA.
6   Apparently contradicting other evidence discussed in Chapter 5.
7   This includes rivers on the Pacific coast of South and Central America that are fed by geothermal groundwater from springs in the Andes. Almost all other locations in Figure 1.1 are groundwater bodies, including springs.
8   For all practical purposes, in dilute solutions μg/L and ppb (or mg/L and ppm) are identical. This is not true, however, for saline waters.

Chapter Two

Hydrogeochemistry of Arsenic

2.1 Introduction

It is remarkable that arsenic occurs widely in rocks and soils, but high concentrations of arsenic in water are rare and unevenly distributed on a global scale. This chapter explains the processes that control arsenic pollution, specifically what causes arsenic in minerals to be released into groundwater (mobilisation) or in reverse, to be removed from water (immobilisation). There are four mechanisms of practical importance that cause arsenic pollution of natural waters. Two occur where arsenic is adsorbed onto metal oxides or clays: under alkaline conditions, arsenic may be directly desorbed, which we refer to as alkali desorption (AD); alternatively, under reducing conditions, the minerals to which arsenic is adsorbed break down and dissolve causing arsenic to be released into solution, which is known as reductive dissolution (RD). The third mechanism is the oxidation and break-down of sulphide minerals containing arsenic (sulphide oxidation, SO). The fourth mechanism involves mixing with geothermal waters, where arsenic was leached from rocks by hot water, either at great depth or in areas of volcanic activity. Evaporation can increase the concentration of arsenic derived from any of these mechanisms, but cannot account for its original presence in the water. In theory, other processes, such as carbonate complexation, might mobilise arsenic, but are not believed to be of practical significance. It is also important to consider the means by which arsenic is immobilised. Two processes dominate: adsorption on metal oxides in oxic waters; and coprecipitation with, or adsorption on, sulphide minerals in reducing waters.

After briefly describing the occurrence of arsenic in minerals and water, we consider the fundamental chemical processes of adsorption and desorption (section 2.3), with special reference to the iron oxide minerals ferrihydrite and goethite. Arsenic sorption becomes weaker at high pH and in the presence of some competing ions. Knowledge of these processes underpins an understanding not only of the causes of arsenic pollution, but also of the behaviour of arsenic in soils, the operation of arsenic-removal plants, and the management of arsenic-contaminated aquifers. We then consider the roles of sulphide minerals (section 2.4) and microbial activity (section 2.5) in controlling the occurrence of arsenic. Having outlined the geochemical foundations, section 2.6 describes the four mobilisation mechanisms and their occurrences. Finally we describe the association of arsenic with other trace elements in groundwater (section 2.7) and briefly consider the association of arsenic pollution with mining activities (section 2.8). A commentary on the methods available for the analysis of arsenic in natural waters is given in Annexe 2.1.

2.1.1   Common arsenic minerals

Arsenic is present at an average concentration of 1.8 ppm in the Earth's crust (Mason, 1966), and is commonly present at five times this level in shales and alluvium. Occasionally, elemental arsenic is found in hydrothermal veins, but more commonly it is found either in primary arsenic-bearing minerals or adsorbed onto various mineral phases such as iron and aluminium oxides, clays and iron sulphides, which as we will discover later, are nature's most important stores of arsenic. The most common primary arsenic minerals are listed in Table 2.1. Other arsenic-bearing minerals include enargite (Cu_3AsS_4), cobaltite (CoAsS), niccolite (NiAs), arsenolite (As_2O_3) and claudetite (As_2O_3). However, these mostly occur as accessory minerals in ore deposits (Mason and Berry, 1978), and are not known to be responsible for any cases of arsenic pollution.

The most important minerals that incorporate arsenic are iron oxides and the common sulphide, pyrite (FeS_2). A wide variety of iron oxides and hydroxides occur in nature, some with indistinct structures or overlapping chemical compositions. Their properties are broadly similar, and it is not essential to know details of each individual phase, which are often grouped under titles such as iron oxyhydroxides or hydrous ferric oxides (HFO). In the literature, it is common to represent this range in terms of a few idealised forms including amorphous iron oxides (or ferrihydrite), goethite (α-FeOOH), haematite (α-Fe_2O_3) and magnetite (Fe_3O_4). With the exception of magnetite, which contains both Fe(II) and Fe(III), these minerals contain Fe(III) and hence are most stable under more oxidising conditions. In general, amorphous iron oxides dominate in recent sediments, but over time are replaced by more crystalline forms such as goethite and haematite, which are more stable, have smaller surface areas, and therefore lower

Table 2.1   Important arsenic minerals

Mineral	Chemical formula	Characteristics	Geological occurrence
Arsenic	As	Light to dark grey, metallic, nodular	Hydrothermal veins in crystalline rock
Orpiment	As_2S_3	Yellow to yellowish-brown, pearly or resinous, transparent prisms	Found in low-temperature hydrothermal mineralisation and at hot springs
Realgar	AsS	Red to orange, resinous prisms. Transparent when fresh	Minor constituent of hydrothermal sulphide veins. Occasionally found with limestone and clay in volcanic terrain
Arsenopyrite	FeAsS	Silver-white to steel-grey, metallic prisms with rhombic cross-sections	The most abundant As mineral, formed at moderate to high temperature, associated with Sn, Au and Ni–Co–Ag ores in
Scorodite	$FeAsO_4 \cdot 2H_2O$	Yellowish-green to greenish brown, bluish green, or very dark green; may be fibrous, granular or earthy	Primary mineral in hydrothermal deposits and secondary mineral in gossans, an intensively oxidized rock capping a mineral deposit

Source: Mason and Berry (1978)

adsorption capacities. Amorphous iron oxides also have solubilities up to five orders of magnitude greater than more crystalline forms (Whittemore and Langmuir, 1975). Thus, the amorphous forms can be expected to represent the behaviour of iron oxides in Holocene aquifers containing reducing water, while goethite and haematite better represent the behaviour of older and oxic aquifers. Manganese and aluminium oxides behave in a similar way to iron oxides, but differ in their abundance and the strength of their attraction for arsenic. Manganese oxides are more easily reduced than iron oxides, and hence their sorbed load may be released and readsorbed by iron oxides. In this manner, iron oxides commonly have a controlling influence on arsenic mobility.

2.1.2   Arsenic speciation in groundwater

The molecular form, commonly termed species, in which arsenic occurs affects both its toxicity and mobility in groundwater, and its removal in water treatment. In water, arsenic occurs in one of two main forms: a reduced form, arsenite, with a valence of +3; and an oxidised form, arsenate, with a valence of +5. These are often referred to simply by their oxidation states as As(III) and As(V). Arsenic also exists in the As^0 and As^{-3} states, but these are of little importance in natural waters (Cullen and Reimer, 1989). Arsenic can also exist in many organic forms, of which the most common are monomethylated acids (MMA) and dimethylated acids (DMA), both of which exist as As(III) and As(V) forms. These only ever occur as trace components in natural waters, but they are important in plant and animal metabolism (Akter et al., 2005a; Chapter 5).

Under oxidising conditions, arsenic usually exists as one of a series of pentavalent (arsenate) forms such as $H_3AsO_4^0$, $H_2AsO_4^-$, $HAsO_4^{2-}$, AsO_4^{3-}, depending on the Eh and pH conditions (Ferguson and Gavis, 1972). The charge on the arsenate ion controls how it behaves in groundwater and water treatment systems, because negatively charged ions are readily adsorbed onto the surfaces of metal oxides, with the strength of sorption depending greatly on the pH. The variation of the proportion of these ions is shown in Figure 2.1, which allows the stable species in groundwater to be predicted. The uncharged $H_3AsO_4^0$ ion is only important in very acid waters, which are rare naturally, but are encountered in acid mine drainage. In the

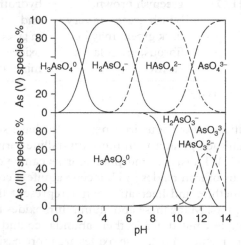

Figure 2.1   Inorganic arsenic species in water. The figure shows the distribution of As(V) and As(III) species as a function of pH at an ionic strength of 0.04 m.
Source: Meng et al. (2000)

range of pH typical of most natural waters (pH 6.5–8.5), both $H_2AsO_4^-$ and $HAsO_4^{2-}$ are likely to be present.

In reducing water, arsenic is present as the trivalent (arsenite) form, which undergoes a similar series of dissociation reactions from $H_3AsO_3^0$ to $H_2AsO_3^-$ and $HAsO_3^{2-}$. The important difference between arsenite and arsenate is that the uncharged ion ($H_3AsO_3^0$) dominates when the pH is less than 9.2, and limits the extent to which arsenite is adsorbed. While Eh–pH relationships help in understanding the qualitative relationships between arsenic species, quantitative use is generally not recommended because of the difficulty of making accurate and representative measurements of Eh (e.g. Langmuir, 1997), and because the phase boundaries depend on the concentrations of other components in the water.

2.2   The Chemistry of Normal and Arsenic-rich Groundwaters

The mobility of arsenic is controlled by oxidation and reduction reactions. Most groundwaters exploited for water supply have a range of pH between about 6.0 and 9.0, but differ greatly in the availability of oxygen, and vary from being saturated with oxygen to being so anoxic that methane is produced. Although it can be measured as Eh, the oxidation–reduction state of an aquifer is best assessed from the dissolved species present. A significant factor in the evolution of any groundwater, and a critical one for arsenic, is the gradual depletion of sources of oxygen. A well-defined sequence of reactions, controlled by micro-organisms, defines this path (e.g. Chapelle, 2001, and references therein). This sequence commences with atmospheric oxygen dissolved during recharge, and is followed by nitrate, which is reduced to nitrogen gas. When oxygen and nitrate are exhausted, the next species to be reduced are manganese (Mn) and iron (Fe). The oxidised forms of both Fe and Mn are normally stable as solids, but the reduced forms occur in solution. Increasing reduction involves the conversion of sulphate to sulphide. If iron is present in solution, the iron sulphide mineral pyrite will be precipitated, until one or other element becomes limiting. If iron is not available, hydrogen sulphide gas is formed.

The various mechanisms that cause arsenic pollution are described later in the chapter, but it is noted here that arsenic normally occurs in groundwater with one of the four chemical associations, each linked to a particular mobilisation mechanism (Table 2.2). The four water types are:

1   **Near-neutral**, strongly **reducing (NNR)** water, rich in bicarbonate, iron and/or manganese, and low in oxidised species such as nitrate and sulphate. Near-neutral reducing waters are dominated by As(III). These waters are associated with the **reductive-dissolution (RD)** mobilisation mechanism.

Table 2.2 Generalised chemical characteristics of arsenic-rich groundwaters*

	Water type			
	Near-neutral, reducing	Alkali-oxic	Acid-sulphate	Geothermal
Mobilisation mechanism	Reductive dissolution	Alkali desorption	Sulphide oxidation	Geothermal
Examples	Bengal Basin; fluvio-glacial aquifers in the USA	Pampean Plains of Argentina; southwest USA	Wisconsin (USA); Perth, Australia	Chile, Tibet, New Zealand
As	Up to a few ppm	Up to c. 10 ppm	Up to a few tens of ppm	Up to 120 ppm
As-species	As(III)	As(V)	As(V)	Mostly As(III)
Temperature	Any	Any	Any	Up to 85°C
pH	c. 7.0	≥8.0	Acid, minimum pH < 6	Variable, usually near neutral
DO	Absent	High (several ppm)	Variable	Low
Cl	Low	Variable	Variable	Positively correlated with arsenic
HCO_3	High	Moderate	Low to moderate	Low to moderate
SO_4	Very low (<5 ppm)	Moderate to high (>10 ppm)	High to very high	Variable
PO_4	High (>1 ppm)	Variable	Variable	Low
NO_3-N	Very low (<1 ppm)	Low to moderate	Variable	Low
NH_4-N	High (0.5–5.0 ppm)	Absent	Absent	Low
DOC	High (>2 ppm)	Variable	Very low	Low
Fe	High (1–10 ppm)	Low to moderate (<1 ppm)	Low to high	Variable
Mn	High to low	Low to moderate	Variable	Variable
F	Low to moderate	Moderate to high (>1.5 ppm)	Low to moderate	Low to moderate

*Descriptions are qualitative and relative. Quantitative data are presented elsewhere in the book.

2 **Alkali-oxic (AO)** waters, with pH$\geq$8.0, containing dissolved oxygen and/or nitrate and sulphate, and low in iron and manganese. Alkali-oxic waters are dominated by As(V). These waters are associated with the **alkali-desorption (AD)** mobilisation mechanism.

3 **Acid-sulphate (AS)** waters, with slightly to strongly acid (pH < 1–6), high sulphate concentrations, and often, high iron concentrations. Acid-sulphate waters are also dominated by As(V). These waters are associated with the **sulphide-oxidation (SO)** mobilisation mechanism.

4 **Geothermal (GT)** waters, distinguished primarily by a temperature well above the background, and usually also correlation of arsenic with chloride.

2.3 Adsorption and Desorption of Arsenic

In both the reductive-dissolution and alkali-desorption mechanisms, which as described in later chapters are also the most important mechanisms, arsenic is initially adsorbed to solid-phase oxides and clay minerals, although the precise processes that release arsenic vary. In the RD case, the solid-phase carrier dissolves, while in the AD case, arsenic is desorbed, leaving the carrier as a solid phase. Adsorption is also the main process that removes arsenic from solution.

2.3.1 Introduction

The basic processes of sorption, studied in the laboratory with simple mineral and water compositions, provide a framework for understanding the more complicated systems that occur in nature. Laboratory test results are often carried out using artificial minerals that may not reflect the behaviour of their geological equivalents, or are conducted under conditions beyond those encountered in normal aquifers. Sorption can be divided into three processes: *adsorption* where a chemical adheres to the solid surface; *absorption* where the chemical is drawn into the solid; and *ion exchange* where the chemical replaces another already on the solid surface (Appelo and Postma, 1996). Because adsorption is related to edge and surface properties, it is most important in minerals with high surface areas, such as clays, fresh oxide coatings, and some kinds of organic matter. In clays, surface charges originate from elemental substitutions in the crystal structure, defects in the structure, and broken or unsatisfied bonds at the edges and corners of crystals; whereas the surface charges in oxides, hydroxides, carbonates and phosphates originate mainly from ionization of surface groups, or surface reactions (Langmuir, 1997). In the latter case, this accounts for their pH dependency, because at low pH the surfaces are positively charged, but become negatively charged at high pH. Thus negatively charged arsenite or arsenate ions can be adsorbed only when the mineral surface is positively charged, as described by the zero point of charge (ZPC), the pH at the point of transition from positive to negative surface charge. The capacity for adsorption can then be expressed in terms of the number of surface sites (N_s) that can hold charged ions.

Adsorption of arsenic onto Fe, Al and Mn oxides, clay minerals and organic matter is critical in controlling the mobility of arsenic in groundwater. Most cases of natural contamination originate with arsenic that is adsorbed onto iron oxyhydroxides, although mobilisation can involve either desorption or dissolution of the host (sorbent) phase. Natural soils almost always contain a variety of oxides, clays and organic matter. Hence the relative importance of each phase is not always clear. However, the consensus in the literature is that arsenic is mainly adsorbed onto iron oxyhydroxides, and to a lesser extent on titanium (Ti) oxides, with the clay minerals kaolinite, illite and vermiculite adsorbing arsenic to a much smaller degree (Violante and Pigna, 2002). Below, we first describe the behaviour of arsenite and arsenate on individual minerals, and then expand this to consider the effects of combined arsenic species and competing anions, such as sulphate, phosphate, carbonate and natural organic acids. The properties of some minerals that may adsorb arsenic are summarised in Table 2.3.

Table 2.3 Sorption-related properties of some common geological materials

Mineral/phase	Surface area (m^2/g)	Surface site density (nm^{-2})	pH^*_{ZPC}
Silica (amorphous)	53–292	4.2–12	3.5–3.9
Calcite	–	–	8.5–10.8
Gibbsite (α-Al(OH)$_3$)	120	2–12	9.84–10.0
Birnessite (α-MnO$_2$)	180	2–18	1.5–2.8
Pyrolusite (β-MnO$_2$)	–	–	4.6–7.3
Ferrihydrite (Fe(OH)$_3$)	250–600	20	8.5–8.8
Goethite (α-FeOH)$_3$)	45–169	2.6–16.8	5.9–6.7
Haematite (α-Fe$_2$O$_3$)	1.8	5–22	4.2–6.9
Kaolinite	10–38	1.2–6.0	≤2–4.6
Illite	65–100	0.4–5.6	–
Montmorillonite (sodic)	600–800	0.4–1.6	≤2–3
Muscovite			6.6
Organic matter	260–1300[†]	2.3[†]	2[‡]

*pH_{ZPC} is the pH at the zero point of charge.
[†]Soil humic material.
[‡]Algae and sewage effluent (bacteria).
Source: Langmuir (1997)

2.3.2 Iron oxides

Ferrihydrite and goethite

Dixit and Hering (2003) investigated the adsorption of arsenite and arsenate, as single anion solutions, on ferrihydrite and goethite as a function of increasing pH (Figure 2.2). Adsorption of arsenite (As^{3+}) on both ferrihydrite and goethite is virtually constant between pH 5.0 and 9.0, and at all initial concentrations. By contrast, adsorption of arsenate (As^{5+}) onto minerals varies with both pH and initial concentration. At high initial concentrations of arsenate, adsorption on both ferrihydrite and goethite declines continuously from pH 4 to pH 10. However, at lower initial concentrations, adsorption of arsenate tends to be uniform on ferrihydrite up to pH 8.0, and on goethite up to pH 9.0. Goldberg (2002) obtained similar results, observing that ferrihydrite

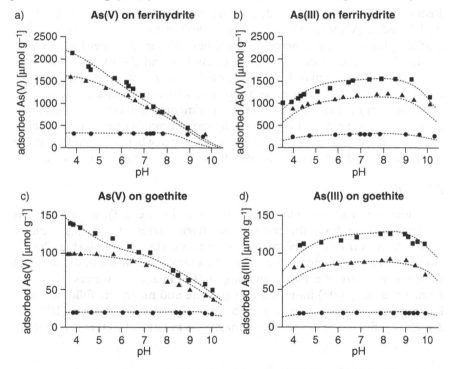

Figure 2.2 Adsorption of arsenic onto ferrihydrite and goethite: (a) As(V) on ferrihydrite; (b) As(III) on ferrihydrite; (c) As(V) on goethite; (d) As(III) on goethite. Experiments were conducted with 0.03 g/L of ferrihydrite and 0.5 g/L of goethite. Symbols represent arsenic concentrations: squares 100 μM (750 ppb); triangles 50 μM (375 ppb); and circles 10 μM (75 ppb). The solutions contained 0.01 m $NaClO_4$. The lines are best-fit surface complexation models to experimental data.
Source: Redrawn from Dixit and Hering (2003)

adsorbed 100% of As(V) from pH 3 to pH 7, and 100% of As(III) from pH 2.5 to pH 10.5, but because of its larger surface area, at any given pH, greater amounts of both arsenite and arsenate are adsorbed onto ferrihydrite. The Dixit and Hering (2003) demonstrated that, contrary to common misconceptions, As(III) is strongly adsorbed and more mobile in neutral and weakly alkaline conditions. Since As(III) and As(V) are sorbed to similar extents between pH 6 and pH 9 on ferrihydrite and goethite, it follows that microbial reduction of As(V) to As(III) will not increase its mobility (section 2.6.2). Although ferrihydrite has a much larger surfa ce area than goethite, and therefore a greater sorption capacity per unit weight, Dixit and Hering (2003) also noted that transformation of ferrihydrite to goethite does not decrease the adsorption affinity for As(V) and, if anything, appears to increase it.

Haematite

Redman et al. (2002) showed that natural haematite effectively adsorbs both As(III) and As(V), while Giménez et al. (2007), who tested both natural and synthetic haematite, magnetite and goethite, obtained somewhat different results. The sorption capacity for both As(III) and As(V) decreases with increasing pH, and at pH < 7, haematite has higher sorption capacities for both As(III) and As(V) than either goethite or magnetite, although at higher pH the differences for As(III) are small. In the experiments, equilibrium was achieved in less than 2 days, which is geologically insignificant, but may be critical in water treatment. Giménez et al. (2007) showed that, when adjusted for surface area, natural and synthetic haematite have similar sorption capacities.

Magnetite

The adsorption of arsenite onto magnetite (Figure 2.3), a mineral that contains iron in both the ferrous and ferric states, differs significantly from adsorption onto ferrihydrite and goethite (Dixit and Hering, 2003). Adsorption onto magnetite rises slowly to a maximum at about pH 9.5, and so should be more effective in retaining As(III) in alkaline waters. However, Giménez et al. (2007) indicated that goethite and magnetite followed similar trends in sorption capacity with increasing pH for both As(III) and As(V). Confirmation of the role of magnetite in natural waters is required.

2.3.3   Aluminium and manganese oxides

Goldberg (2002) tested adsorption of single and mixed solutions of As(III) and As(V) onto amorphous aluminium oxide (Figure 2.4a). She found that Al oxides achieved 100% adsorption of As(V) from pH 3 to pH 9, before reducing rapidly in effectiveness beyond pH 10.0. However, the mass of arsenic adsorbed per unit mass of oxide is much less than for iron oxides.

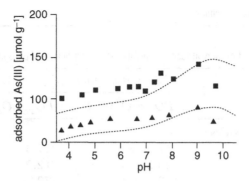

Figure 2.3 Adsorption of arsenic onto magnetite. The experimental conditions and legend are the same as Figure 2.2.
Source: Redrawn from Dixit and Hering (2003)

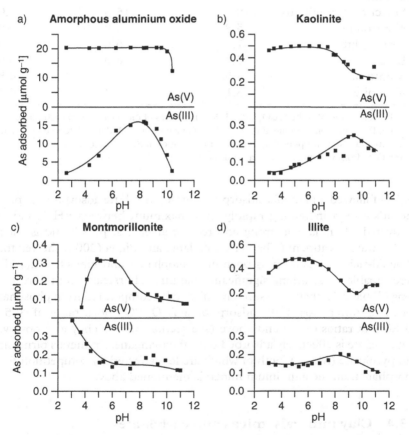

Figure 2.4 Adsorption of arsenic onto aluminium oxide and clay minerals: (a) amorphous aluminium oxide; (b) kaolinite; (c) montmorillonite; and (d) illite. All experiments were conducted with 20 μM/L (1300 ppb) of arsenic. The suspensions contained 1 g/L of aluminium oxide and 40 g/L of each clay mineral.
Source: Redrawn after Goldberg (2002)

Table 2.4   Arsenate adsorption on various minerals under the influence of phosphate

Mineral	AsO_4 sorbed ($\mu mol/g$)		R_f^*
	$PO_4:AsO_4 = 0.0$	$PO_4:AsO_4 = 1.0$	
Oxides and hydroxides			
Birnessite	17.3	17.3	2.10
Pyrolusite	23.2	12.2	1.25
Goethite	152	72	1.00
Boehmite (AlOOH)	n.d.	166	0.58
Allophane	113	10	0.05
Gibbsite	151	60	0.37
Clay minerals			
Smectite (ferruginous)	18.9	15.8	0.93
Nontronite	5.8	4.9	0.89
Vermiculite	7.5	6.6	0.90
Illite	7.4	6.0	0.87
Montmorillonite	8.5	7.2	0.83
Kaolinite	8.1	5.3	0.45

* R_f, the molar ratio of sorbed AsO_4/sorbed PO_4, measures of the selectivity of each mineral for arsenate. Pure solutions contained 0.1 mmol/L of arsenate, and all data relate to experiments at pH 7.0 and results for phosphate with 1:1 molar ratios. n.d., not determined.
Source: Data from Violante and Pigna (2002)

As(III) followed a parabolic adsorption curve, with little adsorption at pH 3, and adsorption increasing rapidly to a maximum between pH 7 and 10. 'Activated' alumina is a strong adsorber of arsenic at pH < 7 and is widely used in water treatment (Chapter 7). Violante and Pigna (2002) showed that, while Al-rich phases such as boehmite, allophane[1] and gibbsite ($Al(OH)_3$) were capable of adsorbing significant quantities of arsenate from pure solutions (Table 2.4), they were severely affected by competition from phosphate, declining from almost 100% adsorption at AsO_4/PO_4 molar ratios of <0.5 to 70–80% at ratios of 1.0 and above (see section 2.3.5). They also observed that arsenate is effectively adsorbed onto the manganese minerals birnessite[2] and pyrolusite (MnO_2), both of which are less affected by competition from phosphate than the aluminium minerals mentioned above.

2.3.4   Clay minerals, micas and carbonates

Clay minerals are ubiquitous in soils, sediments and weathered rock, but vary greatly in their adsorptive properties (Tables 2.3 and 2.4). Goldberg (2002) found that sorption of As(III) and As(V) on kaolinite, illite and montmo-rillonite[3] follows similar trends to those for iron oxides (Figure 2.4), although in all cases the mass of arsenic adsorbed per unit mass of mineral is much less. Maximum adsorption of arsenate occurred at pH 5, and of arsenite at pH 8–9. However, the adsorption affinity of clays for arsenic is less than that of oxides, and only kaolinite achieved 100% adsorption, at pH 5. Adsorption of As(V) onto kaolinite declines above pH 7.0, whereas adsorption of As(III) actually increases from pH 6.0 to a maximum at pH 9.5. Illite behaves similarly to kaolinite: adsorption of As(V) reduces significantly above pH 6.0, whereas adsorption of As(III) is relatively insensitive to pH, but is at a maximum at pH 8.0. The behaviour of montmorillonite is more complex: adsorption of As(V) is strongly pH-dependent, with a maximum at pH 4.5 and a minimum at pH 9.0. Adsorption of As(III) on montmorillonite, on the other hand, is relatively insensitive to pH.

Lin and Puls (2003) examined the adsorption and desorption of As(III) and As(V) on six types of clay: halloysite, two types of kaolinite, illite, an inter-layered illite-montmorillonite and chlorite[4]. In the pH range 5.5–7.5, all the clays adsorbed more As(V) than As(III), except for illite–montmorillonite at pH 7.5. Halloysite adsorbed almost 100% of As(V), but adsorbed As(III) weakly. Only chlorite adsorbed both As(III) and As(V) strongly. On all the clays, As(V) adsorption was greatest at pH 5.5, and As(III) adsorption was greatest at pH 7.5. In experiments with phosphate solutions at pH 5.5, As(V) was more readily desorbed than As(III). Desorption of As(V) was greatest from halloysite and kaolinite (the 1:1 clays), and least from chlorite. The retention of sorbed arsenic increased after the clays had been 'aged' for 30–75 days between sorption and desorption, suggesting that geologically aged clays will also retain arsenic relatively strongly.

Micas are structurally similar to clay minerals and might be expected to display a similar range of adsorption characteristics related to their iron content, which will be high in biotite and low in muscovite. Based on field studies in Bangladesh, Breit (2000) showed that weathered micas may be enriched in arsenic, and suggested that micas may be a source of arsenic pollution, although it is presently uncertain how important this is.

2.3.5 Competitive adsorption and desorption

Phosphate

Negatively charged ions such as phosphate, sulphate, silica and carbonate potentially compete with arsenic for adsorption sites. Most attention has been given to phosphate, which certainly affects the behaviour of arsenic. Despite their opposed toxic and life-supporting natures, the chemistries of arsenate

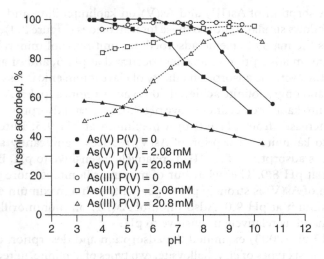

Figure 2.5   Influence of phosphate on adsorption of arsenic onto ferrihydrite. Experiments conducted in solutions containing 2.08 mm (156 ppm) of As(III) or As(V) and with an ionic strength of 0.1 M and 2 g/L of ferrihydrite. Phosphate concentrations were 0, 2.08 or 20.8 mM (1980 ppm).
Source: Redrawn after Stollenwerk (2003)

and phosphate have much in common. Jain and Loeppert (2000) found that phosphate reduces As(III) adsorption onto ferrihydrite at low pH, but that the effect becomes insignificant at pH 9.0 (Figure 2.5). At pH 7.0–8.0, conditions typical of waters in which arsenite is dominant, the sorbed load could be reduced by 20%. The effect of phosphate on As(V) adsorption follows the opposite trend, where adsorption decreases rapidly above about pH 6.0, and by 60% at pH 9.0. However, these experiments were conducted at much higher concentrations than are normal in nature, and so the effect will be small in most practical situations. Dixit and Hering (2003) also showed that, in the presence of phosphate, As(III) is sorbed preferentially to As(V) over the pH range of 4–10. Phosphate has similar effects on adsorption by both goethite and ferrihydrite (Manning and Goldberg, 1996). It is possible that high phosphate concentrations might reduce the adsorption of As(V) in alkaline-oxic waters but have only a small effect in near-neutral, reducing waters.

Violante and Pigna (2002) showed how phosphate variably reduces the adsorption of arsenate (but not arsenite) on a variety of oxides, clays and soils in the range pH 4–8. Tested alone, most minerals adsorbed similar quantities of arsenate and phosphate; however, Fe, Mn and Ti oxides and iron-rich clay minerals (such as smectite and nontronite) retained arsenate more strongly than phosphate. On the other hand, Al-rich minerals such as gibbsite, boehmite, amorphous Al hydroxide and the clay minerals allophone, kaolinite and halloysite retained phosphate more strongly than arsenate. Tests on natural soils showed that large applications of phosphate displaced highly variable quantities of arsenate, pointing to the complexity of competition from phosphate and the importance of establishing the soil mineralogy. Acharyya et al. (1999, 2000) suggested that phosphate fertilisers might be a cause of arsenic pollution in the Bengal Basin, although this was subsequently rejected as a significant cause of arsenic mobilisation by Ravenscroft et al. (2001).

Carbonate

Some authors have suggested that arsenic is mobilised by high carbonate and bicarbonate concentrations, both from sulphides in Palaeozoic sandstones in Michigan (Kim et al., 2000) and alluvium in the Bengal Basin (Appelo et al., 2002; Anawar et al., 2004). However, laboratory experiments (Neuberger and Helz, 2005), column experiments with iron-coated sand (Radu et al., 2005), and field data from West Bengal (McArthur et al., 2004) do not support these interpretations. In batch experiments on a Pleistocene sand from Bangladesh, Stollenwerk et al. (2007) also found that bicarbonate had no significant effect on arsenic sorption.

Silica

Silica is found at concentrations of a few ppm to a few tens of ppm (as SiO_2) in most groundwaters. Silicate decreases the adsorption of As(III) on ferrihydrite between pH 4 and 10 by as much as 35%, and also decreases the adsorption of As(V) above pH 6 by as much as 60% (Swedlund and Webster, 1999). However, in natural waters these effects may be partly counteracted by magnesium and, in particular, calcium, which increases As(V) adsorption on ferrihydrite at pH 9 (Wilkie and Hering, 1996; Smith and Edwards, 2005). In water treatment trials with ferric chloride, Meng et al. (2000) found that increasing the silica concentration from 1 to 10 ppm (as Si) reduced the adsorption of both As(III) and As(V) from 90% to 45%, although in the presence of Ca and Mg the effect on As(V) was much reduced, but not on As(III).

Other ions

Other ions that could affect arsenic sorption include sulphate, nitrate, chloride, calcium and magnesium. Jain and Loeppert (2000) showed that sulphate has almost no effect on the adsorption of As(V) on ferrihydrite at any pH. Sulphate does, however, reduce adsorption of As(III) between pH 2 and pH 6, but the effect is negligible between pH 7 and pH 10. Therefore sulphate will not normally be a significant control on arsenic sorption in sedimentary aquifers. Smith, Naidu et al. (2002) reported that chloride and nitrate have insignificant effects on adsorption of As(V).

Calcium increases the adsorption of As(V) on Al oxides, which are inherently more sensitive to silica interference than ferrihydrite. However, Smith and Edwards (2005) showed that adsorption of arsenic increased in the presence of calcium, but only in the first few hours, and hence it is important in water treatment but not at hydrogeologically significant timescales.

Natural organic matter

Natural organic matter (NOM) acts in three ways to influence the behaviour of arsenic in the presence of iron and manganese oxides. First, organic matter is a potential sorbent; second dissolved organic carbon (DOC) competes for sorption sites; and third high DOC can cause the oxide minerals to which arsenic is adsorbed to dissolve (section 2.6.1). Since high concentrations of DOC are more common in reducing groundwaters, where As(III) is dominant, the interaction of DOC with As(V) tends to be less important. Natural DOC is extremely complex, and experimental studies either use natural samples, the relevance of which may be site-specific, or use purified solutions of humic, fulvic[5] or citric acids. Thus inference from experimental results, especially to other locations or regions, must be made with caution.

The effect of NOM on arsenic adsorption depends on the oxidation state of arsenic, the composition of the NOM, and the type of iron mineral present. Grafe et al. (2001, 2002) simulated the effects of DOC on As sorption on goethite and ferrihydrite using solutions of humic acid (HA), fulvic acid (FA) and citric acid (CA), as shown in Figure 2.6. The influence of DOC is greater, but also more complex, on goethite than ferrihydrite, and the effects depend strongly on the specific iron phase, the form of arsenic and nature of the DOC. When ferrihydrite is the sorbent, the trend of As(III) adsorption with increasing pH shown is reduced by citric and fulvic acids across the pH ranges 3–7 and 8–11, but not at all by humic acid. However, As(V) adsorption on ferrihydrite is not affected by humic or fulvic acids at any pH, but is reduced by citric acid below pH 6.0 (Grafe et al., 2002). When goethite is the sorbent, As(V) adsorption is reduced by a small to negligible degree at all pH values. As(III) adsorption on goethite is reduced by all three acids in the order CA > HA > FA. The reductions are pH-dependent: the effect of citric acid becomes negligible at pH 8, for fulvic acid at pH 9, and for humic acid only at pH 10. Humic acid significantly reduces As(III) adsorption on goethite across the full range of pH encountered in normal groundwater. The effect of organic matter on other oxides may differ, and hence correlations with DOC measurements should be treated with caution. Stollenwerk (2003), citing earlier studies, reported that fulvic acid reduces adsorption of As(V) on Al oxides at pH values <7.

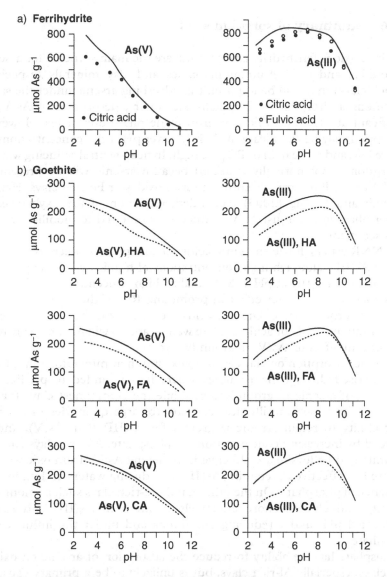

Figure 2.6 Influence of dissolved organic carbon (DOC) on adsorption of arsenic onto (a) ferrihydrite and (b) goethite. The dashed lines illustrate the effects of different forms of dissolved organic matter (HA, humic acid; FA, fulvic acid; CA, citric acid) on the adsorption of As(III) and As(V) onto both ferrihydrite and goethite; the solid line represents the base case of no DOC added. Points represent experimental measurements. All solutions contained 1.0 mm of DOC and 1.0 mm (75 ppm) of As(III) or As(V).
Source: After Grafe et al. (2001, 2002)

2.3.6   Summary of sorption studies

The iron oxides ferrihydrite and goethite are the main sorbents for arsenic in aquifers and soils. Aluminium oxides and clay minerals (especially Fe-rich clays) may also be important in adsorbing arsenic under the same conditions as iron oxides. In alkali-oxic waters, desorption of As(V) is significant at pH > 8.0, whichever iron oxide phase dominates. However, desorption may be significant at slightly lower pH if the concentrations of Ca are low, and those of Si or PO_4 are high. In near-neutral reducing waters, desorption is not normally expected because arsenic will be present as As(III) and will be strongly sorbed to iron oxides or Fe-rich clays. Hence, as Dixit and Hering (2003) concluded, reduction of the oxyhydroxide carrier phase and not just As(V) reduction is required to mobilise arsenic from sediments.

In NNR waters, fulvic and citric acids do not appear to decrease adsorption of As(III), although high concentrations of humic acids may promote desorption of As(III) at pH 7–8. In reality, high concentrations of organic acids may have a greater effect in promoting RD of the iron oxides that carry the sorbed arsenic. Organic acids are unlikely to be present at high concentrations in AO or acid-sulphate waters, and so will not normally have a significant effect on As(V) in groundwater.

Arsenic adsorption on clays is complex, and their mineralogy should be characterised through field studies where it is intended to predict the transport of arsenic in groundwater. While the commonest clays (kaolinite, illite and montmorillonite) can adsorb large quantities of arsenic, their ability to retain arsenic is greater for As(III) than As(V), and is reduced by increasing concentrations of phosphate. Al-rich clays such as kaolinite and halloysite are effective in removing As(V) from oxic waters, but are less effective in retaining As(III) in reducing waters and under the influence of phosphate. On the other hand, Fe-rich clays such as montmorillonite and chlorite more effectively retain both As(III) and As(V) at elevated pH, under reducing conditions and under the influence of phosphate.

Phosphate has the ability to reduce the adsorption of arsenic on oxides and clays, especially Al-rich clays, but is unlikely to be a primary cause of mobilising arsenic. Silica reduces the adsorption of both arsenic species, especially As(III), although Ca and Mg tend to counteract this effect. Therefore silica will have the greatest effect on As(V) mobilisation in sodic groundwater, but may also be relevant to mobilising As(III). Despite some suggestions that carbonate promotes desorption of arsenic, there is currently little field evidence to support this idea.

2.4   The Role of Sulphur in Strongly Reducing Groundwater

2.4.1   Sulphate reduction and pyrite formation

The behaviour of arsenic in groundwater is closely connected with that of sulphur. Metal sulphides are often rich in arsenic, and hence their oxidation can be a source of dissolved arsenic (see section 2.6.3). In anaerobic systems, sulphate reduction, aided by bacteria (e.g. Chapelle, 2001, and references therein), leads to the precipitation of minerals such as pyrite, which act as sinks for arsenic by incorporating arsenic into their structure, and which can also adsorb arsenite onto their surface. Depending on the availability of iron, the process can produce hydrogen sulphide or sulphide minerals. Initially, hydrogen sulphide is formed by the bacterial reduction of sulphate by organic matter (Appelo and Postma, 1996):

$$2CH_2O + SO_4^{2-} \rightarrow 2HCO_3^- + H_2S \tag{2.1}$$

Pyrite formation takes place in a two-step process (Appelo and Postma, 1996) as follows:

$$2FeOOH + 3HS^- \rightarrow 2FeS + S^0 + H_2O + 3OH^- \tag{2.2}$$

where dissolved sulphide reacts with iron hydroxide, producing black precipitates of an iron monosulphide (mackinawite or troilite), which is then slowly converted to pyrite as follows:

$$FeS + S^0 \rightarrow FeS_2 \tag{2.3}$$

Pyrite, mackinawite and troilite all have the capacity to remove arsenic from solution, and the limits to their growth can therefore determine whether As contamination will occur. Low sulphate concentrations are ubiquitous in the As-affected alluvial aquifers of South Asia and the glacial aquifers in the USA, and where sulphate reduction is commonly assumed to occur. Nickson et al. (1998) demonstrated that pyrite is a sink for arsenic in the Bengal Basin. Arsenic contamination occurs in NNR waters only when the capacity of sulphides to remove it is exhausted. Kirk et al. (2004) demonstrated the relation of sulphate reduction to As mobilisation in the Mahomet Buried Valley Aquifer of Illinois (Figure 2.7). Where DOC is >2 ppm, sulphate is virtually absent and methane is abundant. Where iron dominates, sulphide concentrations remain close to detection levels. While iron and sulphur reduction are active, organic species in water are rapidly consumed, inhibiting the growth of methanogens. In the Mahomet aquifer,

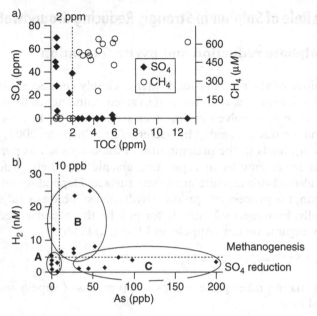

Figure 2.7 Arsenic and sulphate reduction in the Mahomet Buried Valley Aquifer. (a) The relation between total organic carbon (TOC), sulphate and methane (CH$_4$). (b) The relation between arsenic and hydrogen concentration, a sensitive indicator of reducing conditions. Group A waters contain little methane, high sulphate and <3 ppm of iron. Group B and C waters contain negligible sulphate, abundant methane and high (1.4–5.9 ppm) iron.
Source: After Kirk et al. (2004)

high As concentrations only develop after sulphate reduction is complete, although curiously the highest concentrations were reported from the sulphate-reducing, and not the methanogenic, section of the aquifer (Kirk et al., 2004).

2.4.2 Adsorption on sulphides

Although less important overall than oxide minerals, under reducing conditions, arsenic may be adsorbed on the iron sulphide minerals pyrite (FeS$_2$), troilite (FeS) and mackinawite (FeS) and, although they are less abundant, other sulphide minerals such as sphalerite (ZnS) and galena (PbS). Bostick and Fendorf (2003) determined that arsenite is adsorbed onto pyrite and troilite (Figure 2.8), where adsorption was minimal at low pH and strongest at pH > 5–6, involving the formation of an FeAsS-like precipitate. Because both Fe and S are incorporated into the precipitate, the

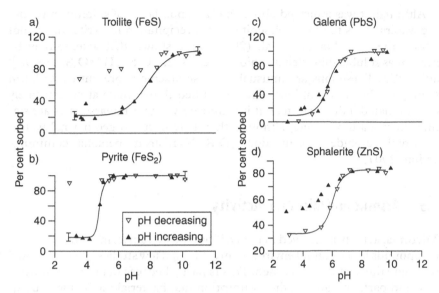

Figure 2.8   Adsorption of arsenic on sulphide minerals: (a) troilite; (b) pyrite; (c) galena; (d) sphalerite. All experiments were conducted with 50 μM (3750 ppb) As, 1 g/L of sulphide and a background electrolyte of 0.01 m NaNO$_3$. The lines are sigmoidal fits to experimental data.
Source: After Bostick and Fendorf (2003) and Bostick et al. (2003)

process changes the nature of the mineral surface, and hence its ability to retain arsenic. Similar experiments on galena and sphalerite found that arsenite is adsorbed at pH > 5 and pH > 4.5 respectively (Bostick et al., 2003). In all cases, increasing sulphide concentrations significantly reduced adsorption of arsenite. Adsorption of arsenate was not considered because it is not normally stable in groundwater in which sulphides are stable and capable of adsorbing solutes. Wolthers et al. (2005) found that adsorption of As(III) on disordered mackinawite (tetragonal FeS), which they consider to be more representative of the Fe(II) monosulphides in natural environments, was not strongly pH-dependent in the pH range 5.5–8.5, but had a maximum of 23% at pH 7.2. However, they found that adsorption of As(V) on mackinawite was strongly pH-dependent, rising rapidly to a maximum at pH 7.4 and then falling even more rapidly to a negligible level at pH 8.5.

Kirk et al. (2004), McArthur et al. (2004) and O'Day et al. (2004) all recognised that the mobilisation and immobilisation of arsenic in reducing groundwaters are determined by the balance between the quantities of Fe, S and organic carbon. Initially, an excess of organic carbon is required to reduce Fe(III) oxides completely and release the sorbed As to solution, whereafter the availability of sulphur controls the sequestration of arsenic by sulphide minerals.

Although it was indicated above that an abundance of sulphur in reducing waters tends to remove arsenite by coprecipitation in pyrite, this is not always the case. Stauder et al. (2005) have shown that arsenic may be present as soluble thioarsenate anions such as $HAsO_3S^{2-}$, $HAsO_2S_2^{2-}$, $AsOS_3^{3-}$ and AsS_4^{3-}. These ions are unusual because arsenic is present as As(V) in strongly reducing conditions. They identified thioarsenate at an extremely contaminated industrial site, but it is unclear whether thioarsenates are significant in natural waters, although they may occur in geothermal waters with high sulphide concentrations (D.K. Nordstrom, personal communication, 2007).

2.5 Arsenic and Microbial Activity

Microbial activity is involved in many, if not most, transformations of arsenic compounds in the natural environment, although few studies have attempted to isolate the bacteria concerned. This is partly because of practical difficulties, and partly because of the assumption that bacterial mediation is ubiquitous. It is of practical importance to know to what extent the presence of a particular organism controls the transfer of arsenic between solid and liquid phases because it may be possible to exploit these organisms to aid remediation or water treatment.

Iron oxides can adsorb both As(III) and As(V). Alluvial sediments probably acquire most arsenic by adsorbing As(V) in oxic environments, where As(III) is not stable. The conventional view of arsenic mobilised by reductive dissolution is that (solid) Fe(III) is reduced to release aqueous Fe(II) and As(V) into solution. Organisms such as *Shewanella alga* can increase the rate of Fe(III) reduction, accelerating the release of As(V) into solution, where other organisms could undertake its reduction to As(III). Attention has focused on whether the transformation of As(V) in the solid phase to dissolved As(III) is a coupled process, and whether microbes can decouple reduction of the iron and arsenic[6]. Zobrist et al. (2000) found that *Sulfurospirillum barnesii* can reduce arsenate to arsenite, both in solution and when adsorbed on ferrihydrite. However, because of the variety of organisms that can perform both the iron-reducing task and the aqueous arsenic-reducing task, Inskeep et al. (2002) considered that prior reduction of Fe(III) oxides will be the most common pathway. Nonetheless, Oremland and Stolz (2003) argued that bacteria that reduce sorbed arsenate on the solid phase may be important in the Bengal Basin. However, as Dixit and Hering (2003) pointed out, arsenite is strongly adsorbed by Fe(III) oxides in near-neutral waters, and so As reduction is probably not the critical step.

Islam et al. (2004) conducted incubation experiments on sediment from an As-contaminated aquifer in West Bengal. Aerobic incubation had a negligible effect, but anaerobic incubation reduced Fe(III) and released small quantities of As(III) after 38 days. Adding acetate, a proxy for reactive organic matter, stimulated the reduction of Fe(III), which was followed, after a distinct delay, by the release of arsenic. Initially As(V) was detected, but later As(III) became dominant. This implies that Fe(III) reduction is decoupled from the release of arsenic to solution, although an abiotic explanation has also been proposed in which arsenic is readsorbed until the adsorptive capacity of the remaining Fe(III) is saturated (Welch et al., 2000; McArthur et al., 2004). The main organism reducing As(V) to As(III) was *Geothrix fermentans* (Islam et al., 2005). Van Geen et al. (2004) conducted incubation experiments on grey and orange-brown sand from Araihazar in Bangladesh. Samples collected during drilling were diluted with local wellwater and incubated for up to 60 days, which mobilised small quantities of arsenic, but only after orange Fe(III) oxyhydroxides had first been reduced to grey-black Fe(II) phases. Adding antibiotics severely inhibited the release of arsenic, confirming that micro-organisms naturally present in the sands can mobilise arsenic. Conversely, adding acetate increased the rate and quantity of arsenic mobilisation by providing a substrate for bacterial growth.

Oremland and Stolz (2005) proposed three mechanisms (Figure 2.9) by which bacteria might mobilise arsenic from Fe(III) oxides through the action of arsenate-resistant microbes (ARM) termed dissimilatory arsenate-respiring prokaryotes (DARP). The ARMs may not actually gain energy through the release of arsenic, but metabolising arsenic allows them to cope with an As-rich environment. In the first mechanism, iron-reducing bacteria such as *Geobacter* reduce Fe(III) and release As(V) directly to solution where it is converted to As(III) by biotic or abiotic means. In the second mechanism, the DARP transforms As(V) to As(III) at the solid surface prior to its release. In the third mechanism, iron-reducing DARPs, such as *Sulfurospirillum barnesii*, directly release both Fe(II) and As(III). As Oremland and Stolz (2005) note, in nature, all three mechanisms may operate simultaneously.

2.6 Arsenic Mobilisation Mechanisms

As noted earlier, there are four basic mechanisms that can mobilise arsenic to groundwater. In the following sections, we explain how the basic processes described above act in different geochemical environments to produce the characteristic water types. We also begin to explore the geological factors that determine where mechanisms are important, although these factors are examined in more detail in Chapter 3, and in the case histories in Chapters 8–10.

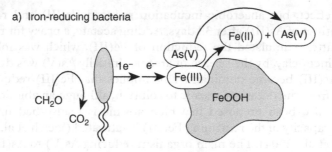

a) Iron-reducing bacteria

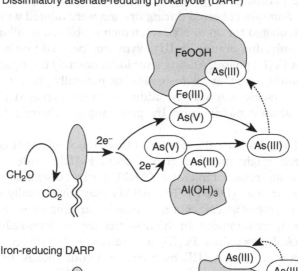

b) Dissimilatory arsenate-reducing prokaryote (DARP)

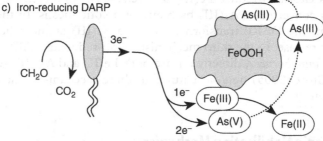

c) Iron-reducing DARP

Figure 2.9 Microbial mechanisms of arsenic mobilisation. The diagram shows three possible mechanisms of microbially mediated arsenic mobilisation in anoxic environments. All the reactions are driven by oxidation of organic matter, where microbes use either Fe(III) or As(V) as the terminal electron acceptor. *Source*: After Oremland and Stolz (2005)

2.6.1   Mobilisation by reductive dissolution

Mechanism

Ferric oxides and hydroxides are ubiquitous adsorbers of arsenic and other trace elements, but will release this arsenic when they are reduced to the ferrous state and dissolve. Hence, the mobility of arsenic depends in large part on the stability of iron oxides. Contrary to some accounts, this mechanism is distinct from those involving desorption of arsenic from solid mineral surfaces. The redox reactions controlling iron in natural waters have been studied in great detail (e.g. Hem, 1977; Langmuir, 1997), and the process of iron reduction by organic matter may be represented by the following equation:

$$8FeOOH + CH_3COOH + 14H_2CO_3$$
$$\Rightarrow 8Fe^{2+} + 16HCO_3^- + 12H_2O \tag{2.4}$$

This reaction requires the operation of a strong redox driver, usually sedimentary organic matter, which consumes all available sources of oxygen. McArthur et al. (2001) proposed that the dominant redox driver in alluvial aquifers is the microbial mineralisation of buried vegetation that accumulated as peat or organic-rich mud in abandoned channels and overbank environments. Arsenic-rich groundwater in strongly reducing conditions has a characteristic chemical signature, and has been described in most detail in the Bengal Basin (e.g. Nickson et al., 2000; Ravenscroft et al., 2001; Harvey et al. 2002; Zheng et al., 2004). The degradation of organic matter generates high bicarbonate concentrations, accompanied by high concentrations of reduced species such as As(III), manganese, ferrous iron, ammonium and DOC, and discharges of methane gas. Conversely, oxidised species such as dissolved oxygen (DO) and nitrate are absent, and sulphate concentrations are usually very low, or at least accompanied by signs of sulphate reduction. Degrading organic matter produces a characteristic N:P ratio of about 16, but the As-rich groundwaters in Bangladesh contain a higher proportion of phosphorus. Like arsenic, phosphate is also strongly adsorbed to iron oxides, and McArthur et al. (2001) attributed the excess P to reductive dissolution. Manganese, which is mobilised under mildly reducing conditions, does not have a consistent relation with arsenic. In some areas, high Mn and As concentrations coexist (e.g. van Geen, Zheng et al., 2003a) and elsewhere they are mutually exclusive (McArthur et al., 2004). On the other hand, increasing concentrations of iron, phosphate and ammonium are all associated with elevated As concentrations, although the correlations are non-linear and far from perfect (Figure 2.10).

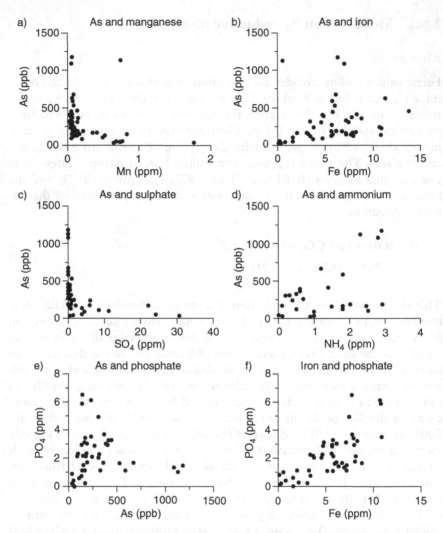

Figure 2.10 Relationships between As and Mn, Fe, SO$_4$, PO$_4$ and NH$_4$ in a shallow arsenic-contaminated aquifer in West Bengal. All analyses are from water wells screened at depths of less than 50 m deep.
Source: Redrawn after McArthur et al. (2004)

A complementary line of evidence supporting the operation of RD concerns the chemistry of the sediments, which has been investigated by selected leaching with solvents ranging from simple water to hot concentrated acid, in order to determine the 'availability' of arsenic. Particular emphasis is given to the quantities of arsenic extracted by solutions of phosphate and oxalate, the latter often being regarded as a measure of arsenic

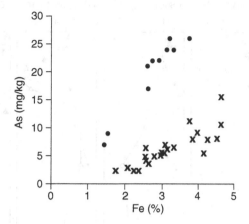

Figure 2.11 Correlation of sedimentary iron and arsenic in Bangladesh and Vietnam.
Note: The Bangladesh analyses (solid circles) were obtained from extractions with hot HCl by Nickson et al. (2000), and the Vietnam analyses (crosses) from extractions with HNO_3 and H_2O_2 by Berg et al. (2001).

bound to iron oxides. Hence, positive correlations between diagenetically available iron and arsenic have been observed in Bangladesh and Vietnam (Figure 2.11), and are considered to be strong evidence that dissolved arsenic was originally adsorbed on iron oxides. Figure 2.12 shows an example of a detailed profile of water, sediment and gas chemistry in an As-polluted alluvial aquifer in central Bangladesh, and demonstrates how various lines of evidence combine to support the interpretation of RD. The peak in dissolved As is only weakly correlated with solid-phase arsenic, but mobilisation by reduction is indicated by the correlation with other parameters in solution. Coincident peaks in ammonium, DOC and methane point to the decomposition of buried plant matter; the near-mirror-image minimum in sulphate concentrations indicates that sulphate reduction is a precondition to high dissolved As; and peaks of calcium and DIC point to dissolution of carbonate minerals.

Iron oxides (As carriers) and organic matter (redox driver) frequently do not occur in the same sedimentary horizons, which therefore requires that DOC migrates before arsenic is mobilised. In alluvium, oxyhydroxides occur mainly as coatings on sands deposited in the channels (i.e. future aquifers), whereas organic matter accumulates in overbank environments (later forming aquitards). The organic degradation products are drawn into the aquifers by groundwater flow, with or without the influence of pumping, as shown in Figure 2.13. Similar relations exist between sands and organic matter within fluvio-glacial sediments, and beneath thick glacial sediments where the redox driver lies within the drift and the oxide

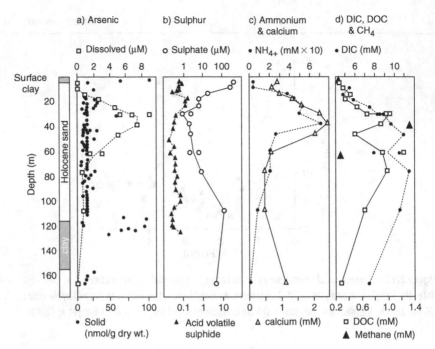

Figure 2.12 Geochemical profiles from an arsenic-affected aquifer in Bangladesh. (a) Dissolved As measured in piezometers and average solid phase As at each depth. (b) Dissolved sulphate and acid volatile sulphide (basically iron sulphide minerals). (c) Dissolved ammonium and calcium. (d) Dissolved inorganic carbon (DIC), organic carbon (DOC), and methane gas in piezometers.
Source: Simplified from Harvey et al. (2002)

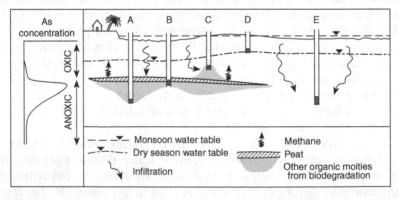

Figure 2.13 Simple model of arsenic pollution in the Bengal Basin. The model applies to sediments hosting organic-rich deposits. Water moving downward under natural and induced hydraulic gradients is intercepted by wells in an area with a discontinuous peat layer. The occurrence of arsenic can be considered in terms of five scenarios (A–E): A, low concentrations of DOC reduce some FeOOH and cause low-level As-contamination; B, high concentrations of DOC reduce much FeOOH and cause severe As pollution; C, DOC is drawn upwards by pumping from the well to reduce FeOOH and mobilise As; D, very shallow wells are safe from As contamination; E, uncontaminated well where concentrations of DOC are low, but there may be a long-term risk due to lateral migration of As mobilised adjacent to the peat.
Source: After Ravenscroft et al. (2001)

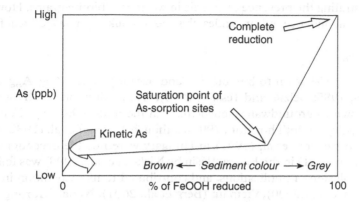

Figure 2.14   The kinetic arsenic model. Kinetic arsenic is that released by the partial reduction of FeOOH and not immediately re-sorbed, where the As concentration reflects the relative rates of reduction and adsorption. Initially, the build up of iron concentrations is accompanied by low concentrations of kinetic arsenic. High As concentrations develop only after sufficient iron has been reduced so that all sorption sites on the residual iron oxides are saturated, and can adsorb no more arsenic.
Source: After McArthur et al. (2004)

carrier-phase is in underlying bedrock, and hence As mobilisation is concentrated near the bedrock surface.

Horneman et al. (2004) and Islam et al. (2004), for example, have commented on the relatively poor correlation between Fe and As concentrations in water (as distinct from the sediments). Almost all As-rich waters contain high Fe, but many Fe-rich waters do not contain high As, because many other factors are involved. McArthur et al. (2004), extending an idea put forward by Welch et al. (2000), explained the absence of a simple relationship through the release and readsorption of what they termed 'kinetic arsenic' (Figure 2.14). The ferric oxyhydroxides coating alluvial sands have a significant buffering capacity, whereby ferrous iron in solution may coexist with ferric oxyhydroxides in the solid phase. When only part of the oxyhydroxide mass has been reduced, its sorbed load of arsenic may be released to solution, and then almost immediately readsorbed onto the residual ferric phase. Under the 'kinetic arsenic' scenario, severe As contamination does not develop until most or all of the iron oxyhydroxides are reduced. During the early stages of iron reduction, if any sulphate is present in solution, some of the arsenic will be incorporated into diagenetic (framboidal) pyrite.

Not all workers agree that iron oxides are the primary control on arsenic mobility in reducing groundwater. Smedley and Kinniburgh (2002) suggested that manganese oxides might be important carriers of arsenic, but in general, the abundance of iron oxides ensures that, even if Mn oxides release arsenic, it is readsorbed onto iron oxides (McArthur et al., 2004). Breit et al. (2005) suggested that micas are important carriers of arsenic, demonstrating the presence of arsenic in weathered biotite grains. However, given the abundance of iron oxides, this seems unlikely to be a critical factor.

Occurrence

Although well-known to limnologists and oceanographers (e.g. Aggett and O'Brien, 1985; Belzile and Tessier, 1990), As mobilisation by RD was not well known to groundwater geochemists in the mid-1990s (e.g. Edmunds and Smedley, 1996; Thornton, 1996), although Matisoff et al. (1982) in the USA and Varsányi et al. (1991) in Hungary were notable exceptions. The description of RD in the Bengal Basin by Nickson et al. (1998) was followed by an explosion of publications, and contributed to its recognition in India (Acharyya et al., 2000), Vietnam (Berg et al., 2001), Nepal (Gurung et al., 2005) and China (Lin et al., 2002). These studies also led to a re-evaluation of As pollution in glacial aquifers in the USA (Kirk et al., 2004).

The geographical distribution of cases of As mobilisation attributed to RD is shown in Figure 2.15a. The most important cases of RD are located along the South and Southeast Asian Arsenic belt (SSAAB) that runs from the Indus in Pakistan, along the southern margin of the Himalayas and Indo-Burman ranges to Taiwan and some of the inland basins of China. Beyond Asia, the other important occurrences are in the Danube and Po basins in Europe, and along the USA–Canadian border. With minor exceptions, it is remarkable how few reports there have been of As contamination from superficially similar fluvial settings in North and South America, Australia and Africa. Almost all cases of RD come from Late Pleistocene to Holocene alluvial or fluvio-glacial sediments. The association with young sediments is readily explained by the reactivity of fresh organic matter, and is confirmed by the young age (to a few decades) of contaminated waters (e.g. Aggarwal et al., 2000; Klump et al., 2006). Sedimentary conditions favourable to RD are discussed further in Chapter 3.

2.6.2   Mobilisation by alkali desorption

Mechanism

As described earlier, sorption of arsenic depends strongly on pH and, to a lesser degree, on the presence of competing ions. The term alkali desorption is used to describe a set of processes that involve an increase in pH that promote desorption of arsenic from iron oxides or other minerals, and hence produce alkali-oxic waters. Alkali desorption has been invoked to explain the occurrence of arsenic in alkali-oxic groundwaters in Argentina, the southwestern and central USA, Spain and other locations where pH is elevated and As mobilisation could not be readily explained by other mechanisms.

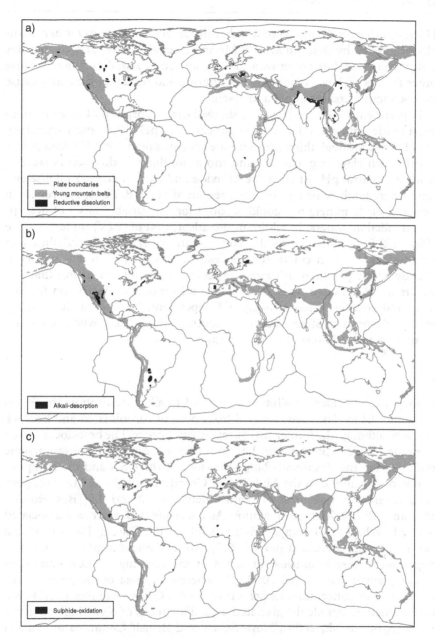

Figure 2.15 Geographical distribution of arsenic contamination by mobilisation mechanism. The figures show the locations of arsenic contamination that have been attributed to (a) reductive dissolution, (b) alkali desorption and (c) sulphide oxidation. See Table 1.2 for identification of reference numbers, Figure 1.1 for the location of all arsenic occurrences, and Chapters 8–10 for details of individual occurrences. The tectonic plate boundaries and young mountain chains are from ESRI (1996).

However, there is dispute as to whether the arsenic in some AO waters actually originated by desorption, and McArthur et al. (2004) argued that this water type alone does not prove a causal connection with desorption because other factors such as evaporation, weathering and residence time may cause independent increases in pH and arsenic.

Experimental data (section 2.3) showed that adsorption of arsenate onto most oxides and clays decreases significantly at pH $\geq$ 8.0, and particularly at pH > 8.5, although this varies with the specific mineralogy. For iron oxides and Fe-rich clays (e.g. chlorite and montmorillonite), this occurs steadily from subneutral pH, whereas for Al oxide and Al-rich clays (kaolinite and illite) there tends to be a peak in the region of pH 6–8. Thus, differences in clay and oxide mineralogy could account for the variable onset of desorption in alkaline waters. In addition, the adsorption of As(V) on ferrihydrite (Figure 2.2) is sensitive to the concentrations of phosphate, silica and organic acids, which could explain desorption of As(V) in oxic waters at slightly lower pH than otherwise expected. It is not surprising that AO waters are dominated by As(V) because adsorption of As(III) on ferrihydrite and goethite is less strongly pH-dependent. In moderately reducing waters, desorption of arsenic, if it occurs, is most likely where there are extreme concentrations of organic acids.

Occurrence

Occurrences of arsenic pollution attributed to alkali desorption are shown in Figure 2.15b. They are reported from both unconsolidated and bedrock aquifers, although the former are of greater significance. The best-documented examples of desorption in alkaline groundwater causing extensive arsenic pollution are the Basin-and-Range Province of the USA and the Pampean Plains of Argentina. In the Middle Rio Grande Basin (New Mexico), peak As concentrations occur at pH values between 8.0 and 9.0 (Bexfield and Plummer, 2003). In Argentina, most As-contaminated waters are associated with pH values in the range 7.5–8.5, while in the Datong Basin of China elevated arsenic occurs at pH 7.8–8.5, and in Finland at pH 7.5–8.0. The Argentinean case is unusual in terms of the very high concentrations of arsenic, which may exceed 1000 ppb, whereas in most of the better documented cases concentrations are <100 ppb As. Other examples of AD-type contamination include the glaciated crystalline rocks of New England in the USA (Ayotte et al., 2003), Nova Scotia and British Columbia in Canada (Bottomley, 1984; Boyle et al., 1998) and southwest Finland (Loukola-Ruskeeniemi and Lahermo, 2004). The AD mechanism is also encountered in consolidated Tertiary sediments in central Spain (Hernández-García and Custodio, 2004; Garcia-Sanchez et al., 2005) and Permian sandstones in Oklahoma (Schlottmann et al., 1998). A pH-related mechanism appears to operate in the alluvial Datong Basin in China (Guo et al., 2003), although RD probably operates simultaneously in different parts of the basin.

The occurrences listed above are associated with four lithologically distinct groups that have little in common: alluvium; Tertiary–Mesozoic sedimentary rocks; crystalline bedrock; and volcanic-loess. In crystalline bedrock, arsenic is expected to be present in either sulphide minerals coating fractures or their weathering products. In alluvium and sandstone, arsenic is expected to occur in oxyhydroxide coatings on sands. In volcanic-loess, arsenic may be directly leached from volcanic glass, but the glass may also have been weathered with arsenic sequestered in oxyhydroxide coatings. Volcanic-loess appears to be critical in generating high-As (and fluoride) groundwater in Argentina. Arsenic has also been linked to volcanic ash in South Dakota (Carter et al., 1998) and Oregon (Whanger et al., 1977). The volcanic material in the Pampean Loess, which has a high alkali (Na+K) content, contains very reactive volcanic glass (Sracek et al., 2007). A more general influence is that oxic weathering of many silicate rocks gives rise to alkaline sodium–bicarbonate waters. In New England, British Columbia and Finland, where the lithology is often granitic, it appears that sulphide mineralisation in veins and coating fracture surfaces is the primary source of arsenic. In such cases, AD requires prior weathering (i.e. sulphide oxidation) to transfer arsenic from sulphide to oxide phases. Thus, it is possible that AD and SO could operate simultaneously in close proximity in the same geological terrain.

Arsenic in AD groundwater in New England, British Columbia and southwest Finland has also been associated with marine transgressions that followed the retreat of the Pleistocene glaciers. Rocks covered by hundreds or thousands of metres of ice subsided many metres. Post-glacial sea-level rise occurred faster than the isostatic rebound of rock masses, inundating lowlying areas that have since re-emerged. Flooding by seawater promoted ion-exchange reactions with clays and iron oxides, which became enriched in sodium and boron, and depleted in calcium and magnesium. When the rocks re-emerged, the processes were reversed. Calcium and magnesium were adsorbed onto mineral surfaces and sodium and boron were released to the porewater. Depending on the lithology, the resultant high-Na and low-Ca waters tend to produce elevated pH, which favours desorption of arsenic.

2.6.3   Mobilisation by sulphide oxidation

Mechanism

The iron sulphide minerals pyrite (FeS_2) and arsenopyrite ($FeAsS$) are the most important stores of arsenic in 'reduced' minerals, and therefore their oxidation can be important sources of arsenic pollution. Pyrite is the commonest sulphide mineral, and is most abundant in marine sediments, igneous rocks and areas of hydrothermal alteration. Pyrite oxidation is commonly associated with mining activities but is also an important natural process. Arsenic in the two previous mechanisms, the mobility of arsenic depends on the behaviour of iron minerals, and hence we first describe the reactions controlling their stability. Pyrite may be oxidised by oxygen, nitrate or ferric iron, and the processes have been studied by many authors (e.g. Appelo and Postma, 1996; Langmuir, 1997). The implications of these reactions can be appreciated by examining the reaction equations, first for oxygen:

$$2FeS_2 + 7O_2 + 2H_2O \Rightarrow 2Fe^{2+} + 4SO_4^{2-} + 4H^+ \qquad (2.5)$$

The reaction consumes large quantities of oxygen, seven molecules of O_2 for every two of iron sulphide. Also, as indicated by the last term of equation (2.5), it produces acidity, accounting for the low pH values recorded in many mining areas. If carbonate minerals are present, the acidity will be quickly neutralised, but in areas of crystalline basement the acidity may be persistent. Where additional oxygen is present, the dissolved ferrous iron is then oxidised to ferric iron, consuming some of the acidity, as follows (Appelo and Postma, 1996):

$$Fe^{2+} + \tfrac{1}{4}O_2 + H^+ \Rightarrow Fe^{3+} \tfrac{1}{2}H_2O \qquad (2.6)$$

The ferric iron will be precipitated as ferrihydrite, which will adsorb at least some of the released arsenic. Pyrite may also be oxidised by nitrate, a process that could be important in areas of intensive farming that overlie sulphide-rich subsoils. This reaction is significantly different to equation (2.5) because it produces nitrogen gas and does not produce such strongly acidic products, and results in different water chemistry. The equation for the reaction with nitrate is:

$$5FeS_2 + 14NO_3^- + 4H^+ \Rightarrow 5Fe^{2+} + 10SO_4^{2-} + 7N_2 + 2H_2O \qquad (2.7)$$

In the absence of free oxygen, nitrate may oxidise ferrous to ferric iron, which is precipitated as ferrihydrite, while the other reaction products are nitrogen gas and acidity[7] (Appelo and Postma, 1996):

$$10Fe^{2+} + 2NO_3^- + 14H_2O \Rightarrow 10FeOOH + N_2 + 18H^+ \qquad (2.8)$$

While pyrite can contain up to 3.8% of arsenic (Ballantyne and Moore, 1988), arsenopyrite contains 46% and is a more potent source of pollution. In New Zealand, Craw et al. (2003) studied the stability of arsenopyrite in calcitic gold-bearing veins in the Otago Schists and the sediments derived from them. Although arsenopyrite can break down readily at pH<4 to generate highly polluting waters containing >400 ppm As, under near-neutral and alkaline conditions its stability is similar to that of pyrite. They found that natural groundwaters in contact with arsenopyrite contained <5 ppb As, and suggested that mine tailings kept saturated and mildly reducing will remain stable in long-term storage. The other arsenic sulphides, orpiment and realgar, are obviously also potential sources of pollution, as are some sulphides of iron (marcasite, FeS_2), copper (chalcopyrite, $CuFeS_2$) and antimony (stibnite, Sb_2S_3), which can all accommodate significant proportions of arsenic in their crystal structure.

Occurrence

Known occurrences of natural arsenic contamination attributed to SO are shown in Figure 2.15c. Pyrite oxidation has received great attention because of its importance in generating acid mine drainage, and is discussed further in section 2.7. Sulphide oxidation can occur wherever sulphide minerals are exposed to oxygenated or nitrate-rich water. Crystalline bedrock often has coatings of sulphide minerals on fracture surfaces, which can be mobilised by infiltrating rainwater, especially where soils are thin and there is little carbonate to neutralise the acidity. Thus, shallow wells are particularly vulnerable to pollution, as in Washington State (USA), Nova Scotia, France, Ghana and central India. Schreiber et al. (2000) described a classic example of severe contamination of Palaeozoic sandstones in Wisconsin (USA) due to the pumping-induced fluctuation of the water table across a sulphide-rich horizon (section 9.2.7). The other classic situation where pyrite oxidation occurs is in the formation of so-called acid-sulphate soils[8], where water-logged peat or mangrove soils are exposed to the atmosphere (e.g. Appleyard et al., 2006). When swamps are drained, pyrite oxidation (at the water table) and RD (beneath the swamp) may operate simultaneously in close juxtaposition (Appleyard et al., 2005). Further details of these occurrences are presented in Chapters 8–10.

2.6.4 Geothermal arsenic

Geothermal arsenic is common in active and former continental-volcanic settings such as in New Zealand, the Andes, southern Italy and the Rockies, and to a lesser extent in oceanic-volcanic terrains. Geothermal resources have received much attention because of their potential for power generation, but are not normally developed for water supply or irrigation. Webster and Nordstrom (2003) identified three tectonic settings in which GT arsenic commonly occurs. The first is at colliding plate boundaries, which includes not only subduction zones such as the Andes and the Indonesian arc, but also continental sutures such as the Qinghai–Tibet plateau. Geothermal arsenic is also encountered at intraplate 'hot spots' where magma chambers rise to shallow levels in the Earth's crust, such as at Yellowstone and Hawaii. The third situation is along rift zones such as the East African Rift Valley and Rio Grande Valley in Colorado and New Mexico. Heat sources for geothermal waters include volcanic activity, metamorphism, faulting and radioactivity. The potential for generating hot As-rich waters was demonstrated through experiments in the 1960s, which showed that not only could elements such as Cl, B and F be leached from country rocks, so too could Li, Rb and Cs, and did not require a magmatic source (Webster and Nordstrom, 2003). These early leaching experiments extracted substantial quantities of arsenic from andesite, and As, Sb, Se and S from greywacke.

Ballantyne and Moore (1988) noted that arsenic, as As(III), is present in geothermal reservoirs at concentrations that range over three orders of magnitude, and which tend to correlate directly with temperature in low salinity waters (<3000 ppm Cl). They also noted that As concentrations vary inversely with the partial pressure of hydrogen sulphide, and took this as evidence that arsenic in high-temperature fluids is regulated by the crystallisation of pyrite. In low-temperature systems, arsenic may be present as either As(III) or As(V). Near the surface, with cooling, pyrite may coexist with native arsenic. However, as conditions become more oxidising, the minerals orpiment and realgar may be precipitated. In many hot springs, GT arsenic is accompanied by high concentrations of other toxic elements such as B, F, Li and Cs.

High As concentrations (e.g. at the ppm, or tens of ppm, level) are common in continental hot springs, but in oceanic settings in Hawaii and Iceland they contain <100 ppb As. The highest known natural As concentration in geothermal (or any other) water is 126 ppm from the Sogdoi spring in the west of the Qinghai–Tibet plateau, in a zone of massive crustal thickening, where the Asian and Indian continents collided (Mianpiang, 1997). In addition, the Sogdoi spring also discharges 1917 ppm of boron and 50 ppm of lithium. In most geothermal waters, there is a positive correlation between As and Cl, even though Cl is probably derived from magma and arsenic from rock leaching. Thus arsenic is higher in neutral, Cl-rich hot springs than in acid-sulphate springs. Webster and Nordstrom (2003) suggested that the As:Cl ratio can be used as a tracer for the dilution of geothermal fluids. At Yellowstone, As and Cl followed a linear decrease to virtually zero from a source estimated to contain 400 ppm of chloride. Here, As(III) predominates at hot springs and geysers, but is rapidly oxidised to As(V) in the receiving streams, a process thought to be catalysed by bacteria.

Arsenic is pervasive in geothermal groundwater, but for various reasons rarely poses a major health risk. Many geothermal regions have low population densities, the flow from many hot springs may be too small for community supply, and there may be a natural reluctance to use such sources for regular drinking water. Of more significance are As-rich geothermal waters that leak into surface and groundwaters of non-geothermal origin. This occurs in the Waikato River in New Zealand, which supplies 100,000 people in the city of Hamilton (McLaren and Kim, 1995) and the Rio Toconce in Chile, which supplies >200,000 people at Antofagasta. Deep geothermal ground-waters, leaking into the base of alluvial aquifers, have been proposed as components of As contamination in the Rio Grande Basin of New Mexico and in Alaska (Chapter 9).

2.6.5   Evaporative concentration

Although not strictly speaking a mechanism for mobilising arsenic to groundwater, evaporative concentration can dramatically increase the concentrations of dissolved arsenic (Gao et al., 2007), and in some situations could cause arsenic concentrations to cross health-related thresholds. The likelihood of evapo-concentration is increased by an arid or semi-arid climate, and in the presence of a shallow water table. The effects of evapo-concentration may be indicated by high values of Cl, EC or TDS. However, a correlation between As and Cl can also indicate GT arsenic. Evapo-concentration may be distinguished by the correlation of arsenic with most major ions in water. If there remains uncertainty, the evaporation of water can be indicated conclusively by analysis of the stable isotopes of water ($\partial^{18}O$ and ∂^2H). Here, the heavy isotopes, which are less easily evaporated, become concentrated in the remaining groundwater. Evapo-concentration of arsenic has been recognised as a factor in the Carson Desert of Nevada (Welch and Lico, 1998), the Okavango delta of Botswana (Huntsman-Mapila et al., 2006) and the Chaco-Pampean plains of Argentina (Bhattacharya et al., 2006).

2.7   Associations of Arsenic with other Trace Elements

In many As-contaminated aquifers, other chemicals may also be of health concern. In many cases, these chemicals are mobilised by the same processes that mobilise arsenic. Studies in the southwest USA (Robertson, 1989) and Argentina (Nicolli et al., 1989) associated AD with high levels of fluoride, vanadium, molybdenum, antimony and selenium. Associations may be found between arsenic and other trace elements in many environments, but as shown in Table 2.5, the link to dangerous concentrations is more common where AD is the dominant process. This is slightly

Table 2.5 Association of arsenic with other trace elements of health concern

Region	Ref	Process	F	V	Mo	Se	U	Sb	Pb	Ba	B	Li	Cr	Ni	Mn	Other
Guideline (ppb):	–		1500	–	70	10	15	20	10	700	500	–	50	20	400	
Basin and Range Province, USA	1	AD	+ve	+ve	+ve	+ve			+ve		+ve					Rb(+ve)
Central Oklahoma Aquifer	2	AD				+ve	+ve						+ve			
Grass Mountain, S. Dakota, USA	3	AD		+ve	+ve											
Chaco–Pampean Plains, Argentina	4, 5	AD	+ve	+ve	+ve	+ve	+ve		+ve		+ve					
Bowen Island, Canada	6	AD	+ve		+ve						+ve					
SW Finland	7	AD	+ve		+ve					-ve		+ve		+ve		
Madrid Basin, Spain	8	AD	+ve	+ve	+ve						+ve		+ve			W(+ve)
Datong Basin, China	9	AD/RD	+ve		+ve											
Inner Mongolia, China	10	RD/AD	+ve												+ve	
Bengal Basin	11	RD			+ve		-ve								+ve	
Vietnam: Red River	12	RD		-ve	+ve				-ve	+ve					+ve	Ga(+ve)
Illinois, USA	13	RD			+ve					+ve						
Wisconsin, USA	14	SO											+ve	+ve	+ve	Zn, Co, Cu (all +ve)
E. Thessaly, Greece	15	SO						+ve								Cu(+ve)
Kutahya, Turkey	16	SO						+ve						+ve		Cd(+ve)
Afyon, Turkey	17	GT									+ve		+ve			Zn(+ve)
Qinghai–Tibet, China	18	GT								+ve	+ve	+ve				Cs(+ve)
Rio Loa, Chile	19	GT								+ve	+ve	+ve				Cs(+ve)
Altiplano, Bolivia	20	GT						+ve			+ve	+ve			+ve	Be(+ve)

Processes: AD – alkali-desorption; RD – reductive–dissolution; SO – sulphide oxidation; GT – geothermal. '+ve/(–)ve' indicate positive or negative correlations. References (1) Robertson (1989); (2) Schlottmann et al. (1998); (3) Carter et al. (1998); (4) Smedley et al. (2002); (5) Bhattacharya et al. (2006); (6) Boyle et al. (1998); (7) Juntunen et al. (2004); (8) Hernández–García & Custodio (2004); (9) Guo et al. (2005); (10) Smedley et al. (2003); (11) DPHE & BGS (2001); (12) Agusa et al. (2005); (13) Warner (2001); (14) Schreiber et al. (2000); (15) Kelepertsis et al. (2006); (16) Colak et al. (2003); (17) Gemici & Tarcan (2004); (18) Mianpiang (1997); (19) Romero et al. (2003); (20) Banks et al. (2004).

Table 2.6 Concentrations of arsenic and other chemicals at selected mining sites*

Country	Mine/area	Ore	Mineralisation†	Maximum As (ppb)	pH	Eh. (mV)	Fe (ppm)	Cu (ppb)	SO₄ (ppm)
Malaysia	Penjom (Peninsular Malaysia)	Au	SZH mesothermal lode (Au–Sb)	2970	2.5		27	<10	
Malaysia	Jugan (Sarawak)	Au	Shale hosted epithermal (Au–As)	2910	2.1	435	655	1020	3484
Thailand	Ron Phibun	Sn	Pegmatite veins	5114	6.6	366	0.02	91	39
Thailand	To Mo	Au	Epithermal (Au–Ag–As–Sb–Ni)	410	5.7		<1	<1	
Philippines	Dizon (Luzon)	Cu, Au	Porphyry	63	2.1	692	434	98,964	5326
Philippines	Diwalwal (Mindanao)	Au	Epithermal (Au–As–Cu)	120	8.4	−180	3.09	101	33
Zimbabwe	Globe and Phoenix	Au	SZH mesothermal lodes	7400	8.2	272	0.51	34,467	9194
Zimbabwe	Iron Duke	Fe, Au	Banded Iron Formation (BIF)	72,000	0.5	634	133,000	20,087	355,000
Argentina	Colo-Colo (San Juan)	Pb, Zn	Mesothermal lodes	140	8.5	196	0.01	<3	211
Argentina	Mendoza	Pb, Zn	Mesothermal lodes	24	8.1	336	0.08	<3	370
Ecuador	Ponce Enriquez	Au	Mesothermal lodes	430	8.1	342	0.16	7277	109
Ecuador	Portovelo	Au	Meso- and epithermal	1200	6.9		<1	27	
Brazil	Passagem	Au	SZH mesothermal lodes (Au–As–Cu)	1700	7.8	209	0.05	<3	5
Brazil	Morro Velho	Au	SZH lode and BIF (Au)	7300	9.0	35	0.05	1820	1038

*Data are summarised from a larger data set of 34 sites given in Williams (2001). Here only the two sites with the highest As concentration in each country are included. The pH, Eh, Cu, Fe and SO₄ concentration apply to the sample with the highest As concentration.

†SZH, shear zone hosted. Epithermal ore deposits are formed from hot waters ascending to shallow depth, at temperatures ranging from 50–200°C, and mesothermal deposits are formed at greater depth, and at temperatures of 200–300°C.

surprising because in both the AD and RD mechanisms the source of arsenic is adsorption onto iron oxides. In many of the cases in Table 2.5 there is not a linear correlation, but there is a clear association between high As concentrations and either elevated concentrations or absences of other elements. The existence of an association, as opposed to a correlation, is likely to result from either a threshold concentration, or multiple sources of the element. The associations with trace elements may also be helpful in elucidating the origins of arsenic in some groundwaters. For instance, the common occurrence of elements forming oxyanions (e.g. V, Mo and Se) in AD waters, and cations such as Ba, Li, Cs and Cr in geothermal waters, appear distinctive.

2.8   Arsenic Pollution and Mining

Although it is not the focus of this book, there is a widely recognised connection between mining and arsenic pollution, especially the mining of gold and base metals, where the ore or gangue minerals are rich in sulphide minerals. Arsenic pollution and health problems associated with tin and arsenic mining in Cornwall have been known for centuries, although this has an impact on soils much more than groundwater (Abrahams and Thornton, 1987; Meharg, 2005). Williams (2001) reviewed pollution associated with gold and base metal mining at 34 mines in Africa, Asia and Latin America (Table 2.6). He found that surface or groundwater contained >50 ppb As at 60% of the sites, and that 30% of the sites had extreme As concentrations of >1000 ppb As. However, only at one site (Ron Phibun in Thailand) was arsenic poisoning of humans confirmed. The popular image is that As pollution from mining is due to the formation of acid mine drainage (AMD), produced where sulphide minerals are oxidised by contact with water and oxygen, such as during infiltration through tailing dams and waste-rock piles or water-table rise through abandoned underground workings. Based on the chemical data (Table 2.6), the AMD model appears to fit the Penjom, Jugan, Dizon and Iron Duke sites, where the water is strongly acid (pH ≤ 2.5) and sulphate is in the thousands of ppm range. At the remaining sites, the water is either subneutral (pH 5.7–7.8) or, at six sites, actually sufficiently alkaline (pH 8.1–9.0) for arsenic to be desorbed. Williams (2001) attributed the high pH to complexation with cyanide used in the mining process. Nonetheless, most samples have high sulphate concentrations and are oxic, suggesting that arsenic was originally mobilised by oxidation of sulphides. Only one of the 14 sites had strongly reducing water (Diwalwal). Iron concentrations range over six orders of magnitude, probably reflecting the extent of precipitation of iron oxides. Williams (2001) suggested that most epithermal, shear-zone hosted and banded-iron-formation ore bodies

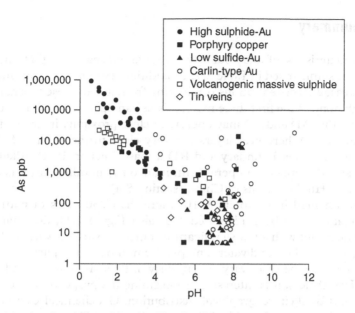

Figure 2.16 Arsenic and pH at mining sites. The pH and As values were mainly measured in anthropogenically polluted surface water bodies, and the data are classified by the type of associated ore deposit. The highest As concentrations occur at low pH and are associated with high-sulphide gold deposits. Volcanogenic sulphide deposits also produce extremely severe acid pollution, but As concentrations are consistently lower at any given pH. Carlin is a location in Nevada where microscopic gold occurs in calcareous rocks. *Source*: After Bowell (2002)

tend to generate acid, high-As waters. High-As waters are also formed at pH 5–8 from skarn (a rock formed by contact metamorphism of carbonate rocks) ore bodies, and some epithermal ores with low sulphide content. He also suggested that low-As waters are generated under acid (pH 1–4) and near-neutral pH at porphyry Cu–Au and alluvial Au deposits respectively. In summary, while the association of arsenic pollution with mining may be justified, its widely perceived link with AMD is a gross oversimplification.

As SO is commonly the dominant geochemical process at mining sites, it is hardly surprising that there is a strong inverse relationship between As concentration and pH, as shown in Figure 2.16. Bowell (2002) showed that, for a wide variety of ore bodies, there is a negative correlation with As concentration between pH 1 and pH 8. Within this group, almost all the grossly polluted waters occur at pH < 5 and especially at pH ≤ 3. Between pH 6 and pH 7.5, many of the waters contain less than, or only slightly exceed, 50 ppb As. However, at pH > 7.5 there is a distinct increase in As concentrations that may be attributable to desorption from iron oxyhydroxides.

2.9   Summary

The characteristics of the four geochemical mechanisms that mobilise arsenic are summarised in Table 2.7. In addition, evaporative concentration may increase As concentrations originating from any of these mechanisms. Although none of the first three mechanisms can operate simultaneously, it is possible that AD and SO may operate in close proximity in areas of crystalline bedrock. Where peat layers are very close to the surface, SO may operate at the upper boundary and RD at base (section 10.4). Alkali desorption and RD appear to operate simultaneously in different parts of the Datong and Huhhot basins of China (section 8.4).

As documented in Chapters 8–10, more than 230 cases of natural As contamination have been identified (see also Figure 1.1), dominantly in groundwater, but with a few significant instances of surface-water pollution fed by geothermal groundwater. The precise number is not particularly significant because the cases vary enormously in their size, impact and continuity. Nevertheless, it is interesting to examine the proportion of cases by process and by their geographical distribution. Geochemical causes of As contamination were inferred in 169 cases, of which 44% were attributed to RD, 23% to GT, 18% to AD and 15% to SO. The distribution of arsenic mobilised by each the four mechanisms, and their geological, climatic and tectonic associations, are discussed further in Chapter 3. When these cases are weighted by the affected populations (Chapter 11), RD is seen to be even more important.

Annexe 2.1   Analysis of Arsenic in Natural Waters

A2.1.1   Laboratory analysis of arsenic

In natural waters, arsenic occurs predominantly in the inorganic forms As(III) and As(V), and in negligible amounts as organic forms (Cullen and Reimer, 1989). Hung et al. (2004) reviewed the many analytical methods for inorganic arsenic in water. Many methods rely on pre-reduction of As(V) to As(III). If determination of the individual species is required, pre-separation must be carried out and the totals of As(III) and As(V) determined separately. Pre-reduction is often done with potassium iodide, but only works in the presence of strong acid (Hung et al., 2004). There are four groups of techniques, and many variants, for arsenic analysis, as listed in Table A2.1.

Hydride generation is the most popular method of converting arsenite and arsenate to volatile (and highly toxic) arsine gas prior to analysis.

Table 2.7 Summary of arsenic mobilisation processes

Name	Description	Requirements	Characteristic Signals
Reductive dissolution (RD)	Produces near-neutral reducing waters. Reduction is driven by decay of organic matter. Arsenic is sorbed onto Fe, Mn or Al oxides, and possibly clay minerals. Arsenic is released as As(III) when the sorbent becomes unstable and dissolves. More than one sorbent may be present, but most commonly, iron oxides are the controlling sorbents	1. Anaerobic, strongly reducing water, generated by the decay of organic matter 2. As sorbed to amorphous or crystalline oxyhydroxides	1. Very low DO, NO_x and SO_4. 2. High HCO_3, DOC, Fe, possibly Mn. 3. Negative Eh 4. Methane gas. 5. Near-neutral pH
Alkali desorption (AD)	Produces alkali-oxic waters. As(V), the stable form of As under oxidising conditions, is desorbed from Fe, Mn and Al oxides at pH $\geq$ 8.0. The pH at which desorption is initiated varies slightly with the type of oxide phase and water chemistry (PO_4, Ca, Si and DOC). The metal oxides remain as stable solids	1. Aerobic, oxidising or weakly reducing water 2. As sorbed to amorphous or crystalline oxyhydroxides 3. Little organic matter present	1. pH $\geq$ 8.0 2. Some DO, plus low to high NO_x and SO_4. 3. High HCO_3 4. Low Fe, possibly Mn 5. Na > Ca 6. High F, V and Mo common
Sulphide oxidation (SO)	Produces acid-sulphate waters. Oxidation of sulphides such as arsenopyrite, pyrite and pyrrhotite occurs under oxic conditions. It requires water and abundant oxygen, and generates much acidity. The process occurs close to the water table, and is normally localised, but is common in mining and mineralised regions	1. Aerobic, oxidising water 2. Fluctuating water table	1. pH < 7 High SO_4
Geothermal arsenic (GA)	Geothermal As waters are formed by high-temperature leaching of silicate rocks in areas of recent volcanicity or where there is rapid and deep circulation of groundwater	1. Heat source 2. Country rock containing As	1. Near-neutral pH 2. Elevated T 3. Positive correlation with Cl

Table A2.1 Major techniques for laboratory arsenic analysis

Spectrometric techniques	Hydride-generation atomic absorption spectrometry (HG-AAS)
	Hydride-generation atomic fluorescence spectrometry (HG-AFS)
	Graphite-furnace atomic absorption spectrometry (GF-AAS)
	Silver diethyl-dithio-carbamate spectrophotometry (SDDC)
Inductively coupled plasma (ICP) techniques	ICP atomic emission spectrometry (ICP-AES)
	ICP atomic fluorescence spectrometry (ICP-AFS)
	ICP mass spectrometry (ICP-MS)
	High-pressure liquid chromatography (HPLC) and ICP-MS
Neutron activation analysis (NAA)	
Electrochemical methods:	Polarographic techniques
	Cathode stripping voltammetry (CSV)
	Anodic stripping voltammetry (ASV)
	Microlithographic fabricated arrays

Source: Hung et al. (2004)

Sodium and potassium borohydrides are routinely used for this process (Hung et al., 2004). Combined with AAS or AFS, reliable As determinations are achieved with levels of detection comfortably below 1 ppb As. In the graphite-furnace technique, there is no hydride generation but arsenic is evaporated from a graphite tube at high temperature. The GF-AAS technique achieves similar or better levels of detection to HG-AAS (Hung et al. 2004). Silver diethyldithiocarbamate (SDDC) spectrophotometry has been widely used in laboratories, but is subject to interference from anions, in particular phosphate (Kinniburgh and Kosmos, 2002), which is common in many arsenic terrains. For this and other reasons, AAS is widely preferred to the SDDC method, despite the higher capital cost, especially where precision below 50 ppb As is required.

Inductively coupled plasma (ICP) techniques involve spraying an acidified sample into high temperature plasma, which atomises and ionises all forms of arsenic present, and does not require the thorough digestion used in HG-AAS. The great advantage of ICP is its ability to analyse a wide range of elements simultaneously, although ICP–AES suffers from lower sensitivity at low As concentrations (Hung et al., 2004). Hence, AAS tends to be preferred when the focus of a survey is primarily on arsenic rather than a range of contaminants. Derivative techniques, such as HPLC with ICP–MS, have specialist applications such as analysing arsenic speciation, and ICP–MS is gaining in popularity.

Neutron activation analysis is a very sensitive technique for analysing arsenic, but it is mainly used as a reference for new methods. Its accuracy is affected by chloride and it is not normally used for surveys. A variety of electrochemical methods have recently received attention in the USA (Feeney and Kounaves, 2002; Melamed, 2004) and Bangladesh (Rasul et al., 2002). Of these methods, anodic stripping voltammetry (ASV) offers a possible alternative to AAS and ICP techniques and is equally sensitive to As(III) and As(V) (Melamed, 2004). The ASV technique involves three steps: first a carbon electrode is coated with a thin film of gold; second the sample is acidified with HCl; and third, after the electrode is put in the solution, part of the arsenic is reduced onto the electrode surface. The amount of current required to oxidatively remove (strip) the arsenic is quantitatively related to its concentration. The ASV technique may find application in small laboratories or dedicated arsenic-testing facilities, being of potentially lower cost than other laboratory methods and better performance than field test kits.

A2.1.2 Arsenic field test kits

Laboratory analysis of arsenic is technically demanding, expensive and time-consuming. In rural areas of less-developed countries, where hundreds of thousands, even millions, of wells need to be tested, it is natural to seek a field test that is rapid, reliable, immediate and preferably also cheap. In recent years, much effort has gone into developing better field kits, and the application of field-testing in water-supply mitigation programmes is discussed in Chapter 6. Most field kits are based on the Gutzeit method, named after the nineteenth century chemist, although the method has been modified since then. Most designs have used zinc powder and an acid to reduce As(V) and As(III) to arsine (arsenic trihydride, AsH_3) by the following reaction

$$As_4O_6 + 12Zn + 24H^+ \Rightarrow 4AsH_3 + 12Zn^{2+} + 6H_2O$$

where

$$Zn + 2H^+ \Rightarrow Zn^{2+} + H_2$$

The reaction takes 10–30 minutes to complete, and the generated gases pass through a paper impregnated with a reagent such as mercuric bromide, producing a stain that changes from white to yellow to brown with increasing As concentration. The colour is interpreted either by eye or with a portable spectrometer. The latest kits claim detection limits of a few ppb, although the reliability of analysis in real groundwater below, and close to, 10 ppb is uncertain, and is discussed further in section 6.3.2. The staining is subject to interference by hydrogen sulphide, and so the gas is first passed through a filter containing either the commercial oxidant Oxone® or lead acetate to remove it. One of the weaknesses of this approach was the use of concentrated hydrochloric acid, which is dangerous to operators. The kits have been refined by substituting solid sulphamic acid for HCl, and also by replacing zinc with sodium borohydride. Because kits based on the Gutzeit method generate arsine (AsH_3) gas, the most toxic form of arsenic, there is a danger to the testers, which increases when testing samples with high As concentration, in large numbers and in confined spaces. Hussam et al. (1999) showed that the quantities of arsine generated may exceed USA health and safety at work guidelines. It is recommended that tests should be conducted in a well-ventilated space, and workers should be provided with gas masks. Recent kits, such as the WagTech Arsenator®, include a scrubbing filter after the indicator paper to remove excess arsine.

There is uncertainty about the prospects for using electrochemical methods in the field. They have the potential to perform quick and accurate determinations of arsenic, but some doubt that the equipment can be made sufficiently robust and cheap for field use (e.g. Kinniburgh and Kosmos, 2002). However, Feeney and Kounaves (2002) successfully used prototype equipment in the field, and Hung et al. (2004) consider that the method can be developed into a rapid and accurate field device. Melamed (2004) reports verification of several portable anodic stripping voltammetry devices by the US Environmental Protection Agency. They achieved minimum detection limits (MDLs) of 7 and 13 ppb, but expressed doubts about their use by non-technical operators. Melamed (2004) noted that microelectrodes are becoming more affordable, but their fragility remains a constraint for use in the field, although he cites the survival of a gold electrode for 30 days in the field as a success. Commercial ASV field kits have been marketed (http://www.mtidiagnostics.com) and claim reliable determination of arsenic at the 10 ppb level and can achieve greater throughput of samples after initial set up, but require more operator training. Further evaluation will be needed before such equipment can be deployed in rural South Asia for example. The reader is advised to monitor the development of commercial electrochemical field kits, and to pay careful attention to field-based evaluations of their 'physical' reliability.

Unusual test methods under development include genetic techniques, in which arsenic-responsive DNA control sequences are linked to an additional gene, called a reporter gene (Melamed, 2004). Stocker et al. (2003) developed strains of *Escherichia coli* labelled with three reporter proteins. In the laboratory, the biosensors routinely detected arsenite in spiked tap water at concentrations of ≥ 4 ppb. A field-test was developed by drying sensor cells onto a paper strip and placing it in the water sample for 30 minutes. They reported that it produces a visible blue colour in arsenite concentrations >8 ppb As. The authors suggested that it offers a realistic alternative for measuring arsenic in potable supplies. However, careful verification must be carried out before such techniques can be applied in practice.

When selecting a field kit, it is essential to test the performance in determining low levels of arsenic in natural waters in the field, similar to those to be surveyed, and not merely in spiked solutions of pure water in the laboratory. This comparison should be done at reference laboratories, and should preferably involve two laboratories in the analysis of blind duplicates. As Kinniburgh and Kosmos (2002) point out, because accuracy at low concentration is increasingly important, trace-level impurities of arsenic in zinc powder can produce erroneous detections (false positives). Therefore, high purity reagents are vital for both the laboratory and field kits. This also highlights the importance of regularly analysing field blanks, which ensures that the 'zero-level' of arsenic is correct and also guards against systematic procedural errors.

A2.1.3   Field testing of soils

Portable X-ray fluorescence devices have been produced to determine concentrations in soils and sediments (Melamed, 2004). A US Environmental Protection Agency draft test method (SW-846-6200) is reported to achieve an interference-free detection limit of 40 mg/kg. This may be useful at industrially contaminated sites, but will have little application at naturally contaminated sites. However, only a modest improvement in detection limits would make this useful in studies of irrigated soils, where impacts are anticipated at the levels of a few tens of mg/kg, as discussed in Chapter 4. The ASV techniques have also been applied to field testing of soils and are reported to determine arsenic concentrations of 1 mg/kg, but require pre-digestion with concentrated acid and hydrogen peroxide.

NOTES

1   An amorphous mineral with the general formula $Al_2O_3 \cdot (SiO_2)_{1.3-2} \cdot 2.5-3 \ (H_2O)$.
2   A complex oxide of manganese, with the general formula $Na_{0.3}Ca_{0.1}K_{0.1}Mn^{4+}$ $Mn^{3+}O_4 \cdot 1.5(H_2O)$.
3   Kaolinite and halloysite are characteristic of highly weathered rocks and soils; illite of shales and some young alluvial deposits; and montmorillonite of alkaline conditions and basic rocks.

4   Halloysite and kaolinite are what are referred to as 1:1 clays, meaning they
    contain alternating sheets of silica tetrahedra and alumina octahedra, and have
    similar chemical compositions, basically $Al_2Si_2O_5(OH)_4$. Illite, montmorillonite
    and chlorite are 2:1 clays, and also contain significant but very variable iron,
    magnesium and manganese contents, imparting greater swelling potential and
    adsorption capacity. The illite group, however, can to some extent be regarded as
    having properties intermediate between the 1:1 and the other 2:1 clays.

5   For example, the term 'fulvic acid' simply defines compounds extracted by a
    certain procedure.

6   The conventional view (section 2.6.1) is that the release of arsenic, its trans-
    formation between As(III) and As(V), and the breakdown of iron oxyhydrox-
    ides are interlinked, or coupled. In a decoupled operation, the processes occur
    separately.

7   Appelo and Postma (1996) observed this reaction in agricultural areas on glacial-
    outwash soils, where nitrate originated from arable farming. Such reactions
    could occur widely in northern Europe and North America.

8   Which are neither strongly acidic nor sulphate-rich until they are drained.

Chapter Three

The Hydrogeology of Arsenic

3.1   Introduction

This chapter places the processes described in Chapter 2 in their geological and hydrological context, and develops these ideas to explain how arsenic moves in the subsurface between its sources and sinks, at scales that range from a few metres to entire sedimentary basins. After summarising As concentrations in rocks, sediments and rivers (sections 3.2 and 3.3), we describe the associations between As contamination and climate, lithology and geomorphological and tectonic setting (section 3.4). Because by far the commonest setting for As-contaminated groundwater is in alluvial basins, in section 3.5 we attempt to explain why some basins are contaminated but others are not. This leads to a more general discussion of the geological conditions under which arsenic pollution is, and is not, commonly found. From the global survey of As occurrence, certain geological themes emerge, including the roles of Quaternary sea-level change, subsidence, and deep weathering of basement rocks in many uncontaminated areas. In addition, the geochemistry of river systems is shown to be a valuable tool in predicting the occurrence of arsenic in alluvial aquifers.

   In section 3.6 we consider the evidence for migration of arsenic in the subsurface and changes in As concentrations over time. In particular, we examine the evidence for wells changing from safe to unsafe levels over time, and consider evidence for the migration of arsenic in groundwater at different scales. This has major implications for water users, and also for monitoring and follow-up surveys. Section 3.7 presents three case histories of the hydrogeology of contaminated aquifers: the first an alluvial aquifer in West Bengal; the second Permian Sandstones in Oklahoma; and the third a watershed study from Switzerland. Finally, section 3.8 considers the prospects for continued groundwater irrigation, the movement of arsenic between aquifers, and movements at the basin scale, and ends by discussing the sustainability of groundwater abstraction in alluvial basins.

3.2   Arsenic in Rocks and Sediments

Table 3.1 shows the typical concentrations of arsenic in a variety of rocks and sediments, but not soils, which are described in Chapter 4. Arsenic concentrations in most rock groups are extremely variable. Most volcanic and metamorphic rocks, and some consolidated sediments, show high degrees of enrichment, probably due to hydrothermal activity. Extreme As enrichment (and variation) is observed in coal and ironstone, the former because arsenic accumulates as authigenic pyrite in swamps, and the latter because arsenic is scavenged by iron hydroxides under oxic conditions. Compared with both general rock types and the global average for river sediments (5 mg/kg), the As contents of sediments from contaminated aquifers in the Bengal Basin and Argentina are unremarkable. As discussed repeatedly in this book, extensive pollution of groundwater can rarely be attributed to source material alone, but depends on the particular conditions under which arsenic is concentrated and mobilised.

3.3   Arsenic in River Water and Sediment

Here we differentiate the suspended and bedload sediment of active rivers from buried alluvium as described above. Mandal and Suzuki (2002) report the average content of modern river sediment to be 5 mg/kg As. Table 3.2 includes analyses of arsenic of water and suspended sediment from some of the world's major rivers, although because of different sampling and analytical protocols not all of the results are necessarily entirely consistent. Most of the major rivers contain dissolved concentrations of 1–3 ppb As, although the Amazon and Niger contain even less arsenic. Some smaller rivers that contain much more arsenic, not listed in Table 3.2, include the Loa (1400 ppb) and Toconce (800 ppb) in Chile, the Waikato (150 ppb) in New Zealand and the Madison (72 ppb) in the USA, and all receive discharges from geothermal springs. Overall, there is a crude correlation between the concentrations of arsenic in sediment and water; however, there is no relation between the concentrations either in sediment or river water and the likelihood of arsenic being mobilised in nearby alluvial groundwater.

Table 3.1 Typical arsenic concentrations in rocks and unconsolidated sediments

Lithology (location)	Arsenic (mg/kg)	
	Mean	Range
Igneous rocks:		
volcanic glass	5.9	2.2–12
granite, aplite*	1.3	0.2–15
andesite, trachyte	2.7	0.5–5.8
basalt	2.3	0.18–113
gabbro, dolerite	1.5	0.06–28
ultrabasic igneous rocks	1.5	0.03–16
Metamorphic rocks:		
phyllites, slate	18	0.5–143
schist, gneiss	1.1	<0.1–19
amphibolite	6.3	0.4–45
Sedimentary rocks:		
shale, mudstone		3–15
sandstone	4.1	0.6–120
limestone, dolomite	2.6	0.1–20
ironstones		1–2,900
coal		0.3–35,000
Unconsolidated sediments:		
alluvial sand (Bangladesh)	2.9	1.0–6.2
alluvial mud (Bangladesh)	6.5	2.7–15
Holocene mud (West Bengal)	7.7	2.8–17
Holocene sand (West Bengal)	5.2	0.3–16
Pleistocene sand (West Bengal)	1.2	0.1–2.3
glacial till (Canada)		1.5–45
loess (Argentina[†])		5.4–18
peat	13	2–36

*Aplite and trachyte are finer-grained equivalents of granite and andesite.
[†]The loess from Argentina is atypical because of its high volcanic ash content.
Source: Summarised from compilations by Mandal and Suzuki (2002) and Smedley and Kinniburgh (2002) plus West Bengal data from McArthur et al. (2004). The average crustal abundance of arsenic is 2 mg/kg (Mason, 1966).

Table 3.2 Drainage basin characteristics and arsenic occurrence in alluvial basins

		Drainage area (km²* 10⁶)	Type (1)	Arsenic polluted	CI	Average temperature (°C)	Runoff (mm/yr)	Sediment					Solute		
Continent	River							Yield (t/km²/yr)	TSS (ppm)	Q:F:R	As (mg/kg)	Load (t/km²/yr)	TDS (ppm)	CWI	PWI
Asia	Ganges-Brahmaputra	1.55	M	Y	8	21.8	737	851	1080	57:21:22	10	97	297	1.11	5.25
Asia	Indus	0.97	M	Y	6	19.8	245	260	2778	43:24:33	13		302	0.35	1.70
Asia	Mekong	0.80	M	Y	8	23.2	590	435	321	70:05:24	27	74	263	2.00	1.80
Asia	Yellow (Huang-He)	0.75	M	Y	4	8.7	65	1170	460	41:34:25	13		55	0.19	5.50
Asia	Irrawaddy	0.43	M	Y	8	23.1	995	620	535	46:04:50		150	201	2.10	1.20
Asia	Red	0.12	M	Y	8	>20		1083		52:12:36		75	428		
Europe	Danube	0.81	M	Y	7	9.4	250	83	313	27:13:60			667	3.00	3.10
Europe	Po	0.05	M	Y	7	11.8	670	280	354	44:11:45			183	1.00	1.40
N. America	Yukon	0.84	M	Y	5	-4.2	249	71	286	49:17:32					
N. America	Rio Grande	0.67	M	Y				30							
Africa	Congo	3.82	P	N?	8	23.6	340	14	32	97:01:02		12	35	0.16	0.02
Africa	Nile	3.00	P	N?	6	24.2	30	37	388	68:10:22		6	10	0.10	0.09
Africa	Zambezi	1.34	P	N?	6	21.3	390	75	80	62:31:07		11	77	0.25	0.15
Africa	Niger	1.21	P	N?	6	27.1	160	33	59	96:03:01	0.7	8	128	0.14	0.13

Continent	River	CI	Catchment type	PWI	CWI	Climate Index	TDS	TSS		Q:F:R					
Africa	Orange	1.02	P	N?	18.0	6	100	147	238	47:08:45		12	59	0.12	0.18
Africa	Limpopo	0.34	P	N?	20.2	6	15	96	520	42:29:29	13		221	2.60	8.80
Asia	Yangtze-Kiang	1.90	M	N?	14.5	7	500	226	400	37:10:53			85	0.34	1.20
Asia	Tigris-Euphrates	1.05	M	N?	20.3	6	45	52	1619		7	53	193		
Asia	Godavari	0.31	P	N?	26.6	6	270	550	453			8	22	0.03	0.07
Australia	Murray - Darling	1.07	M/P	N?	17.8	6	21	30					600	1.40	0.42
Europe	Rhine	0.17	M	N?	8.1	7	190	4		65:10:25			565	3.30	16.00
Europe	Rhone	0.09	M	N?	10.2	7	530	340	339	41:16:43	12		216	0.54	0.66
N. America	Mississippi	3.27	P	N?	11.0	7	150	107	862	62:12:26	15	40			
N. America	Colorado	0.64	P	N?	13.3	4	28	190		63:21:16			44	1.00	1.00
S. America	Amazon	6.15	P	N?	24.1	8	100	81	182	85:03:11	6	1.00	44	0.59	0.56
S. America	Orinoco	0.99	P	N?	25.6	8	1100	152	132	93:01:06	7	0.59	25	0.33	0.03
Asia	Yenesei	2.57	P	?	-4.6	5	229	5	23			0.33	112	0.19	0.07
S. America	Parana	2.87	P	?	21.2	8	189	32	139		4	0.19	86	5.40	22.00
S. America	Magdalena	0.29	M	?	23.4	8	843	773	928	55:08:37		5.40	118		

Sources: Amorosi et al. (2002); FAO (2005); Gaillardet et al. (1999); Huang et al. (1988); Ludwig and Probst (1998); Milliman and Syvitski (1992); Pasquini et al. (2005); Potter (1978, 1994); RivDIS data: http://www.eosdis.ornl.gov/rivdis; Seyler and Martin (1990); Thomas (1994); Yang et al. (2004).

CI – climate index. CWI – chemical weathering index. PWI – physical weather index.

Catchment type: M – mountain; P – plateau. Q:F:R – quartz: feldspar: rock ratio. TDS – total dissolved solids; TSS – total suspended solids.

The indices of chemical and physical weathering are taken from Gaillardet et al. (1999), and are normalised to the composition of the Amazon.

Climate Index: 4. Temperate-Dry; 5. Tundra and Taiga; 6. Tropical-Dry; 7. Temperate-Wet; 8. Tropical-Wet

3.4   Geo-environmental Associations of Arsenic in Groundwater

3.4.1   Climate

Some general relationships can be identified between climate and the mobilisation mechanisms for natural arsenic contamination of groundwater. To identify these associations, the climate of each As occurrence was categorised by mean annual temperature and average annual rainfall. Temperature was divided into three groups: cool, temperate and warm, with boundaries at 10° and 15°C. Rainfall was also divided into three groups: dry, moist and wet, with boundaries at 600 and 1600 mm. In Table 3.3, 158 occurrences of arsenic contaminated groundwater are classified in a matrix of rainfall and temperature. The absolute numbers should not be considered important because the individual instances vary enormously in terms of area and number of people affected. Overall, there are far fewer instances

Table 3.3   Arsenic mobilisation and climate

Annual temperature	Process	Annual rainfall		
		Dry	Moist	Wet
Cool (<10°C)	AD	2	0	0
	RD	3	0	0
	SO	0	0	0
	GT	4	0	0
	Unknown	3	0	0
Temperate (10–15°C)	AD	1	5	2
	RD	4	14	5
	SO	0	6	0
	GT	1	5	5
	Unknown	1	15	2
Warm (>15°C)	AD	8	4	1
	RD	5	1	15
	SO	4	3	4
	GT	9	0	4
	Unknown	13	5	4

AD, alkali desorption; RD, reductive dissolution; SO, sulphide oxidation;
GT, geothermal.
Source: Temperature and rainfall were assigned using data from ESRI (1996).

in cool climates (12) than in temperate (66) or warm (80) climates, while overall there are roughly equal numbers of instances in dry, moist and wet climates. Three climatic associations dominate the matrix shown in Table 3.3. The most important is the temperate–moist association (45), where reductive dissolution (RD) is the principal mechanism. Almost as important is the warm–dry association (39), where alkali desorption (AD) and geothermal (GT) causes are the most common mechanisms, but none dominates. The third is the warm–wet association (28) where reductive dissolution dominates. Reductive dissolution appears to be favoured by increasing rainfall and temperature, which both favour the growth of vegetation. Both alkali desorption and sulphide oxidation (SO) appear to be favoured by increasing temperature.

3.4.2 Tectonic and geomorphological setting

The same data set was reclassified in terms of the tectonic and geomorphological setting, as shown in Table 3.4. Forty cases were assigned to

Table 3.4 Arsenic mobilisation and morpho-tectonic setting

Morpho-tectonic setting	AD	RD	SO	GT	Unknown	Total
Deltas or coastal plains	3	15	2	7*	3	30
Alluvial plains (inland)	6	10	0	1	0	17
Foreland basin[†]	4	9	0	2	0	15
Rift valley	0	0	0	0	1	1
Tertiary orogenic belts	4	2	6	15	13	40
Mesozoic–Tertiary sedimentary basin	2	2	1	1	7	13
Cratonic (Precambrian–Palaeozoic)	3	9[‡]	7	0	7	26
Uncertain	1	0	1	2	12	16
Total	23	47	17	28	43	158

AD, alkali desorption; RD, reductive dissolution; SO, sulphide oxidation; GT, geothermal.
*Mostly in streams originating from hot springs in the Andes.
[†]Elongate basins adjacent to mountain chains and principally filled by alluvial deposits, such as the Indus, Ganges and Brahmaputra alluvium, and the Basin-and-Range Province in the USA.
[‡]A significant number of the cases of reductive dissolution in cratonic areas are associated with fluvio-glacial sediments in North America, and not the underlying bedrock.

areas of Tertiary mountain building (orogens), where arsenic may be encountered in sedimentary, igneous or metamorphic bedrock, or in inter-montane alluvial basins. In Table 3.4, the term 'craton' denotes both Precambrian basement and Palaeozoic basins located in stable intracontinental settings or on passive plate margins. Overall, it is seen that As contamination may be encountered in almost any tectonic or geomorphological setting, but is more common in some than others. For instance, more than 40% of all cases occur in alluvial basins, of which approximately 60% can be attributed to reductive dissolution. Alkali desorption occurs preferentially in alluvial basins, but is also significant in bedrock aquifers. Sulphide oxidation, on the other hand, is common in both young mountain chains and areas of ancient rock, and is associated with intense mineralisation. Geothermal arsenic, predictably, is most common in areas of recent mountain building. Viewed at a global scale (Figure 2.15), a high proportion of As occurrences are located along, or immediately adjacent to, young mountain belts (foreland basins). This is particularly true of geothermal arsenic, but also of many of the AD occurrences and the non-glacial RD occurrences.

3.4.3   Lithology and depositional environment

In Table 3.5, the most important occurrences of arsenic pollution[1] are classified according to their geological and climatic associations and geochemical mobilisation process. Some important occurrences (e.g. in Mexico) had to be omitted because the geology of the aquifers is poorly known. The range of As concentrations varies greatly between the examples cited, but is generally higher in alluvial than bedrock aquifers, although no general distinction can be made on the basis of climate. Table 3.6 shows average concentrations of arsenic and other parameters from a representative range of polluted aquifers around the world. The different mobilisation processes produce major differences in water chemistry, especially in the mobilisation of iron and manganese, even where the lithologies are similar. This is illustrated by the similarities between groundwaters from the Bengal Basin, the northern USA and Hungary, where reductive dissolution dominates; and their difference from alluvial groundwater in China, the southwestern USA and Argentina. The tell-tale characteristics of the RD waters are the high iron and low sulphate concentrations, and near-neutral pH; AD waters are distinguished by elevated pH, low iron, and parameters indicating oxic conditions such as nitrate and sulphate.

The dominance of reductive dissolution in alluvial aquifers is greatest in the South and Southeast Asian Arsenic belt (SSAAB) that extends from

Table 3.5 Important occurrences* of groundwater arsenic related to geology and climate

Aquifer/geology	Cool-temperate		Humid: tropical and subtropical		Arid and semi-arid: warm–hot	
	Occurrence	Process	Occurrence	Process	Occurrence	Process
Alluvium: deltaic; fluvial; lacustrine; aeolian	Waiotapu valley, New Zealand	GT	Assam, Manipur and Tripura, India	RD	Basin-and-Range province, southwest USA	AD
	Fukuoka and Sendai prefectures, Japan	AD	Bengal Basin and Ganga Plains: India and Bangladesh	RD	Inner Mongolia, China	RD, AD
	Danube Basin: Hungary, Croatia and Romania	RD	Chittagong coastal plain, Bangladesh	RD	Shanxi province, China	AD, RD
					Xinjiang province, China	AD, E
	Fukui, Osaka and Takatsuki prefectures, Japan	RD	Mekong plains and delta, Vietnam and Cambodia	RD	Sindh and Punjab provinces, Pakistan	RD
	Wairu Plain, New Zealand	RD	Red River Delta, Vietnam	RD	Okavango Delta, Botswana	RD, E
			Irrawaddy delta, Myanmar	RD	Carson Desert, Nevada, USA	RD, E
			Hat Yai, Thailand	RD	Perth, Australia	SO, RD
			Northeast and southwest Taiwan	RD	Rio Verde basin, Mexico	SO
			Terai; Nepal	RD	Rio Loa and Rio Elqui, Chile	GT, E
			Citarum river, Indonesia	GT	Altiplano, Bolivia	GT, E
					Qinghai-Tibet Plateau	GT, E
Alluvial-volcani-clastic	Willamette Basin, Oregon, USA	AD			Cordoba, Santiago del Estero, La Pampa, Tucuman, Argentina	AD, E

(cont'd)

Table 3.5 *(cont'd)*

Aquifer/geology	Cool-temperate Occurrence	Process	Humid: tropical and subtropical Occurrence	Process	Arid and semi-arid: warm–hot Occurrence	Process
Glacial, and fluvio-glacial sediments	Alaska, USA	RD				
	Minnesota, Iowa and NandS Dakota, USA	RD				
	Ohio, Illinois and Michigan, USA	RD				
	Saskatchewan, Canada	RD				
Alluvium and limestone			Ogunstate, Nigeria	?	Zimapán, Mexico	AD
Tertiary, intra-continental sediments					Madrid and Duero basins, Spain	AD
					Emet-Hisarcik, Turkey Kurdistan, Iran	SO ?
					Qinghai-Tibet, hot springs	GT, E
Tertiary–Recent, Volcanic	S. Dakota, USA	AD	Lake Ilopango, El Salvador	GT	Etna, Stromboli, Vulcano and Vesuvius, Italy	GT
Palaeozoic–Mesozoic-sedimentary	Oklahoma, USA	AD			East Caucasus Mts, Russia	?
	English Midlands, UK	AD			S. Mangyshlak, Kazakhstan	?
	Bavaria, Germany	?				
	Wisconsin, USA	SO				
Palaeo-Mesozoic igneous and metamorphic	Bowen Is. and Sunshine Coast, Canada	AD			E. Thessalonika, Greece	SO
PreCambrian– Palaeozoic crystalline bedrock	Washington State, USA	SO	Iron Quadrangle, Brazil	SO	Chhattisgarh, India	SO
	Nova Scotia, Canada	SO			Southwest Ghana	SO
	New England, USA	AD			Yatenga, Burkina Faso	SO
	southwest Finland	AD				
	Lapland, Finland	SO				

AD, alkali desorption; RD, reductive dissolution; SO, sulphide oxidation; GT, geothermal; E, evapoconcentration.
*Locations are shown in Figure 1.1, and described in detail in Chapters 8–10. Occurrences where the geology of the aquifers is not well documented are omitted.

Table 3.6 Chemistry (means) of arsenic-contaminated groundwater in different lithologies

Aquifer and Location	Process	As (ppb)	pH	Fe (ppm)	Mn (ppm)	HCO$_3$ (ppm)	SO$_4$ (ppm)	Cl (ppm)
Alluvium, Faridpur, Bangladesh	RD	95	6.9	5.6	0.66	536	3	9.3
Alluvium, Barasat, West Bengal	RD	188	7.0	3.7	0.87	583	5	51
Duna–Tisza interfluve, Hungary	RD	50	7.6	0.80	ND	330	ND	4.6
Fluvio-glacial sediment, Mahomet Buried Valley Aquifer, USA	RD	37	7.2	2.0	0.02	587	<0.1	63
Deep alluvium, Huhhot Basin, Inner Mongolia, China*	AD/RD	128	7.9	0.38	0.19	409	14	87
Alluvium, Datong Basin, Shanxi Province, China	AD/RD	366	8.2	0.09	0.09	580	107	200
Alluvium, Middle Rio Grande Basin, New Mexico*	AD	23	8.2	0.03	0.002	174	92	13
Alluvium and loess, Santiago del Estero, Argentina	AD	743	7.6	4.6	0.57	581	446	221
Madrid Basin (Tertiary), Spain	AD	25	7.9	0.03	0.02	185	56	28
Triassic Sandstone, Bavaria, Germany	?	19	7.3	0.24	0.11	298	36	31
Crystalline bedrock, New England, USA	AD/SO	5.5	7.6	0.20	0.09	116	15	32
Crystalline bedrock, Pirkanamaa, Finland	AD/SO	10	7.4	0.35	0.12	124	21	14

ND, no data.

*Median concentrations.

Sources: DPHE/MMI/BGS, 1999; Ayotte et al., 2003; Bexfield and Plummer, 2003; Varsányi and Kovács, 2006; Bhattacharya et al., 2006; Smedley et al., 2003; McArthur et al., 2004; Juntunen et al., 2004; Guo and Wang, 2005; Warner, 2001.

Pakistan to Taiwan, along the southern margin of the Himalayan and Indo-Burman ranges. The association between alluvium and reductive dissolution is partly climatic, but the causal relationship lies in the abundance of fresh organic matter. Where organic matter is abundant, the potential for AD is less because iron oxides tend to be dissolved, and also because the decay of organic matter has a buffering effect on pH. Thus RD may operate in arid environments where local factors, such as deposition in lakes or swamps, preserve organic matter. In some semi-arid areas (e.g. the Datong Basin of China), alkali desorption and reductive dissolution, although distinct processes, appear to operate in the same basin. Contaminated glacial and fluvio-glacial aquifers of Quaternary age are restricted to cold and temperate climates but, curiously, all are in North America and all are attributed to reductive dissolution, presumably due to the abundance of peat beds interbedded with permeable sand and gravel, especially in younger glacial deposits (Erickson and Barnes, 2005b; Kelly et al., 2005). Another factor influencing glacial aquifers is that the low temperature at the time of erosion means that there is limited chemical alteration of the source material prior to or during glacial transport, which leaves the sediment susceptible to chemical weathering by percolating waters under a later, temperate climate.

Sulphide oxidation does not appear to be of great importance in polluting alluvial aquifers, despite the common oxidation of pyrite in acid-sulphate soils (e.g. Appleyard et al., 2004). This is probably because the reaction products only percolate a few metres due to the presence of either a shallow water table or low permeability clays at the base of peat basins (e.g. Brammer, 1996). Sulphide oxidation only appears to be an important cause of aquifer pollution in crystalline bedrock that has been enriched in sulphides by hydrothermal alteration[2]. Where sulphide minerals are weathered by aerated water near the water table, arsenic may be transferred to iron oxide coatings. Consequently, alkali desorption and sulphide oxidation may also operate in close juxtaposition, but not simultaneously.

Alkali desorption is encountered in a wide range of geological settings. In alluvial aquifers, AD-type waters are found mainly in drier areas, but in bedrock AD waters are found in all climates, and in rocks ranging from Tertiary sediments to Precambrian metamorphic rocks. In terms of impact, the most important occurrence occurs beneath the Chaco-Pampean plains of Argentina, for which there is no comparable occurrence elsewhere in the world[3]. Apart from the high pH, all researchers attribute great importance to the volcanic component of the loess, but differ in the degree to which they consider arsenic is mobilised by direct weathering of volcanic glass (e.g. Nicolli et al., 1989; Sracek et al., 2007) or, indirectly, by way of iron oxides (e.g. Smedley et al., 2002; Bhattacharya et al., 2006).

Lastly, it is appropriate to comment on the areas where As contamination has not been identified, and to ask whether this is evidence of absence or simply an absence of evidence. Some of the largest areas with no arsenic recorded are the vast areas of tundra and taiga[4], and in large areas of Africa, South America, India and Australia. Arsenic is notably rare in the major alluvial basins in North and South America, Europe (excepting the Danube and Po), and Africa, and also in fluvio-glacial sediments outside North America. In the following sections, we examine possible explanations for these absences, which are considered further in Chapters 8–11.

3.5 Geochemical Processes in their Geological Context

3.5.1 The rarity of arsenic pollution in tropical basement terrain

There are very few reports of As pollution from the vast areas of South America, Africa, Australia and peninsular India that once formed the ancient supercontinent of Gondwanaland. In plate-tectonic terms, these areas now lie within, or adjacent to, passive continental margins, characterised by gentle uplift or downwarping. In contrast to the volcanically and/or tectonically active Alpine–Himalayan–Indonesian arc and the Andean Chain, over much of the tropics, rivers drain non-orogenic terrain underlain by ancient crystalline rocks that are covered by thick ferrallitic and fersiallitic weathered mantles (or saprolite)[5]. These areas originated with the 'dismantling of ancient weathering profiles as a consequence of Early Cainozoic uplift' (Thomas, 2003), where stores of kaolinitic saprolite have been the main source of alluvial sediment during the Quaternary. This includes sediments such as the Continental Terminal of West Africa and the Barreiras Formation of the Amazon Basin. Feruginous soils and iron-crusts, 'almost omnipresent in Africa south of the Sahara' (Boulet et al., 1997), were formed by hydrolysis reactions which result in iron, aluminium and part of the silica accumulating *in situ* to form goethite and gibbsite, while most other elements are removed. These soils have a typical vertical sequence as described by Boulet et al. (1997). The lowest horizons of coarse saprolite contain primary quartzo-feldspathic minerals, above which the saprolite becomes finer and quartz is absent, but goethite and/or haematite are present. The middle of the sequence is mottled with haematite nodules and kaolinitic clay. Approaching the surface, an increasingly iron-rich 'carapace' is succeeded by nodular or massive haematite. All of these minerals have some ability to adsorb arsenic. Gibbsite and kaolinite have modest adsorption capacities, adsorbing As(V) but not As(III) in acidic to neutral waters, but release As(V) at pH $\geq$ 8.0 (Chapter 2). Haematite can adsorb arsenic, and if abundant, which is likely, it will have the ability to readsorb arsenic released during the early stages of reduction.

Primary sources of arsenic are manifold, but whatever the source, weathering in a ferrallitic soil profile will reduce these mineral assemblages to a residuum of iron and aluminium oxides and kaolinite. Arsenic from the source rock will either be flushed away or trapped firmly in the mass of haematite, ensuring the non-availability of arsenic in the saprolite. Similar weathering processes are observed beneath the Pleistocene Madhupur and Barind surfaces in Bangladesh (Brammer, 1996), where deeply weathered red and grey clays are underlain by brown sands that are free from As contamination. These generalisations do not apply to all locations; notable exceptions do occur, particularly in areas of intense, but shallow, sulphide mineralisation such as in Chhattisgarh (India) and southwest Ghana. Nevertheless, the long history of weathering in tropical basement terrains is a general reason for the rarity of arsenic pollution in such regions.

3.5.2   Arsenic in alluvial basins

Many of the most As-affected aquifers are found in the middle and lower reaches of the great alluvial systems of Asia: the Ganges–Brahmaputra, Mekong, Irrawaddy, Red, Yellow (Huang-He) and Indus. Here, groundwaters are strongly reducing and arsenic is mobilised by reductive dissolution, driven by decomposition of organic matter. The headwaters of these rivers originate on the Tibetan Plateau. It is remarkable how few major rivers[6] outside Asia are severely affected by arsenic, although notable exceptions are the Danube and Po rivers in Europe. As contamination has been detected in two other alluvial settings. The first is where rivers drain active geothermal provinces, such as in Chile, New Zealand, Indonesia and Yellowstone Park (USA), where cause and effect are self-evident. The second, and potentially more significant, is the Basin-and-Range Province of the southwest USA, where arsenic is mobilised by alkali desorption. The climate is semi-arid, the groundwaters are oxic, and run-off from adjacent mountains is an important component of recharge.

Catchment types

Discussing fluxes of sediment from tropical watersheds, Thomas (2003) distinguished between rivers draining mountains and those draining plateaus. Plateau catchments have long channels with low gradients and slow sediment delivery to the ocean. Upper catchments in plateau watersheds produce fine-grained sediment derived mainly from saprolite and existing floodplains. The upper catchments are extensively weathered, as discussed above. Other features of the plateau watersheds that drain the remnants of Gondwanaland may limit arsenic contamination. Most rivers are developed in hard rock terrain that resist incision, and as Goudie (2005) notes, a large part of the coast of Africa is upwarped, creating a 'hypsometry' where only a small proportion of the basin is located at low elevation. Consequently, little accommodation space was created during sea-level low stands for the deposition of Quaternary alluvium. Further, because gradients and sediment loads are lower, a higher proportion of the accommodation space was filled by marine sediments, which have not subsequently formed exploitable aquifers.

Mountain catchments of the SSAAB and the Basin-and-Range Province have similarities in their upper catchments, but profound differences in their lower catchments, primarily related to climate. The upper catchments are significantly drier and/or colder than the lower reaches, such that physical weathering dominates. The upper catchments are steep, favouring rapid delivery and accumulation of iron-coated sands in the lower catchments. This is also why these basins do not have major saprolite stores in their upper reaches. Although both have warm climates, the lower catchments differ fundamentally in their depositional or chemical weathering environment. The humid SSAAB catchments will tend to be fully saturated, organic-rich and anoxic, promoting reductive dissolution of iron oxides. Basin-and-Range type catchments will have deep water tables, lack organic matter, and therefore groundwater will evolve along oxidising geochemical pathways (Chapter 2). The key similarity, however, is the rapid delivery of the relatively unweathered rock to the alluvial basins in the lower catchment.

Sediment and water characteristics

The downstream products of upstream processes differ greatly. Sediment transported out of the mountain catchments is rich in lithic or mineral grains with little alteration. Sands are deposited with iron-rich coatings produced in the early stages of chemical weathering that may adsorb any arsenic released. For example, sands deposited by the Ganges and Brahmaputra contain abundant biotite, which can be a source of arsenic. However, in humid plateau catchments, biotite and other ferromagnesian minerals tend to be destroyed in the soil zone. Hence, in the Niger Delta the dominant minerals are quartz and kaolinite with only small quantities of smectite, illite, feldspar and limonite (Oomkens, 1974; Olorunfemi et al., 1985). The composition of river sands may be characterised by the ratio of quartz to feldspar to rock fragments (QFR). In the Amazon, the QFR ratio changes from 47:8:45 near the Andes to 85:3:11 near the mouth, showing the effects of chemical weathering and dilution by plateau sediment (M.F. Thomas, 1994).

Given that both the AD- and RD-type mobilisation mechanisms are related to weathering and diagenetic changes, As occurrence should be related to the sediment and water quality in rivers (Table 3.2). In Figures 3.1 and 3.2, sedimentary, weathering and water quality parameters of major rivers have been classified according to the presence or absence of As contamination in their alluvial deposits. Sands from As-affected basins have a limited range of quartz content (40–65%) but a wide range of suspended load. However, all the rivers with very high loads (>400 t/km²/year) are As-affected basins from the SSAAB, whereas the Amazon, Orinoco, Niger and Congo plot far outside the range of the As-affected basins. The As-affected basins are characterised by higher indices of both physical and chemical weathering. Viewed from the perspective of QFR ratios of the river sands, it is observed that the Amazon, Orinoco, Niger and Congo are almost pure quartz sands, while other unaffected mountain watersheds are rich in rock fragments and plot close to the 'Andean' field of Potter (1994). Sands from the As-affected basins, however, plot in a triangular area of intermediate composition with a tendency towards increasing feldspar content. The degree of chemical weathering is also reflected in the chemistry of the river water. River water from As-affected basins has a distinctive anionic composition, dominated by bicarbonate and containing < 10% of silica. However, water from the unaffected tropical watersheds has a much higher proportion of silica, reflecting the advanced state of chemical weathering[7].

Potter (1994) suggested, from the perspective of plate tectonics, that the three great families of modern sands in South America (Andean, Brazilian and Transitional; see Figure 3.2 and Chapter 10) are representative of three global families. He proposed that the Andean-type represents the debris of active and suture margins, the Brazilian of cratonic, passive margins, and the Transitional family of molasse aprons surrounding active margins. Although there is no direct causal relationship, there is an indirect connection between the geochemical processes that determine sand mineralogy and those that mobilise arsenic. Potter's classification of sands has a parallel in Thomas' (2003) classification of watersheds, but with the important difference that Potter recognises an intermediate category, relating to recycled orogenic materials, where there has been significant but incomplete weathering. This analysis suggests that plate tectonic setting and climate can provide a basis for first-order prediction of As occurrence, and can be correlated with the tectonic zones (see Figure 2.15).

Influence of Quaternary sea-level change

As shown in Table 3.5, most severe cases of As pollution involve mobilisation by reductive dissolution in Quaternary, and predominantly Holocene, alluvium. This requires the juxtaposition of sources of organic matter (in mud or peat) and sands (potential aquifers) with iron-rich coatings that

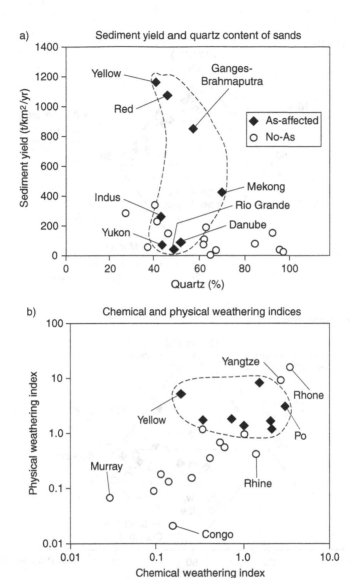

Figure 3.1 Relation of sediment yield, sand composition and weathering rates to arsenic occurrence in alluvial basins. (a) Sediment yield and quartz content of sands. (b) Chemical and physical weathering indices. The physical and chemical weathering indices represent the suspended solids and total solute loads of the rivers, normalised relative to the Amazon, which therefore plots at 1.0, 1.0 on the graph. The symbols indicate whether arsenic polluted groundwater is known to be present in the alluvium of the basin, or is thought to be absent.

Source: Data from Potter (1978, 1994); Ludwig and Probst (1998); Gaillardet et al. (1999); and Borges and Huh (2006)

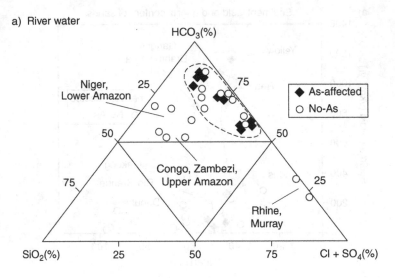

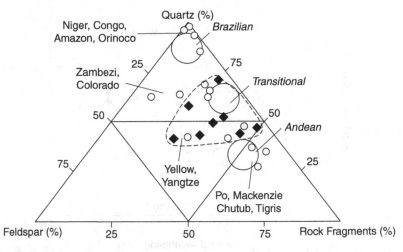

Figure 3.2 Relation of river water chemistry and sand composition to arsenic occurrence in alluvial basins. (a) River water, anions; (b) sand composition. The symbols are the same as in Figure 3.1, except that large circles represent the Great Sand Families of Potter (1978).

Sources: Data from Potter (1978, 1994), Gaillardet et al. (1999), Yang et al. (2004), Pasquini et al. (2005) and Borges and Huh (2006)

have arsenic adsorbed to them (Ravenscroft and Ahmed, 1998). Further, the sands and organic material must be in hydraulic continuity. In the affected basins, tectonic subsidence or channel incision create accommodation space for young sediments and also maintain a shallow water table with slow flushing and reducing porewaters. The As-affected parts of these basins were not glaciated, but were profoundly influenced by glacio-eustatic sea-level changes, especially in deltaic regions (e.g. Ravenscroft et al., 2001, 2005). By lowering the water table, incision of the major channels created conditions favourable for immobilising arsenic in remnant Pleistocene sediments, while porewater conditions in the Holocene sediments that filled the incised channels were favourable for reductive dissolution. There were many glacial cycles in the Pleistocene, however, we concentrate on the Last Glacial Maximum (LGM; 30–18 ka), which was not only the most recent but also had the lowest sea level for at least the past 130,000 years (Lambeck et al., 2002), and therefore had the greatest impact. At the LGM, when global sea level stood 120–130 m below its present level, rivers incised channels into the soft alluvial sediment, leaving terraces in the interfluvial areas. In many regions, especially along the front of the Himalayas, monsoonal rainfall was greatly reduced at this time (e.g. Dawson, 1992). In the interfluves, the water table fell many tens of metres permitting deep, oxidative weathering of the sediments, destroying organic matter and forming crystalline ferric oxides and kaolinite. Under these conditions, dissolved arsenic was either flushed away or became tightly bound in haematite or goethite.

After 18 ka, sea level rose rapidly till about 7 ka. Initially, elongate estuaries invaded the incised channels, but with the return of monsoonal circulation, fluvial aggradation and prograding deltas rapidly filled the estuaries, pushing back the coastline. The channel-fill sediments were largely sands, but locally interbedded with organic-rich mud. When the rising sea level reached the surfaces of the Pleistocene terraces, enormous areas were flooded by seawater, and changed the pattern of sediment transport and deposition. Instead of being transferred to the oceans, following the 'conveyor-belt' model of Blum and Törnqvist (2000), fine sediments accumulated in wide, shallow bays. Channel-sands formed only a small proportion of the sediment deposited near the coast. The mid-Holocene climatic optimum resulted in greatly increased rainfall, river discharges and warmer temperatures, encouraging the growth of extensive peat basins, until they were eventually overlapped by coalescing delta plains (e.g. Goodbred and Kuehl, 2000a,b). After 7 ka, sea level fluctuated by only a few metres. The low topographic gradients of the modern deltaic plains ensured that groundwater flow was sluggish, with limited flushing of shallow aquifers. These sedimentary processes thus created conditions suitable to juxtapose fresh organic matter and sand with amorphous iron coatings with adsorbed As. Shifting channels (now aquifers) locally cut through peat layers, or are separated by only a few metres of poorly consolidated mud. First, under the natural flow regime, and later exacerbated by pumping, DOC produced by the degradation of organic matter leaked into the sand layers, creating reducing conditions, and subsequently mobilising arsenic.

The Bengal Basin serves as a model for all alluvial basins that were open to the oceans during the LGM. Interpreting the three-dimensional structure of Quaternary units in deltas will provide a basis for predicting the occurrence of arsenic, planning surveys, and developing mitigation plans. However, even in the SSAAB, significant differences may occur due to the specific geological structure and history of the basin. For instance, in the Mekong delta, shallow bedrock prevented deep incision of the river (Morgan, 1970) and therefore limited the accommodation space for Holocene sands. In the Chao Phraya delta of Thailand, the Holocene sequence at Bangkok is almost entirely marine (AIT, 1981) so there are no recent sands from which to mobilise arsenic, the older sands having been flushed during the LGM lowstand.

Although less significant than for reductive dissolution, Quaternary sea level changes also influenced As-mobilisation by alkali desorption in glacial lowlands. As discussed in Chapter 2, post-glacial inundation promoted ion-exchange reactions that tended to increase pH, and therefore promote desorption of arsenic after isostatic rebound lifted the rocks above sea-level. Such phenomena have been recorded in Finland, New England and British Columbia.

3.6   Behaviour of Arsenic in Aquifers

3.6.1   Temporal changes of arsenic concentrations in groundwater

Arsenic concentrations in well-water and aquifers may be expected to change over time, and over different timescales. Temporal changes in concentration at wells result from lateral or vertical migration of arsenic through aquifers at a variety of scales. Changes in the first few minutes or hours of pumping will be related to the microenvironment of the well and are important for sampling. Of more profound importance are changes over weeks to a few years that lead to effectively permanent changes in the average quality of water withdrawn. Over periods of months to many years, such pumping-induced changes grade into bulk changes in the water quality of entire aquifers.

The United States of America

In fluvio-glacial aquifers in Minnesota containing iron-rich RD-type water, Erickson and Barnes (2006) showed that the As content of 40% of municipal

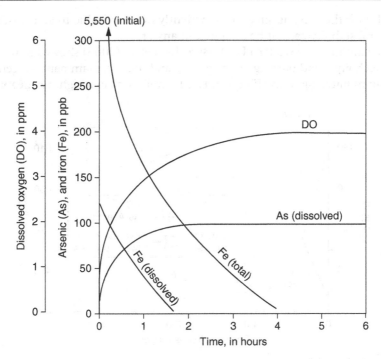

Figure 3.3   Pumping-induced changes in water chemistry in the Basin-and-Range aquifers, Arizona. The trends of elemental concentration represent the general behaviour of deep water-supply wells, installed with steel casing in alluvial aquifers in various parts of the Basin-and-Range province.
Source: After Robertson (1989)

wells increased from just below, to just above, 10 ppb As during the first hour of operation. Within 4 hours of stopping the pump, As concentrations showed a reciprocal decline. They attributed these changes to adsorption on iron oxides in, and immediately surrounding, the borehole. Robertson (1989) showed comparable behaviour in AD-type waters in Arizona (Figure 3.3). When pumped, the As concentration rose over 2 hours to stabilise at 100 ppb As. In parallel with the changes in arsenic, dissolved oxygen rose but iron fell rapidly, before stabilising after about 4 hours.

In granitic terrain in Washington State (USA), Frost et al. (1993) found that As concentrations varied seasonally by a factor of between 1 and 19. At Fallon, Nevada, in a typical Basin-and-Range aquifer where As concentrations ranged from below detection to 6200 ppb As, Steinmaus et al. (2005) found that over periods of 1 to 20 years, As concentrations in most wells remained stable over time. They concluded that 'a limited number of measurements per well can be used to predict arsenic exposure over many years'. This may be valid for the Nevada site, but is evidently not applicable to all areas, and temporal stability cannot be assumed in any area.

At a landfill in the western USA, Barcelona et al. (2005) showed how sampling technique and purging affect arsenic and other contaminant concentrations in monitoring wells (Figure 3.4). The wells, one in a high-permeability,

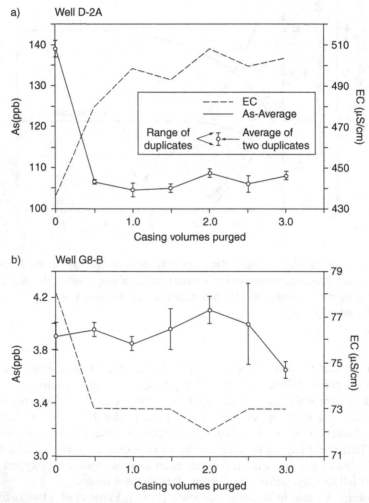

Figure 3.4   Effect of purging on arsenic concentrations in monitoring wells at a landfill in the USA. (a) Well D-2A is screened in a low-permeability horizon. (b) Well G-8B is screened in a high-permeability horizon. Both wells were sampled using low-flow pumping with continuous monitoring of redox-sensitive parameters. Although well D-2A takes longer to stabilise, it is ready for sampling after two casing volumes have been withdrawn.
Source: After Barcelona et al. (2006)

and the other in a low-permeability, stratum, were sampled by low-flow pumping with a bladder pump. Measurements of Eh, pH, DO, EC and temperature were taken in a flow-through cell. In both cases, As concentration increased during the first one to two casing-volumes purged, by which time redox-related parameters, EC and drawdown also stabilised. They argued that, for general survey and monitoring purposes, the use of low-flow pumps, and the stabilisation of drawdown and redox-sensitive parameters, provides an appropriate basis for reliable sample collection.

The Bengal Basin

There has been some controversy about temporal changes in the As content of tubewell-water in the Bengal Basin. When As contamination was discovered in Bangladesh, there were no historical data to indicate whether it had always been present, whether it had increased over time, and what might happen in the future. Although some agencies believed there was no alternative but to wait and monitor wells for 5 to 10 years, others showed that statistically valid inferences, vital for policy makers, could be drawn from current As concentrations and the age of wells (DPHE/MMI/BGS, 1999; McArthur et al., 2004). This analysis was based on the results of surveys of thousands of tubewells, and the assumption that, on average, hand tubewells pump at the same rate, and hence well-age is a proxy for the total volume of water pumped. Because As concentrations spanned four orders of magnitude, the data were processed as percentage of wells from each year group exceeding various concentration thresholds. The results (Figure 3.5) show a general trend for wells to increase in concentration over periods of 10–20 years. This trend is independent of the threshold concentration, and was observed in all affected regions, but not in wells deeper than 150 m. Less than 25% of new wells exceeded 50 ppb As, but the proportion increased to around 40% in wells more than 10 years old.

Attempts have been made to measure long-term changes. Cheng et al. (2006) monitored 20 hand tubewells in Araihazar (Bangladesh) for 3 years, and showed little change, giving the impression that concentrations remain stable over time. The timespan of these measurements was too short to reach sound conclusions, and they ignored the inferences based on well-age in the same areas and elsewhere (Sengupta et al., 2006b; Ravenscroft et al., 2006).

Other countries

In Nepal, NASC/ENPHO (2004) reported a weak correlation between arsenic and well-age on the Terai. In Cambodia, Polya et al. (2005) indicated there were insufficient data to determine unequivocally whether As concentrations were increasing. Under different conditions in the semi-arid

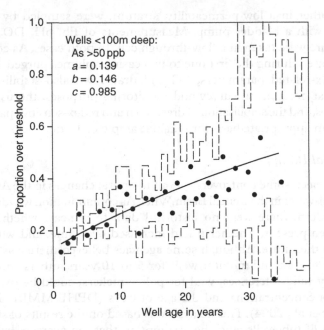

Figure 3.5 Temporal trends of arsenic in groundwater in Bangladesh. The graph shows the increasing proportion of wells <100 m deep that exceed the 50 ppb drinking water standard with increasing age, and hence increasing cumulative abstraction. The trend of arsenic concentration with well age is represented by a model (solid line) showing the proportion of wells exceeding a threshold concentration with as a function of time, fitted numerically by the function [proportion over threshold] = $b-(b-a)c^{-t}$ where a is the intercept, b is the plateau value, c is a constant and t time in years. The solid circles show the proportion of wells exceeding 50 ppb in each year group, and the dashed lines represent the confidence limits.
Source: After McArthur et al. (2004)

Puna de Atacama region of northern Argentina, Concha et al. (2005) reported fluctuations in the range of 140–220 ppb As in well-waters over a 10-year period, but no overall trend was observed.

In summary, present understanding indicates that wells tested as safe cannot be assumed, or even expected, to remain safe, and should be monitored on a timescale of 1–2 years.

3.6.2   Migration and attenuation of arsenic in groundwater

While changes in concentration over time in a well indicate that arsenic is moving through an aquifer, this alone tells us little about how far, how fast, or from where it has moved. Direct evidence of the scale and rate of As movement in aquifers is largely absent. Höhn et al. (2006) measured movements of a few metres in a period of weeks in a fluvio-glacial sand as described below. Apart from temporal changes, indirect evidence of arsenic movement can be inferred from geochemical profiles and geological reasoning. In the Joypur, Ardivok and Moyna (JAM) aquifer in West Bengal (section 3.7.1), an arsenic front was observed to move 1–2 m downwards over a period of 18 months, and downward movements of 10–30 m over 6000 years were inferred.

Attenuation processes

The migration of arsenic is primarily controlled by the advective flow of groundwater[8]. Diffusion is of secondary importance compared with dispersion in permeable aquifers, although convective flow may be important in geothermal systems (Ingebritsen and Sanford, 1998). Geochemical processes limit the migration of arsenic within the constraints imposed by the groundwater flow paths[9]. The velocity of groundwater flow is the effective upper limit for the migration of arsenic. Therefore, to understand the migration at any site it is essential to understand the hydraulics of the aquifer first. Within a defined flow system, As concentrations may be modified by one of four main processes: (a) adsorption onto, or coprecipitation with, metal oxides or clays; (b) coprecipitation with, or adsorption onto, sulphide minerals[10]; (c) dilution by leakage from adjacent strata; and (d) evaporative concentration in the vicinity of a shallow water table. The most important process that retards arsenic migration is adsorption, and the most important sorbents are iron oxides (Chapter 2). The way that adsorption retards the transport of arsenic, and many other contaminants, can be expressed in a simplified way by the distribution coefficient[11] (K_d) which describes its partitioning between the solid and liquid phases (Langmuir, 1997), and is defined as:

$$K_d = s/C \tag{3.1}$$

where s is the concentration sorbed to the soil (in µg kg[1]) and C is the concentration dissolved in water (ppb). The value of K_d relates the velocity of the contaminant (v_c) to the velocity of the water (v_x) through a parameter known as the retardation factor (R_f), as defined by the following equation (Fetter, 1999):

$$R_f = 1 + (\rho_b/\theta) \cdot K_d \tag{3.2}$$

Table 3.7   Experimentally determined arsenic distribution coefficients (K_d) for selected minerals*

Mineral	As (III) [L/kg] 0.01 M	0.1 M	Not specified	As (V) [L/kg] 0.01 M	0.1 M	Not specified
Alumina (α-Al₂O₃)	520	42				760
Gibbsite (Al₂O₃·3H₂O)						133
Ferrihydrite[†] (Fe₅OH₈·4H₂O)	399,000	120,000		175,000	>1,000,000	
Goethite (α-FeOOH)			32		192	1800
Lepidocrocite (γ-FeOOH)			35			1000
Haematite (Fe₂O₃)			21		34	25
Birnessite (δ-MnO₂)	46,000[‡]			57,500		
Illite			98			
Kaolinite			19			760
Bentonite (montmorillonite)			30			
Quartz					2	

*All estimates relate to pH 7 and do not involve the effect of competing ions.
[†]Ferrihydrite is roughly equivalent to the terms HFO and amorphous iron hydroxide.
[‡]Average of five determinations. The K_d was thought to have been affected by oxidation to As(V).
Source: Summarised data from Smedley and Kinniburgh (2002)

where ρ_b is the dry bulk density and θ is the porosity. Hence the velocity of the contaminant can be expressed as:

$$v_c = v_x/R_f \tag{3.3}$$

Thus an R_f of 10 means that the contaminant moves ten times slower than the water. Relatively, bulk density varies little between lithologies, while porosity is typically 0.2–0.3 in granular aquifers, and of the order of 0.01 in fractured rock aquifers. Table 3.7 lists distribution coefficients for arsenic determined for minerals relevant to its migration and attenuation in groundwater. The values of K_d vary enormously between minerals, underlining the importance of characterising the mineralogy of vulnerable aquifers

(Lin and Puls, 2003). Values of K_d are sensitive to ionic strength, but even more sensitive to the effect of competing ions. For example, the values quoted for ferrihydrite in 0.1 M solutions are from Swedlund and Webster (1999) who showed that, in the presence of 62 ppm silica, the K_d of As(III) is reduced by an order of magnitude, and that for As(V) by two orders of magnitude. The extreme values for ferrihydrite were determined for freshly formed precipitates, and are relevant to water treatment, but less so to aquifers where more crystalline forms dominate. The high values of K_d for most oxides indicate their high attenuation capacity, and hence the mobility of arsenic depends strongly on stability of the oxides present.

The K_d approach is convenient because groundwater velocity can usually be determined with reasonable confidence, and uncertainty in K_d estimates can be assessed using sensitivity analysis. For example, considering the example of the JAM aquifer described below, the groundwater velocity, ahead of an As(III)-rich plume, was estimated to be 30 m/year. The aquifer contains crystalline iron oxides and clay minerals, and hence suggest a K_d of about 30. Assuming a porosity of 0.25 and a bulk density of 2.0 g/cm³, this results in an R_f of 241, or in other words arsenic would migrate more than 200 times slower than flowing groundwater (about 10 cm/year). Although the retardation factor approach has serious limitations for predicting long-term attenuation, especially for the ultimate 'clean-up' of aquifers (Bethke and Brady, 2000), which warrant approaches such as surface-complexation adsorption modelling (e.g. Sracek et al., 2004), it is useful for assessing the semi-quantitative potential for attenuating arsenic in aquifers. As suggested by the wide range of K_d values in Table 3.7, the main difficulty with this approach arises from the shortage of field-determined K_d estimates, and the effect of competing ions. Smedley and Kinniburgh (2002) noted that most field determinations from contaminated aquifers have very low K_d values, which reflects the mobility of arsenic therein, although it is of greater importance to determine K_d in the receiving strata. It will also be helpful to use groundwater from investigated sites for batch tests to account for the effect of competing species.

Plume behaviour

Understanding the fate of a potentially mobile plume of arsenic requires understanding the hydraulics of the system, the characteristics of the plume, and the water chemistry and mineralogy of the aquifer into which it migrates. Table 3.8 illustrates the scenarios resulting from an As plume mobilised by each of the four mechanisms migrating into groundwater bodies with different redox characteristics (but all with no dissolved arsenic), some of which are more likely than others. The degree of attenuation depends largely on the contrast between pH and redox conditions of the plume and the receiving water.

Table 3.8 Factors influencing the migration of arsenic-rich plumes in aquifers

Process in plume	Characteristics	Typical aquifers	Character of (As-free) Receiving Water		
			Oxic DO, NO_3 present	Mildly reducing no DO, low NO_3 ± Mn	Strongly reducing Fe, NH_4, CH_4 present; low SO_4
Reductive Dissolution	As(III); anoxic; neutral; high Fe, Mn, NH_4, HCO_3 and DOC; low SO_4	Alluvium and glacial sediment. Example: Bengal Basin.	Unlikely Strong retardation by iron oxides, enhanced by precipitation of ferrihydrite, and if Fe:As>20. Mn oxides may be precipitated.	Likely Limited precipitation of ferrihydrite, but modest adsorption onto goethite or haematite. Mn remains in solution.	Likely Possible adsorption of As(III) onto sulphides, or precipitation where excess of S^{2-} leads to pyrite formation.
Alkali-Desorption	As(V); alkaline; low Fe, Mn & DOC; some NO_3 or SO_4	Alluvium, sandstone, volcanic and crystalline rock. Example: Argentina	Likely As-mobility high if pH >=8.0, but adsorbed on iron oxides at pH <8.0.	Likely Similar to the oxic case (left), but more likely to result in near-neutral pH, and hence As adsorbed by iron oxides.	Unlikely As attenuated by sulphate reduction and coprecipitation in pyrite.
Sulphide-Oxidation	As(V); acid; high SO_4; high to low Fe; no DOC.	Mineralised bedrock. Example: Wisconsin (USA)	Likely As(V) mobile if not adsorbed by iron oxides. Acidity neutralised by carbonate minerals.	Likely As(V) mobile if not adsorbed by iron oxides. Acidity neutralised by carbonate minerals.	Unlikely Reduction of As(V) and sulphate reduction leads to coprecipitation in pyrite. Acidity neutralised by carbonate minerals.
Geothermal	As(III); no DOC; High chloride ± sulphide	Volcanic or tectonically active terrain. Example: Andean Altiplano.	Likely Oxidation of As(III) and adsorption onto iron oxides. Sulphide oxidised to sulphate.	Likely Possible oxidation of As(III). Sulphide oxidised to sulphate (by NO_3). Some adsorption of As on iron oxides.	Unlikely As(V) reduced to As(III) and attenuated by coprecipitation in, or adsorption onto, pyrite.

The aquifer material is assumed to contain Fe, Mn, Al and Si, and therefore, depending on conditions, their weathering products in the form oxides and clays.

Where a reducing plume, rich in As(III), ferrous iron and DOC, migrates into a reducing aquifer, arsenic may remain relatively mobile, but may still be attenuated if the adsorption capacity of iron oxyhydroxides for As(III) is not saturated. However, where a reducing plume migrates through an oxic aquifer with little dissolved iron and significant concentrations of oxygen, sulphate and nitrate, arsenic will be strongly attenuated by adsorption onto both existing and freshly precipitated iron oxyhydroxide coatings. For the arsenic front to advance, the Fe(III) oxide coatings must be substantially reduced, at least to the point where all As(III) sorption sites are saturated (McArthur et al., 2004). This requires a continuous supply of DOC and explains why arsenic lags far behind the flow of water.

Where an oxic plume, whether mobilised by alkali desorption or sulphide oxidation, moves into a reducing aquifer containing dissolved ferrous iron, precipitation of iron oxyhydroxides and consequent adsorption strongly retards arsenic. If the plume contains sulphate and the receiving porewaters are sufficiently reducing, sulphate-reducing bacteria will promote crystallisation of (framboidal) pyrite, which can accommodate arsenic in its structure or adsorb it on its surface. However, where an oxic plume migrates through an oxic aquifer, the mobilisation mechanism will determine the attenuation of arsenic. Where the plume was mobilised by alkali desorption, arsenic will only be adsorbed by oxide phases at pH ≤ 8.0. However, where the plume is mobilised by sulphide oxidation, arsenic can be adsorbed onto oxides and clays.

Modelling and batch testing

Theoretically, all of the retardation processes can be simulated using geochemical models such as PHREEQ (Sracek et al., 2004), but it is rarely practical to calibrate models reliably. Calibration requires time-series monitoring of piezometer nests, followed by supplementary studies to justify extrapolation to areas with fewer data. An example of the work required to calibrate such a model was given by Stollenwerk et al. (2007) using piezometer nests and batch-testing on core samples at a site 20 km west of Dhaka (Bangladesh). The site was underlain by two aquifers: an upper grey Holocene sand extending to 50 m and containing ≤ 900 ppb As, and a lower brown Pleistocene sand containing <5 ppb As. Sand from the lower aquifer was equilibrated with synthetic groundwater that had been spiked with varying quantities of arsenic, phosphate and silica. Thus, they were able to define the adsorption isotherms and capacities applicable to retardation of the downward migration of polluted water from the Holocene sediments that can be expected as abstraction wells are deepened to avoid shallow arsenic. It was shown that the lower aquifer has substantial capacity to remove arsenic from groundwater and that, as water is drawn from increasingly

deeper wells, a large part of the shallow arsenic will be permanently sequestered in the brown sands.

A tracer test at Cape Cod, USA

Höhn et al. (2006) conducted a natural-gradient tracer test to investigate the
movement of oxic groundwater containing As(V) into an anoxic, sandy aquifer in Massachusetts (USA). The injected water contained 500 ppb of As(V)
plus dissolved oxygen and nitrate to ensure the water was initially oxic, plus
bromide added as an inert tracer. The receiving groundwater had pH 6.5,
and contained no nitrate but high iron (13.8 ppm) and 10 ppb of As(III). The
plume was monitored for 3.5 months at piezometers 1–5 m away from the
injection well. The sand had a permeability of about 80 m/day and the flow
velocity was estimated to be 0.3–0.4 m/day. Within 10 days, oxygen and
nitrate reacted to precipitate iron hydroxides, which then adsorbed the As(V),
but injection was continued until As(V) broke through at the nearest piezometer. Seven days after injection ceased, the groundwater became anoxic
again, and As(III) concentrations began to increase. During the monitored
'reducing' period, both As(III) and As(V) were transported, indicating significant retardation of both species, although the adsorption of As(V) was
greatest. In the reducing period, the rise in Fe(II) concentrations lagged
behind that of As(III), which was attributed to adsorption of Fe(II). This
study shows that reduction and oxidation of arsenic species can occur on a
timescale of days (i.e. rapid compared with groundwater flow), and also demonstrates the complexity of the geochemical processes by which arsenic and
iron species are transformed and transferred between solid and liquid phases.

3.7   Case Histories of Arsenic-affected Aquifers

3.7.1   The JAM alluvial aquifer in West Bengal

Few studies of arsenic mobilisation in the Bengal Basin (Chapter 8) have
integrated geochemistry and hydrogeology. An exception is the study of the
contiguous villages of Joypur, Ardivok and Moyna (JAM) near Barasat,
20 km north of Kolkata (McArthur et al., 2004, 2008). The JAM study
shows how extreme lateral and vertical concentration gradients can be
explained, elaborates the migration pathways, and shows how aquifers
might be protected from contamination.

Geology and hydrogeology

The JAM site is located on the floodplains of the Ganges delta. Holocene
silt covers the area to a depth of 10–25 m, overlying a shallow aquifer formed

Table 3.9 Simplified lithostratigraphy of the Joypur, Ardivok and Moyna aquifer, West Bengal

Unit	Depth range (m b.g.l.)	Geology
VI	3–15	Holocene grey coarse sand (at one site only, within Unit V)
V	0–20	Holocene (c. 8–2 ka) overbank muds and peat; grey-green to black; low permeability
IV	6–30	Terminal Pleistocene to Holocene (c. 23–7 ka) channel-fill sand; grey to brownish-grey; high permeability
III	20–23	Pleistocene (>23 ka) stiff brown clay; laterally correlatable and virtually impermeable.
II	23–45	Pleistocene (>>23 ka) fluvial sands; brown to grey-brown; high permeability
I	>45	Grey clay

Source: After McArthur et al. (2004)

of Holocene and Pleistocene sands that extend to about 45 m (Table 3.9 and Figure 3.6). A discontinuous, but low permeability, brown clay, crosses the area at a depth of 20 m. This clay is a palaeosol formed during the Late Pleistocene, and separates the post-LGM sediments from weathered brown sands below. The hydrogeology of the area can be visualised in terms of two profiles: a channel-fill sequence and a palaeointerfluve sequence. In the palaeointerfluve sequence, thick dark grey muds are hydraulically separated from the underlying aquifer by the palaeosol. In the channel-fill sequence, the palaeosol has been eroded and the resultant channel filled by Holocene sands, which form elongate, trench-like aquifers that provide vertical conduits for the flow between the surface and the more laterally extensive Pleistocene aquifer. In the villages, households draw water from hand-pumped wells, 20–50 m deep, while larger volumes of water are pumped from beneath the adjacent agricultural fields to irrigate rice and vegetables.

Arsenic concentrations in private wells range from below detection to >1000 ppb over distances of a few hundred metres. Arsenic pollution occurs mainly in the Holocene channel-fill sands, while brown sands generally contain <10 ppb As. However, some grey Pleistocene sands are polluted adjacent to the channel-fill deposits, where organic-rich groundwater has migrated into and reduced the brown sands. The differences in the chemistry and hydraulic behaviour between the interfluve and channel-fill sequences, which are critical to understanding the distribution of arsenic at the JAM site and elsewhere in the Bengal Basin, are illustrated in Figure 3.6. At the interfluve site (DP), silt and black peat, rich in sulphur and organic matter,

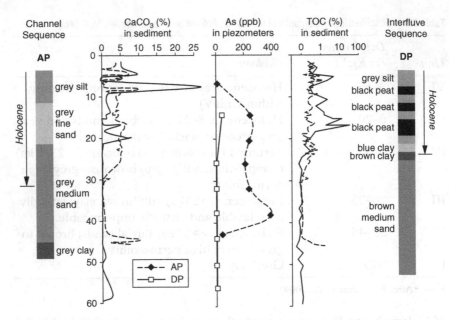

Figure 3.6　Hydrogeochemical profiles of the Joypur, Ardivok and Moyna (JAM) aquifer, West Bengal. Site AP is typical of a channel-fill alluvial sequence, where Holocene and Pleistocene sands are in continuity. The base of the Holocene sediment is marked by a rapid drop in the content of carbonate and total organic carbon (TOC). In the low-As interfluve sequence, the boundary is located at the top of the brown clay (palaeosol) horizon.
Source: Modified after McArthur et al. (2004)

overlie the palaeosol, below which there are 30 m of brown sands with very low sulphur, carbonate and OM contents, and where groundwater contains <5 ppb As. At the channel-fill site (AP), 6 m of Holocene silt overlie 24 m of grey sand and 15 m of brown sand. Here, groundwater contains several hundred ppb of arsenic, except in the lowest 5 m, where the reducing waters have not yet reached. The total As contents of the sediments are summarised in Table 3.10, which shows the higher concentrations of both arsenic and iron in the Holocene sands. The aquifer beneath the palaeosol is more strongly confined than in the channel-fill sequences.

Arsenic migration

Figure 3.7 shows a conceptual model of shallow groundwater flow based on a flow-line through AP and DP. The combination of the aquifer geometry, topography and pumping generates a circular flow cell. Groundwater is pumped for irrigation from the brown sands beneath the palaeosol. Part of this water percolates through the paddy soils, creating a mound at the water

Table 3.10 Mean* arsenic and iron concentrations of lithostratigraphic units in the Joypur, Ardivok and Moyna aquifer, West Bengal

Lithostratigraphic unit	Channel-fill sequence (FP)			Interfluve sequence (DP)		
	Number	As (mg/kg)	Fe (wt%)	Number	As (mg/kg)	Fe (wt%)
V Holocene silt	8	10.7 (4.6)	1.5 (0.54)	18	5.6 (2.1)	0.32 (0.14)
IV Holocene sand	13	7.3 (3.7)	1.2 (0.42)	0	–	–
III Pleistocene clay	0	–	–	3	3.5 (0.31)	0.11 (0.05)
II Pleistocene sand	9	1.7 (1.0)	0.60 (0.11)	18	1.2 (0.79)	0.06 (0.03)

*Standard deviations are given in parentheses.
Source: Data from McArthur et al. (2008)

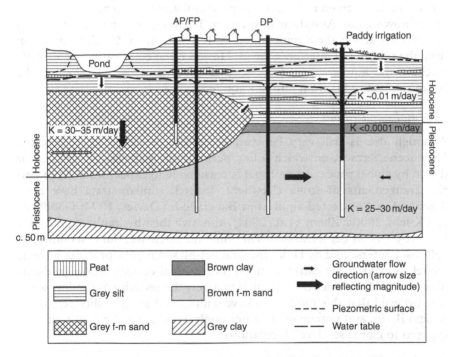

Figure 3.7 Conceptual model of flow in the shallow aquifers of the Bengal Basin. Note the figure is based on the Joypur, Ardivok and Moyna (JAM) site but is believed to represent, in principle, processes operating over wide areas of the Bengal Basin. The vertical dimension is approximately to scale, but horizontal dimensions will vary widely. The reference to AP/FP represents the Holocene channel-fill condition, and DP represents the interfluve condition.

table that drives shallow groundwater back toward the village and the channel-fill sequence. When this flow reaches the point where the palaeosol has been eroded, it moves down through the Holocene sands and into the Pleistocene sands. Direct rainfall-recharge also moves down to the aquifer along this pathway. Here, part of the infiltrating groundwater is abstracted by hand tubewells for potable supply, but the remainder is drawn back toward the irrigation wells, completing the cycle.

Although arsenic mobilisation began a few thousands years ago, the flow cell described above drives its ongoing mobilisation and migration. Reductive dissolution is driven by the decay of organic matter in the Holocene mud and peat. As DOC migrates down into the aquifer, it reduces iron oxide coatings in the aquifer and releases arsenic. At JAM, arsenic pollution has reached almost to the base of the channel-fill sequence, and in at least one location As-polluted groundwater has migrated laterally beneath the palaeosol horizon. Although sand colour can be a guide to the short-term safety of wells[12], the long-term security of safe wells in the JAM aquifer depends on the position of the well screen relative to the palaeosol and the attenuation capacity of the brown sands. As indicated by Figure 3.7, as organic matter within, and immediately above, the channel-fill sands is depleted, DOC will be drawn in from the peat in the interfluvial areas. However, the concentrations of DOC reaching the aquifers will decrease over time, progressively slowing the advance of the redox front into safe aquifers.

Regional implications

Although details will vary between areas, the existence of a dissected Pleistocene terrace, on which a low permeability palaeosol developed, is driven by global processes, and so it is reasonable to expect similar geometric arrangements of strata elsewhere. Indeed, similar strata have been described in As-affected aquifers in Bangladesh (Davies, 1994; Goodbred and Kuehl, 2000a; Zheng et al., 2004), although their hydraulic significance has not yet been demonstrated. The thin and extensive, but discontinuous palaeosol, intersected by Holocene channel-fill sediments, provides a viable model to explain the extreme lateral and vertical concentration gradients observed, and a framework in which to assess the security of shallow wells. It is believed that this model will have widespread applicability across the Bengal Basin, and potentially to other unglaciated alluvial basins that were exposed to global sea-level fluctuations.

3.7.2   The Central Oklahoma Sandstone Aquifer

The Central Oklahoma Sandstone Aquifer (COA) is formed by ancient alluvial deposits of the Permian Garber Sandstone and Wellington

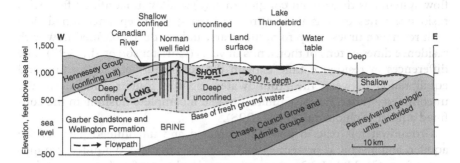

Figure 3.8 Hydrogeological section through the Central Oklahoma Aquifer. Arsenic is mobilised by desorption along deep flow paths in the confined aquifer, where ion-exchange reactions dominate the groundwater composition in a zone of partial flushing of ancient saline water.
Source: Smith (2005)

Formation, and contains concentrations of up to 232 ppb As in the deeper and confined parts of the aquifer (Figure 3.8). In the COA, groundwater flow, on a scale of kilometres horizontally and hundreds of metres vertically, exerts a primary control over arsenic mobilisation. The diagenetic history of the Permian rocks (Breit, 1998) is such that the occurrence of arsenic in relation to depth and the age of groundwater is the opposite of that in the Bengal Basin. In the COA, fresh organic matter (the critical redox driver in the Bengal Basin) has either been destroyed or is of low reactivity. Shortly after deposition, silicate minerals were dissolved and carbonates and iron oxides precipitated, probably sequestering arsenic in the latter. During the Mesozoic era, the rocks were inundated with seawater, precipitating dolomite, barite, quartz and more iron oxides, and also leading to local accumulations of selenium, uranium and vanadium. Uplift and erosion during the Tertiary and Quaternary initiated flushing of saltwater from the aquifer, also dissolving silicates and dolomite, but precipitating Fe- and Mn-oxides and kaolinite (Breit, 1998). Flushing, however, remains incomplete, and the bottom of the flushed-freshwater zone forms the effective base of the aquifer (Smith, 2005).

Figure 3.8 shows a hydrogeological section through the COA near the city of Norman, which obtains about 20% of its water supply from 24 wells in the aquifer (Smith, 2005). The Garber Sandstone and Wellington Formation dip gently to the west beneath the Hennessey Group mudstones. Norman straddles the confined–unconfined boundary of the aquifer. Although domestic and agricultural wells are normally completed in the top 100 m, municipal wells are typically completed at depths of 180–250 m in both the confined and unconfined parts of the aquifer. The groundwater flow system has three main components: (a) shallow unconfined flow with residence times of tens to hundreds of years; (b) deep unconfined flow with residence times of up to 5,000 years; and (c) deep confined flow with residence times of tens of thousands of years (Christenson et al., 1998). The differences in residence time explain the advanced state of flushing and equilibration between the groundwater and the aquifer minerals in the unconfined aquifer, but disequilibrium and incomplete flushing in the confined aquifer (Schlottman et al., 1998).

Groundwater is oxic in both the confined and unconfined parts of the aquifer, and arsenic is present as As(V). In the unconfined aquifer, groundwater is a Ca–Mg–HCO$_3$ type, whereas in the confined aquifer it is a Na–HCO$_3$ type. Schlottman et al. (1998) attributed the increasing sodium content to cation exchange whereby Ca and Mg are exchanged for Na that was adsorbed onto clay minerals when the rocks were buried beneath the sea. In parallel with these changes, as water passes along deep, confined flow-paths, carbon dioxide, dissolved in the soil zone, is exhausted, driving up the pH to >8.5 and facilitating desorption of arsenic, chromium and selenium. Not only is the COA a convincing example of arsenic being mobilised by desorption from iron oxides at high pH, it also demonstrates how the long-term hydrogeological evolution of an aquifer has determined the distribution of As contamination. The Mesozoic history ensured not only that arsenic could not be mobilised by reductive dissolution because reactive organic matter was consumed, but also that the deeper parts of the aquifer were conducive to developing alkaline groundwater due to reactions with saline waters.

The COA stands in distinct contrast to modern alluvial basins in that high As concentrations are found in strata and groundwater that pre-date, and are deeper than, any natural or pumping-induced water level lowering. The practical consequence for Norman is that deep municipal wells are affected more than shallow private wells. Since 1990, the city authorities have stopped drilling wells in the confined aquifer, and concentrated on drilling in the deep unconfined aquifer to the east. Continued pumping from the deep confined aquifer would probably continue to mobilise arsenic, but it is hoped that by concentrating abstraction in the shallower and unconfined parts of the aquifer, As-polluted groundwater will remain relatively stationary, and not be drawn towards pumping wells in significant quantities. Schlottman et al. (1998) and Smith (2005) have also shown that individual sandstone layers have relatively predictable concentrations of arsenic and other toxic elements that allow for differential screening of aquifer horizons to improve the quality of water abstracted. Thus, in order to predict, and avoid, arsenic in individual wells, it is necessary to understand both the basinal scale hydrogeological regime and the small-scale lithological differences between strata.

3.7.3   The Malcantone Watershed, Switzerland

The study of the small, mountainous and forested Malcantone catchment in southern Switzerland is special because Pfeifer et al. (2004) identified almost all the major processes of As mobilisation and attenuation within a single watershed of just 200 km². The climate is sub-Mediterranean, with an average annual temperature of 10°C and rainfall of 2000 mm. Bedrock comprises granite and high-grade metamorphic rocks with sulphide mineralisation containing Fe, As, Sb and Au, all overlain by complex fluvio-glacial deposits. Streams contain 1–10 ppb As, and oxygenated groundwaters in the upper and middle catchment contain 10–90 ppb As, while reducing groundwater in alluvial aquifers in the lower catchment contains 40–300 ppb As and affect water supplies to the population of 5000. Figure 3.9 illustrates the succession of chemical processes that control the distribution of arsenic in the catchment. Arsenic is initially released by oxidation of sulphide minerals but regulated by adsorption on iron oxides, and to a much lesser extent by aluminium phases. Alkaline-oxic waters percolate through granular soils to discharge through As-rich springs, but lower in the catchment the soils are waterlogged and the underlying fluvio-glacial and deltaic sands are interbedded with organic-rich glacial-lake sediments. Here, the highest As-concentrations are encountered due to reductive dissolution of iron oxides. However, arsenic in this water is precipitated where it seeps into larger, regional rivers at the bottom of the catchment.

3.8   Implications of Long-term Pumping of Arsenic Contaminated Groundwater

3.8.1   General considerations

In most cases, large quantities of As-contaminated groundwater have been pumped for only a few decades, and in almost all cases, there are insufficient data to reconstruct historical changes in water quality, let alone predict future trends. In the following sections we consider whether the (bulk) As concentrations of aquifers will increase or decrease over time, how much more arsenic will be mobilised, whether it will migrate in the subsurface, or be added to the surface environment.

As groundwater is abstracted and replaced by fresh recharge, future concentrations will depend on whether this fresh recharge mobilises As from minerals in the aquifer. Where As is mobilised by reductive dissolution, the continued input of arsenic depends on the quantity of As adsorbed to the sands and the influx of dissolved organic carbon. Both are finite sources,

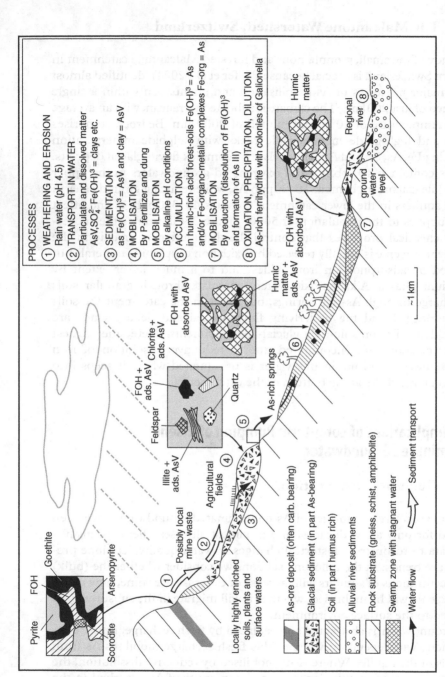

Figure 3.9 Hydrogeochemical processes in the Malcantone catchment, Switzerland. The figure demonstrates the diversity of geochemical mobilisation and immobilisation processes that can occur within a single watershed, from the oxidation of sulphide ore deposits in the upper catchment to the alluvial plain of the Tresa River. FOH, ferric oxyhydroxides; ads, adsorbed.

Source: Pfeifer et al. (2004)

PROCESSES

① WEATHERING AND EROSION
  Rain water (pH 4.5)

② TRANSPORT IN WATER
  Particulate and dissolved matter
  As,SO_4^{2-} $Fe(OH)^3$ = clays etc.

③ SEDIMENTATION
  as $Fe(OH)^3$ = AsV and clay = AsV

④ MOBILISATION
  By P-fertilizer and dung

⑤ MOBILISATION
  By alkaline pH conditions

⑥ ACCUMULATION
  in humic-rich acid forest-soils $Fe(OH)^3$ = As
  and/or Fe-organo-metalic complexes Fe-org = As

⑦ MOBILISATION
  By reduction (dissolution of $Fe(OH)^3$
  and formation of As III)

⑧ OXIDATION, PRECIPITATION, DILUTION
  As-rich ferrihydrite with colonies of Galionella

Humic matter

Regional river ⑧

ground water level

FOH with absorbed AsV

⑦

Humic matter + ads. AsV

As-rich springs

⑥

FOH + ads. AsV   Chlorite + ads. AsV

Feldspar

Quartz

⑤

Illite + ads. AsV

Agricultural fields

④

③

② Possibly local mine waste

① Pyrite   FOH   Goethite

Arsenopyrite   Scorodite

Locally highly enriched soils, plants and surface waters

~1 km

As-ore deposit (often carb. bearing)

Glacial sediment (in part As-bearing)

Soil (in part humus rich)

Alluvial river sediments

Rock substrate (gneiss, schist, amphibolite)

Swamp zone with stagnant water

Water flow   Sediment transport

but different outcomes will follow depending on which is in excess, and their spatial arrangement. For instance, where there is a peat layer within or immediately adjacent to the aquifer, concentrations are likely to be near their maximum at the start of pumping, and decline thereafter. However, where the peat layer is some metres above the aquifer, high concentrations of DOC may not reach the aquifer until after pumping starts, and hence there will be a delay before pollution reaches abstraction wells. Subsequently, concentrations will rise to a maximum before going into long-term decline. In these scenarios, although the position and length of well screens[13] will not change the overall outcome, they will modify the temporal response in individual wells. The greater the distance between the well screen and the peat layer, the greater the lag time before the peak As concentration.

Where arsenic is mobilised by alkali desorption, complex trends in As concentrations may be anticipated. As with the RD case, desorption will be limited by the quantity of adsorbed As on the sediment[14]. However, in practice the release of arsenic will depend on whether the recharge that replaces the pumped water continues to have high pH.

3.8.2   The Bengal Basin scenario

A simple model of groundwater irrigation

In the Bengal Basin (Chapter 8), As-polluted groundwater is largely confined to the upper 50 m of alluvial deposits. Although it is the main source of drinking water, about 90% of all groundwater pumped is used for irrigation, and mostly for growing rice. Below, we illustrate the issues associated with long-term abstraction using simple calculations for a hypothetical aquifer profile based on the JAM aquifer described earlier (section 3.7.1). Our hypothetical aquifer has a surface area of 1 m², and comprises 20 m of silt overlying 30 m of sand, with a water table 5 m below ground. The sand contains 3 mg/kg of arsenic, adsorbed to iron oxides, and has a porosity of 0.3. All solid organic matter is in the silt, but DOC has penetrated to the aquifer, which is perfectly mixed, with an initial concentration of 200 ppb As. A single crop of rice, irrigated with 1000 mm of groundwater, is grown over 65% of the area. The root zone (topsoil) extends to 150 mm and has an initial content of 10 mg/kg As. The soil and underlying sediment have a bulk density of 1800 kg m⁻³. The fields are bunded so there is no surface runoff, and the aquifer is fully recharged by rainfall every year. Water percolating through the surface aquitard acquires DOC, which mobilises arsenic when it enters the aquifer.

Consider the consequences of irrigating a rice crop every year into the indefinite future. There are no other sources of abstraction or lateral flows of water, so that all arsenic in irrigation water accumulates in the soil (i.e. without leaching or methylation[15], and with negligible crop uptake). In this scenario[16], the column of water in the aquifer is replaced every 14 years. If no more arsenic were mobilised from the aquifer, irrigation would raise the As content of the topsoil from 10 to 19 mg/kg. Unfortunately, it is almost certain that arsenic will continue to be mobilised[17]. If the supply of DOC were unlimited, high concentrations of arsenic in groundwater could be maintained for over 1000 years. After 50 years, arsenic in the soil would rise to around 40 mg/kg, and after 100 years to around 70 mg/kg As. Such soil-As concentrations raise grave concerns for both human exposure through food and for toxicity to crops (Chapter 4). In reality, groundwater concentrations are more likely to decline gradually, and hence soil-As would increase more slowly. The point of these calculations, however, is simply to provide a perspective on the size of the arsenic stores in the aquifer. The main implication is that, so long as there is a redox driver, the aquifer sediments could release arsenic to groundwater for many decades, and possibly centuries, to come, and irrigation with this water will continue to add arsenic to soils.

Changes at the basinal scale

Moving to a larger scale, we now consider the relationship of pumping groundwater from both As-contaminated and adjacent uncontaminated aquifers, which approximate the Holocene and Pleistocene strata. Figure 3.10 shows an idealised hydrogeological section through the lower Bengal Basin, and includes four hypothetical abstraction wells. The lower aquitard is absent inland, but thickens towards the coast where the deep aquifers tend to become increasingly confined. The mechanism and quantity of recharge to the deep aquifer are uncertain, but involve a combination of vertical leakage and lateral inflow from further inland. The figure also shows the main water quality hazards: arsenic throughout the shallow aquifer, and salinity in the coastal sections of both aquifers, and in the lower aquitard further inland. Each well in Figure 3.10 involves a particular risk scenario:

Well A   Pumping from the inland shallow aquifer is endangered by lateral migration of shallow arsenic, and if polluted, this will affect both drinking water and irrigation. This scenario is equivalent to the hypothetical aquifer profile described above.

Well B   Well B is similar, but also faces a salinity risk. To avoid pollution, abstractors will first deepen wells and later, switch to the deeper aquifer. The extracted water will also be partly replaced by lateral inflow from the coast, although this quantity will be small because the aquifer is not open to the sea.

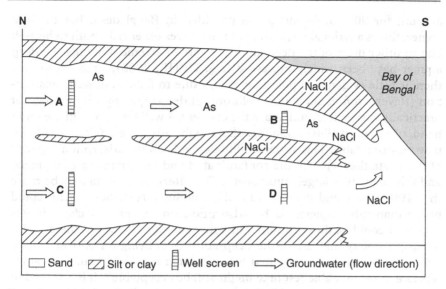

Figure 3.10   Schematic hydrogeological section through the lower Bengal Basin. Although not to scale, the vertical dimension is of the order of 300 m, and the horizontal dimension of the order of 100 km. Both the upper and middle aquitards become increasingly confining towards the coast. Salinity and organic matter also become increasingly common in the lower parts of the basin. The top of the middle aquitard often coincides with the Holocene–Pleistocene boundary.

Well C   Pumping will draw shallow arsenic into oxidised Pleistocene sands. These strata will attenuate arsenic, but there is a risk that wells pumping from the deep aquifer may eventually be polluted. Because well C is recharged mainly by lateral flow, increased pumping from deep wells further inland may reduce the through-flow of groundwater and induce either leakage from above or inflow of saline water from the coast.

Well D   Pumping at well D is similar in principle to that at well C. However, in practice, because chloride is not retarded, if pumping is not sustainable, the well will probably be salinised long before it is contaminated by arsenic. In scenarios B and D, the closer the well is to the coast, the greater will be the risk of salinisation.

Human responses to hydrological changes

As people become aware of the risks described above, they will change their water use, either by switching to surface water or, more likely, by drilling deeper wells, as is already happening. As noted in Chapter 6, deep wells account for 90% of As mitigation provided in Bangladesh. For the well owner, this is a rational response, but introduces other risks both to himself and to other users of the deep aquifer. Fears of arsenic polluting the deep aquifer have been widely expressed (e.g. DPHE, 2000), although to date there is little evidence of pollution except due to failures of well construction (Ravenscroft et al., 2005). Pollution of deep aquifers will be slow, but practically irreversible, and hence the concern is well founded. On the other hand, use of deep alluvial aquifers offers many advantages (Chapter 6) and may be sustainable. This sustainability depends on the adsorption capacity of the strata that separate the contaminated and uncontaminated aquifers, and this capacity is largely unknown[18]. The intervening strata may be more than 100 m thick, and so there is a real possibility that shallow arsenic could be permanently sequestered by adsorption on oxides and clays. If this occurs, it could be the optimum mitigation solution. However, there is also a real possibility that use of the deep aquifers is living on borrowed time before these sources are polluted too. Although exploitation of deep aquifers as a non-renewable resource might still be acceptable[19], it is essential to know how fast and with what concentrations arsenic is migrating downwards in order to have time to develop long-term alternatives such as treating deep groundwater[20] or long-distance surface water transfers. Presently, there is insufficient information to answer these questions, and only by instigating extensive investigations, and long-term monitoring of multilevel piezometers, can appropriate courses of action be identified.

3.9   Summary and Conclusions

Arsenic concentrations in rocks are extremely variable and a poor indicator of groundwater contamination. The availability of arsenic is more important than its total quantity. Classified by mobilisation mechanism, arsenic has some relation to climate. Reductive dissolution, the most important pollution mechanism, occurs preferentially in alluvial and fluvio-glacial sediments and under moist–temperate and warm–wet conditions, where organic matter production is high. Alkali desorption occurs in both alluvium and bedrock aquifers, and mainly in drier and, to a lesser extent, warmer climates. Both these mechanisms, and geothermal arsenic, are strongly concentrated within or immediately adjacent to young orogenic belts, especially in foreland basins. Only sulphide oxidation occurs preferentially in ancient bedrock aquifers.

Large areas where arsenic contamination is (apparently) absent have some common characteristics. The most important are the areas of weathered basement and associated alluvial deposits developed on the remnants of the ancient supercontinent Gondwanaland. The long weathering history and stable tectonic conditions in these areas have generally removed arsenic from the near-surface environment. The chemistry of the river sediments and water, which reflect this history, provide important clues for identifying areas where As contamination is more, and less, likely to be found, guided by parameters such as suspended load, quartz content of sand, and silica content of water.

Although there are few long-term monitoring data, As concentrations increase over time in a significant proportion of wells. Caveats can be expressed, but the implications are clear: in the absence of evidence to the contrary, safe wells cannot be assumed to remain safe; and monitoring must be integral to any mitigation plan. There is also a dearth of evidence documenting As migration in aquifers. There is an important need to develop validated numerical models of As transport in aquifers to evaluate, *inter alia*, risks to existing safe wells, and the flushing of aquifers. Potentially suitable models exist, but their application is severely inhibited by the shortage of calibration data. More tracer tests (e.g. Höhn et al., 2006) and sorption studies (e.g. Stollenwerk et al., 2007) should be conducted to understand the flushing of reducing aquifers, *in situ* arsenic removal, and migration of anoxic As(III)-rich waters into deeper aquifers. Such studies should be replicated in aquifers across South and Southeast Asia and elsewhere. Selected sites, where geochemical investigations have already been conducted, should be monitored for many years and the results integrated with calibrated models of groundwater flow. Such sites can become foci for developing national research capacity and testing mitigation technologies.

Case histories from India, the USA and Switzerland demonstrate the importance of groundwater flow in the mobilisation and movement of arsenic, and highlight the need for integrated studies of hydrogeology and geochemistry. Many of the examples described later (e.g. the Huhhot and Datong Basins in China, New England, Spain and Argentina) might well have clearer explanations if the hydrogeology of those areas was better understood.

From a regional perspective, large-scale transfers of arsenic should be expected. Where As-polluted groundwater is used for irrigation, arsenic will be transferred to the soil. Concentrations of a few hundred ppb will raise As concentrations in paddy soils by 1 mg/kg every 1–2 years. Even without further release from the aquifer minerals, arsenic will be added for decades to come. However, the magnitude of such changes is not being monitored. While current groundwater irrigation has the effect of transferring arsenic from shallow aquifers to soils, the use of deep wells[21] may have the opposite effect, drawing arsenic down toward deeper, uncontaminated aquifers. Such developments raise profound questions of sustainability that involve both threats and opportunities. Current irrigation practices are leading to the progressive degradation of agricultural soils, over decades to centuries.

Pumping groundwater from deeper aquifers, on the one hand, risks pollution of deep aquifers by shallow arsenic but, on the other hand, may contribute significantly to the clean-up of shallow aquifers and provide long-term, possibly permanent, sources of low-As water, and moreover contain low iron concentrations and have better microbiological status. Pumping from deep aquifers is increasing rapidly, but to know whether the outcome will be beneficial or harmful can be determined only by urgently implementing monitoring of multilevel piezometers supported, in the longer run, by modelling studies.

NOTES

1   A semi-quantitative judgement intended to express either the number of people and/or water sources affected.

2   Arsenic pollution in Mexico may be an important exception, but presently there are insufficient published accounts of the hydrogeology of the affected regions there to be certain (see Chapter 9).

3   Although there are some similarities with the Willamette Basin of Oregon, described in Chapter 9.

4   Areas of coniferous forests found throughout the high northern latitudes, also referred to as boreal forest.

5   Ferrallitic soils are rich in iron and aluminium. Fersiallitic soils are similar, but are the products of less intense weathering and retain some silicate minerals.

6   We refer here only to active river systems and not to ancient glacial channels such as the Mahomet Buried Valley Aquifer in Illinois (USA) as described in Chapter 9.

7   It was the stimulus of these relationships that led to our identifying information confirming As contamination in the alluvial aquifers of the Po Basin in Italy (Chapter 9).

8   The simple movement of the dissolved constituent (As) without considering the effects of diffusion or dispersion.

9   Measurement of flow directions and rates are described in standard texts such as Fetter (2001).

10 Carbonate minerals may also adsorb As (e.g. Román-Ross et al., 2006), although it is uncertain how important this is in practice

11 Theoretically, longitudinal dispersion could cause As to move faster than water, but this requires there is no retardation at all, which is extremely unlikely.

12 Sand colour has been advocated as a tool for safe well design by von Brömssen et al. (2006), as discussed in Chapter 6.

13 The well screen is the slotted pipe or filter through which water enters the well from the aquifer.

14 The availability of As can be estimated by sequential extraction techniques. The amount of As held by iron oxides is usually considered to be the oxalate-extractable arsenic content (Raiswell et al., 1994).

15 Methylation is the least well-defined of the attenuation processes, and could be important, especially at lower As loadings, and in low-lying irrigated fields that are more saturated and contain more organic matter.

16 Annual groundwater abstraction is 650 L, and adds 0.48 mg/kg As to the top-soil each year. The aquifer column comprises 9000 L of water, which contains 1.8 g of arsenic in the porewater in the aquifer, and a load on the sand of 162 g (i.e. a mass ratio of 90:1).

17 If not, As concentrations would now be declining significantly in large areas that have been intensely irrigated for 30 years or more, and there is no evidence to support this.

18 The study by Stollenwerk et al. (2007) is a model for the type of investigation needed.

19 If, for instance, they are expected to provide safe water for 30 years or longer.

20 Treating deep groundwater would be easier and cheaper than treating shallow groundwater.

21 Deep wells have been the dominant form of water-supply mitigation to date, and a possible future trend in irrigation.

Chapter Four

Soils and Agriculture

4.1 Introduction

Drinking contaminated water is not the only means by which people can ingest excessive amounts of arsenic. Food crops can absorb arsenic from soils, which in turn is ingested by people eating contaminated crops or foods prepared from them. Some soils contain large amounts of arsenic, either naturally or as a result of pollution from industrial, urban or agricultural sources. The most important source of agricultural contamination today, on which this chapter focuses, is groundwater irrigation. An important characteristic of irrigation is that the addition of arsenic is gradual and continuous. The cumulative effect is to threaten the sustainability of agriculture in affected areas (Heikens, 2006; Heikens et al., 2007).

Plants vary in their tolerance of soil-arsenic. Moreover, plant tolerance limits are different in waterlogged soils, such as where paddy rice is grown, from aerated soils used for dryland crops such as wheat and vegetables.[1] Thus there is no one level of arsenic in soil that is toxic to plants. Additionally, different plants – even different crop varieties (cultivars) – take up arsenic in different amounts. Therefore, the relationships between arsenic in irrigation water, soils and plants are complex, and they are not yet fully understood, particularly in the case of paddy soils. In this chapter we consider only the uptake of arsenic into crops. How this translates into human exposure through food is described in Chapter 5.

This chapter examines the information on soil-As contents; the factors that influence As mobilisation and leaching in soils; As availability and toxicity to plants; and various measures that might be used to mitigate problems of arsenic in irrigation water and soils. We describe experience of irrigation with As-contaminated groundwater in Bangladesh and West

Bengal, which should serve as a model for other tropical areas underlain by As-contaminated alluvial aquifers. The final section outlines research and development needs. To facilitate comparison of data and readability, As concentrations in water are presented in parts per billion (ppb), in soils as mg/kg, and in plant materials and food as μg/kg.

4.2   Arsenic in Soils

4.2.1   Definitions

This chapter deals entirely with cultivated soils. Such soils generally comprise three main layers or horizons (Brammer, 1996).

- *Topsoil:* the surface soil horizon that is disturbed by ploughing and other cultivation operations. In paddy soils, it comprises two subhorizons: the *cultivated (or plough) layer* in which soil is dispersed (puddled) by ploughing when wet; and the *ploughpan*, the underlying layer compacted by ploughing and trampling by work-animals and cultivators when soils are ploughed wet. Under small-farmer conditions, the cultivated layer is generally about 10 cm thick and the ploughpan about 5 cm thick.
- *Subsoil:* the layer below the topsoil where soil-forming processes have wholly, or almost wholly, destroyed alluvial stratification or rock structure. This horizon commonly extends to a depth of 50–100 cm, but it may be thinner or absent in young and eroded soils, and in soils over a contrasting sandy or hard rock substratum (see below).
- *Substratum:* the little-altered alluvial or rock layer below the soil.[2] This layer may or may not be similar in texture to the overlying soil. In shallow soils, it may occur directly below the topsoil.

In paddy soils, rice roots generally do not penetrate deeper than 20 cm. In aerated soils, roots of annual dryland crops – including rice grown as a dryland crop – penetrate to 30–50 cm or deeper.

4.2.2   Soil safety standards

Two kinds of soil safety standard are used, but they are not always clearly differentiated. One relates to the health hazard for people (especially children) eating soil directly, inhaling dust blown from contaminated soils, and eating soil that remains on the leaves or roots of vegetables. The other relates to levels of soil-As that interfere with satisfactory plant growth and crop yields. These standards are derived mainly from tests on mining, industrial and urban wastes, not on natural soils. In addition, standards are required for soil concentrations that lead to excessive uptake of arsenic into the edible parts of plants.

Health hazard to humans

In the UK, the Environment Agency's soil guideline value for residential and allotment sites is 20 mg/kg As of dry soil (DEFRA and EA, 2002a,b). Standards in Canada and The Netherlands range between 10 and 20 mg/kg (Duxbury and Zavala, 2005), while Germany allows 25 mg/kg for children's playgrounds (Norra et al., 2005). Naidu et al. (2006a) report a recent revision of Australian thresholds for the assessment of acceptable risks to 100 mg/kg for residential soils, 200 mg/kg for land used for recreational purposes, and 500 mg/kg for land used for industrial or commercial purposes. These national standards can be regarded only as guidelines because of the many factors that influence the bioavailability of soil-As and the exposure of people or animals to risks. They are appropriate for site screening, but should be supported by a site-specific risk assessment where there is doubt.

Plant toxicity

It is more difficult to establish a safe standard for soil-As in relation to plant growth. *Inter alia*, that is because of variations in As tolerance between plant species and cultivars, and the greater availability of arsenic to plants in waterlogged paddy soils than in aerated soils where dryland crops are grown, and on which most studies have been carried out (section 4.4). Warren et al. (2003) quote a UK guideline value of 50 mg/kg for soil in which fresh food produce is grown (MAFF, 1993). Ant et al. (1997) give a standard of 25 mg/kg in Ontario, Canada. Norra et al. (2005) cite international references ranging from 20 to 50 mg/kg, and Naidu et al. (2006a) quote a similar range of threshold values for Australia. These standards apparently apply to dryland soils. For wetland soils, Norra et al. (2005) cite a German guideline of 50 mg/kg As for reduced soils. However, major yield reductions have been observed in rice in Bangladesh below this concentration (Duxbury and Panaullah, 2007). Huang et al. (2006) refer to limits of 30 mg/kg in China for paddy soils with pH <6.5 and 25 mg/kg for soils with pH 6.5–7.5. All these levels apparently refer to total As, not to plant-available As. The latter is only a minor fraction of the total, so total arsenic data are an imperfect indicator of actual risk (section 4.2.3).

4.2.3   Arsenic levels in soils

Total arsenic

Arsenic concentrations in uncontaminated natural soils generally reflect the arsenic contents of the rocks or sediments from which they were derived (Chapter 3). High soil-As contents are particularly associated with carbonaceous shales, some volcanic materials and rocks containing mineral ores. McLaren et al. (2006) indicate that As-contents of uncontaminated soils worldwide range from 1 to 100 mg/kg, but state that they are mainly below 10 mg/kg and often below 5 mg/kg. These levels compare with 'safe' soil-As guidelines of 20–50 mg/kg generally established for plant production, as described above.

O'Neill (1995) states that silty and clayey soils generally contain more arsenic than sandy soils. Huang et al. (2006) found significant correlations between arsenic content and both clay and silt contents in a wide range of Chinese soils used for vegetables, but not in paddy soils. Mahimairaja et al. (2005) cite earlier studies reporting that 'calcareous soils can be expected to have higher levels of arsenic than noncalcareous soils.' The available evidence indicates that natural topsoils generally contain less arsenic than subsoils, except where irrigated with As-rich water (section 4.3.2). Arsenic concentrations found in irrigated soils in Bangladesh and India are described in section 4.3.2.

Plant-available arsenic

Plant roots can absorb only a very low fraction of the total soil-As. Huang et al. (2006) cite literature suggesting that the proportion ranges between 0.1 and 1.8%. The low availability reflects the strong As-adsorption capacity of clays and iron oxyhydroxides in aerated soils generally used for agriculture. However, flooding of soils reduces ferric iron to the ferrous state, which greatly increases As availability. The factors influencing As availability to plants are discussed in sections 4.2.4–4.2.6.

4.2.4   Soil diversity and complexity

Soil diversity

Even in a country as small as Bangladesh, there are considerable differences between the soils formed in different physiographic regions (Brammer, 1996), and these soils, irrigated with As-contaminated water, have widely varying availability of arsenic to plants. Within a physiographic region, considerable soil

Table 4.1   Soil properties within typical soil associations of four physiographic regions in Bangladesh*

Property	Ganges River Floodplain[†]	Jamuna River Floodplain[‡]	Old Meghna Estuarine Floodplain[§]	Ganges Tidal Floodplain[§]
Soil series (number)	9	7	6	5
Flooding depth (cm)	0–>90	0–>180	<90–>180	0–90
Topsoil clay (%)	11–73	18–59	12–44[¶]	23–68[¶]
Topsoil OM(%)	0.69–9.29	0.92–2.5	1.44–3.10	1.3–2.6
Topsoil pH	6.1–7.9	4.8–7.3	5.0–5.9	4.8–7.8
Topsoil $CaCO_3$ (%)	0–9.6	0	0	0–2.5

*Data relate to the example soil association only. They do not indicate the full range in properties within the physiographic region.
[†]Brammer (2000). [‡]Brammer (2004). [§]FAO (1988).
[¶]Taken from the soil survey reports indicated in FAO (1988).

and environmental differences can occur within an individual village, even within a shallow tubewell (STW) command area. Table 4.1 shows the range in soil properties that occur within four typical regions on Bangladesh's floodplains. Typically, topsoils on floodplain ridges contain less clay and organic matter (OM), have a higher pH, and are flooded less deeply and for a shorter period than soils in adjoining depressions. On the Ganges River Floodplain, topsoils on the ridges contain up to 10% lime, but those in adjoining depressions can be strongly acid, with lime found only at some depth in the subsoil. Soil patterns on river meander floodplains are generally more complex than those on estuarine and tidal floodplains.

Soil complexity

In addition to natural soil differences, human use of soils can create differences in properties between fields and within fields resulting from field levelling, cultivation practices, differences in amounts of fertilisers used, irregular fertiliser/manure distribution, incorporation of stubble and roots of previous crops, and burrowing activity of soil animals (Brammer, 2000).[3] Differences can occur at a microscale, too: e.g. differences in redox potential between decomposing plant remains and iron-plaque remnants in topsoils, and probably also between soil coatings, grey mottles and yellow/brown mottles in subsoils. Differences can also occur within a year: e.g. between the oxidised condition of topsoils in the dry season and their reduced condition when submerged by floodwater or irrigation water. On a longer timescale, it is probable that topsoil organic matter contents are gradually increasing with time in irrigated paddy soils that were formerly dry in the dry season. In areas irrigated with As-contaminated water, soil-As contents can vary considerably within STW command areas (section 4.3.2).

Seasonal flooding

There can be considerable regional, local and interannual differences in the depth and duration of seasonal flooding on floodplains, and therefore in the duration of periods when topsoils are oxidised and reduced. Contrary to a common misconception, most of Bangladesh's floodplains are flooded by ponded rainwater and local run-off; flooding by silty river water is confined to areas close to active river channels (Brammer, 2004). Therefore, most of the country's floodplain soils do not receive regular increments of new alluvium as some authors assume (e.g. Polizzotto et al., 2005). In fact, most young floodplain areas receive new alluvium only during exceptional floods, and some older areas have not received new alluvium for several centuries or possibly for thousands of years (Brammer, 2004).

Implications for soil investigations

Diverse and complex soil conditions affect the availability of arsenic to plant roots at regional, local and microscales. Availability also varies within and between years (section 4.4). These observations have important implications for planning arsenic investigations and interpreting results. Evidence of regional, local and temporal variations should be taken explicitly into account, not only in Bangladesh but wherever arsenic investigations are undertaken.

4.2.5   Arsenic transformations in the soil

Arsenic species

Arsenic occurs in different chemical 'species' in different soil environments. These differences affect arsenic mobility and availability to plants. The chemical processes relating to arsenic in soils are essentially the same as those described in Chapter 2. This section focuses on those aspects that influence the movement of arsenic in soils and its availability to plants. The two most common arsenic species in soils are the inorganic forms arsenate, As(V), and arsenite, As(III). Other species are the organic forms monomethylarsonic acid (MMA^V) and dimethylarsinic acid (DMA^V). At high doses, arsenite is much more toxic to humans than arsenate, which in turn is much more toxic than MMA^V or DMA^V (Chapter 5). Arsenobetaine (AsB) and arsenocholine (AsC) found in some animal and plant foods are considered to be of very low toxicity. Arsine gas that can be produced by methylation in soils is highly toxic if inhaled.

Factors influencing arsenic transformations

The solubility and plant availability of arsenic in soils are influenced by several factors, including pH, redox potential (Eh), clay content, clay type, organic matter and phosphorus contents, iron, aluminium and manganese oxide concentrations, and microbial activity (Chapter 2). As(V) is the main species found in aerated soils and is readily adsorbed by ferric iron. As(III) is mainly associated with reducing conditions where iron, in the ferrous form, binds arsenic less strongly. The two species are transformed in top-soils that alternate between oxidised and reduced states, such as in seasonally flooded soils and flood-irrigated rice paddies. Soil microbes – especially bacteria, which are particularly active under reducing conditions – help to transform As(V) to As(III). Bacteria and algae in reduced soils, and fungi and algae in aerated soils, also convert inorganic As to organic forms by methylation, leading to loss of arsenic to the atmosphere by volatilisation (section 4.2.9). The transformation from As(V) to As(III) is not instantaneous, so both species may coexist in topsoils that become flooded as conditions change from oxidised to reduced (O'Neill, 1995), and presumably vice versa when submergence ends; see also section 4.2.6.

Distribution of species within the soil

As(III) and As(V) can occur in different horizons of the same soil. In seasonally flooded soils in Brahmanbaria, Bangladesh, Breit et al. (2005) found that arsenic was present in the subsoil as As(V), associated with ferric oxides, and as As(III) in the underlying saturated substratum. This is consistent with observations that seasonally flooded soils have a grey mottled yellow or brown subsoil in which air is entrapped in soil voids during the period of submergence, and that the substratum is uniformly grey and permanently saturated below about 1–2 m (Brammer, 1996). However, grey or dark grey coatings (gleyans) on the faces of structural units and pores in the subsoil may also be reduced during the period of submergence, and the grey or dark grey topsoil in such soils is reduced during the period when it is submerged. The surface 1 mm of submerged soils also fluctuates between oxidised and reduced conditions with alternations between aerated and stagnant conditions in the overlying water; and bacteria and algae living and decomposing in and on this surface soil 'skin' cause further arsenic transformations, including changes to organic forms through which arsenic may be lost by volatilisation (section 4.2.9). The nature and scale of these changes in irrigated paddy soils deserve study, and their influence on As uptake by plants and on toxicity needs to be assessed.

4.2.6   Iron plaque formation

Rice and other wetland plants growing in reduced soils 'pump' oxygen from the air and discharge it through their roots, forming ferric iron coatings (plaque) around the roots. Liu et al. (2006a) found that the amount of plaque deposited varied considerably between six rice varieties (range 55–168 g/kg) and was composed of 81–100% ferrihydrite and up to 19% goethite. By adsorbing arsenic, the iron plaque acts as a filter. In pot experiments in China with a phosphate-deficient soil, Hu et al. (2005) grew three rice varieties under saturated conditions, with and without phosphate (P) application. They found that the iron plaque was strongest in the untreated soil and that adding phosphate greatly decreased plaque formation. In pot experiments with a soil–sand mixture, Hu et al. (2006) found that adding sulphur (S) increased iron plaque formation. The effects of phosphate and sulphur addition on As uptake are discussed further in section 4.4.6. Iron plaque formation ceases when plants stop growing, and plaque remnants form yellow or brown mottles in topsoils until the iron is gradually reduced during the next period of submergence.

The fact that rice plants contain arsenic indicates that the As-filtering mechanism of an iron plaque is not wholly effective. The effect of iron plaque on the uptake of arsenite and arsenate by rice roots is discussed in section 4.4.4. Observations in Bangladesh that rice growing in permanently-wet-depression soils with high organic matter contents has white roots suggests that an iron plaque may not form in strongly reducing soils. Iron toxicity in rice was observed in such sites, but it is not known whether As toxicity also occurs. These observations suggest that there might be significant differences in iron plaque formation and its As-filtering effect in different soils within floodplain toposequences and STW command areas.

Experience with arsenic removal in water treatment (Chapter 7) shows that efficiency of As removal is strongly dependent on the Fe:As ratio of the water. Thus the effectiveness of iron plaque in filtering arsenic may also depend on the Fe:As ratio of the soil water. Since the Fe:As ratios of shallow groundwater in Bangladesh vary by several orders of magnitude, it seems probable that the As-adsorption capacity of iron plaques will also vary considerably within and between command areas. These effects require further study.

4.2.7   Interaction of phosphorus and arsenic

Arsenic in phosphatic fertilisers

Rock phosphate fertiliser may contain 8 to 18 mg/kg As depending on the source (EFMA, 1999; O'Neill, 1995). Applied at 150 kg/ha (*c.* 50–60 kg/ha of P_2O_5), rock phosphate containing 10 mg/kg As would add 1.5 kg of arsenic per hectare, equivalent to 0.015 mg/kg mixed in 10 cm of topsoil. That amount would generally be considered negligible, even where added twice a year. However, it could be of greater significance where it adds to the amounts of arsenic being applied from irrigation water, and if the added phosphate also displaces arsenic from the soil as discussed below. Manufactured fertilisers such as triple superphosphate do not contain arsenic.

Competition between phosphorus and arsenic

Phosphate and arsenate, As(V), are chemically similar and compete for anion exchange sites in soil (section 2.3). Therefore, soils with a high phosphate content may have fewer sites for As adsorption. Competition between phosphate and arsenate may be particularly acute in sandy topsoils with a low organic matter content that have few available exchange sites. In principle, addition of phosphate might displace arsenic from the soil exchange complex into the soil solution and make it available for plant uptake. This is less likely to apply, however, in reduced soils where arsenic is in the arsenite form, As(III), but interactions in soils that are alternately reduced and aerated need to be studied.

Smith, Naidu et al. (2002) described how phosphate affects adsorption of both As(V) and As(III) in four Australian soils. Phosphate displaced more arsenic from two Alfisols (Lixisols) containing low-activity clays than from either a Vertisol with high-activity clays or an Oxisol (Ferralsol) with finely divided ferric iron.[4] In the Oxisol, phosphate displaced As(III) more effectively than As(V). The results demonstrate the strong binding capacity of iron oxides and high-activity clays. In pot experiments with rice grown under saturated conditions in samples from a highly weathered red soil from Hubei Province in China, Hu et al. (2005) found that phosphate fertilisation did not significantly affect the As concentration in rice shoots harvested after 4 weeks. In pot trials in Bangladesh, Talukder (2005) reported that adding phosphate decreased As toxicity in rice grown under reduced soil conditions, but Jahiruddin et al. (2005) reported that phosphate aggravated the adverse impact of arsenic (added at a rate of 20 mg/kg) on Indian spinach although not on red amaranth (both presumably grown in aerated soil). The role of phosphate in the differential uptake of arsenite and arsenate by rice roots in the presence and absence of an iron plaque is discussed in section 4.4.4.

4.2.8   Leaching of arsenic

Vertical leaching

There is little evidence that arsenic added to soils in irrigation water or As-rich wastes is leached to the subsoil or groundwater in significant

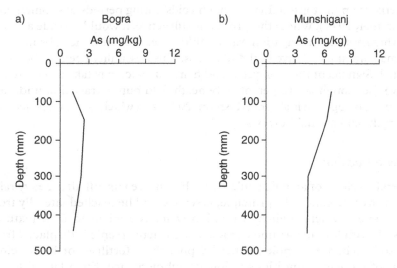

Figure 4.1   Variation of arsenic with depth beneath two irrigated paddy soils in Bangladesh. (a) Shallow tubewell (STW) command area at Bogra in northwest Bangladesh irrigated with groundwater from a STW containing <1 ppb As. (b) Shallow tubewell command area at Munshiganj in south-central Bangladesh irrigated with groundwater from a STW containing 320 ppb As. Both profiles were sampled during the dry season. *Source*: Saha and Ali (2006)

amounts. Permeable soils on which dryland crops are grown are aerated and oxidised, so that arsenic is quickly immobilised by ferric iron. In impermeable soils, arsenic might only reach lower layers where water or topsoil material is carried through soil voids such as animal holes or cracks that are open at the time of heavy rainfall, irrigation or flooding. The risk of leaching is higher in those acid-sulphate soils in which extreme acidity occurs in the topsoil. Figure 4.1 illustrates the distribution of arsenic with depth in paddy soils irrigated by two STWs in Bangladesh, one with low-As water (Bogra, <1 ppb As) and one with high-As water (Munshiganj, 320 ppb As). Differences between the arsenic levels in subsoils from the two locations reflect differences in mineralogical characteristics between Pleistocene (Bogra) and Holocene (Munshiganj) sediments.

In Bangladesh, paddy soils have a strong ploughpan at the base of the cultivated layer which reduces percolation losses in soils that would otherwise be permeable (Brammer, 1996). Also, subsoils below the ploughpan are partially oxidised (except in perennially wet depressions), which would quickly immobilise any arsenic leached from the topsoil. However, the prominent grey or dark grey coatings in the subsoil suggest that reduced soil material from the topsoil flows through voids during periods of submergence (Brammer, 1971). Where this process is still active, it would provide a means by which arsenic in irrigation water could be leached into the subsoil, albeit in small amounts relative to the soil mass. This possibility needs to be investigated. Significant flows of water, and hence arsenic, may take place laterally above the ploughpan to percolate beneath field bunds (raised boundaries) where the ploughpan is absent (Rushton, 2003) and which are often penetrated by cracks and animal burrows.

Lateral leaching

Lateral leaching of arsenic could occur by surface run-off after heavy rainfall or over-irrigation. In principle, arsenic could be leached laterally from topsoils: e.g. where high-As irrigation water is applied to light-textured topsoils with low adsorption capacity, and where arsenic is displaced from the soil exchange complex either by phosphate fertiliser or by development of reducing conditions following submergence. Such lateral leaching could increase arsenic levels in soils and water bodies on lower sites. However, lateral leaching seems unlikely to occur on a significant scale because of immobilisation by coprecipitation with ferric iron in aerated flowing water; field studies are needed to confirm this. Mazid Miah et al. (2005) reported that ponds, rivers and canals in a contaminated part of northwest Bangladesh contained between 2 and 63 ppb As, and suggested that high levels were caused by losses from irrigation systems. On the other hand, Sanyal and Nasar (2002) reported that surface-water bodies are largely free of arsenic in parts of West Bengal where irrigation water is contaminated, and O'Neill (1995) observed that the As content of a poorly-drained Gleysol was similar to a better drained Grey Luvisol occurring upslope. These studies need to be supplemented by surveys that take account of the range of climate, topography, soil and As concentrations in irrigation water.

4.2.9   Loss of arsenic by volatilisation

Losses from aerated soils

The ready adsorption of arsenic on ferric compounds in aerated mineral soils might suggest that loss of arsenic by volatilisation in such soils will be low. However, Bolan et al. (2006) state that fungi and algae play an important role in loss of arsenic to the atmosphere by volatilisation in aerated soil environments, and O'Neill (1995) reported arsine being given off by lawns and moist soils. In a 7-year study in the USA, Woolson and Isensee (1981) measured the effect of three arsenical agrochemicals applied at three rates to a bare soil before planting soyabean and radish. They reported annual As losses of 14–15%, most of which they attributed to volatilisation. They also found interannual variations, which they attributed to differences in weather. These findings indicate the need for studies to determine the scale of As losses by volatilisation in soils irrigated with As-contaminated groundwater, both from soils growing irrigated dryland crops and from paddy soils during periods of the year when they are not flooded.

Losses from reduced soils

Kabata-Pendias (2001, cited by Norra et al., 2005), stated that microbial methylation of arsenic in reducing soils releases arsine gas. In principle, under weather conditions where there is little air movement, arsine gas released to the atmosphere by methylation from paddy fields and swamps could accumulate to toxic levels, especially in depressions. However, the lack of reports of adverse impacts suggests that the risks are low, which may be explained by the rapid oxidation of arsine in strong sunshine (McLaren et al., 2006). O'Neill (1995) concluded that 'the universality of microbial methylation reactions and the degree to which arsenic compounds are mobilised by conversion to gas-phase or solution phase still require to be determined.'

The magnitude of methylation losses in paddy soils is particularly uncertain. Reed and Sturgis (1936), in trials with rice grown under flooded conditions on soils treated with calcium arsenate pesticide, reported considerable loss of total As that was not accounted for by crop uptake and which they attributed to loss by volatilisation under strongly reducing soil conditions. Algal species, which are important in nitrogen fixation in Bangladesh's paddy fields (Catling, 1993), may be important in As methylation. In pot experiments in Bangladesh, Shamsudhoha et al. (2006) showed that a green alga (*Pithospora sp*) could assimilate up to 1400 mg/kg As from a nutrient solution to which arsenic had been added. They also showed that, after mixing the algae in soil, a test plant (*Ipomea aquatica*) could assimilate arsenic in direct proportion to the amount of arsenic applied. However, it is extremely difficult to relate laboratory studies to field conditions. Therefore, quantitative studies are needed of algal assimilation and methylation of arsenic in irrigated paddy fields. Subsequent studies could then investigate whether changes in irrigation or cultivation practices could significantly increase As losses by volatilisation without at the same time reducing crop yields. Such studies should take into account the many environmental variables in paddy fields noted earlier as well as the amount of light reaching water and soils at different crop growth stages.

4.3 Irrigation with Arsenic-contaminated Water

4.3.1 Groundwater irrigation in Bangladesh and West Bengal

This section focuses on experience with groundwater irrigation in Bangladesh and West Bengal where the most serious problems of As contamination of soils and crops have been identified, and where most research into the impacts and possible remedies have been carried out. About 85–90% of the groundwater pumped in Bangladesh and West Bengal is used for irrigation, and mainly for rice (Ravenscroft, 2003). About 85% of the area irrigated in Bangladesh is under *boro* paddy, the rice crop grown during the dry season.[5] Due to the growth of tubewell irrigation since the 1960s, some 2.5 M ha were irrigated with groundwater by 2005 (Jahiruddin et al., 2005), and *boro* rice now accounts for more than half of Bangladesh's national rice production. Fortunately, a large part of the *boro* crop is grown either in the northern areas where As contamination is least, or where it is irrigated with surface water, but Ross et al. (2006) estimated that 7% of the *boro* crop is grown with water containing >100 ppb As. Large differences in the amounts of arsenic added to soils result from variations in groundwater As-concentrations and irrigation water requirements. In Bangladesh, the irrigation requirement for *boro* rice typically ranges between about 400 mm and 1500 mm (BADC, 1992), while Norra et al. (2005) quote figures of 1144–1775 mm for rice and 238–400 mm for wheat in West Bengal.

Figure 4.2 is an attempt to show the distribution of risk resulting from using As-contaminated groundwater for irrigation in Bangladesh. The maps combine upazila-level information on gross groundwater abstraction and the proportion of wells that exceed 50 ppb As. It should be emphasised that this map is only a general indication of risk, and a number of important caveats should be applied. First, upazila-average data provide relatively coarse resolution; second, the boundaries between the risk classes are arbitrary; and third, the arsenic statistics are mostly from domestic wells (although they mainly tap the same aquifer as irrigation wells). Nevertheless, Figure 4.2 indicates where, other things being equal, arsenic accumulation in soils is likely to be greatest. The intensities of irrigation pumping and arsenic contamination are almost mirror images of each other. Abstraction is greatest in the northwest and centre of the country, and arsenic levels greatest in the south and east. Thus high intensities of groundwater irrigation and arsenic mainly coincide across the centre of the country. Only 15 upazilas fall into the very high risk category, while 360 (78%) are assigned to the low risk class. However, local

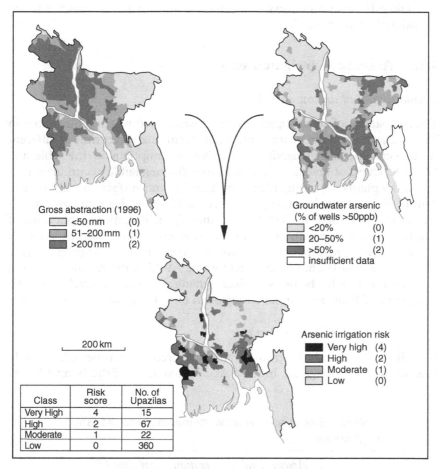

Gross abstraction (1996)
- <50 mm (0)
- 51–200 mm (1)
- >200 mm (2)

Groundwater arsenic (% of wells >50ppb)
- <20% (0)
- 20–50% (1)
- >50% (2)
- insufficient data

200 km

Arsenic irrigation risk
- Very high (4)
- High (2)
- Moderate (1)
- Low (0)

Class	Risk score	No. of Upazilas
Very High	4	15
High	2	67
Moderate	1	22
Low	0	360

Figure 4.2 Distribution of the arsenic hazard from groundwater irrigation in Bangladesh. The proportions of wells containing >50 ppb As were calculated on an upazila basis from 12,500 new and existing laboratory analyses reported by DPHE/MMI/BGS (1999) and DPHE/BGS (2001). Gross abstraction was calculated from the DAE 1996 Minor Irrigation Inventory and water usage data from UNICEF/DPHE (1994). Rice water requirements and deep percolation used upazila-specific estimates, but non-rice crops were assigned a standard water requirement of 200 mm. Arsenic contamination statistics are compiled from 12,000 project and pre-existing laboratory analyses, applying a minimum requirement of five analyses per upazila. Each map was classified with low, medium and high ratings (scored 0, 1 and 2) and then multiplied to produce an irrigation risk factor. This map does not represent the risk at individual wells, only the proportion of wells that are likely to be affected.

variability is such that very few upazilas in the latter group can be considered entirely 'safe'.

4.3.2   Arsenic in irrigated soils

Accumulation of arsenic in soils

The As loading of soils irrigated with contaminated water is illustrated in Table 4.2, which shows how arsenic might accumulate over time at different As concentrations in irrigation water. Key assumptions in the table are: (a) no leaching of arsenic to groundwater; (b) negligible accumulation of arsenic by plants; (c) negligible methylation; (d) no surface run-off; (e) soil density of 1500 kg m³, porosity of 0.3 and a 10-cm active root zone, which are widely applicable in Bangladesh; and (f) an irrigation application of 1000 mm. Irrigation with 1000 mm of water containing 100 ppb As adds 1 kg of arsenic per hectare per annum, an increment of 0.56 mg/kg per year when mixed into 10 cm of cultivated topsoil. At this concentration, it could take several decades before significant changes in soil-As levels could be differentiated from an original background of 5–10 mg/kg As.

Arsenic losses in irrigation channels

Not all of the arsenic in groundwater delivered from tubewells actually reaches the fields irrigated. In most As-affected areas of the Bengal Basin,

Table 4.2   Effect of concentration and time on arsenic loading of soils from irrigation water

Years of irrigation	Arsenic load in irrigation water (ppb)		
	100	250	500
	Arsenic addition to soil (mg/kg)		
1	0.56	1.39	2.78
5	2.78	6.94	13.9
10	5.56	13.9	27.8
20	11.1	27.8	55.6
50	27.8	69.4	138.9

The cells have been shaded according to the following tentative interpretative guide: <5 mg/kg – below background;
5–15 mg/kg – loading is indistinguishable from background;
15–50 mg/kg – marginal probability of distinguishing from background;
and >50 mg/kg – probably distinguishable from background.

groundwater is rich in iron which is oxidised and precipitated as hydroxides on exposure to the air, and then adsorbs arsenic. Hossain (2005) reported As concentrations in irrigation water at one Bangladeshi tubewell site decreasing from 136 ppb at the well-head to 68 ppb at the end of the 100-m distribution channel, with most of the loss in the first 30 m. At another site in Bangladesh, Roberts et al. (2007) showed a decrease from 397 to 314 ppb in a 152-m-long channel. For these reasons, the As concentration in water measured on delivery from a tubewell is not a reliable indicator of the amounts of arsenic actually added to soils in different parts of the command area.

Arsenic loading of paddy soils

Most of the arsenic added to paddy soils from irrigation water remains in the topsoil, and the amounts leached to the subsoil or groundwater appear to be small (section 4.2.8). In a survey of 270 STWs distributed more or less evenly across Bangladesh, Mazid Miah et al. (2005) found topsoil concentrations ranging between 0.2 and 67.5 mg/kg As, although the majority contained <20 mg/kg As. Mean concentrations in the topsoil (0–15 cm) were generally higher than in subsurface layers (15–30 and 30–60 cm), and significantly higher in irrigated soils than in non-irrigated soils. Norra et al. (2005) reported similar trends in a paddy soil in West Bengal, with arsenic levels decreasing more-or-less regularly from 38 mg/kg at the surface to 11 mg/kg at 1 m. In an adjacent wheat field, arsenic decreased from 17.5 mg/kg at the surface to 11.9 mg/kg at 10–15 cm, but levels varied irregularly between 10.6 and 16.4 mg/kg in deeper layers. The authors attributed the differences between the paddy and wheat topsoils to more intensive irrigation of the paddy field, despite the higher As concentration in the irrigation water used on the wheat field (782 vs 519 ppb). They attributed higher As levels in the lower layers of the wheat soil to seepage from an irrigation channel only 8 m from the sampled site.

At the Bangladeshi STW sites referred to above, Hossain (2005) reported a range in topsoil-As levels between 61 mg/kg in a field near the well-head and 11 mg/kg in an outer field. Dittmar et al. (2007) at their site showed a decrease in topsoil-As levels from 33 mg/kg at a field inlet to 11 mg/kg at the far end of the field. Duxbury and Zavala (2005) reported that total As in the uppermost 15 cm of soils was >10 mg/kg at 48% of 456 STW sites studied in Bangladesh, and Huq et al. (2003) reported that 21% of samples from a 24-upazila study had >20 mg/kg As. Huq et al. (2003) reported a high level of 81 mg/kg As in a topsoil at one site in Bangladesh that had been irrigated for more than 10 years.

In West Bengal, Norra et al. (2005) calculated an annual addition of 1.1 mg/kg As to a paddy topsoil irrigated with water containing 519 ppb, and noted that water standing in the field overnight had decreased to 16 ppb As. Roychowdhury et al. (2005) reported arsenic deposition ranging from 2 to 9.81 kg/ha in 1 year at four STW sites in Murshidabad District where applied water contained 19–120 ppb As (at the well-head), equivalent to 0.02–1.2 mg/kg mixed in 10 cm of topsoil. In neither example from West Bengal could the As loading of soils be related directly to the As content of the water actually reaching the fields, and the loading rates in the two studies appear inconsistent. More measurements are needed of the number of years that irrigation has been practised at individual STW sites, As levels in water actually delivered to individual fields and soil-As levels within fields in different parts of command areas. In the latter respect, soil samples from known localities stored by national soil survey organisations might provide information on soil-As levels before tubewell irrigation began.

Arsenic loading of dryland soils

Irrigated dryland crops generally receive only about 20–25% of the amount of water applied to rice, so As accumulation in affected soils is correspondingly slower. Norra et al. (2005) calculated that groundwater containing 782 ppb As added 0.45 mg/kg As in 1 year to the uppermost layer of a wheat soil studied. The topsoil of the field studied contained 18 mg/kg As, and the authors calculated that the site had been irrigated for 23–28 years. In Bangladesh, dryland crops are mainly irrigated in the northwest of the country where As concentrations in groundwater are generally low. Nonetheless, soils irrigated with water containing less than the 50 ppb drinking water standard will still accumulate arsenic over time, which may affect following monsoon-season rice crops. These factors should be kept in mind when planning monitoring and mitigation programmes.

4.4   Arsenic Uptake by Plants

4.4.1   Relevant analytical methods

Arsenic is normally determined on dried soil samples. This is satisfactory for aerated soils in which dryland crops are grown, but the availability of arsenic to plants differs under reduced soil conditions, and the puddled topsoil of paddy soils is essentially a soil-water suspension. Therefore, methods are needed to directly determine available As in paddy topsoils, or wet soil samples should be preserved prior to laboratory analysis to determine how much arsenic is actually available to rice roots. The results need to be correlated with As contents of rice grown on the sampled sites. Correlation with rice yields would also be useful.

4.4.2   Fluctuating soil-arsenic concentrations

The content, bioavailability and phytotoxicity of arsenic in paddy soils is further complicated by variations during the rice-growing period. Irrigation water is typically added every 3–7 days to maintain about 5–10 cm of standing water in the field up to the time of crop heading. The As concentration in the soil solution may vary from day to day as water in fields stagnates or is aerated by wind or rain-drops, is evaporated, absorbed by soil and plants, and replenished by irrigation or rainfall. These fluctuations between aerobic and anaerobic conditions may be accompanied by transformations in the As species which also influence plant uptake. Similar fluctuations may occur in response to diurnal variations in respiration rate of algae living in the water and on the soil surface. Studies are needed to quantify these fluctuations, which should also be considered in soil sampling and assessing phytotoxicity.

4.4.3   Occurrence in plants

Differences between plants

Plants vary considerably in their tolerance of arsenic and in the amounts of arsenic that they can take up from soils and water. O'Neill (1995) provides an example of grasses containing up to 3460 mg/kg As dry weight on spoil material from old arsenic mines in southwest England which contained up to 26,530 mg/kg As, whereas similar grasses contained a maximum of 3 mg/kg when growing in natural soils containing 20 mg/kg As (Mahimairaja et al., 2005). Ma et al. (2001) reported a hyperaccumulating fern, *Pteris vittata* (brake fern), growing on a contaminated site in Florida, USA, that contained 3280–4980 mg/kg As in the fronds (dry weight). Pot studies showed that this fern accumulates arsenic rapidly and has potential for reclaiming contaminated soils (section 4.5.5). Sheppard (1992), citing earlier work, noted that some plants can rapidly evolve tolerance to As, and that this process is influenced by mycorrhizal fungi.

Differences between plant parts

Many studies have shown a general pattern of arsenic accumulation in different parts of plants where root > stem > leaf > grain. For example, in Bangladesh, Das et al. (2004) reported rice containing 2400 μg/kg As in roots, 730 μg/kg in stems and leaves, and 140 μg/kg in grain. Likewise potato and other root crops accumulate more arsenic in the skins than in the flesh (see Table 4.5). The preparation and cooking of food plants can result in major changes to the amount of arsenic that is actually eaten by humans

(Chapter 5). If discarded plant parts or cooking water rich in arsenic are fed to livestock, this may be harmful both to them and to people consuming meat, milk or eggs produced by them (section 4.4.8).

4.4.4 Occurrence in food crops

Although O'Neill (1995) stated that the As content of edible plants is generally low and often close to the limits of detection, recent studies in Bangladesh and West Bengal have reported significant As concentrations in a large number of crops, as well as differences between individual crops from different areas. The latter observation implies that use of averaged data could lead to misleading interpretations. It also implies that soil and plant samples should be taken from the same site if meaningful correlations are to be made. The As contents of different crops also need to be interpreted in relation to the quantities that are eaten. This is because, despite the high As content of some vegetable and tuber crops, their contribution to the total daily intake of arsenic in many Asian countries is much less than that of rice (e.g. Williams et al., 2006; see also Chapter 5).

Arsenic in rice

In a study of 330 uncooked rice samples from markets across Bangladesh, Williams et al. (2006) found considerable variations in As contents both between and within districts (Table 4.3). Their sample included As-affected as well as unaffected areas. They sampled dry-season *boro* rice which is normally irrigated, and late-monsoon *aman* rice which receives little, if any, irrigation. These crops are widely, but not everywhere, grown in rotation; thus arsenic added to soils in irrigating *boro* is potentially accessible to a subsequent *aman* rice crop grown in the same field. Both *boro* and *aman* samples probably included several varieties. The variables indicated above could account for the wide range of As contents of both *aman* and *boro* rice in Table 4.3. For both *aman* and *boro* rice, the range within some districts is almost as great as the national range. Some international data on the total As content of rice grain are summarised in Table 4.4.

Arsenic in dryland crops

Williams et al. (2006) analysed 114 samples of 37 commonly grown vegetables, pulses and spices from farmers' fields in eight districts of Bangladesh. Very few of these crops are normally irrigated. Total As contents were highest in radish leaves (790 µg/kg), arum stolons (740 µg/kg), spinach (620 µg/kg) and cucumber (620 µg/kg). The lowest As concentrations (<200 µg/kg) were

Table 4.3 Arsenic contents of *aman* and *boro* rice in Bangladesh

Region	District	Aman			Boro		
		Range (μg/kg)	Mean (μg/kg)	Number of samples	Range (μg/kg)	Mean (μg/kg)	Number of samples
Northwest	Bogra	100–220	140	5	130–170	150	2
	Dinajpur	60–110	8	5	130–170	150	3
	Rangpur	NA	NA	0	140–240	190	5
	Thakurgaon	110	110	2	NA	NA	0
	Naogaon	NA	NA	0	120–170	140	4
	Natore	80–180	120	6	110–200	170	5
	Rajshahi	90–230	160	4	140–150	140	2
North-central	Jamalpur	110–140	130	2	NA	NA	0
	Mymensingh	40–180	110	15	210–360	170	4
	Sherpur	70–130	120	8	130–230	170	2
	Tangail	NA	NA	0	180–330	250	2
Central	Dhaka	90–150	110	3	120–230	180	3
	Gazipur	NA	NA	0	180–330	240	7
South-central	Barisal	100–320	160	14	170–440	250	4
	Faridpur	NA	NA	0	440–580	510	2
Southeast	Brahmanbaria	150–310	220	3	210–310	260	3
	Chandpur	130–400	220	13	40–910	280	8
Southwest	Chuadanga	100–480	240	6	150–180	320	27
	Jessore	60–250	130	12	NA	NA	0
	Khulna	<40–320	120	24	140–200	170	2
	Kushtia	70–280	190	15	120–230	180	8
	Magura	130–290	210	5	210–310	180	2
	Meherpur	60–420	180	16	150–840	290	18
	Satkhira	80–920	360	23	190–620	380	14

NA, not available.
Source: Williams et al. (2006)

found in all pulses and most fruits, vegetables and spices. Das et al. (2004) found great variability in eight vegetables from three As-affected districts of Bangladesh: nine samples of arum leaves contained 90–3990 μg/kg, and five samples of potatoes contained 70–1390 μg/kg As. Roychowdhury et al. (2002) analysed 30 crops and food items from three villages in Murshidabad (West Bengal), which are compared with market-basket data from Bangladesh in Table 4.5.

Table 4.4 International comparison of arsenic in uncooked rice grain

Country	Number of samples	Mean (µg/kg)	Range (µg/kg)	Reference
Bangladesh		340	<80–1010	Islam et al. (2005)
Bangladesh	300	190	<40–920	Williams et al. (2005, 2006)
China (Beijing)	32	120	70–190	Williams et al. (2005, 2006)
India	16	37		Duxbury and Zavala (2005)
India (*basmati*)	34	239	43–443	Roychowdhury et al. (2002)
Italy	10	50	30–70	Williams et al. (2005, 2006)
Japan	7	158		Duxbury and Zavala (2005)
Philippines	–	40		Watanabe et al. (2004)
Spain	22	70	0–250	Williams et al. (2005, 2006)
Taiwan	12		290–410	Laparra et al. (2005)
Thailand	10	135		Schoof et al. (1998)
Thailand	9	93		Duxbury and Zavala (2005)
USA	15	100	60–140	Williams et al. (2005, 2006)
USA	22	181		Duxbury and Zavala (2005)
Venezuela	4	303	196–462	Schoof et al. (1998)
	12	84		Duxbury and Zavala (2005)

Table 4.5 Arsenic concentrations of selected crop and food items in West Bengal (Roychowdhury et al., 2002) and Bangladesh

Crop/Food	As-content (µg/kg)			
	West Bengal		Bangladesh	
	Mean	Range	Mean	Range
Rice, raw	226	43–443	NA	18–310
Rice, cooked	374	290–490	NA	NA
Potato, flesh	5.47	<0.04–29	380	50–890
Potato, skin	293	59–690	NA	NA
Spinach	55	<0.04–120	620	620
Green papaya	196	156–237	400	110–690
Onion	1.28	<0.04–5	60	<40–150
Lentil	3.90	<0.04–16	40	<40–90
Coriander	335	290–379	490	100–980

NA, not available.
Source: Williams et al. (2006)

Correlation between soil and crop arsenic

In only one of the three studies cited above could the food samples be linked to the soils on which the crops were grown. Here, Roychowdhury et al. (2005) reported good correlations between As-contents of irrigation water, soils and plants at four STW's in Murshidabad District. On the other hand, at ten agricultural sites in central India, where samples of rice (144–432 µg/kg As) and soil (8.8–252 mg/kg As) were taken from the same fields, Patel et al. (2005) found little correlation between the As-content of rice and the soil on which it was grown.

Islam et al. (2005) presented coincident measurements of arsenic in water, soil and rice-grain at 456 STW's in five upazilas of Bangladesh, as summarised in Table 4.6. However, no useful correlations can be drawn from the aggregate data, which supports the view that As accumulation is determined by complex local factors. Using the same data set, Jahiruddin et al. (2005) showed that the total arsenic content of soils is positively correlated with the contents of both clay and iron oxides, but not of organic matter, and also that the phosphate and oxalate-extractable concentrations are strongly correlated, suggesting that 'available' arsenic is bound to iron oxides. Loeppert et al. (2005) identified the main reactive minerals in these soils as biotite, high-Fe vermiculite, smectite, Fe-chlorite, and Fe-oxides

Table 4.6 Mean concentrations of arsenic in irrigation water, topsoil (0–15 cm) and rice in five upazilas of Bangladesh

Medium	All areas	Brahmanbaria*	Faridpur[†]	Paba[†]	Senbagh*	Tala[‡]
Soil (total, mg/kg)	12.3	6.5	19.6	7.2	4.7	19.4
Soil (oxalate extractable, mg/kg)[§]	6.6	4.8	9.4	2.6	2.5	11.5
Soil (PO$_4$ extractable, mg/kg)[§]	2.8	1.9	4.7	1.2	0.8	4.3
Water (ppb)	100	110	100	20	140	150
Grain (µg/g)	340	420	480	70	440	330

*Old Meghna Estuarine Floodplain.
[†]Ganges River Floodplain.
[‡]Ganges Tidal Floodplain.
[§]The phosphate and oxalate-extractable concentrations provide a perspective on the 'available' arsenic.
Source: Islam et al. (2005)

(goethite, lepidocrocite and ferrihydrite). Further studies are needed to establish the links between arsenic in soil, irrigation water and plants for different crop types and varieties, and in different environments.

4.4.5 Differences between rice types and varieties

The arsenic levels in rice shown in Tables 4.3 and 4.5 are consistent with those reported by other researchers working in Bangladesh and India, including Meharg and Rahman (2003), Norra et al. (2005) and Patel et al. (2005). However, As contents also vary between rice varieties and between the kinds of rice grown in different countries. Meharg and Rahman (2003), for example, report As contents of rice grain ranging between 0.058 and 1.84 µg/kg in 13 different varieties tested in Bangladesh, with higher values generally (but not uniquely) in modern varieties than in traditional varieties. They also reported comparative figures of 200–460 µg/kg As for raw rice in the USA and 63–200 µg/kg As in Taiwan. Duxbury and Zavala (2005), quoting data from 15 countries, reported low mean As concentrations of 32–46 µg/kg for aromatic rices from Bangladesh, Bhutan, India and Pakistan, and high mean values in the USA (181 µg/kg) and Spain (186 µg/kg). The highest concentration, 753 µg/kg As, was reported from Texas, USA. However, the authors pointed out that arsenic toxicity is much higher in Bangladeshi rice than in USA rice (section 4.4.4).

4.4.6 Arsenic species in plants

Inorganic As species are more toxic than organic forms found in plants. The proportion of inorganic As in rice varies considerably between countries. Meharg (2005) stated that arsenic in USA rice is predominantly present as dimethylarsinic acid (DMA^V), whereas most of the arsenic in Bangladeshi rice is present as arsenite. Williams et al. (2005) reported that, for many of the 37 commonly grown crops in Bangladesh that they examined, all the arsenic present was inorganic, but they did not differentiate between arsenite and arsenate. However, they reported an average of 81% inorganic As in Bangladeshi rice compared with 37% in a Chinese variety grown under comparable conditions, adding 'the only other country reported that has a low percentage of inorganic in comparison to total-As is the USA'.

Chen et al. (2005) found that the presence of an iron plaque on rice roots increased the uptake of arsenite but decreased the uptake of arsenate. Addition of phosphate did not significantly affect arsenite uptake, irrespective of whether iron plaque was present or not. However, when plaque was present, phosphate resulted in a slight increase in the uptake of arsenate. This study was carried out under highly artificial conditions and needs to be followed up by studies under diverse field conditions.

Ma et al. (2001) reported that the hyperaccumulating fern *Pteris vittata* contained predominantly inorganic arsenic in all parts of the plant, and that the proportion of As(III) was greater in the fronds (47–89%) than the roots (8.3%), indicating that As(V) is reduced during transport from roots to fronds.

4.4.7   Bioavailability and transfer coefficients

Bioavailability

According to O'Neill (1995), in soils with similar total-As contents, plants grown on clays and silts take up less arsenic than plants grown on sandy soils, reflecting the higher activity of Fe and Al oxides and Fe-rich clays. In south-east China, Huang et al. (2006) found poor correlations between total soil As and total As in rice and the edible parts of eight of 16 vegetables studied, but found significant positive correlations in the other eight vegetables. They concluded that food risk assessment based on total soil-As contents was therefore unsafe.

In paddy fields, algae growing in surface water and on the soil apparently take up and recycle arsenic. During algal growth, some arsenic is lost to the atmosphere by methylation, but after death, the remainder returns to the water and soil through decay. Two studies in Bangladesh showed that a green alga (*Pithospora* sp.) took up significant amounts of arsenic (1400 mg/kg As in algal dry matter) after 90 days in a solution containing 5 ppb As, and that this passed into soil material and thence to a plant grown in it (Shamsuddhoha et al., 2006; Huq et al., 2006). However, neither the mass of algae nor methylation were measured, and field studies are needed to determine the significance of algae in influencing the availability and losses of arsenic in paddy fields.

Transfer coefficients

Variations in As uptake from soil are expressed in terms of the transfer coefficient (TC), which is defined as the total As content in the edible parts of the plant divided by the total As content of the soil. Transfer coefficients reported by Warren et al. (2003) for six common vegetables grown on four heavily contaminated sites in southwest England ranged from 0.00015 in potato flesh to 0.0316 in radish skins. In a study of rice and 16 vegetables grown on agricultural soils at six sites in Fujian Province (southeast China), Huang et al. (2006) found the highest median TC in rice (0.020) with much

Table 4.7 Total and available arsenic transfer coefficients for selected crops

Crop	Transfer coefficient (total) Median	Range	Transfer coefficient (available) Median	Range
Celery	0.0074	0.0014–0.0284	0.035	0.006–0.119
Water spinach	0.0059	0.0008–0.0158	0.043	0.010–0.086
Leaf mustard	0.0057	0.0003–0.0266	0.024	0.004–0.120
Garlic	0.0057	0.0010–0.0059	0.017	0.010–0.078
Onion	0.0049	0.0010–0.0139	0.033	0.009–0.070
Pakchoi	0.0037	0.0004–0.0157	0.02	0.003–0.074
Taro	0.0033	0.0028–0.0070	0.028	0.015–0.033
Lettuce	0.0023	0.0004–0.0092	0.019	0.005–0.059
Rice	0.002	0.006–0.036	0.179	0.068–0.440
Chinese cabbage	0.002	0.0003–0.0146	0.019	0.003–0.068
Cowpea	0.0011	0.0003–0.0083	0.016	0.0001–0.078
Cauliflower	0.0011	0.00004–0.0023	0.009	0.001–0.017
Radish	0.0007	0.0002–0.0024	0.053	0.003–0.022
Bottle gourd	0.0006	0.0001–0.028	0.004	0.002–0.008
Eggplant	0.0005	0.0001–0.0020	0.003	0.001–0.012

Source: Adapted from Huang et al. (2006)

lower values in vegetables (Table 4.7), and reported better correlations with the 'available' arsenic in soils.[6] Median values for TC (available) were again higher for rice (0.179) than for all the vegetables studied, but the wide range of TC values should be noted.

4.4.8 Influence of soil amendments

Iron

The addition of various forms of iron to adsorb arsenic and decrease plant uptake has been tested on contaminated soils. In field trials in Britain, Warren et al. (2003) found that ferrous sulphate solutions providing 0.2% Fe oxides in the top 10 cm of soil reduced As uptake by 22% in seven crops. Other studies (e.g. Mench et al., 2006) have produced broadly similar results. However, the relevance of these studies for irrigated paddy soils is questionable because the reducing conditions would decrease As adsorption on iron oxides (section 4.5.3).

Phosphate

In pot experiments, Hu et al. (2005) found that adding phosphate to a severely P-deficient soil in China had no significant effect on the As contents of shoots harvested at 4 weeks but it significantly reduced the As content of roots in two of three varieties tested. In pot trials in Bangladesh, Talukder (2005) found that adding phosphate reduced the adverse effect of arsenic on the growth and yield of rice plants. He also found that growing rice plants in saturated soil conditions reduced the effects of arsenic for all levels of added phosphate compared with growing plants under flooded conditions. Signes-Pastor et al. (2006) found, in pot trials in West Bengal, that addition of phosphate fertilisers up to 600 mg/kg soil increased As solubility under reducing soil conditions, with solubility greater at pH 5.5 than at 8.5. Since phosphate fertilisers are widely used on irrigated rice soils, their impact on As uptake by plants and on crop yields needs to be tested widely under field conditions to discover whether or not there are short-term or longer-term benefits.

Sulphur

Signes-Pastor et al. (2006) concluded that arsenic has a strong affinity for sulphur under reducing conditions, forming insoluble As-sulphide minerals. However, these sulphides might release arsenic again on reoxidation, as in floodplain soils that alternate between anaerobic and aerated conditions. In pot experiments in China, Hu et al. (2006) found that the addition of S to soil considerably decreased the As content of rice shoots but much less so the contents in roots. These reports are of interest because some paddy soils in south and southeast Asia are deficient in sulphur, and rice requires S fertilisation in order to obtain high yields. The possible benefits of adding S fertilisers in restricting As uptake need to be tested widely under field conditions.

4.4.9   Phytotoxicity

Toxicity levels

O'Neill (1995) pointed out that the uptake of arsenic varies greatly between plant species, and toxicity thresholds vary with soil texture and As species (from about 40 mg/kg in sands to 200 mg/kg in clays). Sheppard (1992) indicated that inorganic As is five times more toxic in sands and loams than it is in clay soils. 'Available' As content is a better indicator of phytotoxicity than total As.

A review by Sheppard (1992) revealed considerable variation in the level of soil-As at which yields are reduced, both between and within crops: in beans between 0 and 414 mg/kg, and in corn (maize) between 0 and 2600 mg/kg As[7]. Under field conditions, plant uptake of arsenic can vary from year to year. For example, Peryea (2002) reported that As concentrations in the leaves and fruit of apples grown on soils containing residues of lead arsenate pesticide varied from year to year, and Warren et al. (2003) reported As concentrations of 6.8 and 0.97 mg/kg in successive years in lettuce grown on contaminated mine spoil in Cornwall, England. This evidence makes clear that there is no single level of soil–plant toxicity: toxicity needs to be related to specific soil and environmental conditions, plant species and sometimes crop variety.

Toxicity symptoms

Various symptoms of As toxicity in rice have been reported. They include: delayed seedling emergence; reduced plant growth; yellowing and wilting of leaves; brown necrotic spots on older leaves; and reduced grain yields (Huq et al., 2006). In the USA and Australia, 'straighthead' disease is considered to be an indicator of As toxicity (Frans, 1988; Williams, 2003; Yan et al., 2005). This disease has a variety of symptoms, including shortened plant height, delayed heading, upright panicles, sterile florets, misshapen grains ('parrot-beak') and reduced grain yields. Frans (1988) reported that in Arkansas straighthead disease is frequently found on sandy loam soils but seldom on clay soils, and often in fields where undecayed vegetation had been ploughed into soils just before planting rice. Williams (2003) reported that straighthead symptoms were observed over a wide range of Australian soils, and were worse in soils low in nitrogen and in those after pasture or where previous crop stubble had been incorporated in soils. However, Williams also reported that yield reductions occur across wide areas in fields with high-As levels without straighthead symptoms being observed, suggesting that the disease symptoms can be stimulated or blocked by other soil factors. Symptoms of straighthead disease have been recognised recently in rice in Faridpur, Bangladesh (Figure 4.3), and are associated with major, and approximately linear, reductions in yield from 9 to 3 t/ha at soil concentrations of between 12 and 58 mg/kg As (Duxbury and Panaullah, 2007).

On soils contaminated by arsenical pesticides in the USA, Yan et al. (2005) found considerable variation in varietal resistance to straighthead disease at different arsenic and nitrogen levels. Yield reductions ranged from virtually none in one Chinese cultivar to 80–96% in four of ten USA cultivars tested. The authors also reported that, in an earlier study of straighthead resistance in 124 Chinese rice varieties, yields were not significantly reduced in 18 out of 109 *indica* varieties and in one out of 15 *japonica* varieties tested.

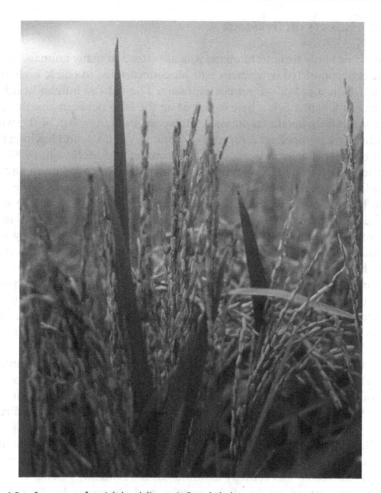

Figure 4.3   Symptoms of straighthead disease in Bangladesh.
Source: Photograph courtesy of Richard Loeppert, Texas A&M University

In hydroponic studies with wheat, Liu, Zhang et al. (2006) found that increasing arsenite concentrations had greater effects than arsenate on seed germination, root growth and shoot height, and that there were significant differences between varieties. They reported that root length and shoot height were more sensitive to relatively low levels of As, and suggested that these characteristics might be used as indicators of As toxicity. The relevance of this technique as a practical field test needs to be investigated, especially for the early detection of As toxicity in rice.

4.4.10   Effects on livestock

Arsenic is not only toxic to humans; it is also toxic to many animals. Also, if arsenic is accumulated by animals and bioconcentrated in edible body parts or products, it may add to human exposure. The risks to human health are described in Chapter 5, but here we focus on the links between arsenic in soil and crops and its uptake in animals. However, in many parts of the world, groundwater is pumped for direct consumption by animals and has long been known to cause disease in livestock (e.g. Grimmet and McIntosh, 1939).

While livestock often feed on pasture, they may also be fed grain and – of particular relevance for parts of south and south-east Asia where rice cultivation, bullock ploughing and small farmers are prevalent – on rice straw. As noted earlier, rice and other grains tend to accumulate arsenic in the order root > stem > leaf > grain, so livestock eating rice straw may be at particular risk. For instance, based on measurements at several hundred sites in Bangladesh, Islam et al. (2005) found that, on average, straw contains seven times more arsenic than rice grain, and Abedin et al. (2002) reported straw from irrigated rice containing up to 91.8 mg/kg As. Nandi et al. (2005) described a wide range of symptoms in cattle reported to be associated with high As intake, and found significantly higher As levels in the hair of cattle in As-affected areas of West Bengal than in non-affected areas.

Sanyal and Nasar (2002) reported that >90% of the As intake by animals in an affected area of West Bengal was from feed sources, with only a small contribution from water. However, O'Neill (1995) stated that the uptake of arsenic from plants by livestock is generally low, and that ingestion directly from soil is a greater danger. Abrahams and Thornton (1983, cited by O'Neill, 1995), reported that 60–75% of As intake by livestock came from soil, but the range (2–90%) was very wide. They also reported that only 1% of the arsenic eaten was actually assimilated, the remainder being excreted. A more widespread study of As uptake and digestion by livestock in As-affected areas is needed, including an assessment of the risks to humans of eating or drinking animal products. Studies should take account of the amounts of straw, domestic waste, leaves, roots, soil and water consumed by livestock in different countries and farming systems.

4.4.11   Effects on aquaculture

Arsenic concentrations in fish and shell-fish are described in Chapter 5. In general, natural surface-water bodies are low in arsenic. However, in many As-affected areas of Asia, ponds are used for fish production, and tubewells are used to top up water levels. Inevitably, if the groundwater is contaminated by arsenic, there will be a risk of As accumulation in the fish. This risk needs to be investigated, therefore. Such ponds are highly profitable and it should be practical to eliminate this risk by use of water treatment or a deeper well.

4.5 Options for Arsenic Management

As described in Chapters 5, 6 and 7, many methods are being tested to reduce the amounts of arsenic that people ingest in food and water. They include As removal, developing surface-water supplies or uncontaminated aquifers, collecting rainwater, and information-based approaches to reduce exposure to arsenic. In this chapter, we focus on methods to prevent or reduce As accumulation in food crops. Several methods have been used to mitigate high-As levels in mining, industrial and urban wastes, and in agricultural soils contaminated with arsenical pesticides or timber preservatives. These methods (section 4.5.5) include soil removal, soil washing, use of Fe compounds and phytoremediation. Few of these methods appear to be practical for small-scale rice farmers, but they could be considered in screening possibilities.

There is a fundamental difference between remediation of industrially contaminated sites, mostly in Europe and North America, and those contaminated by groundwater irrigation, which are mostly in the developing world. In the former, there are clear financial and regulatory drivers whereby the objective is merely to achieve 'clean-up' at least cost, and where timescales of decades may be considered acceptable. However, small farmers operate on a different timescale and have no one to claim against for contamination losses (Chapter 8).

4.5.1 Alternative irrigation sources

Water treatment

Both the simple filtration methods used for rural water supplies and the more sophisticated methods used for treating urban supplies appear to be impractical for treating the enormous quantities of water for irrigation because of the cost, institutional needs and engineering. This is especially true for the near-subsistence rice farmers in Asia who most need the water. The costs must either be very low or be heavily subsidised. In the meantime, therefore, it will probably be more practical to focus on alternative sources of irrigation water.

For rice irrigation, the only treatment method that appears to have potential is to exploit and enhance the oxidation of iron that occurs along irrigation channels. Precipitation of iron oxyhydroxides along such channels is very common, and Hossain (2005) has demonstrated that this process can remove significant quantities of arsenic (section 4.3.2). Potentially, these processes could be enhanced by methods such as increasing turbulence, increasing the distance from the well to the field, using a settling pond, and adding ferric material to the channels or settling ponds. It would also be important that the precipitates are not carried in suspension to fields, and that accumulations are periodically disposed of by simple means such as incorporation into earthworks. Systems using overhead tanks could be adapted to remove iron sludge before irrigation water is distributed to fields. Such treatments may not achieve potable standards, but where groundwater is severely contaminated, a three- to fivefold reduction in As level may be achievable and would greatly reduce the rate of accumulation in soils. That approach is also attractive because the required technology exists in every village, but it will require considerable awareness-raising and education to implement. The cultivation of water hyacinth, a known As hyperaccumulator, in settling ponds also deserves investigation (see section 4.5.5).

Deep aquifers

In most affected parts of Bangladesh and West Bengal, the most practical alternative source of irrigation water appears to be deeper aquifers. To obtain water meeting potable standards, it is often necessary to drill to below 150 m or even 200 m. However, As concentrations often decrease rapidly below about 50 m (Chapter 8), so there may be an important trade-off between improved irrigation water quality and reduced cost by drilling wells of intermediate depth. Deeper wells may not be economic without subsidy, however, and they introduce the risks of drawing down arsenic from the upper aquifer(s) or inducing saline intrusion at the coastal end of the deep aquifer[8]. In addition, the deep aquifer is not of uniformly good quality: apart from salinity, it locally contains high levels of boron and manganese. In all countries and regions, therefore, prior surveys of groundwater availability and quality are needed before initiating deep-aquifer development programmes.

Surface water

Close to rivers, it is possible, in principle, to replace tubewells with irrigation from surface-water sources. In practice, most of the reliable and easily developed irrigation sites on minor rivers and ponds have already been exploited in Bangladesh, West Bengal and probably many other affected areas. In the past, diversions from major rivers in the Ganges–Brahmaputra basin have been fraught with problems such as channel siltation, bank erosion, excessive seepage losses, waterlogging, land acquisition, farmer organisation, cost-recovery, and provision of funds for operation and maintenance (Brammer, 2004).[9] In addition, further large withdrawals from rivers could have adverse environmental and political impacts downstream. Comprehensive impact assessments and rigorous comparison with all alternatives are essential prerequisites. Notwithstanding these reservations, surface-water diversions need to be assessed where they appear feasible.

In parts of India, Nepal and other areas with sparsely populated upland tracts, it may be feasible to build reservoirs in valleys to irrigate floodplains downstream. However, the areas of land that could be irrigated in this way appear to be small in relation to need. Potential problems with valley reservoirs include displacement of population, rapid siltation, decomposition of organic residues and, in some regions, the risks of dam breaching by floods, earthquakes and landslides.

4.5.2 Crop substitution

Arsenic is most commonly a problem in anaerobic soils where arsenic bound to soil minerals or added in irrigation water becomes available for uptake by plants under reducing conditions. Under aerobic conditions, arsenic is bound to iron oxides and is not readily available to dryland crops. Dryland crops also require less irrigation water than rice. Therefore, switching from rice to wheat or maize cultivation could greatly reduce the problem of As contamination. However, for the majority of farmers in south and southeast Asia, rice is by far the preferred crop option, culturally and economically, and much of the land currently irrigated is better suited to paddy rice than to dryland crops. Irrigation of dryland crops would still add arsenic to soils, but the rate of As accumulation would be significantly reduced. The effect of irrigating dryland crops on the availability of arsenic to a subsequent monsoon-crop in flooded paddy fields needs to be investigated in cooler areas of north India and Nepal where irrigated wheat or other dryland crops are grown in the dry winter season and followed by a partially- or non-irrigated monsoon rice crop.

4.5.3 Changing soil and irrigation management

Dryland rice

Experiments have been made in Bangladesh to grow rice in aerated soils: e.g. direct-seeded instead of transplanted, and on raised beds (Lauren and Duxbury, 2005). This not only reduces the amount of irrigation water used, and thereby As soil loading, but the arsenic is less available to the crop in the aerated soil environment. However, the authors reported that, contrary to expectations, rice grown under experimental aerobic conditions in two districts of Bangladesh showed no difference in As contents from rice grown under anaerobic conditions. In addition, rice grown as a dryland crop usually produces lower yields and remains longer in the field than transplanted rice, so that weeding costs are higher and there might not be enough time to grow two (or three) rice crops per year in some areas. It is too early yet to say whether dryland cultivation methods will prove economic and farmers be willing to adopt them, especially for the high-yielding *boro* rice crop.

A system of rice intensification (SRI) is promoting the substitution of dryland rice for paddy rice in several Asian and African rice-growing countries that, *inter alia*, will save irrigation water and reduce drought impacts (Stoop et al., 2002). Evaluations are needed to find out if SRI is economically worthwhile and useful in reducing soil-As accumulation. If successful, it could have widespread application across northern India and Nepal where wet-season rice and dry-season wheat are grown in rotation. Apart from reducing irrigation costs and soil-As loading, it would obviate the need to puddle the topsoil for rice cultivation and would thus leave it in better condition for the subsequent wheat crop. Increased wheat yields would help compensate for the possibly reduced yields of dryland rice.

Soil amendments

Research has been conducted in several places to reduce plant uptake of arsenic by adding iron to soils (Williams, 2003; Lauren and Duxbury, 2005; Yan et al., 2005; Mench et al., 2006). The addition of amendments such as ferrous sulphate, iron grit or other ferric materials is most suitable for aerated soils. It needs to be investigated whether such materials would be beneficial on seasonally flooded and flood-irrigated soils during the early part of the dry season before irrigation begins. The use of crushed brick and burnt soil deserves to be tested, since they would be much cheaper than imported Fe materials. The addition of iron to adsorb arsenic is likely to have greatest benefit on sandy soils low in iron and used for growing As-susceptible vegetables, because the arsenic will be adsorbed by the iron oxides and so not be readily available for plant uptake. The addition of iron oxides to irrigated paddy soils may not be effective because As adsorption will not take place if the iron is reduced. Nonetheless, iron (or brick) grit, because of its coarse particle size, could provide As-adsorption sites for part or all of the rice-growing season in reduced topsoils.

Possible adverse knock-on effects of increasing As adsorption in the topsoil also need investigation. This has two dimensions: a short-term effect where the adsorbed As is released to the soil in the following monsoon season when the soil is flooded and reduced; and a possible long-term effect of continuing As release after iron applications cease or as topsoil organic matter contents increase with continuing paddy cultivation.

4.5.4   Changing crop agronomy

Plant breeding

Observations that rice varieties differ in As uptake and that some are resistant to straighthead disease (sections 4.4.3 and 4.4.7) provide plant breeders with the opportunity to develop As-tolerant rice varieties. Indeed, tolerant varieties are becoming available in some countries, and seem likely to become more widely available in the next few years as a result of ongoing agronomic research. However, this is not a panacea. The substitution of As-tolerant crop varieties will not reduce the rate of As-accumulation in soils. Continued addition of arsenic from irrigation water must eventually raise soil-As to toxic levels, and arsenic will still be available to a following less-tolerant crop. Arsenic-tolerant varieties may be a valuable component within an overall As-mitigation strategy, but, pursued alone, may be just a means to buy time until a long-term solution can be introduced. Also, As-susceptible dryland crops grown in rotation with As-tolerant rice varieties would remain exposed to high-As levels. In such cases, the substitution of As-tolerant pulses, spices, fruits and vegetables might be appropriate.

Other practices

Other mitigation practices reported by Williams (2003) – such as reducing additions of nitrogen and organic matter, or allowing rice fields to dry out completely for 10–14 days prior to the panicle initiation stage – also reduce potential crop yields, which may not be acceptable to small farmers. Additionally, allowing paddy soils to become dry may be practicable for much of a dry-season rice crop but not for a subsequent monsoon rice crop in areas submerged by floodwater between rice planting and heading. The potential benefits of adopting these techniques need to be assessed in terms of the total exposure of annual agricultural production to arsenic.

4.5.5   Rehabilitation of contaminated soils

Even where an As-free irrigation supply can be provided, it will be desirable to reduce As concentrations in affected soils to restore crop yields and/ or reduce crop uptake of As. High As levels will persist in contaminated soils for many years because of the low rates of leaching and other losses (sections 4.2.8 and 4.2.9). In irrigated soils that are permanently aerated, some of the methods used to reclaim industrially contaminated soil might be appropriate. However, the methods tested to date were intended for large-scale commercial farming or for non-agricultural use, and their applicability to subsistence farmers in Asia and elsewhere seems highly questionable.

Alternative irrigation supply

For contaminated paddy soils, the most effective way of continuing satisfactory crop cultivation is to provide low-As water. Addition of low-As irrigation water should dilute the As concentration in the puddled topsoil during the growing season and enable normal rice production to be resumed immediately. However, irrigation with low-As water will reduce the soil-As content very slowly (section 4.2.9). These suppositions need to be tested under field conditions, alone and in combination with one or more of the methods described below. The benefits of substituting low-As water may not be revealed by analysis of dried soil samples, but only by analysing changes in As concentrations in plants and in rice yields.

Topsoil removal

The quickest way to remove the As-hazard in contaminated paddy soils is to remove the topsoil. Although seemingly drastic, this is a simple and speedy solution, and could be undertaken by affected farmers themselves, possibly with government or non-government organisation (NGO) support. The thickness of topsoil that needs to be removed is small: in paddy soils under small-farmer conditions, the heavily contaminated layer is usually no more than 10–15 cm thick (section 4.3.2).

In Bangladesh, farmers commonly sell soil for brick-making. Apart from the immediate cash benefit, this practice may benefit them by lowering land levels to make the depth and duration of seasonal flooding more secure for monsoon-season paddy cultivation. Soil is also widely removed for building road and flood embankments, footpaths, raised house plinths and house walls. After soil removal, farmers generally add farmyard manure, compost or dry water hyacinth to help restore fertility and a looser soil tilth for ploughing, and add fertilisers to the following crop. The cultivation of jute and deep-rooting legumes such as *Crotalaria*, *Sesbania* and pigeon pea (*Cajanus*) also help to restore soil tilth; and puddling soils for paddy cultivation – especially by bullock ploughing – quickly restores a ploughpan, which helps to hold water in and on the topsoil within bunded fields.

This practice is only appropriate for silty and clayey soils in which topsoil removal does not expose a more permeable layer unsuitable for irrigated paddy cultivation. It will be most appropriate where the soil material removed is used for a purpose such as brick-making that locks the arsenic in a form that will not be leached. This would be a suitable subject for appropriate-technology research by NGOs working in As-contaminated areas, and governments could consider subsidising soil rehabilitation by such means.

Soil amendments

As noted above, iron-rich soil amendments may be unnecessary for irrigated dryland crops and ineffective in paddy soils. Nonetheless, the use of coarse iron or brick grit (section 4.5.3) and sulphur fertilisation (section 4.4.6) both deserve investigation. Sulphur, like iron, is reduced in anaerobic soils. Therefore, it needs to be established whether the decreased uptake of arsenic in the presence of sulphur reflects temporary or permanent immobilisation of arsenic, or whether the arsenic might be released to a subsequent monsoon rice crop. Investigations are also needed to assess the knock-on effects of continuing sulphur application on irrigated paddy soils, together with possible environmental impacts of sulphur leached laterally from paddy fields into adjoining depression soils or water bodies.

Hyperaccumulators

The practicality of using hyperaccumulating plants such as brake fern (*Pteris vittata*) to remove arsenic from contaminated paddy soils deserves testing.[10] Wei et al. (2006) reported that several other fern species are also As hyperaccumulators. Indian mustard (*Brassica juncea*) is also reported to accumulate arsenic (Mahimairaja et al., 2005). Water hyacinth (*Eichhornia crassipes*) is a known hyperaccumulator, but it roots in water, so it could only be used to remove arsenic from irrigation water, not from soils.

The use of hyperaccumulators might be considered where it is impractical to provide a low-As irrigation supply. Ma et al. (2001) reported that brake fern took up large quantities of arsenic very quickly. In pot trials in Florida, USA, they found that, at a soil-As concentration of 6 mg/kg, fern fronds contained 755 mg/kg As after 2 weeks and 438 mg/kg after 6 weeks; at 50 mg/kg soil As, they found 5131 mg/kg As in the fronds at 2 weeks and 3215 mg/kg after 6 weeks. The authors did not give figures for the biomass produced at these arsenic levels. Assuming production of 10 tons/ha (perhaps an optimistic assumption after 6 weeks' growth), fern fronds containing 3215 mg/kg As could remove 32 kg/ha As from the soil. That is equivalent to many years addition of arsenic from contaminated irrigation water in STW command areas. However, plant-As concentrations achieved in pot trials are probably much higher than would be attained in the field, and brake fern could be grown only under dryland conditions. Trials are needed to see how effective this, and perhaps other, ferns are in removing arsenic from soils if periodically substituted for a dry-season rice crop or if grown as a short-term crop early in the dry season before an irrigated rice crop is planted. Indian mustard might be tested under similar conditions. However, unlike ferns, mustard accumulates arsenic mainly in the roots (Mahimairaja et al., 2005), so the whole plant would need to be removed from fields in order to remove the arsenic.

The feasibility of using hyperaccumulating plants for paddy soil rehabilitation needs to be tested. The environmental limits to the effective cultivation of such plants in different countries and regions need to be determined. A solution would need to be found to the problem of safe disposal of large quantities of plant residues with high As contents after removal from the fields. Possible health risks to children, livestock and wildlife eating the plants or inhaling ash from burnt material would also need to be investigated.

4.6 Research and Development Needs

Most studies of soil processes and remediation methods have been carried out on industrial, mining and urban wastes and on soils contaminated with agrochemical products: i.e. where arsenic is a historical residue. Much less work has been done on soils irrigated with As-rich groundwater: i.e. where arsenic is continuously being added.

Where rice is the principal crop and is irrigated with high-As groundwater, the most urgent need is to stop adding arsenic. The most practical alternatives to irrigation with contaminated groundwater will vary between areas and they need to be evaluated systematically. After additions of arsenic from irrigation water have ceased, remedial measures identified in section 4.5 can then be tested for relevance, and if appropriate, demonstrated to farmers. For governments and aid donors, the urgent needs are as follows.

1 *To identify STW sites where soils are already seriously As-contaminated, so as to identify areas requiring immediate interventions.* Such surveys will also establish a valuable data base for research and monitoring. In countries suffering widespread actual or incipient soil and crop contamination, a considerable expansion and strengthening of field survey and laboratory institutions for water and soil testing will probably be needed.

2 *To inform farmers where irrigation water is contaminated with arsenic at levels dangerous to soils, crops and food.* This information should probably include semi-quantitative guidelines that reflect the concentration and potential rate of As accumulation in soil.

3 *To seek alternative irrigation sources for each area and, where appropriate, to fund the provision of such supplies.* This involves complex water-resource decisions, since new supplies must not (in the case of deep groundwater)

unreasonably jeopardise safe drinking water sources and must (in the case of surface water) be carefully weighed against ecological damage. However, the mere possibility of adverse effects must not become an excuse for not thoroughly evaluating their potential.

4   *To increase research to find methods of crop cultivation that minimise the addition of arsenic to soils and/or the uptake of arsenic by crops.* This is especially needed in areas where it is impractical to provide alternative sources of irrigation water in the near future.

5   *To test and demonstrate appropriate mitigation or rehabilitation techniques as quickly as possible in areas where potentially suitable alternative practices have been identified for particular environmental conditions.* Where it is considered appropriate to purchase soil for reuse in bricks or earthworks, it is essential that programmes be accompanied by strong technical support for planning and monitoring, or else a great waste of resources could occur.

Agricultural researchers need to obtain more information on soil–water–plant–As relationships and how they can be manipulated to reduce As accumulation in soils and crops, and to speed agricultural rehabilitation. While pot and hydroponic studies help to understand the processes of soil chemistry and plant-availability, and to screen possible remedial treatments, such studies – carried out with pure chemicals and water in a controlled environment – are not sufficient to predict performance in farmers' fields. Therefore, far more field trials need to be carried out to provide practical recommendations. Variations in environmental conditions and As uptake by plants between years warrant trials being continued for several years so that robust recommendations are given to farmers.

A widely overlooked problem with field studies and trials, and one that has sometimes led to oversimplistic and erroneous interpretations, is the regional and local complexity of the environmental conditions under which farming is practised (section 4.2.4). This variability must be recognised and taken into account in sampling soils and crops, designing field studies, and in interpreting and extrapolating results. Equally, reports of trials and investigations must adequately describe soil and environmental conditions at study sites so that their significance can be properly assessed and taken into account in comparing information between sites. In rice-growing areas, methods of laboratory analysis should be used that are appropriate for the wetland conditions under which paddy rice actually grows.

NOTES

1   Paddy rice is grown in saturated soil which, between transplantation of seedlings and crop heading, is usually submerged under 5–10 cm of water in irrigated fields and by up to *c.* 90 cm of floodwater under natural conditions; some deepwater

rice varieties can tolerate up to 3–4 m of floodwater. Rice can also be grown as a dryland crop in aerated soils, when seed is usually broadcast sown or drilled, but seedlings are transplanted in some cultivation systems.

2   In some floodplain soils, the substratum is a buried older soil which may or may not have properties similar to the surface soil. On old landforms, the substratum may be the deeply and strongly weathered rock or alluvial material in which the current soils have developed.

3   In Bangladesh, fields average <0.1 ha in area.

4   Smith et al. used the US Soil Taxonomy names for these soils (Soil Survey Staff, 1999). The bracketed names are those used in the FAO classification (IUSS Working Group WRB, 2006). The name Vertisol is common to both classification systems.

5   Bangladesh's two other seasonal rice crops, *aus* and *aman*, are grown respectively in the first and second halves of the summer monsoon season, and are predominantly rain-fed or irrigated from surface-water sources.

6   Determined by NaH_2PO_4 extraction.

7   The concentration at which no yield reduction was reported in some studies presumably refers to hydroponic studies in which plants responded positively to small additions of arsenic to the growing medium. Miteva (2002) reported an elongation of roots and increase of stem height of tomatoes with additions of 15 and 25 mg/kg of As over the zero As level, but growth reductions at 50 and 100 mg/kg.

8   Unlike arsenic, salinity may not pose a risk to the irrigation well owner, but more likely to affect down-gradient wells used for drinking water.

9   Most of these schemes have also included flood protection.

10   This terrestrial fern is variously referred to as brake fern, Chinese brake fern, ladder brake and ladder fern by Mahimairaja et al. (2005).

Chapter Five

Health Effects of Arsenic in Drinking Water and Food

5.1 Introduction

The consequences of exposure to arsenic for human health are potentially grave, and may extend from general malaise to death. There is a huge literature on the medical effects of arsenic, derived from its use as a poison, its use in medicine, its inclusion in manufactured products, and accidental exposure from industrial and natural pollution of soil and water. Although most clinical effects are independent of the source of exposure, this chapter concentrates on the impacts associated with exposure to arsenic in water, both directly and through food, and on their geographical variation, and how understanding this feeds back into managing natural arsenic pollution. The term arsenicosis pervades the literature, but as Guha Mazumder (2003) points out, there is no standard definition, although the term is used widely to characterise the various clinical manifestations caused by chronic arsenic toxicity due to prolonged ingestion of arsenic.

After a brief account of its history (section 5.2) and toxicity (section 5.3), the chapter considers natural sources of exposure to arsenic in some detail (section 5.4), especially indirect exposure through the food chain, a complex process linked to the water used in irrigation and cooking, and through consumption by animals. The uptake of arsenic by plants from the soil links this chapter to Chapter 4. Acute arsenic poisoning can be fatal, but sudden death hardly ever originates from environmental sources, and so is described only briefly (section 5.5). The health effects of chronic poisoning may be divided into three main categories: dermatological manifestations, carcinogenic effects and systemic non-carcinogenic effects (sections 5.6–5.8). Often, only the first can be linked unambiguously to arsenic poisoning in individuals, the others being inferred from epidemiological studies.

The major causes of death associated with chronic arsenic poisoning are various cancers and cardiovascular and lung disease. A fourth group of effects are social and psychological impacts (section 5.9). Dermatological symptoms have been described in almost all areas with high As concentrations in water; whereas some, such as Blackfoot Disease, are almost unique to one area (southwest Taiwan), other symptoms vary geographically, but by degree (section 5.11).

Unfortunately, there is no cure for chronic arsenic poisoning (section 5.12). The principal recommendation is to remove exposure, supported by symptomatic treatment of skin lesions, dietary supplements, and surgery in extreme cases. The final sections of the chapter examine the beneficial effects of removing exposure to arsenic in drinking water (section 5.13), and close with a case history of long-term arsenic exposure in Murshidabad District in West Bengal (section 5.14).

5.2   A Short History of the Health Effects of Chronic Arsenic Poisoning

Awareness of the diversity of health effects has grown rapidly over the past 50 years or so. The effects of acute poisoning were well known long before the 20th century, and it would have been intuitively recognised that drinking water with arsenic in it was best avoided where possible. However, recognition and confirmation of some of the specific manifestations of chronic poisoning took longer, and in some cases is still ongoing. Some of the landmarks of arsenic epidemiology related to drinking water are listed below:

- *1898, Poland.* Earliest known report of arsenic poisoning from well-water, which produced skin cancer (Mandal and Suzuki, 2002).
- *1920s, Cordoba, Argentina.* 'Bel Ville' disease, a form of skin cancer, is linked to naturally contaminated groundwater (Bado, 1939; Niccoli et al., 1989).
- *1935, Ontario, Canada.* Well-water identified as a cause of arsenic poisoning and death (Wyllie, 1937).
- *1950s, Japan.* Important information that arsenic causes lung and other cancers comes from a case in which waste from a mineral smelter polluted water supplies from 1955 to 1959 (Pershagen, 1983).
- *1960s, Taiwan.* Blackfoot Disease (BFD), a peripheral vascular disease, is linked to drinking well-water (Chen and Wu, 1962). In 1965, close associations are found between BFD and hyperpigmentation, keratosis and skin cancer (Tseng et al., 1968). Follow-up studies from the late

1960s to the early 1980s also link arsenic exposure to lung and bladder cancer.

- *1960s, Antofagasta, Chile.* High levels of arsenic in the municipal supply produce widespread and severe arsenicosis (Borgono et al., 1977).

- *1975, north-central India.* First cases of arsenic poisoning due to drinking water discovered, and associated with non-cirrhotic portal fibrosis (Datta and Kaul, 1976).

- *1980, Xinjiang, China.* First report of extensive arsenicosis in Xinjiang in the far northwest of China (Sun, 2004). Arsenicosis is subsequently identified in 18 other provinces of China.

- *1983, West Bengal, India.* Contaminated tubewell-water is identified as the cause of arsenical skin lesions (Garai et al., 1984), leading to the discovery of one the world's worst cases of arsenic poisoning, and a decade later to the discovery of arsenic in the adjoining areas of Bangladesh and Nepal.

- *1996–98, South America.* Evidence from ecological studies indicate that long-term exposure to arsenic in drinking water in Argentina (Hopenhayn-Rich et al., 1996) and Chile (Smith et al., 1998) is responsible for large numbers of bladder, lung, kidney and skin cancers.

- *2001, Vietnam.* Extensive arsenic contamination of groundwater discovered in the Red River Delta in the north, and later in the Mekong Delta in the south, and adjoining areas of Cambodia (Berg et al., 2001, 2006b).

- *2004, Bangladesh.* Children's intellectual development is shown to be impaired by arsenic in drinking water (Wasserman et al., 2004).

5.3 Toxicity of Arsenic Compounds

Reviews of arsenic toxicity (e.g. Thomas et al., 2001; Hughes, 2002; ATSDR, 2005) have considered a wide variety of organic and inorganic arsenic compounds (or arsenicals), but many are artificial or do not occur in natural waters. The structures of the toxicologically most relevant compounds are shown in Figure 5.1. In groundwater, water supply and soil–plant systems, two arsenic species are of predominant importance: the dissolved inorganic ions arsenate and arsenite. In natural waters, concentrations of organic arsenic compounds form a negligible percentage of the total arsenic present (Cullen and Reimer, 1989). However, in mammals these species may be transformed into the stable mono- and di-methylated forms MMA^V and DMA^V.

The toxicities of some important arsenic compounds are listed in Table 5.1, and these highlight the critical importance of arsenic speciation in assessing acute toxicity. The lethal dose for humans is estimated to be 1–3 mg/kg. Acute poisoning has many metabolic effects, including stomach

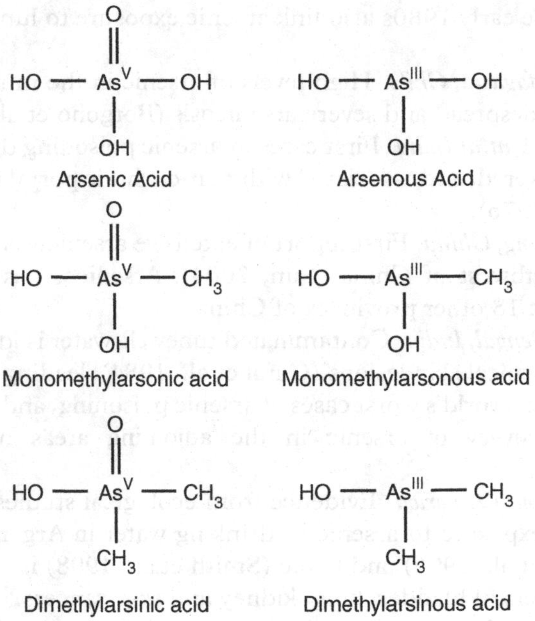

Figure 5.1   Structure of some toxicologically important arsenic compounds.
Source: Hughes (2002)

Table 5.1   Acute toxicity of arsenic in laboratory animals

Chemical	Species	Route	Median lethal dose (LD$_{50}$) [mg As/kg]
Arsenic trioxide	Mouse	Oral	26–48
Arsenic trioxide	Rat	Oral	15
Arsenite	Mouse	Intramuscular	8
Arsenite	Hamster	Intraperitoneal	8
Arsenate	Mouse	Intramuscular	22
MMA^{III}	Hamster	Intraperitoneal	2
MMA^{V}	Mouse	Oral	916
DMA^{V}	Mouse	Oral	648
TMAO^{V}	Mouse	Oral	5500
Arsenobetaine	Mouse	Oral	>4260

LD$_{50}$ is measured in mg As per Kg of body mass.
Source: Hughes (2002)

pain, diarrhoea, vomiting, bloody urine, anuria, shock, convulsions, coma and death (section 5.5). It was previously thought that organic forms are less toxic than inorganic forms, and hence that methylation was a simple detoxification mechanism. However, while DMA^V, the main arsenic compound excreted by humans, is less toxic than inorganic arsenic, MMA[III] is more toxic than arsenite (Hughes, 2002). It is often stated that (in drinking water) trivalent arsenite is more toxic than pentavalent arsenate, and while this may be correct for acute poisoning, it makes little difference to chronic exposure through water and food because arsenate and arsenite are readily interconverted in the human gut (WHO, 2001).

The toxicity of pentavalent arsenic in arsenate is due to its similarity to phosphate (Hughes, 2002). For instance, arsenate substitutes for phosphate in reactions with glucose and gluconate, and also interferes with the ion-exchange system in red blood cells. Perhaps of greatest significance, arsenate substitutes for, and hence interferes with, phosphate in adenosine triphosphate (ATP), which is fundamental to the release and storage of energy in muscles. The trivalent form, arsenite, operates differently, reacting with molecules containing thiol or sulfhydryl[1] groups such as enzymes, receptors or coenzymes, and can therefore affect a wide variety of critical biochemical processes (Hughes, 2002). Trivalent arsenicals react readily with glutathione and cysteine, and inhibit pyruvate dehydrogenase (PDH) which plays a vital role in the citric acid cycle and may therefore explain the depletion of carbohydrates observed in laboratory animals exposed to As(III). Arsenic is also one of the most potent of carcinogens (Smith and Hira-Smith, 2004). Arsenic appears to act in various ways to affect the 'signalling' mechanisms of cells through oxidative stress, damaging DNA by both hypo- and hypermethylation, affecting whether or not DNA is transcribed (Hughes, 2002). It also appears that arsenic inhibits the repair of DNA[2].

The quantity of arsenic absorbed by a body depends on the exposure pathway and the form of arsenic. Inorganic As in food and water is readily absorbed from the gastrointestinal tract, but absorption occurs more easily if the arsenic is already dissolved. Hence, a given quantum of arsenic in water is potentially more toxic than as a solid in food. Around two-thirds to three-quarters of ingested arsenic is excreted as urine within a few days to a week (WHO, 2001). Arsenic metabolism in the human body is controlled mainly by two types of reactions: (a) reduction of As(V) to As(III) and (b) oxidative methylation of As(III) compounds. In humans, both arsenate and arsenite are readily methylated, to produce DMA and MMA, both of which are excreted in urine.

Although such indications have been identified in livestock, there is no evidence that any level of dietary intake of arsenic, however small, is beneficial to human health (Smith et al., 1992). There is some evidence, such as the notorious Styrian 'arsenic-eaters' (Przygoda et al., 2001), that the human metabolism can, to a degree, adapt to arsenic exposure, although the precise mechanisms, which probably involve increased rate of conversion of inorganic to organic forms of arsenic, are not well understood (Squibb and Fowler, 1983).

5.4   Environmental Exposure to Arsenic

5.4.1   Exposure pathways

Before considering the effects of chronic arsenic exposure on human health, we first consider how arsenic may enter the body, and in what forms. At the simplest level, exposure can be classified as respiration, ingestion in food or water, and absorption (dermal contact). At the next level of analysis, we may ask in what situations are these processes important. Although this book is primarily concerned with natural arsenic pollution, it should be remembered that natural and anthropogenic exposure might coexist. A good example is in agriculture, where crops may extract arsenic directly from the soil, be irrigated with As-rich water, have As-rich phosphate fertiliser applied, and be sprayed with arsenical pesticides. After harvest, the crop may be cooked over As-rich coal in As-rich water, and washed down with As-rich drinking water. Another situation where sources may be confused is where airborne particles from smelters or power stations are sources of respiratory As exposure, but also fall to the ground, to be washed into water bodies, giving rise to exposure through drinking water. Common sources of exposure to arsenic are as follows.

1   Respiratory/airborne pathways:
   - Industrial emissions from coal-burning power stations, smelting of non-ferrous ores
   - Domestic fuel (especially coal) combustion
   - Aerial pesticide spraying
   - Cigarette smoking
   - Paint and wallpaper
2   Dermal pathways:
   - Non-aerial pesticide application
   - Washing, bathing and swimming
   - Working in water bodies, notably standing in paddy fields
   - Contact with soil
   - Waterborne effluents
   - Phosphate detergents
3   Ingestion:
   - Drinking water
   - Food
   - Cooking water
   - Medicines

Point sources of dermal or respiratory exposure are normally self-evident and localised, although extensive exposure through domestic coal burning occurs in Guizhou Province of China (Ding et al., 2001). Uptake of arsenic through respiration depends on (a) the particle size, which determines whether it is deposited and (b) very strongly on the solubility of the particular form of arsenic, which determines whether it is actually absorbed. No generalised percentages can be quoted for respiratory exposure, but contents vary between high and low depending on the particular circumstances. Only a small proportion of inorganic arsenic is absorbed through the skin (Webster et al., 1993; Lowney et al., 2005). Tests on monkeys resulted in 2–6% uptake, and experiments with detached human skin resulted in 1–2% absorption over 24 hours.

Globally, the most important source of arsenic exposure comes from natural water sources, either consumed directly or extracted from soil by plants. Proof of exposure to arsenic by ingestion comes from measuring the arsenic content of hair, nails, blood or urine as biomarkers. Urine is the most reliable biomarker, and is a better measure of total exposure than analysis of drinking water (Concha et al., 2006). However, hair, nails and urine respond to arsenic exposure over different time periods and each has specific advantages. Arsenic in water may coat the skin or hair, and can confound interpretations of biomarkers.

Epidemiologists and toxicologists use standardised measures of exposure that combine the total mass of arsenic taken up by the body, independent of whether it is from air, food or water. This is then adjusted to a standard time, normally a day, and also adjusted for body mass. Thus, exposure from all three sources combined is expressed as micrograms of arsenic per kilogram of body mass per day (μg As/kg/day). Adjustment for body weight also allows scaling-up results of animal experiments to human equivalents, and helps in developing drinking water standards that reflect differences in body weight and water consumption between populations.

Another important aspect of exposure is its duration, particularly when developing safety standards for food and drink, where a lifetime exposure (70 years) is commonly assumed. This allows standards to be set simply in terms of a concentration. However, because there is a long lead-time before symptoms of arsenic poisoning develop, cumulative exposure is very important, and so epidemiological studies often measure exposure as the product of time and concentration (with units of 'mg/L.years') or simply the total mass of arsenic ingested.

5.4.2 Arsenic exposure from drinking water

Exposure to arsenic in drinking water is assessed in terms of arsenic concentrations and volumes of water consumed. The proportions of As(III) and As(V) present in groundwater vary greatly, but drinking water standards

Table 5.2   Time-weighted arsenic exposure equivalents in drinking water

Arsenic concentration (ppb)	Cumulative exposure (mg/l.years) according to number of years exposed			
	1 year	5 years	10 years	20 years
10	0.01	0.1	0.1	0.2
50	0.1	0.3	0.5	1.0
100	0.1	0.5	1.0	2.0
250	0.3	1.3	2.5	5.0
500	0.5	2.5	5.0	10.0
1000	1.0	5.0	10.0	20.0

are specified only in terms of the total quantity of arsenic. Exposure to arsenic in drinking water varies with age, gender and lifestyle. Exposure assessment should take account of both deliberate treatment and incidental changes in water chemistry between the water source and actual consumption. Epidemiological studies often assume that arsenic concentrations have remained constant over time (Steinmaus et al., 2005), however, this is not a sound assumption (e.g. Ravenscroft et al., 2006). The health effects of arsenic depend on cumulative exposure, and hence, as shown in Table 5.2, it is convenient to express exposure from water in equivalent cumulative doses.

5.4.3   Drinking water standards

Currently, the World Health Organisation (WHO) and Food and Agriculture Organisation (FAO) recommend a maximum daily intake (MDI) of inorganic As of 130 μg/day. However, average daily intakes (ADIs) recommended in some economically advanced economies vary quite significantly: USA, 53 μg/day; UK and Australia, 63 μg/day; Japan, 182 μg/day (WHO, 2001). As discussed below, the MDI is often greatly exceeded in areas of As-contaminated groundwater, where ADIs of >1,000 μg/day are not uncommon. Extreme exposure data were calculated from the tragic case of accidentally contaminated milk powder in Japan in the 1950s, where ADIs were in the range 1300–3600 μg/day, and resulted in the deaths of 130 infants (WHO, 2001). Dakeishi et al. (2006) report that even 50 years later, 600 surviving victims still suffer from symptoms including mental retardation and neurological diseases.

Until 1993, when the WHO guideline value for arsenic in drinking water was reduced from 50 to 10 ppb, most national standards were set at the same value (WHO, 1993). Since 1993, there has been considerable debate about the appropriate standard. Germany adopted a 10 ppb standard in 1996, while the EU decided to adopt the guideline in 1998, and this became effective at the end of 2003. Australia has adopted an even lower standard of 7 ppb. Guidelines for safe concentrations of chemicals in drinking water are based on assumptions of lifetime exposure, physiological characteristics and water consumption[3]. While the concept of a safe concentration is convenient in practice, standard values may not be applicable to all situations.

Consumption of drinking water increases for people living in hot climates and amongst manual labourers, and decreases in people consuming bottled drinks. Hence, many tens of millions of agricultural and other labourers in the arsenic-affected areas of Asia typically consume 3–4 L of water a day, and mostly from tubewells (Watanabe et al., 2004; Uchino et al., 2006). For these people, drinking water containing 50 ppb As considerably exceeds the MDI without any contribution from food.

In the USA, the history of the setting of standards to regulate arsenic levels in public water supply has been protracted and highly politicised. In 1962, the US Public Health Service (USPHS) recommended a 10 ppb standard, but not until 2000 did the Environmental Protection Agency (EPA) announce that the 50 ppb standard would be replaced by a more stringent standard (Table 5.3). This delay reflected the markedly increased cost of compliance, but was also a measure of the need to trade off the reliability of epidemiological evidence against the cost of implementing it. By the early 1990s, data had accumulated to justify an association between cancers and ingestion of arsenic, and to discount confounding factors such as smoking and diet. The delay led to a position in which the standard for arsenic at 50 ppb As was associated with a cancer risk of 1300–1650 per 100,000. The risk of contracting cancer from drinking water containing 50 ppb of arsenic is more than 100 times greater than for any other chemical contaminant at its respective standard (Smith, Lopipero et al., 2002).

Setting standards is complicated. First, dose–response curves are usually only available at relatively high levels of concentration and cancer risk, and therefore require extrapolation to the lower risk levels at which it is prudent to set standards for public health regulation. As Smith and Hira-Smith (2004) note, '... there is probably no population in the world sufficiently large, and with sufficient numbers of people exposed to such concentrations for the necessary decades of exposure required to establish whether ... [an] estimate is valid or not'. This means that at low concentrations and socially acceptable levels of sanctioned risk, dose–response curves are highly uncertain, confidence intervals are very wide, and potential bias in risk estimates

Table 5.3   History of USA standards for arsenic in drinking water

Date	Action
1942	US Public Health Service sets interim drinking water standard of 50 ppb As
1962	US Public Health Service identifies 10 ppb As the goal
1975	US Environmental Protection Agency adopts the interim standard of 50 ppb As set by the US Public Health Service in 1942
1986	Congress directs US Environmental Protection Agency to revise the standard by 1989
1988	US Environmental Protection Agency estimates that ingestion of 50 ppb As results in a skin cancer risk of 1 in 400
1992	Internal cancer risk estimated to be 1.3 per 100 persons at 50 ppb As
1993	World Health Organisation recommends lowering arsenic in drinking water to 10 ppb As
1996	Congress directs the US Environmental Protection Agency to propose a new drinking water standard by January 2000
1999	US National Research Council estimates cancer mortality risks to be about 1 in 100 at 50 ppb As
2000	US Environmental Protection Agency proposes standard of 5 ppb As, requests comment on 3, 10 and 20 ppb As
2001 (January)	Clinton US Environmental Protection Agency lowers the standard to 10 ppb As
2001 (March)	Bush US Environmental Protection Agency delays lowering the standard
2001 (September)	New US National Research Council report concludes that US Environmental Protection Agency underestimated cancer risks
2001 (October)	US Environmental Protection Agency announces it will adopt the standard of 10 ppb
2002 (February)	The effective date for new standard of 10 ppb As
2006	New arsenic standard implemented

Source: Smith, Lopipero et al. (2002)

increases. A common uncertainty, and one that affects arsenic, is whether there is a hormesis, or threshold effect, below which there is no adverse health effect.

Providing risk estimates appropriate for public health regulation is to enter the realm of what Weinberg (1972) termed trans-science, where the cost of acquiring the necessary evidence outweighs the benefits of knowing the answer (indeed, where the cost may be unconscionable). It has been argued that the non-linearity of dose–response relationships at low concentrations is such that alternatives are necessary to determine risk levels (Schoen et al., 2004). Such alternatives include biology-based modelling and require *in vitro* and *in vivo* (animal) experiments, but the resulting evidence is complex and often contradictory. Smith and Hira-Smith (2004) pointed out that there may be subpopulations with high susceptibility to arsenic poisoning, which implies that standards acceptable for the general population may impose unacceptable risks on subpopulations. Susceptible groups may be genetically disposed to As-induced cancer, and hence randomly distributed. However, susceptibility may be linked to malnutrition, which may be addressed through parallel public health programmes.

Finally, there is the question of the affordability of mitigation. In Bangladesh alone, the exposed populations at the 50 and 10ppb As levels are of the order of 25 and 50 million. Illness and death are not hypothetical 'risks' but are occurring in large numbers already. There is increasing evidence of clinical symptoms at concentrations of <50ppb As (e.g. Ahsan et al., 2006). The financial cost and logistical demands of mitigation are massive. Because most clinical effects follow dose–response relations, the case for risk- (i.e. concentration) based prioritisation is very strong. Some commentators have argued that it would be misguided to adopt a lower standard until the existing standard is widely achieved, fearing that scarce resources might be misdirected. An alternative case for retaining the 50ppb standard is based on the proposition that the risk from arsenic in drinking water should be proportionate to other risks to life, health and livelihood. For instance, in Bangladesh, risks from diarrhoeal disease, road accidents, loss of income, flooding and air pollution are all much higher than international averages. On the other hand, other commentators (e.g. Mukherjee et al., 2005a) allege that such arguments involve blatant double standards – essentially denying poor countries a right to good health. The case for adopting a lower standard is also supported on objective grounds where there is significant additional exposure from food. We believe that some of the arguments confuse objectives with means. The evidence to support a 10ppb standard is sufficiently strong that there is no reason to delay its adoption. However, the standard must be introduced in a carefully phased manner and on a realistic timescale.

Investments in water supply are normally assessed by cost-benefit analysis that requires placing a value on the health effects of arsenic pollution.

Maddison et al. (2005) have estimated that in Bangladesh arsenic will cause 6500 fatal cancers and 2000 non-fatal cancers[4] a year, and that this equates to an aggregate willingness-to-pay to avoid these impacts of about $2.7 billion annually using purchasing power parity (PPP) exchange rates. In the absence of the necessary studies in Bangladesh itself, this estimate was based on age-adjusted mortality rates for each additional ppb of arsenic, derived from a study by Chen and Wang (1990) in Taiwan, and on estimates of the value of a statistical life (VOSL) in India[5]. However, as Maddison et al. (2005) emphasise, it is important not to equate this annual cost of arsenic contamination with the benefits of large-scale mitigation projects, since the latency of cancers arising from their delayed development after continuing exposure to arsenic in drinking water implies that such benefits are likely to be deferred. The degree of such deferral is unknown, and would significantly influence the cost-benefit ratio.

5.4.4 Arsenic exposure from food

Arsenic in raw foodstuffs

Where shallow groundwater is contaminated, it is likely that arsenic is present in bioavailable forms in soil and irrigation water. When considering arsenic in food, two practical points of reference are the FAO/WHO MDI of 130 µg/day and the maximum hygiene standard[6] of 1000 µg/kg applied in the UK and Australia. Table 5.4 shows typical As concentrations in foodstuffs, based on market surveys in the USA. Apart from seafood, the foods

Table 5.4 Arsenic concentrations* in common foodstuffs in the USA

Foodstuff	As (µg/kg)	Foodstuff	As (µg/kg)
Beef, muscle	20	Carrots	30
Beef, liver	30	Potatoes	10
Chicken, muscle	80	Lettuce	20
Chicken, liver	80	Flour (wheat)	<10
Pork, muscle	20	Rice	160
Pork, liver	20	Corn meal	40
Eggs	30	Finfish	1470
Milk	20	Shrimp	670
Tomatoes	30	Oyster	80

*All analyses relate to uncooked food obtained from market-basket surveys.
Source: Jelinek and Corneliussen (1977)

analysed were all low in arsenic compared with the UK and Australian standards. Seafood differs from most other foods in that arsenic is mostly present as arsenobetaine, which has low acute and chronic toxicities (see Table 5.1), and is rapidly eliminated in the urine (WHO, 2001). In many As-affected areas of Asia, freshwater fish is an important component of diet. Fish kept in ponds where shallow groundwater is contaminated may be at higher risk of bioaccumulating arsenic. Liao et al. (2003) found that Tilapia kept in ponds in southwest Taiwan bioaccumulate arsenic in different fish body parts in the order: intestine > stomach > liver > gill > muscle. The bioconcentration factor for the intestine was 2270, but as they point out, simply trimming and discarding the viscera significantly reduces the health risk.

As shown in Table 5.4, rice contains higher levels of arsenic than other staple foods[7]. Rice is also central to the economies of many of the most severely arsenic-affected countries, and hence we examine this issue in detail. The proportion of inorganic As in rice differs between countries and varieties. In Bangladesh, Smith, Lee et al. (2006) reported that arsenic was 87% inorganic in rice and 96% inorganic in vegetables, while Williams et al. (2005) reported that the inorganic-As content of *aman* rice was 85–94% and *boro* rice[8] was 91–99%. However, Chinese rice with a similar total arsenic content (220 μg/kg) contained only 37% inorganic As. Williams et al. (2006) found that As concentrations in other foodstuffs, even though predominantly inorganic, were generally lower than in rice, and when adjusted for dietary intake make a small contribution to arsenic exposure. In the USA, the As content of rice varies regionally: in the south-central area, where soils were extensively polluted by arsenical pesticides, the median grain content was 270 μg/kg compared with 160 μg/kg in California (Williams et al., 2007).

Arsenic exposure from cooked rice

Cooking rice can either increase or decrease exposure. The As concentrations in rice grain are highest where the concentrations in water are also high, and this has knock-on implications for exposure through eating cooked rice (Misbahuddin, 2003). Two key factors are the As concentration of the cooking water and whether the rice is cooked in an excess of water. Some cultures add only a minimum quantity of water to the cooking pot, while others (e.g. large parts of Bangladesh and West Bengal) add an excess of water which is discarded after cooking. For example, Bae et al. (2002) noted water to rice weight ratios of 3.2:1 to 4.0:1 in Bangladesh, compared with only 1.3:1 in Japan. Because raw rice always contains significant amounts of arsenic, a simple matrix of outcomes (Table 5.5) defines the potential for

Table 5.5   Exposure outcomes of cooking rice

Volume of water added	Arsenic in cooking water	
	Present	Absent
No excess	Maximum exposure, equal to sum of arsenic in raw rice and initial water added	Exposure same as content in raw rice
Excess	Arsenic exposure may be increased or reduced relative to raw rice	Arsenic content in consumed food may be significantly reduced

cooking to either exacerbate or mitigate arsenic exposure. Below, we examine the evidence that seeks to quantify these effects.

In West Bengal, Roychowdhury et al. (2002) found the average As concentrations of 27 samples of raw rice and 18 samples of cooked rice were 259 and 569 µg/kg respectively, implying that cooking more than doubled exposure. The differences were seen in all four villages surveyed and suggest that cooking has a major adverse impact on As exposure. In northwest Bangladesh, Bae et al. (2002) asked villagers to cook local rice (IRRI-20) in their normal way, but carefully monitored the quantities and arsenic contents of water and rice. Raw rice containing 173 µg/kg cooked in water containing 223 to 372 ppb As, increased in arsenic content by 57% to 84% after cooking.

In Bangladesh, Rahman, Hasegawa et al. (2006) demonstrated the effects of parboiling[9] and cooking on arsenic consumption for two common rice varieties (BRRI-28 and BRRI Hybrid) collected from high-As (Satkhira) and low-As (Sreepur) areas. The As content of raw rice varied more between areas than either between varieties or with the effect of parboiling. Both the rice and the tubewell-water used for cooking from Satkhira (630 µg/kg and 130 ppb As) contained much more arsenic than in Sreepur (225 µg/kg and 10 ppb As). In the laboratory, 50 g of rice was cooked in either 100 ml of water that was entirely absorbed, or in 250 ml water, of which 100 ml was discarded as gruel. The results (Table 5.6) proved that rice cooked in limited water gains arsenic, but rice cooked in excess water always loses arsenic. However, the results differed between the high-As and low-As areas. In the low-As area, the changes were small, but in the high-As area the changes were dramatic but could be either beneficial or harmful, depending on the cooking method. The effect of parboiling also differed between the high- and low-As areas. In the low-As area, parboiling slightly reduced the As-content of rice, but in the high-As area, it added to the As-content of rice.

Table 5.6   Average arsenic concentrations* in raw and cooked rice and gruel in Bangladesh

Area	Pre-treatment	Raw rice	Cooked in limited water[†]	Cooked in excess water[†]	Gruel
		Arsenic concentration (µg/kg dry wt)			
Low-As water area (10 ppb)	Parboiled	230	250	220	280
			109%	96%	
	Not parboiled		290	230	350
			126%	100%	
High-As water area (130 ppb)	Parboiled	630	990	490	1470
			157%	78%	
	Not parboiled		920	420	1680
			146%	67%	

*Each number is the average of BRRI28 and BRRI hybrid samples from the same area and pre-treatment.
[†]Percentages express the As content of cooked rice relative to raw rice.
Source: Data from Rahman, Hasegawa et al. (2006)

If it is assumed that the arsenic in rice was 85% inorganic, and that adults consume 350 g of parboiled rice a day, the ADI from rice alone in the low-As area would be around 80% of the MDI. In the high-As area, the ADI from rice would be 221 or 442 µg/day As (three times the MDI) depending on the cooking method. These findings suggest that cooking with excess water, even As-polluted water, substantially reduces As exposure, provided that the gruel is discarded. Cooking As-rich rice with As-free water, such as pond water, should reduce human exposure even further, and as a practical measure Sengupta et al. (2006b) have already demonstrated a new rice cooker that combines energy efficiency with the benefits of reduced arsenic content.

5.4.5   Combined exposure from food and water

The physiological and dietary habits assumed in determining food and water safety standards may not be appropriate to all cultures. The standard WHO calculation scheme, based on a 60 kg adult drinking 2.5 L of water a day, will underestimate exposure for manual labourers in hot countries. In Bangladesh, the ADI of rice in rural areas has consistently been around 480 g/day, but has declined to 380 g/day in urban areas (Hossain, Khan et al., 2005). Consider the case of an agricultural labourer in Bangladesh who drinks 4 L/day of As-free water and eats 480 g/day of rice that is half

$aman$[10] (152 µg/kg) and half $boro$ (219 µg/kg) rice, where the arsenic is 85% inorganic. With no transfer to or from cooking water, the ADI from rice would be 89 µg/day (68% of the MDI). However, if our hypothetical labourer lives in a severely As-affected area and drinks contaminated water (200 ppb As) and eats local rice ($aman$ 357 µg/kg; $boro$ 475 µg/kg), his As intake from rice alone would be 200 µg/day (154% of MDI) and from drinking water 800 µg/day. If the rice was cooked in a limited volume of this water, his arsenic intake would be over 1000 µg/day, more than ten times the MDI.

Case history 1: West Bengal

Uchino et al. (2006) investigated the total dietary intake of arsenic in 37 families from Murshidabad District. They analysed the As content of rice and vegetables eaten by each family, and water from the 14 tubewells used. Hair and urine samples were analysed to confirm actual exposure, and a dermatologist examined each person to identify arsenical skin manifestations (ASM). To calculate total exposure they assumed that adult males drank 4 L of water a day, adult females 3 L, and children 2 L. Adults were assumed to eat 750 g of rice[11] and 500 g of vegetables a day; and children to eat 400 g and 300 g respectively. Arsenic in rice was assumed to be 70% inorganic[12]. While this analysis is based on a snapshot and may change over time, it probably gives a reasonable picture of the general pattern of exposure, except that in the long run, As concentrations in rice will increase but will decrease in groundwater (Chapter 3).

Initially, Uchino et al. (2006) assumed that drinking water would be the main source of exposure and, indeed, found a correlation between arsenic in water in both urine and hair. However, while the relation between arsenic in water and the prevalence of ASM was statistically significant, they were surprised to detect arsenicosis in 29% of people drinking water with <10 ppb As. In fact, they determined that food contributed 67% of the total arsenic intake (Table 5.7). The ADI for people with ASM was 424 µg/day and of

Table 5.7   Arsenical skin manifestations (ASM) by total daily intake* in West Bengal

	Daily intake of inorganic arsenic (µg/day)			
	<130	130–250	250–500	>500
Number of persons	27	54	40	26
Number showing ASM	2	17	15	16
Incidence of ASM	7%	31%	38%	62%

*Average daily intake was calculated as the sum of inorganic As in rice, vegetables and water.
Source: Uchino et al. (2006)

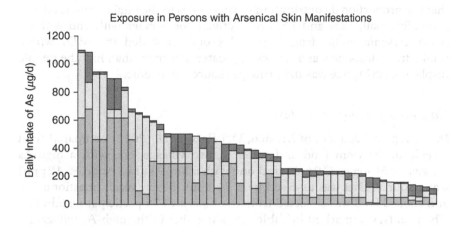

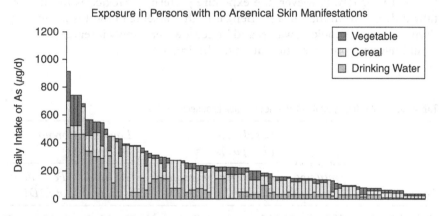

Figure 5.2   Contributions of food and water to arsenic exposure in West Bengal. The stacked bars sum to the total daily intake of arsenic from vegetables, cereal and water. The upper graph shows the higher level of current exposure in people displaying skin lesions, while both show the importance of exposure from food. *Source*: After Uchino et al. (2006)

those without was 245 μg/day. The lowest ADI consumed by an individual with ASM was 112 μg/day, close to the FAO/WHO MDI of 130 μg/day.

The combined effect of arsenic intake from water and food is further illustrated in Figure 5.2, which shows the intake from each source for each person examined, with the individuals being classified according to whether or not they displayed ASM. Although the highest intakes all included a major contribution from drinking water, in most cases the contribution from food is higher than that from water. Uchino et al. (2006) also found that the proportional contribution of vegetables to the intake from food was generally small, 12% and 16% respectively for persons with and without ASM. Arsenic intake from vegetables only exceeded the MDI where intake from drinking water was even greater. For more than half the people displaying ASM, rice was the principal source of arsenic.

Case history 2: northern Mexico

In the region Lagunera of Mexico, Del Razo et al. (2002) compared total arsenic intake from food and water in two villages, one with a high-As (Lagos de Moreno, 410 ppb) and one with a low-As (Los Angeles, 12 ppb) water source. Diet was assessed by a 24-hour dietary recall questionnaire, and cooked food was collected from the houses of 25 participating adults[13]. The results, summarised in Table 5.8, show that in the high-As village, As intakes from both food and water greatly exceeded the FAO/WHO guideline of 130 µg/day. However, the exposure pattern in Mexico is fundamentally different from that in West Bengal in that arsenic in food is principally derived from the cooking water, and hence a water-supply intervention here would have a more dramatic public health impact.

Table 5.8   Total dietary intake of arsenic in Region Lagunera, Mexico

Food stuff	Daily food consumption (g)	Los Angeles (12 ppb As)		Lagos de Moreno (410 ppb As)	
		As intake (µg/day)	Percentage of MDI	As intake (µg/day)	Percentage of MDI
Pinto beans	400	12	9	244	188
Tortillas	221	20	15	75	58
Eggs	52	1	1	8	6
Potato	112	2	2	18	14
Sauce	28	1	1	10	8
Pasta soup	99	3	2	80	62
All food	912	39	30	435	335
As-intake from water and drinks (µg/day)		24	19	666	512
Total Arsenic intake (µg/day)		63	49	1,101	847

MDI, the WHO/FAO recommended maximum daily intake of 130 µg/day.
Source: Del Razo et al. (2002)

Case history 3: northern Chile

Diaz et al. (2004) undertook a study of total dietary intake of arsenic in the village of Chiu Chiu in northern Chile, near the confluence of the Rio Loa and the Rio Salado (see Chapter 10). People had consumed water containing 600–800 ppb As for many years, and there was known to be a high prevalence of skin lesions amongst men. Sampling of foods and dietary surveys were carried out before and after the water supply was switched from a source containing 572 ppb As to a tankered supply containing 41 ppb As. Raw food was collected and cooked in the laboratory according to local practice, with distilled water and both the old and new water supplies. In nearly all the major foods, arsenic was >80% inorganic. Their results show that, despite variations in the As-content of raw foods, the effect of cooking with different qualities of water is significant. Table 5.9 confirms that cooking in distilled water reduced the arsenic content of food, and cooking in contaminated water increased it, except where vegetables (e.g. potato, carrot and beetroot) were peeled before boiling. The maize results were surprising in that cooking with the slightly contaminated water produced negligible change, but the highly contaminated water produced a massive increase in arsenic. Beans were only sampled in the second round, but resulted in a large proportional increase in As content. By comparison with the findings for Pinto beans in Mexico noted above, this suggests

Table 5.9   Effect of cooking (by boiling) on arsenic content of food in northern Chile*

Food	Water (ppb As)	Total As (µg/kg)	Inorganic As (µg/kg)	Inorganic As† (%)	Gain in cooking (%)
Beans	0	7	7	100	−70
	41	57	48	84	109
Maize	0	30	30	100	200
	0	89	70	79	−36
	41	117	107	91	−3
	572	1580	1420	90	14,100
Potatoes	0	04	04	100	−83
(peeled)	41	11	12	109	−50
	572	110	90	82	0

*First sampling, before change in water supply; second sampling, after change in water supply.
†Percentages >100% are artefacts of the analytical procedures.
Source: Diaz et al. (2004)

Table 5.10   Total dietary intake of arsenic in a village in northern Chile

Age group	Source	Period 1 (Water: 572 ppb As)		Period 2 (Water: 41 ppb As)	
		Total As (μg/day)	Inorganic As (μg/day)	Total As (μg/day)	Inorganic As (μg/day)
13–15 years	Food*	56	47	34	30
	Food + water	1435	1443	132	125
>20 years	Food	69	58	39	38
	Food + water	1400	1378	131	125

*This figure is assumed to be the contribution of raw food.
Source: Diaz et al. (2004)

that beans cooked in contaminated water contribute significantly to As-exposure in Chile also.

Diaz et al. (2004) assembled the data on food quality and consumption and water use (2.3 L/day) in order to assess total dietary intake of arsenic. The data were classified according to age group, although little difference was apparent, and are shown in Table 5.10. Under the pre-existing water supply, the ADI was more than ten times the FAO/WHO MDI. However, the improved water supply resulted in an order of magnitude reduction. Dangerous levels of arsenic were derived predominantly from water, but both by direct consumption and through cooking.

5.5   Acute Arsenic Poisoning

Acute arsenic poisoning is not normally associated with environmental exposure through food or water, and is much more commonly associated with accidents or deliberate poisoning. Acute poisoning takes two forms: acute paralytic syndrome and acute gastrointestinal syndrome (WHO, 2001). Acute paralytic syndrome involves either cardiovascular collapse or depression of the central nervous system, and can cause death within hours. Acute gastrointestinal syndrome, which is more common, involves violent vomiting, diarrhoea, dehydration and internal ruptures, and may be followed by failure of multiple organs. Death is likely to follow, but can be slow, and may be prevented by gastric and bowel irrigation and chelation therapy. Vantroyen et al. (2004) described the survival of a 27-year-old woman who had ingested 9 g arsenic trioxide and developed symptoms including gastrointestinal cramps, vomiting, diarrhoea and disturbed liver function. She was treated by gastric irrigation and intestinal cleansing with sodium bicarbonate and polyethyleneglycol, followed by chelation therapy to enhance methylation of arsenic. A year later, her symptoms were limited to polyneuropathy.

5.6   Dermatological Manifestations

The most common and readily diagnostic features of arsenic poisoning are various forms of keratosis or hyper- and hypopigmentation (ATSDR, 2005). Keratosis is an overgrowth of the outermost layer of the skin that produces corn-like elevations on the hands and feet, typically 0.4–1.0 cm across and nodular (Tondel et al., 1999). Some of these symptoms are illustrated in photographs of victims of arsenic poisoning from West Bengal in Figure 5.3. Each of the symptoms has been classified into subcategories by Saha (2003).

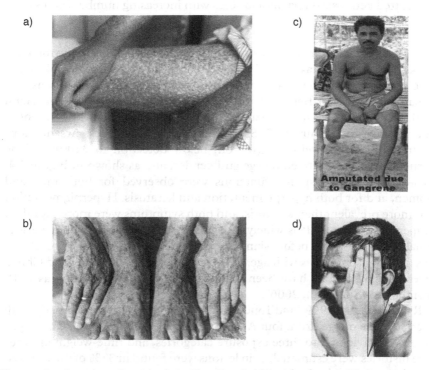

Figure 5.3   Symptoms of arsenicosis in West Bengal: (a) leuco-melanoma; (b) dorsal keratosis; (c) amputation due to gangrene; (d) multiple squamous cell carcinoma.
Source: All photographs courtesy of Dr Dipankar Chakraborti, SOES, Jadavpur University, Kolkata, West Bengal, and with the expressed permission of the individuals.

Hyperpigmentation, which is especially marked on the unexposed parts of the body, takes the following common forms:

- melanosis
- leucomelanosis
- diffuse melanosis on palms
- spotted melanosis on trunk ('raindrop' pigmentation)
- generalised melanosis

Keratosis takes the following forms, generally associated with both increasing exposure and discomfort:

- diffuse keratosis on palms and soles
- partial keratosis, only on the soles of the feet
- severe keratosis, on both the soles and palms
- dorsal keratosis, on the upper parts of the hands or feet
- spotted keratosis on palms and soles with increasing numbers and size of nodules

Bowen's disease[14], a pre-cancerous form of skin lesion only in the top layer of skin, is commonly associated with advanced stages of arsenic poisoning. The association between arsenic in drinking water and skin lesions was documented in West Bengal in the early 1980s by Saha (1984) and Garai et al. (1984). Later, Guha Mazumder et al. (1998) derived dose–response relationships by examining 7683 persons from 57 villages. Arsenic concentrations in 644 wells ranged from below detection to 3400 ppb. The participants were stratified by age and gender, and as shown in Figure 5.4, well-defined dose–response functions were observed for both men and women, and for both hyperpigmentation and keratosis. Hyperpigmentation was more prevalent than keratosis, and both symptoms were more prevalent in men than women. It is widely recognised that there is a latency period, usually of 2–10 years, before skin lesions are developed, and the prevalence of skin lesions increases with age. However, in both West Bengal and China, arsenical skin lesions have been diagnosed in children as young as 6–18 months old (Sun et al., 2006).

Rahman et al. (1999) and Tondel et al. (1999) examined 1595 people, all over 30 years of age, from four As-affected areas of Bangladesh. The population was divided into three exposure categories, and time-weighted exposure histories were estimated. Skin lesions were found in 33% of the exposed population, roughly double the prevalence of keratosis or hyperpigmentation observed by Guha Mazumder et al. (1998) in West Bengal (although in the latter study, 60% of the population were under 30). Here also, the age-adjusted prevalence of skin lesions was greater in men (30.1%) than in

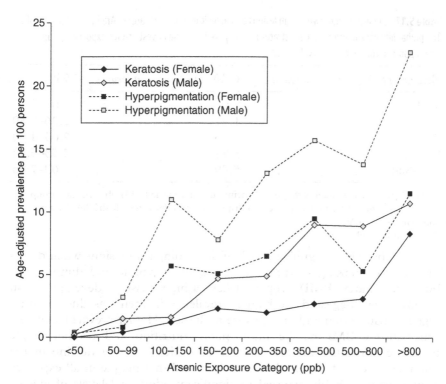

Figure 5.4   Prevalence of keratosis and hyperpigmentation in West Bengal. Keratosis (see Figure 5.3b) is a more severe condition than hyperpigmentation. Both conditions are more prevalent at all concentrations in men than in women.
Source: Data from Guha Majumder et al. (1998)

women (26.1%), and followed a dose–response relationship that was independent of gender.

Rahman, Vahter et al. (2006) found lower prevalence of skin lesions when they surveyed the entire population (166,934 people) of Matlab upazila, 50 km southeast of Dhaka. Groundwater was highly contaminated, with 61% of hand tubewells containing >50 ppb and 9% >500 ppb As. Nevertheless, the crude prevalence of lesions was only 0.3%. Although no dose–response function was reported, they found that hyperpigmentation and keratosis were more prevalent in men than women, and at a maximum (0.61%) in the age range 35–44 years. It should be noted that this, and the other studies cited above, considered only exposure through drinking water and not total dietary exposure.

The most detailed assessment of skin lesions in Bangladesh was a cross-sectional analysis of a population of 11,746 in Araihazar by Ahsan et al. (2006). As shown in Table 5.11, there is not only a strong dose–response

Table 5.11   Association between skin lesions and arsenic in drinking water in Araihazar, Bangladesh. The probability of skin lesions in each stratum is compared with the lowest arsenic exposure group (< 8.1 ppb): CI, confidence interval

Arsenic (ppb) in drinking water	Odds ratio* for skin lesions	95% CI
<8.1	1.0	1.0
8.1–40	1.91	1.26–2.89
40–91	3.03	2.05–4.50
91–175	3.71	2.53–5.44
175–864	5.39	3.69–7.86

*An odds ratio of 1.91 means that people drinking water in the 8–40 ppb exposure group were almost twice (1.91 times) as likely to display skin lesions as people drinking water containing <8 ppb As.
Source: Ahsan et al. (2006)

function, but also a significant risk of developing skin lesions when drinking water containing <50 ppb As. Males, older people and thinner (low body mass index; BMI) people all have a higher risk of developing skin lesions. They suggested the higher prevalence in men was due to either higher consumption and/or exposure to the sun. Higher prevalence in persons with low BMI may be due to poorer nutrition, and in older people might be attributed to less effective detoxification or a decline in the immune system. It should, however, be noted that people in all exposure groups were probably exposed to significant additional levels of arsenic from food.

In China, Yang et al. (2002) reported different prevalences of skin lesions between Xinjiang and Inner Mongolia provinces (Figure 5.5). In all cases, there was a well-defined, and nearly parallel, dose–response trend. In Xinjiang there was a threshold concentration of about 200 ppb As. However, in four out of five studies in Inner Mongolia, although the dose–response data project towards the origin (suggesting no threshold), no symptoms were identified at concentrations of <50 ppb As. In the Chifeng study, the data indicate no threshold, and imply an additional source (food?) of As intake. Guo et al. (2006) compared the prevalence of skin lesions in two villages in Inner Mongolia, finding that for persons drinking water with 51–100 ppb As, the odds ratio (OR)[15] for developing skin lesions was 15.5, for water with 101–150 ppb it was 16.1, and for water with >150 ppb the OR rose to 25.7. Also in Inner Mongolia, Lamm et al. (2006b) identified thresholds of 30 to 50 ppb As for the onset of skin lesions, but noted that skin cancers were detected only in persons who had been exposed to >150 ppb As and had developed either hyperkeratosis or hypopigmentation.

Summarising many studies, ATSDR (2005) concluded that the appearance of skin lesions is the most appropriate indicator for establishing a chronic

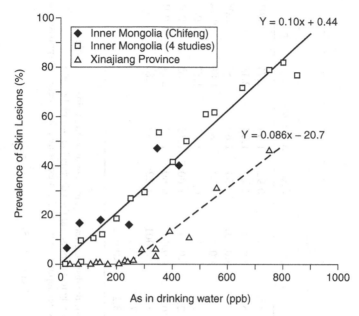

Figure 5.5   Prevalence of skin lesions in Inner Mongolia and Xinjiang Provinces, China. Four of the five studies from Inner Mongolia showed similar results and have been pooled, while the fifth (Chifeng) is plotted separately.
Source: Yang et al. (2002)

minimum risk level (MRL), and that vascular, hepatic and neurological disease have similar thresholds. Based mainly on a study of 17,000 people in Taiwan by Tseng et al. (1961), they derived a chronic MRL of inorganic arsenic of 0.3 μg/kg/day, equivalent to 18 μg/day for a 60 kg adult.

5.7   Carcinogenic Effects

There is a large amount of evidence that long-term exposure to arsenic in drinking water causes a wide variety of cancers. Ingested arsenic has been suspected as a cause of lung cancer since as early as 1879, and of skin cancer since 1888 (Smith et al., 1992). In the BFD-endemic areas of Taiwan, Chen et al. (1988) followed a cohort of 871 BFD patients from 1968 to 1984, and found that standardised mortality rates (SMR) from lung, liver, kidney, bladder and skin cancers were elevated compared with the Taiwanese population. Wu et al. (1989) monitored residents of 42 villages from the 1960s, classified the villages by arsenic concentration, and obtained causes of death from death certificates. They found that the age-adjusted mortality

Table 5.12 Standard mortality ratios (SMR) for various cancers in Taiwan, Chile and Argentina

Cancer	Sex	Taiwan (Blackfoot Disease endemic area)				Chile (Antofagasta)*		Argentina†			
		<300 ppb	300–599 ppb	>600 ppb	p	SMR	p	Low	Medium	High	p
Lung	M	2.5	5.2	5.4	<0.001	3.8	<0.001	0.92	1.54	1.77	<0.001
	F	3.9	6.4	12.9	<0.001	3.1	<0.001	1.24	1.34	2.16	<0.001
Liver	M	1.7	2.4	3.1	<0.05	–	<0.001	1.54	1.80	1.84	0.06
	F	2.4	2.7	3.6	NS	–	<0.001	1.69	1.87	1.89	0.14
Kidney	M	7.6	17.2	23.0	<0.05	1.6	0.012	0.87	1.33	1.57	<0.001
	F	3.8	21.6	64.4	<0.001	2.7	<0.001	1.00	1.36	1.81	<0.001
Bladder	M	7.3	19.7	29.9	<0.001	6.0	<0.001	0.80	1.28	2.14	<0.001
	F	18.3	40.7	79.5	<0.001	8.2	<0.001	1.22	1.39	1.81	<0.001
Skin	M	2.0	13.4	35.0	<0.001	7.7	<0.001				
	F	1.1	6.7	10.1	<0.001	3.2	<0.001				

NS, not significant.

*Although not classified by concentration, almost all exposed persons obtained the drinking water from a common municipal source that contained around 850 ppb As between 1958 and 1970, which dropped suddenly to 110 ppb, and then declined to 40 ppb by 1988.

†The high exposure group was assigned a concentration of 178 ppb As, and water supplies in the medium exposure group were >120 ppb As. No clear relation with skin cancer was identified.

Sources: Chen et al. (1988); Wu et al. (1989); Hopenhayn-Rich et al. (1998); Smith et al. (1998)

rates for lung, liver, kidney and bladder cancers correlated with exposure for both men and women. Increased cancer rates have been associated with As ingestion in Chile and Argentina (Bates et al., 2004). Table 5.12 compares the analyses from Taiwan, Chile and Argentina. However, when comparing the data, it is important to appreciate the significance of the different methods. The Chilean data set is from a single city with a single source of water supply. The Argentinean analysis was based on a compilation of county data (section 10.2.1). The Taiwan data set differed again, being derived from actual exposure information. Thus while the data are expressed in similar statistical form, the chemical and demographic bases of the classes differ significantly. Thus the comparison should be treated with caution. These reservations aside, the dose–response effect appears to be particularly strong in the Taiwan data set.

Evaluating all available cancer studies in order to justify a possible change to the USA drinking water standard, NRC (1999, 2001) concluded that a linear dose–response curve should be adopted, and that the risk of death from cancer is approximately 1 in 500 at 10 ppb, 1 in 100 at 50 ppb and 1 in 10 at 500 ppb As (Smith at al., 2007).

The epidemiological studies of lung and bladder cancer in Taiwan were updated by Lamm et al. (2006a), who found that results from some townships were confounded by non-arsenic related causes of cancer, and by selection bias towards areas where BFD was endemic. After removing the confounding data, they found better defined dose–response relationships for both lung and bladder cancer (Figure 5.6). The prevalence of both cancers was higher amongst men than women. Because the existence of a threshold (hormesis) effect had been considered controversial (e.g. Smith, Lopipero et al., 2002), it was significant that the new dose–response relationships defined distinct threshold effects for both cancers. The upper As concentrations corresponding to no increased risk of bladder cancer were 125 ppb for men and 163 ppb As for women; and for lung cancer were 117 and 217 ppb respectively.

Studies of cancer epidemiology have not yet been completed for Bangladesh or West Bengal. However, using dose–response data from Taiwan, Chen and Ahsan (2004) estimated that there will be at least a doubling of lifetime mortality from liver, bladder and lung cancers (230 vs 104 per 100,000 population) for the whole of Bangladesh due to arsenic in drinking water. This estimate is a warning both of the consequences of inaction, and also of the delayed burden of disease that is likely to develop in coming decades. This is also a warning for countries such as Nepal, Myanmar, Cambodia and Vietnam where exposure is high but only mild symptoms of arsenicosis have been recorded. In these countries, the low prevalence of disease is believed to be due to the short duration of exposure, and may disguise the future cancer burden.

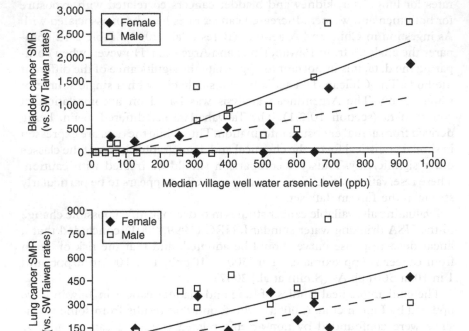

Figure 5.6   Dose–response relationships for lung and bladder cancer by gender in Taiwan. (a) Bladder cancer: males $-Y = 2.75X + 243$, $r^2 = 0.68$, $p = <0.001$; females $-Y = 1.33X + 117$, $r^2 = 0.49$, $p = 0.001$. (b) Lung cancer: males $-Y = 0.536X + 37.5$, $r^2 = 0.40$, $p = 0.003$; females $-Y = 0.371X + 19.4$, $r^2 = 0.52$, $p = <0.001$. SMR, standardised mortality ratio. Both graphs show data after removal of confounding data. The solid line is the best-fit to the male data, and the dashed line is the best-fit to the female data. *Source*: Lamm et al. (2006a)

5.8   Systemic Non-carcinogenic Effects

Arsenic exposure has been linked to a wide range of non-dermatological and non-carcinogenic medical conditions, albeit sometimes with less certainty (Guha Mazumder, 2003) and with widely varying degrees of severity. These ailments may be found preferentially in As-exposed populations but can also be caused by unrelated factors. Below, we review the impacts of some of the more important or better-defined[16] ailments that have been causally associated with As-exposure, including peripheral vascular disease, respiratory illness, cardio- and cerebro-vascular disease, diabetes mellitus, peripheral neuropathy, neurosensory effects and effects on pregnancy. Early stages of arsenic poisoning are widely associated with muscular weakness, lethargy and anaemia. Arsenic has also been linked to other effects that are not described here, but include conjunctivitis, keratitis (inflammation and swelling of the cornea), rhinitis (inflammation of the mucous membranes of the nose), gastrointestinal disease, haematological abnormalities, dysosmia (disorder in the sense of smell), perceptive hearing loss, cataracts, hepatomegaly (enlargement of the liver) with portal zone fibrosis, nephropathy (damage to or disease of the kidney) and solid oedema of the limbs (excess fluid between tissue cells). For more information the reader is referred to the compilations by NRC (1999, 2001), UN (2001), WHO (2001) and ATSDR (2005).

5.8.1   Peripheral vascular disease

The best known vascular disease associated with arsenic is Blackfoot Disease (BFD), characteristic of the As-affected area of southwest Taiwan, but hardly recognised in other As-affected regions[17], including northeast Taiwan (WHO, 2001). According to Chen et al. (1994), BFD starts with spotted discolouration on the skin of the extremities, especially the feet, which change from white to brown and to black. The skin then thickens, cracks and ulcerates, often ending with amputation to save the victims' life. Blackfoot Disease was first recorded in southwest Taiwan in the 1930s and peaked between 1956 and 1960 as groundwater use increased, with prevalences of 6.5–19 per 1000 being recorded in affected villages (Tseng, 2005). In a population of >40,000, Tseng (1977) identified 428 cases of skin cancer and 370 of BFD. Sixty-one people had both conditions, whereas if the conditions were unconnected the expected number would be only four. Chen et al. (1988) reported a significant dose–response relation, and a relation to nutritional status where the risk of BFD is inversely related to the frequency of eating eggs, meat and vegetables, but directly related to consumption of sweet potato. Tseng et al. (1996) also reported a dose–response relationship in well-waters containing up to 1100 ppb As. The odds ratio for cumulative exposure of 1–19 mg/L.years was 3.1, and for >20 mg/L.years was 4.8.

Because BFD is absent in northeast Taiwan, it was suspected that other factors operate in the endemic area. Lu (1990) suggested that BFD was caused by fluorescent humic substances in water, from which he isolated organo-metallic complexes containing As, Fe, Mn, Pb, Cd, Cu, Zn and Ni. Later, Chen et al. (1994) determined that although Co, Cr, Fe, Hg, P, Pb, Sb, Zn, Na, K and Ba are all more abundant than in non-endemic areas, only manganese exceeded drinking water guidelines, and thus rejected the suggestion of Lu (1990), concluding that arsenic was 'still the primary suspect'. The debate continues (Tseng, 2005).

Table 5.13　Dose–response relationship for microvascular disease in Taiwan

	Prevalence of microvascular disease per 100	
Arsenic in drinking water (ppb)	Non-diabetic persons	Diabetic patients
<100	7.51	16.41
100–300	6.59	15.85
300–600	8.02	21.69
>600	11.82	28.31

Source: Chiou et al. (2005)

Other vascular diseases are also associated with As exposure. In southwest Taiwan, Chiou et al. (2005) found a significant relationship between arsenic and microvascular diseases that affect the fine blood vessels and capillaries, leading to loss of sensation and foot ulcers. As shown in Table 5.13, the relationship is even stronger in diabetic patients. Also, Pershagen (1983) noted high prevalences of peripheral vascular diseases in Antofagasta (Chile), which included Raynaud's symptom and acrocyanosis[18], and affected 31% of patients with ASM.

5.8.2　Respiratory illnesses

An increased risk of lung cancer resulting from exposure to arsenic was noted in section 5.7. Guha Mazumder et al. (2000) and von Ehrenstein et al. (2005) investigated the assumption that lung carcinogens also cause chronic respiratory disease. They conducted interviews with, and clinical examinations of, the same group of 7,683 people in West Bengal who had participated in the earlier study of skin lesions (section 5.6). After excluding 819 smokers, and having already classified dermatological symptoms and analysed the drinking water, the participants were divided into two groups: the first having skin lesions, and the second having normal skin and drinking water with <50 ppb As. Thus, by reference to the frequency of coughs, shortness of breath and chest sounds[19], they confirmed the chronic damaging effects of arsenic on the lungs (Table 5.14). By conducting physical tests, they also demonstrated that the lung function of men with skin lesions was very significantly reduced. These results are important because they are risk factors for more serious forms of lung disease. Other studies (e.g. Steinmaus et al., 2003) have found increased cancer risks amongst people drinking As-contaminated water who also smoke. Smoking is both a confounding factor in attributing cause, and a contributory factor to developing respiratory illnesses. Smith, Marshall et al. (2006) have demonstrated that, in Chile, even childhood exposure can cause fatal bronchiectasis in adults.

Table 5.14 Prevalence of respiratory illness in West Bengal

	Male		*Female*	
Symptom	*Odds ratio**	*95% CI*	*Odds ratio**	*95% CI*
Cough	5.0	2.6	7.8	3.1
		9.9		19.5
Chest sounds	6.9	3.1	9.6	4.0
		15.0		22.9
Shortness of breath	3.7	1.3	23.2	5.8
		10.6		92.8

CI, confidence interval.
*The odds ratio (OR) is the ratio of ratios of affected and unaffected persons in each group. In practice, an OR of 2 means that people in the studied group are twice as likely to be afflicted as in the control group.
Source: Guha Mazumder et al. (2000)

5.8.3 Cardio- and cerebrovascular disease

Cardiovascular disease (CVD), the leading cause of death worldwide, is underlain by arteriosclerosis (hardening of the arteries), and As-exposure is considered to be a risk factor for arteriosclerosis. In Taiwan, increases in CVD were identified in both affected areas, but a dose–response relationship was found only in the non-BFD endemic area, where the relative risk of ischaemic heart disease rose to 3.3 for a cumulative exposure of 10–20 mg/L. years, and 4.9 at >20 mg/L.years (WHO, 2001). In a cross-sectional study in Bangladesh, Rahman et al. (1999) found a similar association with hypertension (high blood pressure) where the prevalence ratio rose from 2.2 for a cumulative exposure of 5–10 mg/L.years to 3.0 at >10 mg/L.years. A review by Navas–Acien et al. (2005) concluded that high exposure data from Taiwan provide strong evidence that As exposure plays a role in arteriosclerosis, even though the quantitative relationship is not well defined. However, they judged that it is 'plausible' that low-level arsenic exposure contributes to arteriosclerosis. Arsenic may cause CVD even after exposure ends. In a retrospective analysis of the Antofagasta incident (Chapter 10), Yuan et al. (2007) concluded that arsenic caused 60% more deaths from heart attacks after the 13-year period of high-exposure (800 ppb) than during it.

Chiou et al. (1997, cited in WHO, 2001) found that in the non-BFD endemic area of northeast Taiwan, the dose–response relationship was even stronger when patients with cerebral infarction were analysed separately (Table 5.15).

Table 5.15   Dose–response relation for cardiovascular disease and cerebral infarction in Taiwan

	Odds ratio	
Arsenic exposure (ppb As)	*Cardiovascular disease*	*Cerebral infarction*
<0.1	1.0	1.0
0.1–50	2.5	3.4
50–299	2.8	4.5
≥300	3.6	6.9

Source: WHO (2001)

5.8.4   Diabetes mellitus

Dose–response relationships between cumulative As exposure in drinking water and the prevalence of diabetes mellitus have been found in Taiwan[20] and Bangladesh. In southwest Taiwan, Lai et al. (1994) determined ORs of 6.6 and 10.0 in diabetes mellitus patients who had consumed 0.1 and >15 mg/L.years of arsenic. In Bangladesh, using the simple test for glucosuria as a proxy, Rahman et al. (1998, 1999) divided the study group into zero, low, medium and high exposure groups (<5, 5–10 and >10 mg/L. years) and also according to whether skin lesions were present or not. Dose–response functions were found in both groups, but for those people displaying skin lesions, the age-adjusted prevalence ratios were 1.1, 2.2 and 2.6. On the other hand, for those who did not have skin lesions, the equivalent ratios were only 0.8, 1.4 and 1.4. Nurun Nabi et al. (2005) confirmed the connection between arsenic and diabetes in Bangladesh, finding that diabetes mellitus was 2.8 times more prevalent in a group of 115 people with an average As exposure of 7.6 years than in a control group.

5.8.5   Peripheral neuropathy and neurosensory effects

Peripheral neuropathy, of which there are more than 100 types, describes damage to the peripheral nervous system, which transmits information from the brain and spinal cord to every other part of the body. Its symptoms range from temporary numbness, tingling and pricking sensations to burning pain, muscle wasting and paralysis (www.ninds.nih.gov). Peripheral neuropathy may be inherited or acquired, and exposure to arsenic is just one of many risk factors. Peripheral neuropathy has commonly been described in cases of occupational exposure to arsenic (ATSDR, 2005), and has also been related to drinking contaminated well-water in West Bengal (Guha Mazumder et al., 1988) and Xinjiang Province of China (Lianfang and Jhianzong, 1994). In Inner Mongolia, to detect the subclinical changes in neurological function that precede peripheral neuropathy, Li, Xia et al. (2006a) and Otto et al. (2006) classified 321 people into three exposure groups: low (<20 ppb), medium (100–300 ppb) and high (400–700 ppb As). They found that exposure to >400 ppb As increased sensitivity to pain at a much lower threshold than indicated earlier (1 000 ppb) by NRC (1999). However, the subclinical effects of neurological function were only observed at exposure levels well above those associated with increased risk for cancer and arsenical skin lesions.

5.8.6   Influence on pregnancy and child birth

The first possible link between arsenic in drinking water and infant deaths was identified by Wyllie (1937) in Canada, where three of four children died immediately after birth in a family where the father died of arsenic poisoning, and the mother showed severe clinical symptoms (Chapter 9). In Hungary, Börzsönyi et al. (1992) found significantly higher incidences of both spontaneous abortions (696 as against 511 per 10,000 live births) and stillbirths (77 compared with 28 per 10,000 live births) in the As-contaminated area compared with a low-As control area. In Bangladesh, Hasnat (2005) reported an increased risk of unintended abortion and still-birth from mothers consuming high levels of arsenic in drinking water, but found no evidence of post-natal harm. In West Bengal, Rahman et al. (2005b) also suggested that exposure to arsenic may be linked to various pregnancy-related problems, including spontaneous abortion, stillbirth, premature birth, low birth weight, and neonatal death. Von Ehrenstein et al. (2006) verified some, but not all, of these effects. They found a sixfold increase in the risk of still birth (OR 6.07; 95% CI, 1.54–24.0) and neonatal death (OR 2.81; 95% CI, 0.73–10.8), but found no association with spontaneous abortion or infant mortality. In Chile, Hopenhayn et al. (2006) compared the pregnancy outcomes of 810 women in two cities: one where the water supply contained 40 ppb As, and the other where it contained <1 ppb As. After adjusting for other factors, they found that the prevalences of anaemia in the exposed and unexposed groups were 49% and 17% respectively, suggesting a moderate association between arsenic in drinking water and anaemia during pregnancy.

At Antofagasta, Chile (Chapter 10), Smith, Marshall et al. (2006) demonstrated that exposure to arsenic in early childhood, and even in the womb, caused deaths from lung cancer and bronchiectasis in adulthood. They compared national mortality rates with those of local residents who were born either before or during the period of peak exposure (1958–1971). Although increased mortality was observed in persons born between 1950 and 1957, the rates for those born between 1958 and 1970 were much higher still. The standardised mortality ratios (SMR) for lung cancer and bronchiectasis for those born before 1958 were 7.0 (CI, 5.4–8.9) and 12.4 (CI, 3.3–31.7); but for those born after 1958 were 6.1 (CI, 3.5–9.9) and 46.2 (CI, 21.1–87.7).

5.9   Social and Psychological Effects

5.9.1   Intellectual function and mental health

In their Araihazar (Bangladesh) study area, the Columbia University medical team (Wasserman et al., 2004, 2006) showed that exposure to arsenic affects children's intellectual development. They examined 201 ten-year-old children (and their mothers) drinking water that ranged from 0.1 to 790 ppb. Actual exposure was confirmed by urine analyses, and general information was collected on social class and maternal intelligence. Intellectual function was assessed using a culturally modified version of the Wechsler Intelligence Scale for Children (WISC-III). This test provides verbal, performance and full-scale (total) scores[21]. They deduced that arsenic significantly reduced the intellectual function of children, and that the relationship follows a dose–response trend that takes effect at concentrations as low as 10 ppb As. Many of the waters in Araihazar also contain high manganese concentrations. After isolating a subgroup exposed to high Mn and low As, they showed that manganese has an independent neurotoxic effect on children. After adjusting for socio-demographic factors, Wasserman et al. (2004) determined that children drinking water with >50 ppb Mn achieved significantly lower scores than children drinking water with <5.5 ppb As. In China, Sun et al. (2006) reported that children exposed to arsenic suffer from cognitive delays, reduced IQ, slowed mental growth and resulted in poor memory.

Little attention has been given to effects of As exposure on mental health. However, Fujino et al. (2004) performed a cross-sectional study at two villages in Inner Mongolia (China) that had similar demographic and socio-economic profiles but differed in terms of As exposure. Using a 30–item version of a general health questionnaire, they concluded that mental health in the As-affected village was worse than in the arsenic-free village (OR = 2.5).

5.9.2   Social impacts

Depending on local cultural conditions, As pollution of private water supplies or arsenicosis can lead to a variety of non-clinical social effects, as have been documented in Bangladesh and West Bengal. At a macrolevel in West Bengal, Sarkar and Mehrotra (2005) confirmed the conventional wisdom that the poor always suffer worse, showing that the prevalence of severe clinical manifestations and the mortality rate were significantly higher among individuals of lower socio-economic status. The reasons, however, may be various. For instance, better-off households find it easier to shift to alternative water sources, while agricultural labourers may have higher intakes of arsenic from both food and water. They also identified nutrition as a likely explanatory factor since severe manifestations were significantly associated with low BMI.

Although women are less likely to develop arsenicosis, the social consequences are worse, especially for young women. Even mild dermatological symptoms, such as hyper- or hypopigmentation, are disfiguring, and can result in young women being unable to get married, being forced to divorce, or adopting the *borkha*, and children not being sent to school, to hide evidence of the disease (Hassan et al., 2005). Women are less likely to seek treatment (Sarkar and Mehrotra, 2005). Irrespective of gender, being diagnosed with arsenicosis or having one's tubewell painted red carries a social stigma that can lead to ostracism and exclusion from social activities because arsenicosis is often perceived to be contagious (Hassan et al., 2005). There is even evidence that burial rites have been refused to some victims (Hassan et al., 2005). Such problems are particularly acute where there is a lack of information about the nature of arsenicosis.

Arsenicosis has an economic impact that feeds back to the health and welfare of both the individual and their family (Hanchett, 2004). The most likely person to develop arsenicosis is an adult male, and as such probably the main bread-winner for the family. If symptoms develop to the point where the man is unable to work because he is either too ill or too weak to work or because he loses employment opportunities because of fear of contagion, then he may be unable to feed his family. In the absence of effective public health and welfare services, this leads to the classic downward spiral of poverty and ill-health. Returning to the macroscale, the cumulative impact of these effects is a massive loss of productive activity in an economy that is already unable to support its most disadvantaged members.

5.10   Effect of Other Toxic and Trace Elements

There is limited information about how arsenic interacts with other trace elements in food and water to influence health outcomes. Squibb and Fowler (1983), citing earlier work, noted that cadmium reduces renal concentrations of arsenic by about 11%, and that the metabolism of copper, an essential trace element, is affected by arsenic. World Bank (2005) and ATSDR (2005) suggested that zinc deficiency can increase the toxicity of arsenic, and proposed that zinc and/or chromium supplements might reduce chronic arsenicosis. However, this has not been tested in humans. As noted above, manganese also acts in As-contaminated waters to impair children's intellectual development (Wasserman et al., 2006). Toxic levels of fluoride are common in some As-polluted aquifers, but neither increase nor decrease the toxicity of arsenic.

Selenium (Se) is an essential dietary trace element but is toxic at higher doses, and co-occurs with arsenic in Argentina. Excess selenium has similar toxic effects to those of arsenic, but is not known to be carcinogenic (Spallholz et al., 2004), while deficiency of selenium is well known in China as a cause of Keshan disease[22]. Remarkably, selenium can detoxify both itself and arsenic, as well as lead, cadmium and mercury, through the formation of insoluble selenides. This knowledge has been applied since the 1930s, when arsenic was used in the USA to counteract selenium toxicity in livestock. The main dietary sources of selenium are animal protein (fruit and vegetables contain little selenium). In Bangladesh and West Bengal dietary intake of selenium is very low, and can be traced directly to both the low consumption of animal protein and the naturally low Se-levels in the soil. In recent years, Spallholz et al. (2004) suggested that selenium deficiency could exacerbate arsenic poisoning in Bangladesh and West Bengal, and hence that dietary supplements could be used in the treatment and prevention of arsenicosis. They cite evidence from China that a population exposed to up to 1 ppm As in drinking water displayed a 75% reduction in arsenicosis symptoms after being given Se supplements for 14 months[23]. In another case, Wang et al. (2001) showed that the As contents of blood, urine and hair in people receiving Se therapy declined significantly, and that they also showed improvements in liver and cardiovascular function.

Organic compounds in the human body, often related to nutrition, can potentially affect the toxicity of arsenic. For instance, methylation is one of the main detoxification processes in the body, and so compounds that interfere with methylation could increase the toxicity of arsenic. ATSDR (2005) indicated that deficiencies of choline, methionine and protein could increase the toxicity of arsenic, and could partly explain the greater impact of arsenic on malnourished populations.

5.11 Geographical Differences in Health Effects

There are many reasons why the prevalence of arsenical symptoms might vary geographically. One factor is differences in water chemistry, not only As concentration and its variation over time, but also other toxic elements (section 5.10). These factors should be primarily related to geology, but may also reflect water treatment and storage. A second group of factors relate to the socio-economic conditions and include malnutrition, diet and cooking methods, lifestyle, access to medical care, and the financial capacity to effect mitigation. A third factor is genetic differences between populations.

Finally, interpretations may be confounded by anthropogenic sources of arsenic and differences in the quality of diagnosis.

Most of the long-term epidemiological evidence concerning the effects of chronic arsenic poisoning comes from Chile, Argentina and Taiwan. Interestingly, each represents a different geochemical mechanism and geological and trace element associations (Chapters 8 and 10). The Taiwan case, associated with BFD (section 5.8.1) is hydrogeologically similar to the Bengal Basin, but only one case of BFD has been diagnosed in Bengal (Saha, 2003). Selenium, which can counteract arsenic, sometimes coexists with it in Argentina. In Chile, arsenic is derived from geothermal sources.

Apart from geology, differences in health impacts might be explained by nutritional factors, either through dietary and cooking habits that result in high As consumption, or through malnutrition and dietary deficiencies that render individuals more susceptible to disease. In the irrigated-rice economies of South Asia, these factors may act together. Pershagen (1983) suggested that malnutrition contributes to the intensity of arsenical symptoms in Taiwan, Argentina and Chile. He contrasted these with the general lack of recorded impacts from studies from Oregon, Alaska and Utah in the USA. In Oregon, one case of multiple basal-cell carcinoma was recorded in an arsenicosis patient, but neither squamous-cell nor basal-cell carcinoma could be related to As exposure (Pershagen, 1983). In Fairbanks, Alaska (average 224 ppb As), no clinical or haematological abnormalities could be related to As intake, and it was suggested that the absence of symptoms might be due to the lower water intake and short duration (<10 years) of exposure. In Utah (average 180 ppb As), neither the frequency of skin lesions nor cancers differed from the control population. Nevertheless, there is more recent evidence (see Chapter 9) that clinical symptoms of arsenic poisoning are present in the American population (Zierold et al., 2004; Tollestrup et al., 2005; Ayotte et al., 2006; Knobeloch et al., 2006; Meliker et al., 2007).

As noted earlier (section 5.9.2), the poor suffer worse symptoms of arsenicosis; and poverty and malnutrition often go hand-in-hand. In an ecological study in West Bengal, Mitra et al. (2004) showed that dietary deficiencies increase susceptibility to skin lesions. Their results, indicate significant correlations with deficiencies of calcium (OR 1.89), animal protein (OR 1.94), folate (OR 1.67) and fibre (OR 2.20). However, given the relatively small increases in the level of risk, they suggested that it would be more 'efficient' to give greater priority to reducing exposure than changing diet. Similarly, in the As-endemic region of southwest Taiwan, BFD prevalence was inversely related to the frequency of eating eggs, meat and vegetables (Chen et al., 1988). These results indicate that poor nutrition, a consequence of poverty, can be a significant factor in explaining higher prevalences of arsenicosis.

Table 5.16 summarises the global distribution of reported arsenical health impacts. The table is derived from studies of extremely variable scope and

Table 5.16 Global distribution of arsenical health impacts; for As occurrences not listed, no health related information could be obtained. Empty cells indicate that there is no information available, and although this may be taken as a presumption of absence, only where 'No' is entered is it known that clinical surveys were conducted, and may be taken as proof of absence. Literature references are cited either in the text of this chapter, or in the relevant sections of Chapters 8 to 10

Country/ region	Arsenic exceedance (% > ppb)	Biomarkers > normal* (Y/N, %)	Patients identified/ exposed population†	Skin lesions‡	Cancers (by type)§	Chronic lung disease	Cardiovascular disease	Blackfoot Disease	Other symptoms	Deaths reported
Indus Valley, Punjab, Pakistan	20% > 10; 3% > 50	Yes	6 M (E10); 2 M (E50)	Yes						
Indus Valley, Sindh, Pakistan	36% > 10; 16% > 50		Yes	Yes(?)						
Chandigarh region (India: Punjab, Haryana, Himachal Pr. and UT)	60% > 50	Yes	Yes	Yes					NCPF	
Chhattisgarh, India	8% > 50		10,000 (E50); 130 (P)	Yes 42%						
Colombo, Sri Lanka	?	Yes	Yes						Nausea, GID, Mees line, Neu. D	One
Ganga Plains (India: UP, Bihar and Jarkhand)	B: 11% > 50 UP: 2% > 50 J: 4% > 50	Yes	Yes	Yes					Neuropathy	
Bengal Basin (Bangladesh and West Bengal, India)	25% > 50; 46% > 10	Yes >80%	Yes 33 M (E50)	Yes	S, Li, Lu, B	Yes	Yes	No	Various, including: NCPF, children's IQ,	Yes

Location									
Brahmaputra Plains 17% > 50 (Assam, India)	17% > 50		No						
NE states of India (Manipur, Arunachal Pr., Tripura and Nagaland)	29% > 50	Yes	No						
Terai, Nepal	24% >10; 3% > 50	Yes	555,000 (E50) 2.5 M (E10)	Yes	No	No	No	Bowen's disease (one case)	No
Irrawaddy delta, Myanmar	21% > 50	Yes	2.5 M (E50)	Yes					
Ron Phibun, Thailand		Yes	15,000 (E50); 1000(P)	Yes					
Mekong river, Cambodia	24% >10; 16% > 50	?	Yes	Yes	No	No	No	No	No
Mekong Delta, Vietnam	13% >10		No	No	No	No	No	No	No
Red River Delta, Vietnam	48% > 50	Yes	No	No	No	No	No	No	No
Inner Mongolia, China	11% > 50	Yes	1.0 M (E50)	16%	S, other	Yes	Yes	PN, Diabetes, mental illness	No
Shanxi, China	52% > 50	Yes	932,000 (E50)	13%	Yes	Yes	Yes		
Xinjiang, China	4% > 50	Yes	143,000 (E50)	1.4%	S, Lu	Yes	Yes	Gangrene, GID Diabetes	
Anhui Pr., China	20% >10; 3% > 50	Yes	87,000 (E50);	0.8%					
Beijing, China	8% > 50	No	60,000 (E50)						
Sichuan Pr., China		Yes	Yes						
Jilin Pr., China	12% > 50	Yes	59,000 (E50)	18%					

(cont'd)

Table 5.16 (cont'd)

Country/region	Arsenic exceedance (% > ppb)	Biomarkers > normal* (Y/N, %)	Patients identified/ exposed population†	Skin lesions‡	Cancers (by type)§	Chronic lung disease	Cardiovascular disease	Blackfoot Disease	Other symptoms	Deaths reported
Qinghai, China	8% > 50	Yes	Yes 12,000 (E50)	9%						
Southwest Coast, Taiwan		Yes	Yes	Yes	S, Lu, Li, B, K	Yes	Yes	Yes	Diabetes,	
Northeast Coast, Taiwan	59% > 10; 39% > 50	Yes	Yes	Yes	S, Lu, Li, B, K		Yes	No		
Fukoka–Kumamoto, Japan	23% > 10		No							
Ghazni City, Afghanistan	76% > 10		No 500,000 (E10)							
Western Anatolia, Turkey		Yes	Yes	33%	S				Fatigue, weight-loss	
Kurdistan province, ? Iran		Yes	Yes	Yes					Gangrene	
Mongolia	10% > 10	Y	Yes	Yes						
Danube Basin: Hungary, Romania, and Croatia	Hungary: 17% > 50	Yes	>700,000 (E50) Yes	Yes	S, other	Yes	Yes	No	GID, Haem., pregnancy	Yes
Finland	3% > 10	Y	Yes	No	B	No	No	No	muscle cramps	
Sweden	4% > 10		No							
Norway	1% > 10		No							
Midlands and northwest England	12% > 10; 2% > 50		No							

Location									
Massif Central, Vosges and Pyrenees, France			No						
Siena, Italy	8% > 10		200,000 (E10); 17,000 (E50)						
Po Basin, Italy	21% > 10; 3% > 50		No						
Thessalonika, Greece			No; 5000 (E10)						
New England, USA	30% > 10		103,000 (E10)	B(?)	No	No	No		
Nova Scotia, Canada	13% > 50	Yes	29%	No	No	No	No		
Ontario, Canada		Yes	Yes; 10(P)		Yes	Yes		Weakness, nephritis, GID, still-birth, Neu.D, PN	1–4
Saskatchewan, Canada	23% > 10		No						
Illinois, USA	19% > 10		No						
Eastern Michigan, USA			Yes		Yes	Yes		Cerebro-vascular, and kidney disease; diabetes	
Wisconsin, USA	20% > 10; 4% > 50		Yes	S	Yes	Yes	Yes	Depression	
Minnesota, Iowa and the Dakotas	26% > 10		No						
Fairbanks, Alaska, USA	40% > 10; 28% > 50	Y	No clinical symptoms	No	No	No	No	No	No
Cook Inlet, Alaska, USA	8% > 50		No						

(cont'd)

Table 5.16 (cont'd)

Country/region	Arsenic exceedance (% > ppb)	Biomarkers > normal* (Y/N, %)	Patients identified/ exposed population†	Skin lesions‡	Cancers (by type)§	Chronic lung disease	Cardiovascular disease	Blackfoot Disease	Other symptoms	Deaths reported
British Columbia, Canada	40% > 10		No							
Washington State, USA	18% > 50	Y	Yes ('hundreds')	Yes					Anaemia, Neu.D, nausea	
Oregon, USA	22% > 10; 8% > 50	Y	Yes	Yes	No	No	No	No	PN; anaemia	No
Basin-and-Range Province, USA		Y	No	?						
Región Lagunera, Mexico	50% > 50	Y	400,000 (E50); 21%(P) 2 M 'at risk'	Yes	S			Yes	GID, gangrene	Yes
Zimapán Valley, Mexico	50% > 50	Y	Yes	Yes				No		
Sebaco–Matagalpa Valley, Nicaragua	37% > 10		Yes 1200 (E10)							
Chaco–Pampean plains, Argentina	96% > 10; 73% > 50		2 M (E50)	Yes	S, Li, Lu, K, B					Yes
Bolivia			Yes 25,000 (E50)	Yes					Neu.D	

Location	‡	† Number exposed	*		S, Lu, K, B				Other	§ Cancers
Andean rivers, Peru		250,000 (E50)								
Pacific Coastal Plain, Chile	c. 100%	500,000 (E50)	Yes		Yes	Yes	Yes	No	Raynaud's syndrome, ischaemia of the tongue, liver disease, chronic diarrhoea	Yes
Iron Quadrangle, Brazil		No	Yes							
southwest Ghana	10% > 10	No	Yes	Yes						
southwest Cameroon		No	No							
		4000 (E50)								
Rift Valley, Ethiopia	7% > 10;	No								
Okavango delta, Botswana	30% > 10	No								
Yatenga, Burkina Faso		Yes		Yes			Yes	Yes		
Waiotapu Valley, North Island, New Zealand		No, but livestock affected								

GID, gastrointestinal disturbance; PN, peripheral neuropathy; NCPF, non-cirrhotic portal fibrosis; Haem, haematological disorders; Neu.D, neurological dysfunction

*> normal' indicates that high As concentrations in hair, urine or nails confirm the uptake of arsenic in humans.

†E10 refers to the number of people drinking water with > 10 ppb As, and E50 to drinking more than 50 ppb As. A number followed by the suffix 'P' refers to the number of patients that have been diagnosed. Where exposure has changed over time, the peak figure is quoted.

‡Where quoted, the prevalence of skin lesions refers to exposed population only, unless indicated otherwise.

§Cancers by type: <S>kin, <Lu>ng, <Li>ver, <B>ladder, <K>idney. A '?' symbol indicates a suspected, but unproven link.

quality, and so must be viewed with caution. Symptoms may have been overlooked or misdiagnosed. Even in intensely studied regions such as West Bengal and Bangladesh, causal links to cancer are not well established, and so the difficulty in establishing causation in less-affected countries should be clear. Table 5.16 includes indicators of the severity of the As hazard, and also whether biomarkers of exposure have confirmed human uptake of arsenic. The most characteristic symptoms of arsenic poisoning are the various forms of skin disease, and in almost all cases, were the basis for patients being identified. However, many instances of As uptake have not resulted in clinical symptoms of poisoning; non-diagnosis of symptoms may simply reflect the absence of detailed epidemiological studies. Indeed it would be surprising if more symptoms are not diagnosed in the future.

The widest ranges of non-specific symptoms have been identified in Taiwan, Chile, Argentina, Hungary, China and Bengal where most research has been conducted. By contrast, the general absence of symptoms in the USA and most European countries appears significant, and may be largely attributed to differences in diet. In Nepal, Myanmar, Vietnam and Cambodia, despite high apparent levels of exposure, non-dermatological symptoms have not been identified. Berg et al. (2006b) suggested this is due to the short duration of exposure. If correct, then a rapid increase in arsenicosis is to be expected in the near future.

Although skin lesions are considered to be key diagnostic symptoms, in New England and Finland arsenic has been tentatively linked to bladder cancer without prior recognition of dermatological symptoms (Kurttio et al., 1999; Ayotte et al., 2006). However, studies of the risk of bladder cancer at low As concentrations (60–80 ppb As) by Steinmaus et al. (2003) and Lamm et al. (2004) concluded that the cancer threshold in the USA population is higher than inferred from studies in Taiwan. This was suggested to be due to higher body mass and lower water consumption in the USA. In addition, Knobeloch et al. (2006) have inferred a causal link to excess skin cancers in Wisconsin (USA).

5.12 Case History of Arsenic Exposure in Murshidabad District, West Bengal

In a series of papers, Dipankar Chakraborti and co-workers at SOES (School of Environmental Studies at Jadavpur University in Kolkata) described a 7-year investigation in Murshidabad, conducted to 'better understand the exact magnitude of groundwater arsenic contamination and its health effects in West Bengal'. In increasing detail, they studied the district as a whole (Rahman et al., 2005), Jalangi Block (Rahman et al., 2005a; Mukherjee, Saha et al., 2005) and the cluster-village of Sagarpara GP

(Rahman et al., 2005b). The team included a dermatologist, neurologist, gynaecologist, pathologist, chemist, biochemist, geologist and civil engineer. Based on 30,000 analyses, they inferred that 54% of the estimated 200,000 tubewells in the district exceeded 10 ppb As, and 26% exceeded 50 ppb. They examined 25,274 people from 139 affected villages and found that 4813 (19%) had arsenical skin lesions. Analysis of 3843 samples of hair, nail, urine and skin confirmed the link between arsenic in water and arsenical skin manifestations (ASM) and other effects, including weakness and lethargy, chronic respiratory problems, gastrointestinal symptoms, anaemia, gangrene and cancer. They also found indications of the susceptibility of pregnant women to spontaneous abortion, stillbirth, premature birth, low birth weights and neonatal deaths.

In Jalangi Block (population 216,000), they tested 1916 wells (estimated to be 31% of all wells) and found 78% >10 ppb, 51% >50 ppb and 17% >300 ppb As. On average, 88% of the hair, nail and urine samples analysed exceeded normal levels. Clinical symptoms of As poisoning were common: 21% of 7221 persons had ASM, and some suffered from Bowen's disease and cancers that they tentatively attributed to the effects of arsenic. In Sagarpara GP, which comprises a group of 21 villages with a population of 24,419, they analysed every working hand pump ($n = 565$), which allowed them to confidently determine the numbers of people drinking different concentrations of arsenic, as shown in Table 5.17.

As biomarkers of exposure, they found that 76% of 303 hair samples, 93% of 382 nail samples and 91% of 176 urine samples exceeded the normal range of arsenic concentrations. The mean As concentrations in these biomarkers were five to ten times the normal range. Clinical examinations

Table 5.17   Arsenic exposure profile in Sagarpara GP, West Bengal

As in tubewell water (ppb)	Number of persons	Percentage of population
<10	3413	14.0
10–50	6477	26.5
50–100	3326	13.6
100–200	2494	10.2
200–300	2276	9.3
300–500	3195	13.1
500–1000	2188	9.0
>1000	1050	4.3
	24,419	100.0

Source: Rahman et al. (2005c)

of 3302 people identified ASM in 21% of people, and in all 21 villages. Skin lesions were found not only in adults, but also in 3.4% of the 500 children examined. At Sagarpara, the following generalised sequence of symptoms was deduced:

1 diffuse melanosis on the palms, or the entire body, was often the first symptom;
2 spotted melanosis (raindrop syndrome), on the chest, back or limbs, was very common;
3 leucomelanosis (black and white spotting) was common amongst people who had stopped drinking contaminated water and had had spotted melanosis earlier;
4 mucous membrane melanosis on the tongue, gums and lips;
5 diffuse and/or nodular keratosis on the palms and soles was an advanced stage of arsenical dermatosis;
6 spotted keratosis, with rough-dry skin and palpable nodules, on hands, feet and legs, was seen in severe cases.

They considered the combination of melanosis and nodular rough skin to be diagnostic of arsenicosis. About 70–75% of patients with ASM also reported severe itching on exposure to sunlight, even in winter. Many patients with ASM also had symptoms that were potentially related to arsenic such as enlargement of the liver and spleen, fluid in the stomach, and non-healing ulcers (suspected skin cancer). They were not, however, able to compile systematic information on internal cancers. They also suspected significant underreporting of skin lesions due to a variety of social reasons.

To estimate the future burden of skin lesions and cancer, assuming no change in exposure, the exposure data from Sagarpara were compared with seven regional and international epidemiological studies. It was predicted that between 6400 and 11,000 (26–45%) of the population would develop ASM, and that between 143 and 415 people would develop cancers specifically due to drinking As-polluted water[24].

5.13 Diagnosis and Treatment of Arsenicosis

Arsenicosis, the widely used term to denote the clinical manifestations of chronic arsenic toxicity, has no standard definition. Therefore, Guha Mazumder (2003) proposed a clinical case definition, whereby a satisfactory diagnosis of arsenicosis combines complementary lines of evidence, including: a source of arsenic; proof of arsenic intake above ambient levels; and characteristic clinical symptoms. The first is normally provided by analysis of well-water, and the second requires analysis of urine, hair or nails as biomarkers. Based on statistical comparisons of background and control populations, Guha Mazumder (2003) proposed the following criteria to prove recent exposure to arsenic.

- Urine >50 µg/L, provided the patient has not eaten seafood in the previous 4 days. Based on evidence in the literature, the 'normal' range is 5–40 µg/L.
- Hair with > 0.8 mg/kg (in West Bengal, hair concentrations of 3–10 mg/kg are common in affected persons). The normal range is 0.08–0.250 mg/kg.
- Nails containing >1.3 mg/kg. The normal range is 0.43–1.08 mg/kg.

As noted earlier, many of the clinical effects can have multiple causes, but hyperpigmentation and hyperkeratosis are considered characteristic of As exposure, and the well-known spotty raindrop pigmentation (distributed symmetrically on the trunk and limbs) is considered particularly diagnostic. On the other hand, the systemic effects are non-specific. Amongst the carcinogenic effects, skin cancers (Bowen's disease, squamous-cell and basal-cell carcinoma) are considered to be major cancer factors, while internal cancers (lung, liver and bladder) are considered minor cancer factors (Guha Mazumder, 2003). Diagnostic criteria for chronic arsenicosis, based on experience in West Bengal and Bangladesh, are listed in Table 5.18.

Table 5.18   Diagnostic criteria for chronic arsenicosis

1   Prolonged (>6 months) intake of water with >50 ppb As or equivalent in food, air, etc.
2   Characteristic dermatological features
    (a) Spotty or blotchy pigmentation of the body
    (b) Diffuse or nodular keratosis of the palms or soles
3   Non-cancer systemic manifestations
    (a) Major: chronic lung disease, hepatomegaly, peripheral neuropathy, peripheral vascular disease
    (b) Minor: weakness, diabetes mellitus, hypertension, ischaemic heart disease, swelling of hands and feet, defective hearing, conjunctivitis, anaemia and other symptoms
4   Cancers
    (a) Major: Bowen's disease, squamous-cell and basal-cell carcinoma
    (b) Minor: cancers of the lung, liver and bladder
5   Biomarker of As exposure: urine >50 µg/L; hair >0.8 mg/kg; and nails >1.3 mg/kg

Source: Guha Mazumder (2003)

Based on thousands of examinations, the dermatologist Dr K.C. Saha, who first diagnosed arsenic poisoning in West Bengal, defined a characteristic sequence of symptoms, divided into four stages, seven grades and 20 subgrades, as summarised in Table 5.19.

Table 5.19 Saha's classification of arsenicosis symptoms

	Stages	Grade	Inference	Duration/ treatment
I	Pre-clinical	0	Pre-clinical	6 months–10
		0a	Labile: As is present in blood and urine. It is excreted as MMA or DMA in urine	years. Remove exposure to arsenic
		0b	Stable or tissue phase: As is detectable in hair, nails or skin, but without symptoms	
II	Clinical	1	Melanosis	Reversible if
		1a	Diffuse melanosis on palms	exposure is removed; possible
		1b	Spotted melanosis on trunk ('raindrop pigmentation)	use of chelating agents
		1c	Generalised melanosis	
		2	Spotted keratosis on palms and soles	Effects from Grade 2 onward
		2a	Mild: 1–6 nodules	are irreversible
		2b	Severe: >6 nodules	
		2c	Large nodules	
		3	Diffuse keratosis on palms and soles	
		3a	Partial – only on soles	
		3b	Severe – on soles and palms	
		3c	Complete	

Table 5.19   *(cont'd)*

Stages		Grade	Inference	Duration/ treatment
		4	Dorsal keratosis	
		4a	On hands or legs	
		4b	On hands and legs	
		4c	Generalised	
III	Complications	5	Hepatic disorder	
		5a	Palpable liver	
		5b	Jaundice	
		5c	Ascitis	
IV	Malignancy	6	Malignancy	
		6a	Single lesion	
		6b	Two lesions	
		6c	More than two lesions	

Source: Saha (2003)

According to Saha (2003), there is no satisfactory treatment for arsenicosis, but avoiding As-contaminated water is viewed as essential, and a diet rich in protein, vitamins A and C, and selenium is recommended. He suggested that symptoms of melanosis and mild keratosis (Grades 1 and 2a) may clear in 2–3 months with this treatment. Beyond this stage, treatments are regarded as largely palliative. For instance, ointments containing salicylic acid can soften keratitic nodules, and scraping can relieve the discomfort of thickened soles. For more advanced conditions, such as large nodules, ischaemic[25] gangrene and some cancers, surgery is required. Antibiotics are used for non-dermatological effects such as bronchitis, ulcers and gangrene.

To study the effects of delayed treatment in Bangladesh, Paul and Tinnon-Brock (2006) employed a questionnaire survey of 663 arsenic patients. They defined treatment delay as the time between identification of the first symptoms and consulting the doctor with the intent to recover. The median delay was 12 months, but ranged from a month to 18 years. Delay is particularly important because the illness is considered to be reversible only in its early stages. Low levels of formal education and perception of threat were significant factors contributing to delay, highlighting the need for better health education in affected areas and targeting of messages to more vulnerable groups (e.g. old, women and poor). Based on interviews (in 2002) at hospitals in Bangladesh with an expressed interest in As mitigation, Caldwell et al. (2004) found that clinical staff were inadequately informed to diagnose and manage arsenicosis, and identified an urgent need for focused training of all medical practitioners.

5.14   Removing Exposure to Arsenic

The conventional wisdom is that to improve health it is essential to remove exposure to arsenic. There is limited reliable information on the long-term improvements in health, although what exists is encouraging as regards skin lesions but more worrying with regard to cancer and heart disease. Methodologically, it is important to separate the improvement of conditions that have already developed when exposure ceases from the delayed, or latent, appearance of symptoms after exposure stops. Guha Mazumder et al. (2003) reported on a cohort of 1074 persons in West Bengal who had been examined in a previous study. They distinguished a large subgroup who had been drinking As-free (< 50 ppb) water for 5 years after they had been diagnosed with arsenical skin lesions. The results (Table 5.20) showed an improvement in the symptoms of 50% of the patients who had skin lesions at the start of the 5-year period. They also found reductions in the incidence of non-dermal manifestations, notably the incidence of chronic lung disease (CLD), which was recorded 4.7 times more commonly in the people who

Table 5.20   Condition of skin lesions 5 years after removal from high-arsenic drinking water (≥50 ppb) in West Bengal

		Percentage	
Condition of lesions	Number	Patients*	All
With skin lesions			
Cleared up	40	20.1	13.1
Decreased	59	29.6	19.3
Same	95	47.7	31.0
Increased	5	2.5	1.6
Without skin lesions			
New appearance	32		10.5
No new appearance	75		24.5

*The 199 people who were previously known to have skin lesions out of the total group ('All') that were exposed to high-As drinking water 5 years earlier.
Source: Guha Mazumder et al. (2003)

were still exposed to high-As concentrations than in those who had been removed from exposure. The differences in incidence of CLD were much more pronounced for men (of all ages) than women. Smaller improvements were also observed in the incidence of neuropathy, cerebrovascular accidents and diabetes, which were 3.9, 2.33 and 1.55 times more common in people still exposed to arsenic respectively.

Similar, but less encouraging results were obtained in China, where Xia and Liu (2004) reported that after changing the water source, 30% of patients improved, 52% showed no change, and 18% deteriorated. Moreover, the prevalence of CVD, diabetes and cancer continued to increase. In Inner Mongolia, Sun et al. (2006) evaluated the impact of providing a piped supply (37 ppb As) to Gangfangying village to replace water supplied from wells that ranged from 1 to 1790 ppb As (mean 130 ppb). After 1 year, inorganic As in urine had dropped by a factor of five, organic arsenic species dropped by factors of 1.3 to 1.8, and the condition of many skin lesions had greatly improved. However, after 5 years, there was no significant overall improvement in the condition of the patients. In southwest Taiwan, Yang (2004) concluded that mortality from kidney cancer declined gradually after contaminated well-water was replaced by a low-As piped supply.

In Chile, Borgono et al. (1977) and Smith et al. (1998) studied the impact of installing an arsenic-removal plant at Antofagasta (section 10.2.3). Between 1958 and 1970, the city water supply contained around 800 ppb As, when commissioning of a treatment plant reduced the concentration to around 50 ppb As. After the treatment plant had been operating for 6 years, Borgono et al. (1977) found that hair and nail clippings from children over 6 years of age had greatly reduced As concentrations, and no skin lesions were found in children less than 6 years old. This proved that exposure had been reduced, and was supported by rapid improvements in the incidence of some of the more obvious symptoms of As poisoning such as skin lesions and ischaemia of the tongue. However, later Smith et al. (1998) identified increased mortality from bladder, lung, kidney and skin cancers resulting from the delayed development of cancers decades after peak exposure. Their results, expressed in terms of SMRs, are given in Table 5.21. Such is the significance of arsenic in drinking water, even more than 20 years after exposure had ended, it was estimated that arsenic accounted for 7% of all deaths among people over 30 years of age.

Smith, Marshall et al. (2006) showed that exposure in early childhood, and even in the womb, could cause deaths from lung cancer and bronchiectasis in adulthood (section 5.8.6). The latency of arsenic in causing cancer and heart disease is powerfully illustrated in Figure 5.7 by a 50–year retrospective analysis of excess deaths in Region II of Chile due to acute myocardial infarction (AMI, basically heart attack) and lung and bladder

Table 5.21   Increased bladder and lung cancer risk in Region II of Chile*

		Mortality	
Disease	Gender	SMR	CI (95%)
Bladder cancer	Men	6.0	4.8–7.4
	Women	8.2	3.0–10.5
Lung cancer	Men	3.8	3.5–4.1
	Women	3.1	2.7–3.7

SMR, standard mortality ratio; CI, confidence interval.
*Most cancers developed after the period of peak exposure (1958–1970)
   had ended, and a new water supply had been developed.
Source: Smith et al. (1998)

cancer. Yuan et al. (2007) showed that during the period of high exposure heart attacks were the main cause of excess deaths attributed to arsenic. For men, AMI mortality remained high for two decades after the peak exposure stopped, but in the second decade after the treatment plant was implemented, was overtaken by lung cancer as the main cause of excess deaths. For women, AMI mortality peaked in the decade after high exposure ceased but then declined rapidly, whereas mortality due to both lung and bladder cancer have continued to rise for 30 years. The different latencies of these three diseases produced a remarkable drop in the number of excess deaths in women in the early 1980s, which then rose again as the number of cancer deaths grew. During the period of high exposure, there were a total of 698 excess deaths due to these three causes, and 3452 excess deaths after the period of high exposure ceased. However, the delayed development of cancer and heart and lung disease in Chile is deeply disturbing, and highlights both the likely future burden of death and disease to be expected in Asia and the urgency of removing exposure even where clinical symptoms have not been diagnosed.

5.15   Summary and Recommendations

Knowledge of the range and severity of symptoms of arsenic poisoning has increased in recent decades. Ingestion of arsenic is a major cause of heart, lung, liver and kidney disease, cancer, diabetes, and certain vascular diseases. Arsenic also appears to contribute to mental illness and impair the intellectual

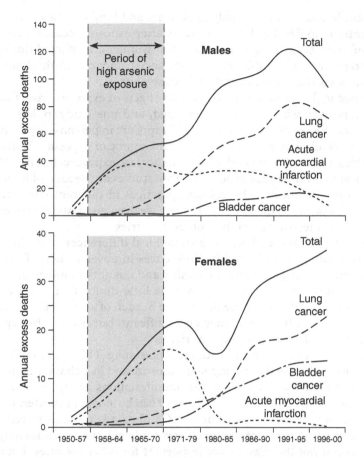

Figure 5.7   Latency of cancer and heart disease in northern Chile. The number of excess deaths attributable to arsenic exposure was determined by comparing mortality data from the exposed region with national statistics. In the main centre of population (Antofagasta), almost the entire population was supplied with water from a single source that, between 1958 and 1970, contained approximately 800 ppb As. After commissioning of a treatment plant in 1971, this was reduced initially to about 100 ppb and later to 40 ppb, and eventually to around 10 ppb As.
Source: Redrawn after Yuan et al. (2007)

development of children. However, the most obvious and diagnostic symptoms are arsenical skin manifestations. The effects of ingested arsenic are cumulative, and all the symptoms have long latencies, ranging from a few years up to decades. Because of the short duration of exposure, some countries have yet to see the full impact of arsenic poisoning. Moreover, where there has been a long period of exposure to high As concentrations, both skin lesions and potentially fatal heart and lung diseases and cancers will continue to develop for many years after exposure ceases. The prevalence of arsenicosis is highest in men, but women are affected during and after pregnancy, and suffer more from social impacts. Both clinical and social impacts disproportionately affect the poor.

It is essential to consider the combined effects of exposure from food and water, especially where crops are irrigated, and one study in West Bengal showed that food was the main source of exposure in persons displaying skin lesions. Globally, rice is the most important source of exposure from food.

Cooking with contaminated water can increase exposure, but if cooked in excess water, it can reduce exposure. More studies are needed of total exposure and its modification by cooking practices in different countries and cultures. Because of dietary differences, western food standards are not necessarily protective of health in other countries.

Interpretation of the observed geographical differences in health effects of As exposure is complicated by differences in poverty, diet, lifestyle, the affordability of mitigation and the quality and quantity of information from different countries. Nevertheless, there is little doubt that measures that reduce poverty will also reduce the disease burden of arsenicosis. Geochemical differences in the waters may be significant, but need to be separated from dietary differences in micronutrients.

Latency is critical to understanding As poisoning. This applies to both the appearance of disease during ongoing exposure and its delayed development after exposure ceases. Arsenical skin manifestations are typically revealed after 5–10 years of exposure, but the period can be longer or shorter. The near absence of arsenicosis in Vietnam and Cambodia is thought to reflect the short duration of exposure. If correct, an epidemic of arsenicosis may soon follow, and if not the reasons are important for other societies. Latency is particularly relevant to cancer, heart and lung disease. Studies in Chile have shown that cancers may develop decades after exposure ceases. In Bangladesh, Chen and Ahsan (2004) predicted that, if unchecked, arsenic exposure will result in a doubling of mortality from liver, bladder and lung cancers.

A major policy issue is whether, or when, to lower the drinking water standard from 50 to 10 ppb As, in line with WHO guidance. Most less economically advanced countries have not revised their standards. Objections to lowering the standard come from fears of unaffordable expense, failing to prioritise mitigation, and uncertainty about clinical effects at low-level exposure. However, there is increasing evidence of harm at concentrations of <50 ppb As, although this is complicated by combined exposure from food. Objectives should not be confused with means, and the 10 ppb WHO guideline should probably be adopted in all affected countries, but implemented in a phased manner within a realistic timescale that takes account of the size of the problem and the resources available.

Although short-term monitoring has indicated symptomatic improvements in conditions such as skin lesions, the limited long-term monitoring is ambiguous. More research is needed on the improvements in health following removal of exposure to arsenic in drinking water, and must also take account of exposure from food.

NOTES

1 Molecular groups characterised by sulphur–hydrogen bonds.
2 There is, however, emerging evidence for the apoptosis-inducing capacity of arsenic trioxide as a treatment for leukaemia (http://www.fda.gov/bbs/topics/answers/ans01040.html).
3 The arsenic exposure dose (ED, in mg/kg/day) for drinking water is calculated from the simple equation: $ED = (C \times DI)/BW$; where C is As concentration (mg/L); DI is daily intake of water (L/day); and BW is body weight (kg). This form of equation is used for developing drinking water standards. The calculations assume that arsenic is entirely in inorganic forms, that As concentrations do not change over time, and assume average DI of 2.5 L/day, BW of 60 kg and exposure over a lifetime of 70 years.
4 Compared with other epidemiological studies, these estimates could underestimate the arsenic-induced cancer burden (see sections 5.7 and 6.2.3).
5 A conservative estimate was used, based on a compensating wage differential study of Indian manufacturing industry by Simon et al. (1999) to give the lower bound of the estimated range from 6.4 m to 13.7 m rupees. This was subsequently adjusted using PPP to 7.6 m rupees and then to US$ 0.35 m. Multiplying the risk per 100,000 individuals per ppb per year by the population average exposure to arsenic in drinking water, and then by the total population and the VSOL, gives the estimated total value of US$2.7 billion.
6 Even though, as will be shown below, this is not adequately protective of health in subsistence rice economies.
7 See also Tables 4.5 and 4.6 for As concentrations in raw rice.
8 *Aman* is the post-monsoon rice grown with little or no irrigated; *boro* is the dry season rice crop and relies heavily on irrigation (see Chapter 4).
9 Most rice in Bangladesh is parboiled in order to preserve the grain during storage.
10 National average data from Williams et al. (2006).
11 This is higher than estimates from Bangladesh which are closer to 500 µg/day, and is presumably the cooked (wet) weight.
12 This is lower than the 80–90% indicated by Williams et al. (2005).
13 Del Razo et al. (2002) separated water consumption in summer and winter. Here we present the arithmetic average.
14 Also known as squamous cell Stage 0 or carcinoma *in situ*.
15 The differences in odds ratios between the studies from China and Bangladesh might be explained by differences in exposure from food. In the former, the low water-As group came from a different village and so may have had lower exposure

from food, exaggerating the difference. In the latter case, the population prob-ably received similar, and elevated, exposure from food, which would tend to blur the difference.

16   In terms of their link to As-exposure.

17   Blackfoot disease has been reported in the region Lagunera of Mexico (Del Razo et al., 2002) and for a single patient in West Bengal (Saha, 2003).

18   Raynaud's symptom is a discolouration of the fingers and/or toes having a char-acteristic white to blue to red colour sequence. Acrocyanosis is a blueness of the hands and feet with mottled discoloration of the fingers, wrists, toes and ankles.

19   Crepitations and/or rhonchi.

20   Either using an oral glucose tolerance test or by where individuals were already receiving insulin.

21   These tests had been used previously to prove the effect of airborne lead on children.

22   Selenium-deficient cardiomyopathy (Oldfield, 2002).

23   A hundred patients received a daily supplement of Se-rich yeast containing 100–200 µg of selenium.

24   These calculations do not take account of As-intake from food, which must increase the disease burden.

25   Where insufficient blood reaches that part of the body.

Chapter Six

Water-supply Mitigation

6.1 Introduction

This chapter is about water supply, but not about water engineering. Arsenic removal could have been described here, but the subject matter is so large that we describe it separately in Chapter 7. Here we focus on two main areas: arsenic surveys and monitoring, and alternative water sources. The overriding objective is to reduce exposure to arsenic, and this can also be achieved through social awareness and educational means (section 6.2). Because there is a higher objective of maximising health benefits, avoiding arsenic must not be achieved at the cost of unreasonably increasing other hazards. Arsenic mitigation should, as far as practical, be integrated with achieving other health benefits through improved sanitation and hygiene. The success of water-supply intervention is therefore measured first in terms of reduced morbidity and mortality, and second in terms of cost, integrated within a framework of risk-benefit analysis. Design of mitigation programmes must be founded on a sound knowledge of the extent and severity of arsenic pollution. Consequently, a major emphasis is given to arsenic surveys, sampling and monitoring (section 6.3), followed by consideration of alternative water sources. Section 6.4 examines the use of safe groundwater within affected areas, while section 6.5 considers the exploitation of surface water. The success of rural water supplies in poor countries depends profoundly on implementation through an institutional structure that is appropriate to the local culture. Hence, in section 6.7 we review examples of experience of socio-economic aspects of arsenic mitigation in Bangladesh. Finally, in sections 6.8 and 6.9 we explore the range of institutional measures and planning initiatives that may be required to support a mitigation programme.

6.2   Approaches to Water-supply Mitigation

6.2.1   Technical approaches

There are three basic technical approaches to removing arsenic exposure:

- treating contaminated groundwater to remove arsenic;
- drawing water from uncontaminated aquifers;
- developing alternative sources of water from rainfall, ponds or rivers.

Non-treatment options depend strongly upon the local geology and hydrology. In practice, technical solutions and the mechanism of their delivery cannot be separated, but in this chapter we address them in turn. The questions of for whom (households, rural communities or municipalities), by whom (government, NGOs, the commercial sector or households) and how this is financed, may well determine the most appropriate technology. Notwithstanding the risk from arsenic, care must be taken to ensure that no other chemical or microbiological hazards are present. Microbiological hazards derive not only from polluted water sources, but may also arise during treatment or storage if they are not properly operated.

6.2.2   Information and educational approaches

Information is fundamental to the design of any mitigation programme and must be shared between technical disciplines and with the affected population. The first requirement is to know which people are exposed to what levels of arsenic and from what sources (section 6.3). Other essential information requirements for effective mitigation include not only technical knowledge such as the hydrogeology and chemistry of groundwater, but also social mobilisation, information dissemination and empowering the exposed population to participate in effecting their own solutions. It has been a common experience that when As contamination is first discovered, governments have tended to deny or suppress this knowledge. Whether due to genuine disbelief, fear of scaring the population or lack of confidence in their ability to solve the problems, the outcome is almost always counterproductive. Blissful ignorance does not protect against arsenic, and delayed response results in avoidable illness and deaths. Governments facing a recently discovered arsenic problem should obtain expert advice on an information campaign at the earliest possible opportunity. In part, this will involve education about the nature of As-related illness in an attempt to reduce the stigma it creates.

The simplest, quickest and cheapest solution is to abandon contaminated wells and switch to an existing safe source (section 6.4.2). The starting point is obviously to make people aware of which water sources are 'safe' or 'unsafe', such as the practice in India and Bangladesh of painting the spouts of pumps red (i.e. danger) or green according to whether or not they exceed the drinking water standard (DWS). This provides encouragement to switch to safe sources. Nonetheless, there are implicit assumptions here, such as understanding the danger, there being safe alternatives within reasonable reach, people being willing to share a safe source, and people making a rational assessment of the risks of switching or not switching. These issues of knowledge and willingness to co-operate become increasingly complex where the general level of education is low, and people's expectations of government (or other benefactors) intervening to solve their problems may be low, or so unrealistically high as to deter initiative.

Where domestic water supply is not provided by a public utility, effecting changes in technology depends on changing perceptions. An example is the expansion of (shallow) hand tubewell installation in Bangladesh. An often overlooked point is that, while the initial expansion was driven by government, whose priority was reducing waterborne disease, the expansion has continued far beyond what health professionals judged necessary (Caldwell et al., 2003). The later stages of expansion were carried out almost entirely by private means in order to have independent water supplies, and by the desire of women to reduce the workload and bother of carrying water from a public tubewell or filtering surface water. Given the popularity and success of tubewells, Caldwell et al. (2003) and others argue against widespread and unjustified abandonment of hand tubewells.

6.2.3 Risk-based approaches

Whatever balance of technical and educational interventions is selected, we argue that the allocation of resources should be risk-based (see section 6.7.3). Prior to the discovery of arsenic, Bangladesh was acclaimed as a success story in safe water provision (e.g. UNICEF, 1998). In the 1970s, Bangladesh suffered terribly from famine and diarrhoeal disease. However, through two decades of state- and donor-supported investment in hand tubewells, together with health education and tubewells for irrigation, the country achieved virtual self-sufficiency in food-grain production and claimed that well over 90% of the population had access to 'safe' water. Unfortunately, 'safe' had been treated as synonymous with water free of coliform bacteria. The burden of morbidity and mortality[1] due to diarrhoeal disease had been enormously reduced (UNICEF, 1998), even if this was not strictly true in terms of compliance with DWSs (Hoque, 1998).

Arsenic pollution came as a huge shock to the water sector. A vast infra-structure of technical and educational interventions had been built around the concept of 'safe water', implying water safe from faecal coliforms. It was thus necessary to redefine the concept of safe water and re-educate a semi-literate rural population to understand the difference between pathogens that can kill in days, but from which a complete recovery is possible, and a slow-acting cumulative poison that debilitates and kills over years.

Risk-based approaches also provide a means to assess other risks such as fluoride, selenium, boron and manganese in drinking water, as well as non-drinking water related risks such as traffic accidents, air pollution and loss of livelihood due to flooding. The Risk Assessment of Arsenic Mitigation Options (RAAMO) study (section 6.7.2) adopted the DALY (disability adjusted life years) as the numeraire for the different risks. Nevertheless, there are additional difficulties where the stakeholders, be they the general public, technocrats or politicians, do not understand the risk assessment process, or perceive that other risks to life and livelihood are as grave as arsenic. The latter perspective is important for people who face serious immediate threats and would accept the risk of future harm to solve today's problem. A source of difficulty is that technocrats accept a model of risk assessment based on the assumptions of objective categories and measur-able probabilities, while the general population bases its risk perceptions on different criteria and concerns (Adams, 1995). This may generate mis-matches between the formulation and implementation of policy as these alternative views come into conflict, unless relevant social surveys are able to bridge the gap. Personal experience, familiarity and differential accept-ance of information from various sources are all major influences on indi-vidual risk perception. Experience of diarrhoeal disease is liable to result in it being perceived as a higher risk than an As-related disease; and suspicion of authority may lead to greater reliance on information from trusted sources even if they are relatively uninformed. Thus, the design of informa-tion and education strategies must be sensitive to these factors in order to optimise the benefits derived from them.

Hossain et al. (2006) highlighted another aspect of perception in relation to experience with arsenic removal plants (ARPs) in West Bengal. Water quality factors such as taste, colour and odour affect people's quality of life, and hence their attitude to risk acceptance. Aside from issues such as how many ARPs were not functioning or did not meet the DWS for arsenic, Hossain et al. (2006) found that after it had been stored for a number of hours, water from 44% of ARPs became coloured by iron precipitation, and 6% had unpleasant odours. Taste and odour influenced people not to use the treated water, and to use 'unsafe' water in preference. Two implications follow: technically, ARPs must remove iron as well as arsenic; and more generally, water must be 'good' as well as 'safe'.

Table 6.1   Relation of cancer risk to arsenic mitigation planning in Bangladesh*

Arsenic (ppb)	Proportion of Wells		Probable Cancer Cases		
	% in class	Cumulative %	Expected number	% in class	Cumulative %
< 10	58.0		84,000	4.9	
10–50	17.0		147,000	8.6	
50–100	8.9	24.9	193,000	11.2	
100–250	9.2	16.0	332,000	19.3	75.3
250–500	5.0	6.8	541,000	31.5	56.0
500–1000	1.7	1.8	368,000	21.4	24.5
>1000	0.1	0.1	52,000	3.0	3.0

*Arsenic data from table 3 in Ravenscroft et al. (2005). See text for explanation, however, these estimates are not intended to be reliable indicators of the future cancer burden, but only to illustrate the benefits of risk-based targeting of mitigation.

The importance of risk-based mitigation programmes is illustrated by simple calculation of the cancer risk in Bangladesh (population 144 million in 2005) using the dose–response estimates cited in section 5.7 and the frequency distribution of arsenic concentrations from a national water quality survey. The probable number of cancers was calculated under the unrealistic, but illustrative, assumption that there is no change in exposure following the survey. For calculation, mid-point concentrations were assigned plus values of 5 and 2000 ppb As to the highest and lowest classes. The indicative calculations in Table 6.1 lead to two important conclusions. First, for the range of concentrations in Bangladesh the presence of absence of a threshold makes little difference to the overall incidence of cancer. Second, and even though the estimates may lack precision, the benefits of risk-based targeting of mitigation are abundantly clear. For instance, mitigating the worst 7% of water sources would remove over half the cancer risk, and action at 16% of polluted wells would remove three-quarters of the risk.

6.3   Surveys of Arsenic Affected Areas

Surveys are a precondition to the design of arsenic-mitigation programmes. This section provides guidance in designing, executing and interpreting an arsenic survey. Methods of arsenic analysis were described in Annex 2.1, and supplementary details of survey procedures are given in Annex 6.1.

Clinical surveys, however, are beyond the scope of this book, and the reader should refer to the relevant WHO publications (e.g. Caussy, 2005).

6.3.1   Sampling design and objectives

Surveys should have a hierarchy of objectives. In addition, constraints of time, budget and personnel normally require a degree of compromise. The first key decision is whether the primary purpose is to assess human exposure, the variation of quality in drinking water sources or the geochemistry of an aquifer. The design of water-supply programmes requires knowledge of all these, but it is difficult to combine all in a single survey. The second decision is whether the survey will be of a reconnaissance or comprehensive nature. An experienced chemist should guide the design of every arsenic survey, but cannot design the survey unaided.

Drinking water surveillance surveys

The first task in planning a surveillance survey is to define the relevant As-concentration thresholds. If the results will be used in epidemiological studies, then arsenic analysis must be accurate over a wide range of concentrations, and so ideally should be carried out in the laboratory. Second, the range of water quality standards, guidelines and minimum detection levels (MDL) must be considered. As a general rule, the level of detection should be at least a factor of three, and preferably ten, below the concentration at which accurate and confident analysis is required. The designer should consider the current legal standard, foreseeable reductions in the standard, and non-regulatory objectives such as reducing the number of persons exposed to water in the range 10–50 ppb As.

Most surveys will adopt a combination of laboratory and field testing. Many field test kits claim levels of detection of 10 ppb As or better. With a supporting quality assurance (QA) system (section 6.3.3), such kits may be suitable for screening at the 50 ppb level, but are currently of marginal suitability at the 10 ppb level. Field test kits should never be used alone for major surveys. The combination of field and laboratory testing also depends on the availability of personnel, their skills, and the capability of laboratories. Depending on the existing hydrochemical database, a subset of the samples should be analysed for other health-related chemicals and microbiological indicators.

Logistical planning is of fundamental importance for large surveys. Surveillance may be conducted as reconnaissance, screening or so-called blanket surveys in which every well is tested (Rosenboom, 2004). Rapid reconnaissance of large areas allows identification and prioritisation of smaller areas for more intensive survey. Before commencing an intensive survey, a pilot study should be carried out in a limited geographical area so that any problems of sampling, analytical requirements and data acquisition can be resolved before full-scale implementation.

Poor chemical quality is only one cause of water-related illness, and consideration should be given to including sanitary inspections, and/or microbiological analysis, but supplementary data collection should not unduly slow the progress of the survey. If field testing is included, a simple time limit follows naturally from the 20 minutes required for the chemicals to react (in the Gutzeit method). However, if arsenic is detected, additional time should be spent to disseminate health education and mitigation advice. It is also important to consider who else will use the results, and how important it is to service their information needs, although this might also be an opportunity for cost sharing. During planning, the designer should hold discussions with concerned ministries, NGOs and research institutions.

Hydrogeochemical investigations

Such investigations are highly specialised and may be site-specific or regional in scale, but some general principles apply. It is essential to study existing information on the geology and hydrogeology, previous surveys, and water use before taking samples. A preliminary conceptual model should be prepared indicating the number and geometry of aquifers, their connection, sources of recharge and water levels. It is also essential to identify human activities such as industry, mining or agriculture that may cause pollution. The investigator should predict what geochemical processes may operate based on the geology and studies in similar areas. Even where there are no arsenic data, inferences can be made from measurements such as EC, temperature, pH, chloride and iron concentrations, colour, taste, odour and gas occurrence. The conceptual model should be used to prepare a sampling plan that represents the range of aquifer conditions, and their relative importance. Time of year might be important, and may warrant resampling selected wells at different times of year. Temperature, pH, redox potential, EC, dissolved oxygen and alkalinity should be measured in the field wherever water samples are collected. Field testing for arsenic can also help select samples for laboratory analysis. Field test kit analyses can also be used to improve the spatial interpolation of As determinations. As a minimum it is important to analyse redox-sensitive species such as reduced and oxidised forms of nitrogen and sulphur, plus iron and manganese[2].

6.3.2 Field testing for arsenic

The ideal arsenic test method is cheap, simple, safe, accurate, precise, reliable and rapid. Unfortunately, no such method exists, and a compromise is required between field and laboratory methods. Laboratory analysis requires preservation of samples, uses expensive equipment, is technically and institutionally demanding and time-consuming, and involves risks of communication failure in returning results to water users. Hence, there is an a priori preference for field methods. In the past 10 years, field test kits have been greatly improved, but there continues to be controversy. Field testing produces results at the time of sampling, so there is no need for sample preservation and storage, and the results can be communicated immediately. The skills required to use field kits are less than for laboratory analysis. Purchased in bulk for large surveys, the cost is of the order of $1 per test or less. Combined with the low cost of skilled labour in many poor countries, this has made field testing very popular. A further reason for their popularity in less-developed economies faced with huge survey needs, is the speed with which surveys can be implemented when the existing capacity of laboratories to meet demand is totally inadequate. On the other hand, disadvantages with field testing include inaccuracy, unreliability, low levels of detection, and poor quality assurance in general.

Early assessments in India and Bangladesh (e.g. DPHE/MMI/BGS, 1999, and references therein) concluded that field test kits used up to 1997 did not reliably identify concentrations of 50–200 ppb in groundwater (as opposed to spiked blanks), although false positives[3] were very rare. Compared with analyses of the same water by ICP or AAS (see Annexe 2.1), field test kits were only reliable for As concentrations of ≥200 ppb As. These early surveys were beneficial in that the wells painted red were certainly dangerous, but unsatisfactory in that many wells declared 'safe' actually posed a serious health hazard. Thus, in villages where some contaminated wells were identified, all the green-painted wells should be retested. Many of the early kits gave 'yes/no' indications of safety, but later kits gave semi-quantitative results and are much to be preferred as the chance of them being in error by more than one concentration band is small.

Since 1998, field test kits have been improved considerably. This is particularly important because many countries have now adopted, or are considering adopting, the 10 ppb WHO guideline. During the period 1998 to about 2002, UNICEF reported satisfactory performance of field test kits at the 50 ppb level (Erickson, 2003). The use of such kits was severely criticised (e.g. Rahman et al., 2002), and this came to a head in a debate between proponents from Columbia University in the USA (van Geen et al., 2005) and opponents at Jadavpur University in Kolkata (Mukherjee et al., 2005b) over the testing of tubewells in Araihazar upazila in Bangladesh. The Araihazar data set is remarkable because, in 2001, all 6000 wells were sampled and analysed by GF-AAS (see Annexe 2.1), and tested again in 2003 by the Bangladesh Government's Bangladesh Arsenic Mitigation Water Supply

Table 6.2   Comparison of laboratory and field kit testing in Araihazar

	Labelled	Number correctly painted (%)	Number wrongly painted (%)
Field kit performance	Safe (green)	405 (50.7)	81 (10.1)
compared with	Not safe (red)	295 (36.9)	18 (2.3)
laboratory analysis			
Adjusted count for	Safe (green)	431 (53.9)	55 (6.9)
10 ppb tolerable error	Not safe (red)	303 (37.9)	10 (1.3)
Adjusted count for	Safe (green)	445 (55.7)	41 (5.1)
20 ppb tolerable error	Not safe (red)	308 (38.5)	5 (0.6)

*Water from 799 wells was tested in the field for compliance with the 50 ppb standard with the Hach kit, and in the laboratory by AAS.
Source: Calculated from data in van Geen et al. (2005*)

Project (BAMWSP) using Hach field test kits, and accordingly painted green or red (>50 ppb). Van Geen et al. (2005) isolated a subset of 799 samples[4] that had been analysed by both field and supplementary laboratory analyses in 2003, which provided an excellent basis for evaluating the field test kits. The Columbia and Jadavpur groups interpreted the same data to reach different conclusions. On the assumption that the laboratory results are correct[5], Table 6.2 summarises the accuracy of well painting. Noting that the Hach kit correctly determined the status of 700 wells, van Geen et al. (2005) stated that 'clearly the Hach Kit should continue to be used to test wells throughout Bangladesh and other countries affected by elevated arsenic in groundwater'.

The Jadavpur group disagreed with the significance, not the accuracy, of the comparison, and rejected this conclusion on the basis that 12.4% is an unacceptable failure rate, especially the 10.1% of wells incorrectly labelled 'safe'. They pointed out that, applied to the 2.36 million wells tested with the Hach kit in Bangladesh, and assuming an average of 24 users per well, these percentages equate to 5.7 million people drinking water that they wrongly believe to be safe. The criticism of Mukherjee et al. (2005b) is basically justified, if a little overstated in terms of impact on health. In terms of risk rather than regulation, the difference between, say, 45 and 55 ppb is almost irrelevant. In other words, small errors can be tolerated. Also in Table 6.2, we have calculated the effect of applying a 'tolerable' error of 10 ppb, and a rather less tolerable error of 20 ppb As. This adjustment improves the apparent performance of the Hach kits, but this still leaves 5–7% of samples significantly exceeding 50 ppb, equivalent to 2.8–3.9

million people living under the false belief that their water is safe. In addition, 2.5% of samples were in error by more that 50 ppb and 0.9% by more than 100 ppb.

Guidance on field test kit performance also comes from controlled laboratory and field evaluations either of individual or multiple kits (e.g. Abbgy et al., 2002a,b; Swash, 2003). Kabir (2005) evaluated nine kits, from seven manufacturers, available in Bangladesh in 2005. The evaluation involved a survey of users, review of technical literature and field testing in two highly contaminated areas, at low (<50 ppb), medium (50–150 ppb) and high (>150 ppb) range wells. Duplicate samples were sent for laboratory analysis. All of the kits were configured to read As concentrations at least as low as 10 ppb As. Measured against the two objectives of accurate analysis at the 50 ppb level and physical performance in the field, only four kits[6] were judged 'more dependable' and came from just two suppliers: Hach (USA) and WagTech (UK).

As more stringent DWSs are implemented, As field test kits will need to improve. Since 2005, a number of field test kits have proven quite reliable at the 50 ppb level, but performance at the 10 ppb level is more problematical. However, a study by Steinmaus et al. (2006) suggests that, with improvements in technology, training and procedures, this may be achievable. Trained scientists tested 136 water sources in Nevada with the Quick Arsenic™ and Hach EZ™ kits, and checked the results by atomic fluorescence spectroscopy (AFS). Both kits are semi-quantitative, but correlated well with laboratory results. However, a small number of serious underestimations (50 ppb versus >200 ppb) were attributed to H_2S interference, and were not corrected for by the manufacturers' recommended procedures. For screening purposes, the proportion and magnitude of false negatives at 10 ppb As is critical. Compared with AFS, the Hach EZ kit produced five false negatives (3.7%), the highest being 14.8 ppb. The Quick Arsenic kit produced three false negatives (2.2%), the highest being 13.4 ppb. From a public health perspective, these errors are acceptable, but more extensive evaluations, particularly in high-iron water, are recommended.

6.3.3 Quality assurance and integrated field and laboratory testing

All good surveys include a quality assurance (QA) programme, but here our concern is limited to aspects that are specific to arsenic surveys. The QA programme must ensure accuracy and reliability, and provide feedback during the course of the survey to correct any problems that emerge. Most laboratories already have a QA system that should meet the requirements for the survey, but preferably would be audited before any samples are delivered. The QA programme should be actively managed during the course of the survey, especially in the early stages, and not simply as a check at the end of a large survey. Where surveys are based on laboratory testing, the QA design should include the following:

- Blind duplicate samples should be sent to the laboratory at the rate of not less than one per sampler per day, in order to determine the consistency of laboratory analysis. Where these samples do not meet the specified criterion, the entire batch of samples should be rejected.
- Trip blanks should also be sent to the laboratory at the rate of not less than one per sampler per day. The blank may be either pure water or water of a known water quality, and the analysis will identify consistent errors in the laboratory.
- On a less frequent basis, blind duplicate samples should be sent to an independent laboratory to ensure that the absolute values of concentrations are correct.

Errors in field testing are less predictable than laboratory errors. Where surveys are based on field test kits, around 10% of samples should be sent for laboratory analysis. A randomly selected subset of, say, 10% of samples should be analysed as blind duplicates, and a trip blank submitted with each batch of samples. Field-test surveys are more vulnerable to human error than laboratories; hence refresher training, supervision, and inter-investigator checks (i.e. 'backs turned' comparisons at the same time and place) can be valuable components of the QA programme.

A cost-effective approach to combining field and laboratory techniques is to use field test kit results to decide which results to check in the laboratory, focusing on potentially problematic results. Thus, if the DWS is 50 ppb, it would be wise to check all samples having any trace of colour up to about 100 ppb As. This will add to the cost of the survey, but will largely eliminate errors. The highest level of assurance is obtained by carrying out both field tests and laboratory analysis at every well. The number of erroneously labelled wells would be an absolute minimum, and the mitigation programme could begin immediately by recommending users to switch water sources until they receive confirmation from the laboratory analysis. The most practical compromise, however, is to use field test kits and collect a water sample at every well. Only a few tens of millilitres are required, so storage of even tens of thousands of (acidified) water samples should not pose a problem. Blanket laboratory testing of any area could then be applied retrospectively at minimum cost at any time. The archive of water samples would also provide a benchmark for assessing changes in water quality over time.

6.3.4　Information dissemination during surveys

As noted earlier, the survey is the first opportunity to pass on information about arsenic, sanitation and hygiene, and is a major advantage of field testing. If arsenic is detected, additional time can, and should, be allocated to disseminating arsenic-awareness and mitigation advice. If only laboratory testing is used, there is a dilemma about how much information to give out during the survey; however, the logistic requirements for return visits are, at least, predictable. Many NGOs in Bangladesh and India have prepared information packs and education materials, rich in graphics and story-telling, for use in villages where levels of literacy and formal education are low (Figure 6.1). While these materials can easily be copied for use in other countries, it is very important to realise that all the better materials have been extensively field-tested and evaluated to ensure that the messages have been tuned to the particular culture of both villagers and extension workers.

6.3.5　Water quality monitoring and access to testing facilities

Formal monitoring and the ability to get water tested for arsenic are closely interrelated because they both require access to laboratories and testing equipment. Periodic monitoring is necessary because it is well established that As concentrations in many wells change over time (section 3.6.1), and so safe wells may not remain safe. Monitoring of public supplies is achievable in most countries, but testing private supplies is much more difficult. Monitoring frequencies for public supplies are normally covered by regulations. Even in the EU, monitoring of private water supplies is often not done on a routine basis.

Detecting change requires a baseline. Even more developed countries may lack a comprehensive inventory of domestic supplies. In developing countries, it is often easier for governments to carry out large, one-off surveys than to allocate resources for routine monitoring. Arsenic surveys are an opportunity to establish a baseline database. This can be complicated by the drilling of new wells (Opar et al., 2007), but governments could use this as an opportunity by offering free arsenic analysis in return for registering details of new wells, updating the database and improving surveillance in a single step. An opportunity could also be offered to retest existing wells on provision of the original survey tag.

The appropriate frequency of monitoring is a compromise between technical issues and logistical constraints. Most groundwater systems change

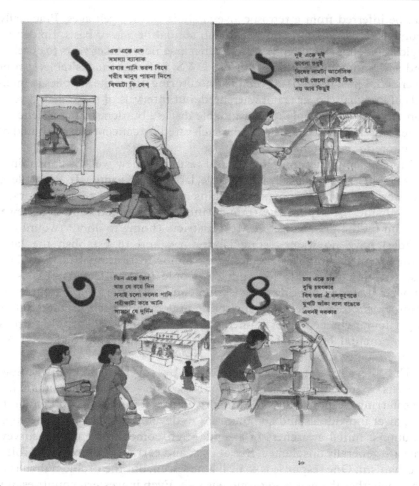

Figure 6.1 Example of arsenic awareness information from Bangladesh. The message is presented in the form of a cartoon story book produced by NGO Forum (2003). The top two scenes establish the link between tubewell-water and ill-health. In the third scene, villagers take water to the local office of the Department of Public Health Engineering for testing, and in the final scene, after arsenic has been detected, the tubewell spout is painted red to show that the water should not be used for drinking or cooking. The story continues with the villagers building a rainwater harvesting system, but continuing to use the red tubewell for washing clothes, and eventually the man regaining his health.

slowly, but hydrogeological principles can be used to prioritise monitoring. Shallow wells tend to change faster than deep wells, fractured-rock aquifers faster than those where intergranular-flow dominates, and wells close to the upper or lower boundaries change faster than wells in the middle of aquifers. Where time-series data are lacking, rates of change of As concentration can be inferred from a retrospective analysis of tubewell ages. Practically, monitoring can be done on a seasonal, annual or *ad hoc* basis. Epidemiological evidence (Chapter 5) indicates that arsenicosis takes years to develop, and so temporary exceedance of the DWS, although undesirable, can be tolerated. Thus, it can be argued that monitoring of private supplies at intervals of less than a year is not warranted, but intervals of more than 2 years run the risk of overlooking an avoidable disease burden. In the absence of other evidence, wells that already have elevated As concentrations should be monitored more often.

In many countries, monitoring and testing of new wells is constrained by inadequate, or practically inaccessible, laboratory facilities. In Bangladesh, for example, the government maintains only four water-testing laboratories outside the capital city (though more are planned) and even fewer are run by the private sector. Most districts (home to about two million people) have no water-testing laboratory, and to establish the large numbers of laboratories required is a major institutional task. Making water-testing accessible to ordinary people in As-affected areas is an important step in fighting As poisoning, and also offers opportunities for improving other aspects of environmental health such as food safety. A particular choice for governments is whether to establish multipurpose environmental health laboratories or to concentrate on dedicated As-testing facilities.

The alternative to formal monitoring by government is to facilitate citizens to test their own water sources. This can be more than just transferring responsibility to the private sector and has potential to empower individuals and communities to develop their own water-supply solutions. Initial awareness of arsenic often comes from one-off surveys that are generally unsolicited, free of cost, and carried out through a project mechanism. One response is to drill a new well, but the problem then is to know whether the new water source is safe. Even in western countries, it is difficult for an ordinary citizen to access water testing, and there may be significant cost. For a poor, possibly illiterate, villager this may be practically impossible. The challenge therefore is to make testing, whether by formal laboratory analysis or with field test kits, available and affordable to ordinary citizens.

6.4 Exploiting Safe Groundwater Sources

6.4.1 The importance of geology

It is a universal experience that successful solutions to groundwater problems are founded on sound geological understanding. The geology of every region is different, and so solutions will differ too. Empirical lessons, such as the advocacy of dug wells in Bengal, are not necessarily transferable to other areas. In alluvium, dug wells usually contain little arsenic, but in fractured rocks, dug wells may contain the highest concentrations of arsenic. The following sections consider options for locating arsenic-safe groundwater in different geological terrains. The first example, the Bengal Basin, serves as a model for alluvial aquifers in humid regions. We then consider alluvial aquifers in semi-arid climates, fluvio-glacial aquifers, and aquifers in crystalline bedrock and other geological settings. In some, the relation of geology (stratigraphy) to aquifers and arsenic occurrence is so obvious that it will be a routine matter for hydrogeologists to classify safe and unsafe locations, but in others, the identification of safe well locations is far from clear.

6.4.2 Alluvial aquifers of the Bengal Basin

Well-switching in partially contaminated aquifers

At the current 50 ppb standard, a large majority of shallow wells in Bangladesh and West Bengal are classified as safe. Even at the WHO guideline of 10 ppb As, the majority of shallow wells are safe. The simplest, cheapest and quickest solution after discovering that one's well is polluted is to take water from a nearby source that has been tested and found safe. In Bangladesh, there are around 10 million hand-pumped tubewells, one for every 10 to 15 people, more than 90% of which are privately owned. This coverage far exceeds health-based targets (typically 100 per well) and suggests that, in principle, well-switching has great potential. Indeed hundreds of thousands, perhaps millions, of people may have already switched sources. However, well-switching involves problems. First, the owners of polluted wells lose control over their water supply, and their wives and children must spend extra time carrying water, and may lead to a reduction in water use. Second, there is a social cost to switching, relating to power in class and kinship relations, which for some disadvantaged groups may amount to exclusion. Third, increased abstraction might endanger the security of safe wells.

Although well-switching is widely practised, it has not been heavily publicised (van Geen et al., 2002). In Araihazar upazila, where half the tubewells exceed 50 ppb As, 90% of the population live within 100 m of a safe well. Van Geen, Ahmed et al. (2003) drew attention to the advantage of 'community wells'. These are basically ordinary wells, although usually a little deeper, but they are known to be safe and are not privately owned, therefore reducing the potential for conflict. At six community wells, the average abstraction was 2200 L/day, with 4 L per person carried to each house. From this they concluded that, in a densely populated village, one community well could supply the potable needs of about 500 people living within 150 m radius.

It is theoretically, but not practically, possible to predict which wells will become contaminated. However, some generalised predictions can be made (Ravenscroft, 2000). For instance, as the number and proximity of contaminated wells increases, the risk to safe wells will also increase. Further, pumping more water must also increase the risk. Hence, it is rational to object to sharing a private well that is close to contaminated wells[7], but this risk may be acceptable for a community well. Well-switching is therefore least applicable where the arsenic problem is greatest, and provides good reason to focus interventions on 'hot-spots', and rely more on public awareness campaigns and promoting well-switching in less-affected areas. In Bangladesh, surveys by the BAMWSP have identified 2316 villages where 100% of wells were polluted, and so switching is not a solution. Nevertheless, it is still preferable in such areas to consume water from wells with lower As concentration as an interim measure. Knowing how long shallow wells will continue to be a safe source of water is fundamental to mitigation. This depends on the local geology, and although prediction cannot replace monitoring, qualitative risk assessments may be possible. In some situations, such as where aquifers are protected by aquitards of very low permeability or high attenuation capacity, wells can remain safe for many years or decades (section 3.6.1).

Redrilling of wells

When redrilling wells in the same aquifer, the knowledge and ability of local drillers to find their own solutions can and should be supported. The occurrence of arsenic can be related to both sediment colour and well depth (Chapter 8). There is anecdotal evidence (e.g. McArthur et al., 2004) that some drillers are already changing drilling depths to avoid arsenic, based on strategies such as avoiding 'black soil' (peat) and favouring screening wells in brown sand. Reinstalling wells as little as 10–15 m deeper, less than 3 m from the original well, can improve water quality from several hundred to less than 10 ppb As. Not all such inferences by local drillers are sound, but the point is that this has been done without expert advice, and highlights an opportunity to help communities. Through knowledge-sharing and access to water testing, drillers and well owners could develop empirical strategies to minimise the As content of tubewell water. A prototype programme was developed in Matlab upazila by von Brömssen et al. (2006), who concluded that positioning well screens based on drillers' lithological descriptions is a reliable indicator of (short-term) well safety. They are developing colour charts, with a Bengali language explanation, to promote the technique. The method is promising and could be spread rapidly, but should be accompanied by monitoring because it does not predict long-term safety. Heuristic methods such as described by von Brömssen et al. (2006) could be supplemented by hydrogeological investigations and modelling at representative sites to develop more theoretically sound guidelines for well design using parameters such as well spacing, discharge and the thicknesses of brown sand. Thus, combined with monitoring, effective mitigation can be achieved with an imperfect understanding of the science.

Dug wells

Use of large-diameter, hand-dug wells for drinking water and irrigation is common in many parts of the world. Dug wells differ hydraulically from drilled wells. When a drilled well is pumped, the effect of water stored inside the well bore lasts for a few seconds until the drawdown is balanced by groundwater flow into the well. When a dug well is pumped, the well bore is the main source of water and pumping continues until the well is nearly empty, when water is allowed to recover to its original level, and the cycle is repeated (Rushton, 2003). Dug wells are constructed to just below the water table, when further digging becomes impossible, and so water is drawn from the uppermost part of the aquifer. Dug wells frequently draw water from strata that are either of too low permeability or are too thin to be exploited by drilled wells. The hydraulic characteristics of dug wells have hydrochemical implications. Dug wells draw in the youngest and most oxygenated groundwater in the aquifer. The interaction between groundwater and air in the well bore is not merely a complication in sampling, but is fundamental to the nature of water withdrawn. Thus, water from dug wells is normally relatively rich in oxygen and oxic species such as nitrate and low in iron and manganese. However, because they are built in villages that rely on on-site sanitation, they are inherently vulnerable to pollution from latrines.

Throughout the Bengal Basin[8], dug wells have much lower As concentrations than drilled wells in the same area, due to reactions with oxygen, either at the water table or inside the well, which precipitate iron oxides and adsorb arsenic. While dug wells provide low-As water supplies, the main concern is faecal pollution from on-site sanitation, as shown in Table 6.3. Bacterial contamination is worse in the wet season, and may be accompanied by ammonium or nitrate. Iron concentrations are low, but manganese is often elevated. The physical quality of water has influenced people's willingness to adopt and maintain dug wells in Jessore district of Bangladesh, where Kabir et al. (2005) found that water from 29% of 69 dug wells was coloured, and 25% had disagreeable odours. In some areas, dug wells have been combined with slow sand filters to reduce faecal contamination, taste,

Table 6.3 Water quality from alternative water sources in Bangladesh

Parameter	DWS	WHO GV	Unit	Dug wells			Pond sand filters			Rainwater systems		
				Wet*	Dry*	Maximum	Wet*	Dry*	Maximum	Wet*	Dry*	Maximum
TTC	0	0	cfu/100 ml	820	47	TNTC	107	37	2200	0	2	640
Escherichia coli	0	0	cfu/100 ml	445	0	3000	5	2	500	0	10	24
pH	6.5–8.5	–	–	7.1	7.1	8.2	7.6	7.6	8.7	9.65	10.75	12.2
EC	–	–	ppm	1380	1350	5290	380	500	7600	115	95	1180
Ammonium	0.5	–	ppm	0.6	0.5	10	0.3	1.1	8.7	0.2	0.7	5.5
Nitrate	50	45	ppm	0.8	1.2	15	0.5	0.1	4.0	0.05	0.5	2.0
Iron	1.0	0.3	ppm	0.1	0.5	2.7	0.02	0.05	0.9	–	–	–
Manganese	0.1	0.4	ppm	–	0.4	2.8	0.02	0.03	0.23	–	–	–
Arsenic	50	10	ppb	0.55	0.8	108	0.5	3	65	0	0.55	6
Zinc	5	3.0	ppm	–	–	–	–	–	–	0.63	1.06	2.5

TTC, thermo-tolerant coliforms; TNTC, too numerous to count; *Escherichia coli,* a bacterium found in faecal waste; DWS, drinking water standard; WHO GV, World Health Organisation guideline value; cfu, colony forming unit; EC, electrical conductivity (a measure of the total amount of dissolved ions).

*Median concentrations for dry and wet season sampling.

Source: Ahmed et al. (2005)

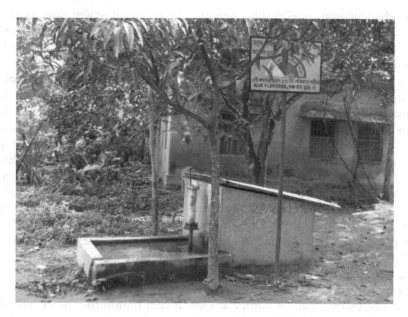

Figure 6.2   Improved dug well in West Bengal, India. Note the excavation, which is lined with concrete rings, is located inside the covered brick structure. Water is withdrawn through the hand pump which discharges onto a well-drained concrete plinth. The sign uses a colour code to indicate the quality of the water. *Source*: Photograph courtesy of Meera Hira-Smith of Project Well and Suprio Das of the Aqua Welfare Society, West Bengal.

colour and odour problems (Kabir et al., 2005). This adds significantly to the capital cost and operation and maintenance burden, but is an alternative to chlorination.

The feasibility of dug wells varies regionally, and observations in West Bengal and Bangladesh indicate that to ensure a good yield to a 1-m diameter well there should be some sand horizons at depths of 5–10 m. However, if there is a large thickness of sand in the first 10 m, a dug well may not be feasible, either because sinking concrete rings becomes impractical or because water levels fall too deep to sustain a year-round supply. On the other hand, if only clay is present to depths of 10–15 m, the yield may be insufficient unless the diameter is increased to about 3 m or more, which results in large increases in cost and land-take.

Despite scepticism in Bangladesh, in West Bengal groups such as Project Well[9] have actively promoted dug wells for arsenic mitigation, premised on the observation of low-As-concentrations and the conviction that the risks of faecal pollution can be managed through improved construction and sanitary protection. Modifications include: installation of concrete rings to provide structural stability; placing sand[10] in the annulus; a masonry wall to control surface drainage; and a metal cover and an insect screen over the concrete rings (Figure 6.2). Water is drawn through a hand-pump (as opposed to a bucket) mounted on a concrete plinth via an offset riser passing through a sealed hole in one of the concrete rings. Use of a flexible rising main reduces the likelihood of drawing in mud or sand when the water table falls. Sanitary protection is also achieved by applying siting criteria so that the well is at least 6 m from the nearest pond and 30 m from any latrine, cattle shed or cultivated fields[11]. New wells commonly have high bacterial counts and are subjected to shock chlorination, and low-level chlorination every month thereafter. The wells are not commissioned until the bacterial count is acceptable, which may take a number of months. 'Organic' odours in new wells disappear over a period of months, probably due to oxidation of buried vegetation exposed during construction. The disappearance of odours and declining coliform counts are parts of a natural 'maturing' process, and exposes a common misconception that because dug wells are an old technology, they are simple. In fact the influence of design, construction, 'maturation' and operation on the quality of water produced by dug wells is complex. Operational monitoring of 11 wells by Hira-Smith et al. (2007) found that coliform bacteria were undetectable in 65% of wells. However, two wells had surprisingly high (61 and 152 ppb) As contents, while the other nine averaged 11 ppb As. The activities of Project Well point to the inadequate level of support given to dug wells in Bangladesh, where simplistic advocacy in the late 1990s has been followed by equally simplistic demands for their abandonment.

Deeper aquifers

By convention[12], deep aquifers in Bangladesh are taken to be those below about 150 m (DPHE, 2000), although in many areas low-As water, underlying contaminated groundwater, can be found at shallower depth. Wells in these deeper aquifers are much less likely to be contaminated by arsenic, and have been the most popular form of arsenic mitigation (APSU, 2005). In a survey of the coastal belt of Bangladesh, only two out of 280 deep wells exceeded 50 ppb As, and the highest concentration was only 100 ppb (DPHE/MMI/BGS, 1999). These wells[13] were originally drilled to avoid shallow salinity, and so fortuitously also avoided arsenic. The probability of As concentrations exceeding 10 or 50 ppb As in Bangladesh varies systematically with depth (see Figure 8.7). The depth of general safety varies greatly from region to region, from as little as 30 m adjacent to the Pleistocene terraces to around 200 m in the rapidly subsiding Sylhet Basin. However, the regional variation is sufficiently predictable to install deep wells with confidence. On the other hand, iron and manganese concentrations, although generally lower than in shallow aquifers, are also problems in parts of the deep aquifers (JICA, 2006). Also, in Jessore District, Kabir et al. (2005) identified a zone where 11% of wells >200 m deep contained >50 ppb As. This zone is not due to overpumping, but is thought to follow a Pleistocene channel of the Ganges, and reinforces the importance of geological understanding in managing groundwater abstraction[14].

Deep alluvial aquifers are not present in all northern regions of Bangladesh, but here arsenic is a lesser problem, while in the south of the delta fresh groundwater may not be encountered within 300 m. A vitally important issue in using deep aquifers for mitigation is uncertainty about the recharge mechanism. Near the coast, the aquifers are overlain by brackish groundwater, and so it follows that they were not recharged by vertical infiltration of rainfall, unless in the geological past (i.e. 'fossil' groundwater). The deep groundwater is more than 10,000 years old (Aggarwal et al., 2000) and was part of an active flow system at the Last Glacial Maximum (LGM), when there was no overlying saline water, and this was later 'plugged' by estuarine sediment during the Holocene transgression. When fresh water is pumped from the deep aquifers, it can be replaced by vertical leakage or by horizontal flow. If there is vertical leakage from above or horizontal flow from the coast, poor-quality water will be drawn towards the well. Only horizontal flow from inland will maintain the potability of the deep coastal groundwater.

There is an important difference in the risks resulting from vertical and horizontal flows. Vertical leakage of salt water or arsenic generates the greatest risk, but it is faced by the abstractor himself, and is therefore self-regulating. Recharge by horizontal flow causes extensive impacts because it is a compound effect of all wells in the aquifer, and the negative impacts are neither evenly nor fairly distributed. The impacts are felt first at the coast and migrate progressively inland. This process will not be self-regulating, and indeed, inland abstractors may not be aware of the consequences of their actions. Determining the direction and magnitude of these flows is critical to assessing the sustainability of abstraction from the deep aquifers, but to date, there has been neither a quantitative study of the deep aquifer resource nor is there effective legislation to regulate abstraction. The requisite studies will require years of field investigation, monitoring and modelling. It is also important to consider the timescale of possible 'failure' of the deep aquifers. If deep aquifers can supply safe water for decades, they will have performed a vital role in reducing human exposure while alternative safe supplies are developed. Even if deep wells become polluted, it will happen slowly, and relatively low-cost treatment could be implemented gradually at pre-existing supply points.

Some insight into the sustainability of deep aquifer abstraction can be gained by examining its performance to date. For instance, at Khulna City, deep aquifers have been intensively exploited since the 1960s, and by the turn of the 21st century the aquifer had neither been salinised nor contaminated by arsenic (DPHE/MMI/BGS, 1999). This was achieved without active management, and points to an inherent resilience in the resource.

Performance data from deep wells must be examined carefully to differentiate between well failures resulting from extensive pollution of aquifers, for which there is little evidence, and those failures due to well construction defects, for which there is widespread evidence. To protect deep wells from arsenic and salinity, the annular spaces of boreholes must be properly sealed, and this is not current practice in Bangladesh, where tubewell construction relies on caving or swelling of clay to form an effective seal. For high capacity wells at least, this must be considered unreliable, and standards should be raised. Hoque (1998) found the incidence of faecal pollution decreased systematically with increasing well depth down to about 80 m, but increased again in wells deeper than about 100 m, which can be explained only by faulty well construction or operation. Improved placement of well casing and grouting should reduce this problem also.

Arsenic mitigation using deep groundwater in Bangladesh has relied on hand-pumped wells, which have a low unit cost and maximise locally available technology and labour. However, manual drilling to several hundred metres often takes weeks, and in some areas gravel or cobble layers make drilling impossible. Although the cost per well is higher, motorised drilling rigs allow rapid installation of power pumps that can support community supplies. This approach should lead to lower costs per person served, faster implementation, and distribution systems with household connections. Nevertheless, installation of high-capacity wells could encourage use of deep groundwater for irrigation, increasing the risk of overexploitation.

6.4.3   Fluvio-glacial aquifers in North America

Geochemical conditions in fluvio-glacial aquifers in the mid-western USA are remarkably similar to those in the Bengal Basin, but the configuration of the aquifers is different (Chapter 9). First, bedrock is present within reach of standard water-well rigs, and second, channel sands are less extensive and thinner. The key similarity is the juxtaposition of sand bodies and organic-rich layers, where natural or pumping-induced migration of dissolved organic matter (DOM) into sand layers causes mobilisation of arsenic. Pumping-induced leakage may be greater in these aquifers because they are thinner and more often pumped by motorised wells. Erickson and Barnes (2005a,b) showed that As pollution is associated with the youngest (Wisconsinan) glacial advance (Figure 6.3). The key to arsenic avoidance lies in not screening wells in horizons into which DOM can easily migrate.

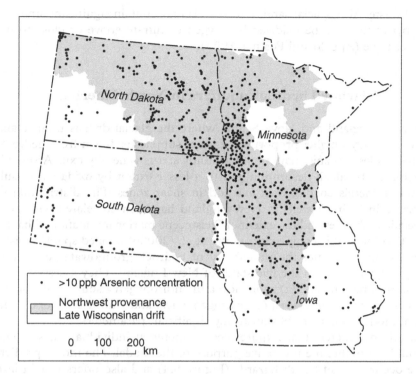

Figure 6.3   Distribution of arsenic contaminated wells in relation to the extent of the Wisconsinan glacial advance, upper mid-west USA. Only the location of wells exceeding 10 ppb As are shown. The figure demonstrates the value of geomorphological mapping in identifying contamination, and as a guide to locating safe wells. Inside the Wisconsinan footprint, 27.7% of private and monitoring wells and 10% of public wells exceed 10 ppb As.
Source: Erickson and Barnes (2005)

Aquifers within or beneath the deposits of the Wisconsinan glacial advance are inherently at higher risk. Wisconsinan sediment potentially can be avoided by drilling deeper. Trade-offs in well design can also reduce the risk of encountering high As concentrations. Longer well screens tend to avoid peak As concentrations by averaging out local extremes. On the other hand, it is even more important to avoid placing screens close to the upper and lower contacts of aquifers, or at the upper contact of bedrock aquifers, where leakage of DOM from aquitards occurs. Where it is not possible to change the screen position significantly, an alternative approach is to reduce the pumping rate to reduce intensive vertical leakage from overlying aquitards. Dug wells might be sources of low-arsenic groundwater, but in practice may not be effective due to the low permeability of glacial tills, annual water fluctuations, and the risks of pollution from microbes, agrochemicals and waste. Also, glacial sands and gravels may contain significant amounts of pyrite that can be oxidised by oxygen or nitrate above or close to the water table (Appelo and Postma, 1996).

6.4.4   Glaciated bedrock aquifers in North America

In New England and Nova Scotia, where the glacial drift is thinner and often absent, a higher proportion of water supplies is drawn from bedrock. There is less organic matter, and groundwater is generally oxic. Arsenic is mobilised by alkali desorption and to a lesser extent by oxidation of sulphide minerals coating fractures and in shear zones. The distribution of arsenic in bedrock wells in New England has been correlated with both specific rock types and the extent of Pleistocene marine inundation (Chapter 9). To address this complexity, Ayotte et al. (2006b) applied spatial logistic regression to predict the probability of bedrock groundwater exceeding 5 ppb at any point in the five states of New England. They assessed three groups of parameters: (a) geological and anthropogenic sources of arsenic; (b) geochemical processes; (c) hydrogeological and land-use factors. Their final model contained 28 statistically significant parameters, but it did not include parameters that require measurements at individual wells, which would contradict the predictive purpose of the model. The model predicts the occurrence of health hazards (Figure 6.4) and also offers insight into the processes controlling arsenic in groundwater. The most important explanatory variables were rock type, high As concentrations in stream sediments, areas of Pleistocene marine inundation, proximity to granitic intrusions, and hydrological factors relating to groundwater residence time. Parameters such as historic pesticide applications, well depth and related variables had no predictive value in the model. This methodology appears to offer potential for other areas of the world, especially for bedrock aquifers, and need not be restricted to glaciated terrains.

6.4.5   Other hydrogeological regimes

Semi-arid alluvial basins

Alluvial aquifers in the Basin-and-Range province of the southwestern USA are extensively contaminated by arsenic (Chapter 9). However, there is little information about the depth distribution of arsenic. Apparently, water utilities have tended to respond by installing centralised arsenic treatment, but there may be potential to reduce the As concentrations by modifying well designs. Detailed hydrogeological investigations should

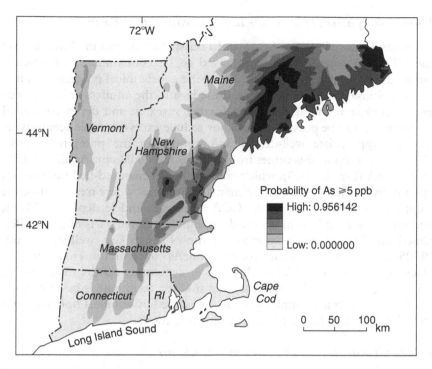

Figure 6.4 Arsenic risk in bedrock wells in New England. The shading shows the relative probability of a well drilled at any point exceeding 5 ppb As based on multiple regression analysis, as discussed in the text. The map should be compared with the distribution of arsenic in wells (Figure 9.10). RI, Rhode Island. *Source*: Ayotte et al. (2006b)

attempt to locate depth ranges or stratigraphical horizons where desorption occurs, and/or where arsenic is subsequently adsorbed by the aquifer minerals.

Volcanic-loessal aquifers in South America

The term 'loessal' aquifer is used here to refer to sequences such as beneath the Pampean Plains of Argentina, where alluvium is interbedded with wind-blown volcaniclastic material. Although the hydrogeology of these aquifers is not well documented, deeper aquifers have lower As concentrations (e.g. Warren et al., 2002, 2005). The age of the loess and its position relative to the water table, which are potentially mappable, are important in determining the risk to groundwater. The same concerns that apply to deep aquifers in the Bengal Basin, that of drawing shallow arsenic downward, apply to Argentina, and must be guarded against by monitoring.

Unmetamorphosed, Palaeozoic–Tertiary sedimentary basins

Complex Tertiary basins in Spain and Triassic Sandstones in Germany and the UK have recently been recognised to be contaminated by arsenic, although relatively little is known about the geochemical processes leading to As mobilisation. However, in all these basins, the aquifers are of considerable thickness, and so, based on further research and depth-controlled sampling, it may be possible to avoid or reduce excessive As concentrations through appropriate well-design and control of the pumping regime. Evidence to support this comes from the Central Oklahoma Aquifer (COA) in the USA (Smith, 2005), which consists of Permian red-bed sandstones, apparently similar to those in Germany and the UK where treatment-based solutions dominate. Wells in the COA aquifer extend to depths of 250 m, and arsenic is found mainly in the deeper and confined parts of the aquifer. Based on detailed depth-sampling at the Norman City wellfield, Smith (2005) was able to draw a plan for reducing As concentrations to acceptable levels by 'zonal isolation', i.e. plugging or cementing off the main arsenic producing horizons. He recommended that the technique is best suited to aquifers where contributing layers are separated by aquitard horizons, and therefore requires detailed geological investigations.

Fractured basement aquifers in tropical regions

This source of As pollution has recently been recognised in Central India and Burkina Faso, and the mobilisation processes are not well understood. Dug wells may not offer a solution because they have occasionally been shown to have the highest As concentrations, probably where sulphide minerals occur in the zone of water table fluctuation (Chakraborti et al., 1999). On the other hand, deep wells may also not provide solutions because the yields of basement aquifers, which are normally low to start with, usually decrease below the zone of surface weathering.

Areas of sulphide mineralisation

Geological mapping should indicate high-risk situations where rocks rich in sulphide minerals are likely to be encountered close to the zone of water-table fluctuation. As indicated by studies in Wisconsin by Schreiber et al. (2000), there are good prospects of avoiding high arsenic and sulphide concentrations by appropriate well construction. In areas with a sulphide hazard, boreholes should be completed to a depth below the deepest historical water level plus an allowance for the drawdown in the well. Where arsenic is mobilised by sulphide oxidation near the water table, dug wells may pose the highest risk, as has been observed in parts of the western USA (Frost et al., 1993).

Aquifers in geothermal regions

The association between arsenic and volcanic or geothermal activity is so common that, quite simply, all aquifers in active, or recently active, geothermal regions should be considered suspect until proven otherwise. It is unlikely that geothermal arsenic will be avoided by drilling to greater depth, but by mapping of temperature and chloride in surface and groundwater there is a greater chance of encountering low As concentrations in shallow groundwater, which may be related to local tectonic features.

6.5 Developing Surface-water Sources

6.5.1 Rivers, streams and ponds

Rivers are also usually sources of low-As water. However, small streams in densely populated areas tend to be polluted and/or unreliable as sources for the whole year. Schemes on large rivers require substantial investment and are normally developed for municipal supply, although they may be exploited for rural supply with centralised treatment and distribution. In less-developed countries there may be inadequate institutional infrastructure for operation, maintenance and revenue collection for such schemes. In the Bengal Basin, the Ganges and Brahmaputra rivers represent the ultimate source of potable supply. However, it would be naïve to imagine that these rivers could offer a general solution to the plight of the arsenic-affected population on a timescale of less than decades. If deep aquifers, currently the main source of mitigation, begin to 'fail' it will probably occur over decades not years. Thus, although such schemes may not be required, it would be prudent, in parallel with monitoring and assessment of deep aquifers, to conduct pre-feasibility studies of the possibility, limitations and environmental impacts of developing the major rivers for potable supply.

In India and Bangladesh there was a tradition of preserving selected ponds for drinking water. However, with increasing population, the use of tubewells and the perception that pond water is not safe, this practice has largely disappeared. Indeed, the massive reductions in mortality and morbidity from diarrhoeal disease are primarily attributed to abandonment of untreated surface water sources (e.g. UNICEF, 1998). Most ponds are unfenced and multipurpose, being used for some combination of bathing, laundry, irrigation, watering and washing animals, fish culture and potable use. Consequently, most pond water is moderately or seriously polluted, and cannot be considered for use without treatment. Nevertheless, for households and small communities, ponds and streams are options for As mitigation. Ponds are generally preferred to small streams because of their

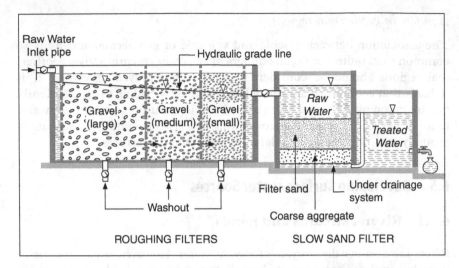

Figure 6.5   Schematic design of a slow sand filter with roughing filter. The roughing filter is added as pretreatment when the water is turbid or has high bacterial content. The pond sand filter is a particular application of the slow sand filter alone where a handpump discharges pond water into the raw water tank. *Source*: Ahmed (2002)

proximity to the point of use, lower turbidity and reliability. These sources may be developed by using the pond sand filter (PSF), a form of slow sand filter (SSF; Figure 6.5), used extensively in Asia. The SSF technology (Huisman and Wood, 1974) relies on a combination of mechanical filtration, oxidation, adsorption and biological growth to purify the water. However, the PSF/SSF technology has a variable performance record and requires a well-organised community (Caldwell et al., 2003). A biological film grows on the surface of the filter, and must be removed after one or two months, which is simple but troublesome. The PSFs are not recommended where turbidity exceeds 30 NTU[15] or the bacterial count exceeds 500 cfu/ 100 mL (Ahmed, 2002). A problem with pond sand filters is that the alternative uses noted above make protection from pollution almost impossible. Ahmed (2002) noted that many PSFs have been abandoned due to difficulties with operation and maintenance or social conflicts over water use. Surveys of water quality in Bangladesh (Table 6.3) show the PSF is effective in avoiding As exposure and in achieving low iron and manganese concentrations, but substitutes microbial risk for that of arsenicosis. More than 90% of water from PSFs contained coliform bacteria. Because of this, it is now recommended to incorporate a roughing filter (Figure 6.5) for more effective removal of bacteria, and to allow use of raw water with greater turbidity. On the other hand, the capital cost increases.

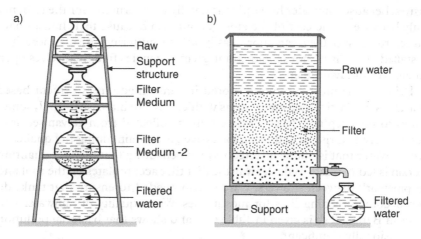

Figure 6.6   Household filters for treating surface water in Bangladesh: (a) three Pitcher ('tin kolshi' filter); (b) small household filter. Both these designs have been adapted for As removal by incorporating iron in the filter medium as described in Chapter 7.
Source: Ahmed (2002)

Surface water sources such as ponds may also be treated at household level using simple filters such as shown in Figure 6.6. Such filters were widely used before the advent of shallow tubewells, and the three-pitcher ('*tin-kolshi*') design has been adapted to remove arsenic by including iron nails in the middle pitcher (Chapter 7). However, the effectiveness of such devices in removing bacteria cannot be taken for granted.

6.5.2   Rainwater harvesting

Rainwater harvesting is used worldwide, particularly where groundwater is saline and in areas of poor aquifer potential. The principles for designing rainwater harvesting systems are given by Ahmed (2002), but always involve significant capital investment in storage facilities. Naturally it works best where rainfall is both high and distributed throughout the year. The advantages of rainwater harvesting are that it is generally, but not always[16], safe from toxic chemicals, is suitable for individual households, requires no energy and can be built by local craftsmen with local materials. The main disadvantages are the high initial cost, preventing pollution, poor taste and lack of mineral content may contribute to deficiencies in diet. For houses with small roof areas and at high-rise developments, the catchment area may be insufficient, while poor houses may be constructed with unsuitable materials such as thatch. As Caldwell et al. (2003) point out, there are equity issues, because rainwater harvesting is chiefly an alternative for the rich, not only because of the cost of the storage, but also because their houses have larger roofs and they can more easily afford guttering. Also, where it is installed at a private household, grant-giving agencies find themselves open to charges of favouritism.

Rainwater is most commonly stored in tanks made from cement-based materials or plastic. Rainwater reacts with cement to increase the pH, sometimes to unacceptable levels. Where rain is collected from galvanised iron roofs, there is a risk of acquiring excessive zinc. Maintaining the quality of stored water that is not disinfected requires ensuring that the first quantum of rain is led to waste to flush away the dirt that accumulates on the roof and in pipework between showers. Care is also needed to ensure that tanks do not become breeding sites for mosquitoes. Water quality of rainwater systems in Bangladesh is given in Table 6.3, and shows that bacterial pollution is occasionally significant.

6.6   Arsenic in Water Distribution Networks

Arsenic-contaminated groundwater in water distribution systems is affected by mixing, reactions during distribution, and disinfection. Where a network is fed by a wellfield, As concentrations can be regulated by blending prior to entry, but only to a small extent within the pipework. Blending affects As concentrations not only by dilution, but also by mixing with oxic waters that promote precipitation of iron hydroxides. In addition, iron oxyhydroxide coatings on the walls of pipes can adsorb arsenic during distribution. Steinberg and Hering (2001) demonstrated these effects at Hanford, California, showing how concentrations vary according to how the system is pumped, and proving that well-head analyses may not represent actual arsenic exposure.

Arsenic-rich groundwaters have particular chemistries that cause them to respond differently to chlorination, due to reactions with bromide and organic compounds to form trihalomethanes such as $CHCl_3$, $CHCl_2Br$, $CHClBr_2$ and $CHBr_3$ that are known or suspected carcinogens. Second, chlorine also reacts with ammonium to form chloramine, which is still a disinfectant, but is a hundred times less effective than free chlorine, resulting in inefficient disinfection of coliform bacteria, viruses and *Giardia* cysts. Disinfection-related risks apply particularly to RD-type waters, but are not related to the As concentration. They can occur in groundwater that has been subject to arsenic removal processes, such as in the Red River delta of Vietnam, where groundwater contains high concentrations of bromide, ammonia and DOC (Duong et al., 2003). In waters where arsenic has been mobilised by other processes, problems due to chlorination by-products are less likely.

6.7   Socio-economic Aspects of Mitigation

Awareness-raising and health education are even more important for water-supply programmes in As-affected areas than elsewhere, which we illustrate below with case histories from rural communities in Bangladesh. The first objective is to make people aware of the danger of arsenic in water, its consequences for health, and in simple terms, its mode of action. Without success at this stage, later activities will be undermined. However, it may be difficult to convince people of the dangers where arsenical symptoms are not present. Recognising the link between arsenic and skin lesions has been much easier to convey than other, potentially fatal, symptoms. The second objective is to make people understand that arsenic avoidance is essential in both preventing and treating arsenicosis. Although messages such as 'do not drink or cook with water from red wells' are simple, this stage introduces two complications. First, the substitution of risks from arsenic and microbial pollution requires a new 'safe-water' paradigm. Second, food can be a major source of dietary exposure, and reducing arsenic intake from food is practically more difficult. Educational campaigns need careful planning and evaluation, and probably progressive elaboration of messages.

Having established awareness, the next stage is to explain the mitigation options and the constraints to their adoption. Aziz et al. (2006) emphasised the important distinction between establishing awareness and taking action to avoid arsenic. Agencies have promoted technologies with very different results in terms of their social acceptability, reliability and affordability. To date, deep hand tubewells have been strongly preferred because they are familiar and require minimal day-to-day maintenance. In South Asia, it has been difficult to organise rural communities to maintain treatment systems without strong support from a sponsor. Fortunately, there has also been a strong reluctance to return to untreated surface water. There is strong interest in piped water supplies, but this is not specific to As-affected areas, and raises equity issues of how to provide for the significant minority who are exposed to arsenic and cannot afford to pay.

6.7.1   Case histories of social investigations from Bangladesh

18DTP public education programme

Hanchett et al. (2002) highlighted some of the obstacles experienced in one of the early mitigation programmes. The 18 District Towns (18DTP) water-supply project started before arsenic was discovered in six of the towns.

In 1998, they tested all the 1384 project-installed wells, and helped in testing other public wells. Using the Merck field test kit[17], they detected arsenic in 55% of wells, and painted them red if they contained >100ppb As, and green if no trace of arsenic was found. If a trace of arsenic was detected, they painted a red question mark ('Red-Q') to signify a 'doubtful' status. In each town, 18DTP organised training, initiated by an 'Arsenic Week', for tubewell caretakers, school teachers and children, and community leaders. People were told that water from red or red-Q wells should not be used for drinking or cooking, but could be used for washing. Users of red-painted pumps were advised to take drinking and cooking water from other sources. They also recommended that an emergency household water treatment method (involving aeration, adding alum, and storage) would no longer be recommended. The evaluation used questionnaire surveys of adults, focus groups, and interviews with school children. The respondents were classified as programme-influenced (PI) or not programme-influenced (NPI). The main findings were:

- The meanings of the red- and green-painted pumps were understood by 80% of PIs, but only 25% of NPIs. The red question marks caused much confusion.
- Painting appeared to have influenced the behaviour of 43% of PIs who had switched their water source, compared with only 15% of NPIs.
- Well sharing was controversial due to the contradiction between the 'need' of the outsiders and the aggravation caused to existing users. Conflict was greatest where safe water was scarcest.
- Many people were confused by the nature of As poisoning. Asked 'what is arsenic?', 38% said a poison and 38% a disease. While professionals see arsenic as an old problem recently discovered, most affected people feel that 'the earth has changed'. However, people were very reluctant to return to drinking surface water, and there was also little enthusiasm for domestic water treatment.
- Despite their leading role in providing water, women's knowledge of arsenic issues was significantly poorer than that of men.
- The economically better-off were better able to connect to the municipal distribution system, whereas poorer people were more likely to continue using contaminated wells, not only because of the cost of the alternative but also because low social status reduced their ability to share safe wells.
- Children effectively took up messages taught in school to promote behavioural change at home.

Arsenic awareness programmes

In 1999, the Bangladesh Rural Advancement Committee (BRAC), the largest NGO in Bangladesh, began an arsenic mitigation project in two upazilas, which involved training water testers, helping communities to choose safe water options, technology demonstrations, identifying patients and promoting safe water use (Hadi, 2003). The programme was evaluated by BRAC through interviews with 600 people in pairs of project-influenced and control villages. Their main findings were:

1   People in project villages had better knowledge of safe water options: 42% could name two safe sources as opposed to only 10% in the control villages.
2   In project villages, 44% of people could list two or more symptoms of arsenicosis compared with less than 8% in the control villages. In project-influenced villages, 43% of people knew arsenicosis is not contagious, compared with only 14% in control villages.
3   In project villages, there were no age differences in knowledge, but in control villages people aged 30–39 years had the best understanding. There was no significant difference between men and women, but knowledge improved with both years of education and land ownership.
4   In all cases, frequent exposure to radio and television increased knowledge of both safe water options and arsenicosis symptoms.

These results are both encouraging and salutary. Although absolute levels of knowledge regarding arsenic were low, considerable progress had been made from a very low base. Ahmed et al. (2005) conducted interviews at several hundred households already using various types of mitigation across the As-affected areas. Almost all respondents (98%) knew about arsenic, and 70% had known about it for at least 2 years. The largest proportion (37%) had learned by 'word-of-mouth', 26% from radio and TV, 21% through NGO activities, and just 9% through tubewell testing. Almost all knew that red-painted tubewells should not be used for drinking and cooking, but 79% did not realise that it is acceptable to use this water for washing. Although recognised to be dangerous, understanding of arsenic poisoning was often unclear: 53% knew that arsenic is a slow poison, but only 44% could name a symptom of arsenicosis, and only 3% knew that arsenic is not contagious.

Household response to arsenic mitigation in Araihazar

The Columbia University studies and interventions in Araihazar upazila commenced with a comprehensive survey in 2001 that showed 53% of wells exceeded 50 ppb As (van Geen et al., 2003a). The results were recorded as actual As concentration on a metal well-tag, thus establishing a reliable baseline. A follow-up survey in 2004 (Opar et al., 2007) of all 6500 households found that awareness-raising had been successful in that the vast majority (89%) of people knew whether or not their well was contaminated.

At the 3410 unsafe wells, 65% of users had changed their source of drinking water. Of these, 55% now used a different private well, 21% had drilled new wells and 16% used community wells. Unsurprisingly, the distance to the nearest safe well was important in determining whether or not people changed their source of water. When the nearest safe well was within 50 m, 68% switched sources, but when it was more than 150 m away, the proportion dropped to 44%. Given a choice of sources within 50 m, people preferred community wells.

A disturbing finding concerned new wells, which had increased in number by about 5% a year, and amongst which 53% contained <50 ppb As, only marginally better than in the original survey (47%). This demonstrates both the urgent need for locally available and affordable arsenic testing, and also suggests that the solution of drilling deeper, into brown sand layers[18], had not been learned by local drillers.

Willingness and ability to pay for arsenic mitigation

To investigate affordability, the Water and Sanitation Program (WSP, 2003) used awareness surveys and contingent valuation methods in affected and unaffected (control) areas. Many more people (87%) in affected areas knew that arsenic was a 'serious' threat to health compared with unaffected areas (53%), but few (35%) understood that the consequences could be as serious as gangrene, cancer or death. In affected areas, 59% of the people with polluted wells had changed their water source, while 41% continued to use water they knew to be contaminated. Only 1% of respondents were unconcerned about As poisoning. Six mitigation technologies were discussed with the affected population: two types of household treatment, community-based treatment, dug wells, pond sand filters and deep tubewells. More than 70% preferred community over household systems, and 76% expressed a preference for deep tubewells over any other technology. The second most popular option (16%) was the three-pitcher household filter (see Figure 6.6). The other four options found little favour. A quarter of households indicated that they could not afford these options. The WSP (2003) also identified a strong preference for piped water systems in all areas, and inferred that the willingness to pay for piped supplies was 40–50% above the estimated cost.

6.7.2   Risk assessment of arsenic mitigation options

Disillusionment with the consequences (arsenic) of the 'solution' (tubewells) to epidemic diarrhoeal disease led some public commentators to advocate a return to surface water. While few technocrats supported this view, it led to the RAAMO study (Ahmed et al., 2005). The RAAMO study

Table 6.4 Performance of arsenic mitigation technologies surveyed in the Risk Assessment of Arsenic Mitigation Options study

| Technology | Number | Average (%) of wet and dry season surveys* | | | | | User satisfaction (%) |
		As > 10ppb	As > 50ppb	TTC (cfu)	Fe > 1.0ppm	Mn > 0.4ppm	
Dug well	36	20	2	89	25	69	87
Deep tubewell	36	0	0	5	51	9	92
Pond sand filter	42	3	1	96	0	6	93
Rainwater harvesting	42	0	0	53	0	–	–

TTC, thermo-tolerant coliforms; cfu, colony forming unit.
*'Wet' and 'Dry' are the median concentrations dry and wet season sampling.
Source: Ahmed et al. (2005)

addressed supply to rural communities across the As-affected areas and evaluated four technologies – dug wells, deep tubewells, pond sand filters and rainwater harvesting – but did not consider arsenic removal plants. Continued use of both polluted shallow tubewells and untreated surface water were considered unacceptable, and therefore excluded. The study focused on risk substitution between options and had three main components: a water quality and sanitary inspection survey; a social acceptability survey; and a quantitative health risk assessment (QHRA). The results of the two surveys are summarised in Tables 6.4 and 6.5. All the technologies are effective in preventing exposure to arsenic at the 50ppb level, although 20% of dug wells exceeded 10ppb As. However, the technologies differed greatly in terms of bacterial contamination. Deep tubewells and rainwater systems provide good quality water throughout the year. Unchlorinated water from both dug wells and pond sand filters was moderately contaminated in the dry season and badly contaminated in the monsoon. Social surveys indicated high levels of satisfaction with all the technologies from the perspective of the user.

The QHRA considered both the chronic effects of arsenic and the acute effects of pathogens including bacteria (*Shigella*), viruses (*rotavirus*) and protozoa (*Cryptosporidium*). Ahmed et al. (2005) combined the water quality survey results with dose–response functions from regional and international sources (mainly Yu et al., 2003). Arsenic concentrations were used directly, but the dose–response functions for pathogens were related to the concentrations of thermotolerant coliforms (TTC). To measure impact, they used DALY[19] to combine mortality and morbidity. They concluded

Table 6.5 Median disease burden associated with arsenic mitigation options

Technology	Pathogenic disease burden (DALY/million population– year)	Arsenic disease burden (DALY/million population)
Dug well	9,400	0.9
Deep tubewell	≤10	0.8
Pond sand filter	2800	0.08
Rainwater	≤10	0.2
Shallow tubewells	≤10	400

DALY, disability adjusted life years.
Source: Data estimated from figures 6.5 and 6.6 in Ahmed et al. (2005)

that the disease burden is dominated by bacterial infection but with a substantial contribution from viruses. The arsenic assessment included skin, lung and bladder cancers, but omitted skin lesions and the other effects detailed in Chapter 5 because of the difficulty of calculating DALYs. The largest cancer burden was due to skin cancers but with a major contribution from lung cancer, and a very small number of bladder cancers. The arsenic and pathogenic disease burdens are compared in Table 6.5, which also includes an estimate for shallow tubewells[20] for comparison with the status quo. Although the precise figures should be treated with caution, and the shallow tubewell estimate is too low because of the excluded effects, the relative magnitude of the DALY estimates leads to clear conclusions. All the mitigation options lead to a dramatic decrease in the arsenicosis burden, but dug wells and pond sand filters lead to an unacceptable microbial risk. The RAAMO study suggests that pond sand filters and/or dug wells could actually make the disease burden worse, and should be promoted only where disinfection, or other verifiable means of microbial risk reduction, can be assured.

The RAAMO methodology can serve as a model for other countries, but must be adapted to the particular local hydrological and socio-economic circumstances. Moreover, there is scope to improve the model by including dose–response data for heart and lung disease[21], which will increase the strength of the argument in favour of replacing polluted shallow wells.

6.7.3 Costs of arsenic mitigation options

Unfortunately, unlike the costs of arsenic removal (Chapter 7), which are relatively independent of location (but not concentration), the costs of

Table 6.6   Indicative costs of water-supply options in Bangladesh

Technology	Technical life (years)	Water output (m³/yr)	Households served	Capital cost ($)	Operation and maintenance cost ($)*	Unit cost ($/m³)
Rainwater	15	16.4	1	200	5	2.13
Pond sand filter	15	820	50	800	15	0.16
Conventional surface water treatment	20	16,400	1000	15,000	3000	0.31
Dug well (8 m)	25	410	25	800	3	0.26
Deep tubewell (300 m)	20	820	50	900	4	0.15
Piped water supply	20	16,400	1000	40,000	800	0.38

*Costs for dug wells, pond sand filters and rainwater systems do not include chlorination, and as such do not offer an equivalent service
Source: World Bank (2005)

alternative water sources vary enormously between areas, and usually not all options will be feasible at any given location. Given these provisos, the cost estimates in Table 6.6 give a general guide to the relative costs of technology options in Bangladesh. Where all options are feasible, deep tubewells and pond sand filters offer the lowest costs, but the latter carry a high microbiological risk (unless chlorinated), and rainwater systems tend to be by far the most expensive. However, these general costs should never be presumed to apply to any given location.

6.8   Policy and Planning Initiatives

6.8.1   National arsenic policies and plans

Conventional wisdom dictates that a good policy is better that a good programme, which in turn is better than a good project. Where As pollution has recently been discovered, a National Arsenic Policy can be a powerful means of mobilising public interest and government action for sectoral programmes and cross-sectoral collaboration. Conversely, bad policies are damaging to good programmes and projects. Bangladesh's 2004 National Policy on Arsenic Mitigation (NPAM) contained four elements: (a) awareness raising; (b) alternative safe water supply; (c) diagnosis and management of patients; and (d) capacity building. In general, the policy correctly comprises short directives that drive programmes and projects, but an unfortunate element of the policy stated that mitigation should 'give preference to surface water over groundwater as a source for water supply' (GOB, 2004). This confuses means (use of surface water) and objectives, which should be to supply 'safe' water by the most socially, environmentally and economically acceptable means. An alternative, and potentially equally effective approach, is to require all sectoral policies, especially water, health and agriculture, to give explicit consideration to the importance of arsenic. In either case, any national arsenic policy should be time-bound, and have the objective of integrating arsenic into all relevant sectoral policies and strategies.

In addition to policy, governments should establish national plans to eliminate dangerous levels of arsenic exposure. The plans should be time-bound, and specify the institutional mechanisms by which mitigation will be carried out. The plans should include quantitative interim targets that incorporate specific exposure levels.

6.8.2   Information policies

Information can help people to understand arsenic poisoning, locate providers of mitigation technology, empower them to develop their own solutions, highlight best practice and expose bad practice. Information has two dimensions: first, its sources of knowledge; and second its means of delivery. Technically, information should be accessed through a web-based database supported by GIS and GPS technology. However, the database should be designed around a framework that allows cooperative development by government and the private sector, not merely creating an official depository of data. Through a flexible geographical design and metadata standards, many agencies can add their own data in a format that can be accessed by all, and allow linking of survey, health, agricultural and mitigation data by researchers and others who seek to design or evaluate projects. To facilitate this process, the lead agency in arsenic mitigation should establish an Information Policy that defines the types of data to be included, responsibilities, and outline procedures for adding and accessing information. While respecting personal privacy, it is recommended that the information policy should involve a presumption of unclassified status for data aggregated above the personal and household level.

6.8.3   Coordination and institutions

Discovery of extensive arsenic pollution raises new challenges that go beyond the individual experience of most professionals and administrators, but not beyond the combined expertise of professionals in different disciplines. Many levels of coordination are required: between disciplines; between government, NGOs and the commercial private sector; between government departments; and between government and the general public.

Arsenic mitigation requires coordination, and this may be achieved either by creating a dedicated organisation or through interministerial committees. The optimal solution is probably specific to each affected country but, in general, the argument in favour of a dedicated agency is stronger where the bureaucracy is less sophisticated, and where the problem is recent and large. Any such organisation should be staffed by a combination of staff seconded from line agencies, NGOs and recognised experts who would disseminate best practice from around the world. The organisation's objectives should be strategic planning, coordination, monitoring and evaluation, and information dissemination, but not implementation. A key function of coordination is to allow national and local government, NGOs and the commercial private sector to operate independently on a day-to-day basis, but in a manner that contributes to a common goal. Any such organisation should have a time-bound existence, wherein redundancy is an objective.

Facing up to As pollution has challenged the knowledge of scientists, engineers and medics. In the most As-affected areas of the world, the great alluvial plains of South and Southeast Asia, groundwater practitioners have operated with a narrow knowledge of geology and almost no training in chemical water quality issues. The educational institutions that trained these professionals reflect the historically perceived needs, and urgently require strengthening to prepare the next generation of professionals to meet the new requirements. In particular, the curricula of water engineering courses need to be expanded in the area of water quality, and reoriented to measure outcomes in terms of 'public health' rather than physical construction.

6.8.4   Technology verification

Although public utilities normally have sufficient expertise to liaise directly with manufacturers, most households and small communities are ill-equipped to procure unproven technologies, and require protection from unscrupulous marketing. Most arsenic removal and some other treatment technologies fall into this category. To meet this need, the Ontario Centre for Environmental Technology Advancement (OCETA; http://www.oceta.on.ca), the

Bangladesh Council for Scientific and Industrial Research (BCSIR) and the BAMWSP project formed a partnership in Bangladesh to establish an Environmental Technology Verification for Arsenic Mitigation (ETV-AM) programme, intended as a '$3.8 million, 30–month, capacity building project to assess, and verify arsenic mitigation technologies for treating contaminated, rural drinking water' (OCETA Annual Report, 1999–2000). The ETV-AM comprised five protocols including: (a) registration of manufacturers; (b) screening of technical, social and fiscal factors; (c) laboratory testing; (d) field testing; (e) verification. The objectives of the ETV-AM programme were worthy, but by January 2006 only four technologies had been approved. This is disproportionate to the scale and urgency of the problem, and suggests that either most technologies are inappropriate or that the ETV-AM programme has stifled the private sector. The West Bengal experience is that performance is much more closely related to operation and maintenance issues than design deficiencies (section 7.6.2). Technology verification should guide, not control, the private sector and the public, and should not overemphasise laboratory benchmarking when factors such as training and support services have an equal or greater influence in the real world.

6.8.5   Water resource and environmental impacts

Effective water-supply solutions are underpinned by sound understanding of the environment of the region. Most, if not all, interventions for arsenic mitigation should have overall positive environmental outcomes due to their impact on health. However, potential negative impacts can be foreseen and should be avoided or minimised. The potential impacts can be considered in terms of the type of intervention.

1   Groundwater treatment:
   - the principal environmental issue is to ensure the safe disposal of As-rich wastes (section 7.6);
   - provided that waste is safely disposed of, treatment can have a positive impact by contributing to clean-up of the aquifer;
   - some household treatment systems remove arsenic but produce such low volumes of water that they are insufficient for good hygiene, although this can be compensated for by using As-polluted wells for washing.
2   Groundwater development:
   - continued use of shallow aquifers may induce lateral migration of arsenic;
   - deep wells may be affected by drawing down arsenic or salinity from above;

- the overpumping of arsenic-safe, and mainly deeper, aquifers may cause saline intrusion that affects abstractions nearer the coast;
- increased pumping from deep aquifers may cause derogation of existing wells due to increased drawdown.

3 Surface water development and treatment:
- the main impacts depend on the reduction of flow in the river or stream that may reduce the availability of water to other abstractors, impair navigation, reduce fish stocks, or cause saline intrusion near the coast – all such negative impacts occur predominantly in the dry season, and depend closely on the proportion of the flow lost;
- where there are multiple schemes on a stream, there may well be additional impacts, of the same type, resulting from upstream developments;
- surface water is vulnerable to pollution by pesticides, fertilisers, hydrocarbons and improper waste disposal.

6.8.6 Social considerations

The mitigation option selected should be the most socially acceptable option that is economically and technically feasible for the particular site. This requires an understanding of the community, its technical capability and, critically, its appreciation of the implications of arsenic to the community. Successfully adopting a new technology depends on awareness of the health issues, the operation and maintenance implications, the ability to organise user groups and the ability and willingness to pay. Awareness is affected by the degree of risk, education level, gender and age. As was clear from the case histories, without an aware and informed population, it is extremely difficult to implement a new water supply and achieve real health benefits (section 6.7). As described earlier, the poor and malnourished suffer worse consequences from arsenic in drinking water. Therefore the design process should explicitly target the most disadvantaged groups to ensure that benefits do not accrue preferentially to the wealthiest members of the community. Hence, social surveys should target women and less-educated members of the community whose voices are not easily heard in public meetings.

6.8.7 Regulation

In general, arsenic mitigation is unlikely to require extensive legislation. However, regulations affecting DWSs and the control of groundwater abstraction may be needed. New DWSs should be enacted in line with guidance from public health experts, but implemented in a timeframe that is achievable (section 5.4.3). Unlimited exploitation of deeper aquifers could result in benefits to irrigation at the expense of DWSs, and benefits to inland users at the expense of coastal communities who are most vulnerable to both saline intrusion and drawing in As pollution (sections 3.8.2 and 6.4.2). There should be a legal basis to control deep well abstraction according to the priority of drinking water over other uses, especially in areas with no alternative source of supply. However, even without legal regulation, abstraction can often be controlled through the supply of financial incentives, such as only offering subsidies for deep wells where the shallow aquifer is unsuitable, and thus 'unnecessary' deep wells will be minimised by financial self-regulation. In general, it is better to apply economic measures first, and legal constraints last, since incentives are likely to be more successful than regulation.

6.9   Monitoring and Evaluation of Water-supply Mitigation Programmes

In poor countries where millions of people are exposed to arsenic, there are profound difficulties in the monitoring and evaluation of mitigation. Monitoring and evaluation must operate simultaneously at multiple levels to reflect a hierarchy of objectives, ranging from chemical changes in aquifers to actual impacts on health and well-being. The basic monitoring measures will be: (a) the range of arsenic and, where appropriate, coliform concentrations in water supplies and groundwater; and (b) the number and operational status of mitigation devices installed[22]. Beyond this, it is necessary to prove the effectiveness and equitable coverage of mitigation through social surveys, and to demonstrate a basis for actual improvements in health through monitoring of arsenic in urine, nails and hair as biomarkers of exposure. This is particularly important where there is significant exposure to arsenic through food. The sampling frame for measuring biomarkers should reflect the age, class and gender structure of the community.

A precondition for monitoring and evaluation is to establish a baseline of exposure, the medical condition of the exposed population and the quality of water. It is easier to determine the initial level of exposure than that after mitigation commences, because knowledge induces change in behaviour. Initial exposure to arsenic is estimated from surveys by assuming no change in water use. As soon as people know the As content of a well, some will begin to change their behaviour, but may do so in many ways. They may switch to existing private or community wells, drill new wells or take up other solutions promoted by NGOs, companies or government. Moreover, these alternatives may not be safer. A complication occurs where government does not take total responsibility, and mitigation is carried out in diverse, and often informal, ways. Hence, assessing the current status may require a triangulation approach. What can be reasonably well known are the 'budgeted' activities of outside agencies: i.e. the number of wells or treatment plants constructed. There follows an iterative process to establish current exposure. Unless reported by water-user groups, the number of people removed from exposure can be estimated from the numbers of devices installed, after adjusting for the average number not functioning. Informal mitigation activities, such as well switching, drilling new shallow wells or household treatment devices, are more difficult to track. Under such a scenario, there can be no presumption of risk-based targeting of high-As wells, and therefore monitoring should explicitly seek out residual pockets of high exposure.

It is obvious from the above that there will always be uncertainty about the status of exposure and the effectiveness of mitigation. An integrated programme of routine monitoring and carefully targeted, periodic evaluations will be required. Monitoring should be conducted at two levels. Individual agencies facilitating alternative water sources should monitor their own activities and supply summarised information to the relevant co-ordinating agency. In the early stages of mitigation, it may be sufficient to track the allocation of devices according to the exposure estimates for each community. Because poorer communities are likely to lag behind in terms of private mitigation efforts, they should be benchmarked by their socio-economic status, using publicly available statistics, so that government can act to ensure that mitigation is targeted equitably.

As mitigation proceeds, it will be increasingly difficult to assess residual exposure in the population, and whether health benefits are being achieved. Periodic evaluations should be conducted to determine (a) the effectiveness of mitigation provided, and (b) how many people are still exposed to arsenic. The latter will require interviews and group discussions, identification of 'red wells' still in use, testing of new wells and analysis of hair, nails and urine. For evaluation purposes, additional information required may necessitate clinical surveys, analysing food, and detailed examinations of water use.

From the water resources perspective, it is important to distinguish local changes in well-water from bulk changes in the aquifer. The latter should be done with purpose-built monitoring wells but may, in practice, have to rely on randomised surveys to provide a baseline. The water quality of safe wells should be monitored, as should contaminated wells, which is best done by testing the source water at arsenic removal plants. The abandonment of wells should also be a basic component of monitoring.

6.10   Summary

Medical evidence makes it clear that the single most important action is to remove exposure to arsenic, and that delay will result in increased disease and death. Surveys underpin arsenic mitigation programmes, and must determine not only the extent and range of As concentrations in water, but also the information necessary to evaluate the impact of interventions on human health and water resources. Where pollution is extensive, compromises may be necessary between the quality and quantity of information obtained at each site, and the cost and time taken to collect it. Arsenic field test kits should play a major role in extensive surveys, but never without a systematic laboratory-based QA programme focused on concentrations close to the prevailing standard. Knowledge, awareness-raising and information dissemination are essential to any arsenic mitigation programme. Understanding the nature of arsenic poisoning, overcoming prejudices and misconceptions, and making people aware of how exposure may be reduced and safe water obtained are preconditions to successful interventions, irrespective of whether led by the public or private sectors.

In general, there are many options for obtaining low-As supplies, both from groundwater and surface water. However, when local geological and hydrological conditions are considered, the range of options will normally be reduced to just a few that are feasible. The alternative water sources described must be weighed against the option of treating contaminated groundwater (Chapter 7). Preferred technical solutions should not be prejudged by national or regional policies, but left to local decisions as to the socially preferred, technically feasible option, where the final judgement is balanced by cost and willingness to pay. A vital issue in developing countries, and one that poses major issues regarding informed choice, is the substitution of risks between arsenic and waterborne pathogens. Where pollution is extensive, interventions must also be assessed for their impact on both the local environment and regional water resources. Some options, such as the use of deeper aquifers, raise important water resources issues that require urgent action.

Where mitigation is not carried out entirely by state investment in municipal and community supplies, monitoring the progress of mitigation raises profound difficulties. Identifying and dealing with pockets of suffering that preferentially affect socially disadvantaged groups can be very difficult. In either case, it is important to measure indicators of actual improvements in public health, and not simply physical and financial measures of the mitigation programme. Last, but not least, water testing facilities should be made available and accessible to communities, so that ordinary citizens can be aware of, and participate in managing and developing their own solutions.

Annexe 6.1   Arsenic Survey Procedures

A6.1.1   Sampling procedures

How water is collected and stored alters the concentration of arsenic that is determined. Suspended particles may carry adsorbed arsenic and other elements that are not part of the 'dissolved' load of the groundwater, but are consumed by users of the well. After drinking, the adsorbed arsenic is likely to be released in the gut. Exposure to air during or after sampling may cause precipitation of iron oxides that adsorb arsenic. In this case, the iron and arsenic are part of the dissolved load of groundwater. The decision on whether or not to filter thus depends on the purpose of sampling. Hydrogeochemical studies seek to determine the condition of the water in the aquifer, and therefore the sample should be filtered immediately and then acidified. However, if the objective is to determine human exposure, then the samples should not be filtered. Nevertheless, in the case of drinking water surveillance, it is essential to know when and how water is used, and in particular whether it is stored before use, and sample collection should reflect actual consumption.

Particles may be removed by filtering through a 0.45 μm filter paper, while minimising contact with the atmosphere. Iron precipitation may be prevented by adding a strong acid (such as nitric, hydrochloric or sulphuric) until the pH is <2. The timescale of iron precipitation on exposure to the atmosphere is notoriously variable, and can be from seconds to days, but is usually minutes to a few hours. Hence, if water is tested immediately in the field, it is not necessary to acidify; otherwise it should be acidified.

Purging of wells prior to sample collection often receives much attention, but again the requirements depend on the objectives of sampling. Much of the literature on groundwater sampling focuses on piezometers, where the rule-of-thumb guide of removing three casing-volumes before sample collection is often applied, but has limited basis in science (Barcelona et al., 2005). If the objective of sampling is a rigorous geochemical characterisation, then it is better to use low-flow pumping equipment and measure sensitive parameters such as pH, temperature, EC and redox potential until they stabilise (Barcelona et al., 2005, and references therein). If, however, the objective is drinking water surveillance, these rules do not apply, and water should be collected under 'typical' conditions. The main provisos are to avoid sampling at times when the well has been idle for a long-time (such as early in the morning) or if the well has been overpumped. Such an approach can be applied to hand-pumped wells or to municipal supply wells. Dug wells are a special case for which the idea of the 'representative sample' does not apply. Interactions between groundwater and the atmosphere are intrinsic characteristics of the dug well, so water should either be collected in the middle of a busy period or sampled on a time-series basis and averaged.

A6.1.2   Sampling and analysis for arsenic speciation analysis

The ratio of As(III) to As(V) in groundwater is sensitive to redox conditions and becomes unstable when the water is removed from removed from the aquifer (e.g. Cherry et al., 1979). Speciation is of interest from the geochemical perspective, and because it affects water treatment and the toxicity of arsenic. Rapid preservation is essential to determine the species present, and hence older studies should be considered suspect unless proper preservation techniques are documented. McCleskey et al. (2004) identified three requirements for sampling for speciation analysis.

1   Samples must be filtered in the field to remove micro-organisms and colloids.
2   Reagents must be added to prevent oxidation and precipitation of dissolved iron and manganese. Suitable reagents include HCl, H_2SO_4 and EDTA, although the latter is not generally recommended because of the high concentrations needed.
3   The sample must be isolated from solar radiation (sunlight).

The exact form of preservation depends on the analytical method to be used and other parameters to be preserved. HCl is preferred for preservation of As, Fe and Se and analysis by HG-AAS, but EDTA preferred if the analysis is to be done by HPLC–ICP–MS, or when organo-arsenic species are to be determined (McCleskey et al., 2004). Determination of As species requires a combination of appropriate separation and detection techniques. While HG-AAS has cost advantages for analysis of As(III), As(V) and common organic species such as DMA, and meets the needs of most groundwater studies, the best technique for routine analysis of As species is liquid chromatography–ICP–MS (Gong et al., 2002; Akter et al., 2005b).

A6.1.3   Supplementary data collection

While collecting water samples or analysing arsenic in the field, much valuable information can be collected. The detail will depend on the purpose of the survey and constraints of time and budget. At the design stage, consideration should be given to at least some of the following, using standard questionnaires to assure uniformity of responses.

1   User and demographic details: the details of the owner, address and administrative classification. Given the low cost and ease of use, location by GPS should be standard.
2   Give each well a unique code and fix a permanent tag at the well site.
3   Water use information: number of users, quantity pumped and purpose. Establish whether and for how long water is stored before consumption.
4   Well construction details: depth and diameter, pipe materials, location of well screen, date of installation, type and capacity of pump and motor, drilling and contractor licensing details.
5   For hydrogeochemical surveys, measure pH, EC, temperature, dissolved oxygen, redox and preferably also bicarbonate potential on-site.
6   Sanitation practices: type, distance to, and depth of, latrines and drains, washing habits.
7   Medical questions: Ask whether water users have, or have seen, symptoms of arsenicosis. Photographs will be useful, but do not imply a clinical diagnosis where the necessary medical training is lacking. Only a referral for proper medical advice should be given.
8   Assess knowledge of arsenic awareness.

NOTES

1   Oral rehydration therapy should also be given great credit for the reduction in mortality, as opposed to morbidity.
2   Arsenic may not be the only hazardous chemical in groundwater, and care should be taken to avoid repeating oversights such as occurred in Bangladesh (see Annex 8.1).
3   A 'false positive' is where the test indicates the water is unsafe, but in truth it is safe. A 'false negative' is where the test fails to identify a dangerous level of contaminant.
4   Made available in digital form as supplementary material with their paper.
5   An assumption that is reasonable here, but not universally so.
6   These were the Hach 5-stage and 'EZ' models and the WagTech VCDK and Digital Arsenator models. The 'Merck Highly Sensitive' and 'Econo-Quick' models gave good analytical performance but were subject to damage in the field.
7   The reason to share the water is moral, not scientific.
8   But not necessarily in other geological settings, as discussed later.
9   Project Well (http://www.projectwellusa.org) was founded by Dr Meera Hira-Smith and operates in the As-affected areas of North 24-Parganas District in West Bengal. Project Well gives much attention to social and organisational issues, as described by Hira-Smith et al. (2007).

10 The sand layer improves the yield of the well, but involves a trade-off against maximum sanitary protection compared with placing an impermeable seal in the annulus.

11 Such criteria have frequently been overlooked with other mitigation options.

12 Some workers have used stratigraphical criteria or required the presence of an overlying aquitard, however, both lead to confusion in practice.

13 The term 'deep well' has caused much confusion in Bangladesh (see Ravenscroft, 2003), where it has different meanings in the irrigation and water-supply subsectors. Here, we use the term for wells deeper than 150 m.

14 This understanding is underpinned by the availability of good quality borehole logs, which in turn requires improved training of field officers of the Department of Public Health Engineering and other government departments.

15 NTU, nepheline turbidity units.

16 In India, Meera and Ahammed (2006) showed that rainwater systems are prone to contamination by heavy metals, trace organics and pathogens.

17 At the time, Merck only rated the kit as suitable for As >100 ppb, although it often gave a weak stain at lower concentrations, whereas the absence of any stain usually corresponded to concentrations of <50 ppb As.

18 Araihazar lies on to the edge of the Madhupur Tract, where brown Dupi Tila sands may be encountered at depths of only 30–50 m.

19 The DALY indicates total disease burden expressed in terms of years per million of population per year, including a statistical range of outcomes (Havelaar and Melse, 2003).

20 The RAAMO study assigns the same microbial risk to shallow and deep tubewells, whereas Hoque (1998) showed unambiguously that shallow tubewells are more contaminated. This will not change the overall conclusions, but makes the argument in favour of abandoning shallow tubewells even stronger.

21 Heart disease was the major cause of death during the period of high exposure in Antofagasta (section 5.14).

22 Noting the findings of the RAAMO study (section 6.7.3), where polluted wells are replaced with alternative sources such as pond sand filters, overall improvements in health should be demonstrated, not assumed.

Chapter Seven

Removing Arsenic from Drinking Water

7.1 Introduction

This chapter describes and compares methods of removing arsenic from contaminated water without regard to the merits of non-treatment solutions (Chapter 6). There are many methods for removing arsenic from groundwater, including oxidation, coagulation-filtration, adsorption, ion exchange, membrane technologies and biological methods, and many more specific technologies that apply them[1]. Aguirre et al. (2006) noted that a web search for 'arsenic treatment' will return several hundred thousand hits and commented that 'most websites offered the 'latest and greatest' solution to arsenic removal, but full-scale experience and commercial availability of many products are non-existent or extremely lacking'. Technologies must be selected that are appropriate to the desired output standard, water chemistry, size of supply, operation and maintenance capability, and socio-economic characteristics of the consumers. Major considerations in selecting treatment technologies are the capacity of the plant and the institutional context, which combine to give a threefold classification: household or small community supplies; large community supplies; and municipal supplies. Large communities are differentiated from small ones by having a piped distribution system, and large communities from municipal supplies by greater institutional support and employment of full-time, skilled operators.

The chapter commences with a discussion of the significance of raw water quality (section 7.2). We then present descriptions of twelve basic methods, and numerous variants, available to remove arsenic from water (section 7.3). Some readers may prefer to skip to section 7.8, which provides guidance on selecting methods and technologies, before returning to read only the subsections relevant to their particular needs. We then consider the radical alternative approach of trying to clean-up contaminated aquifers (section 7.4), and the environmental issues related to disposing of wastes generated by treatment (section 7.5). This is followed by comparative evaluations and case histories that illustrate the effectiveness of treatment technologies in different settings (section 7.6). Finally we summarise the available information on the costs of treatment (section 7.7) and the attempt to develop technical and cost-based guidance that reflects both the variation of water quality and the institutional setting (section 7.8). The chapter closes with a hypothetical assessment of the treatment requirements in Bangladesh if that country's mitigation were to be based entirely on arsenic removal (section 7.9).

7.2   Water Quality Issues

7.2.1   Water quality objectives

The objectives of water treatment are determined primarily by national drinking water standards. In recent years, the European Union, the USA and other countries have lowered their arsenic standards from 50 to 10 ppb As, whereas most As-affected countries continue to use 50 ppb. The literature should be read with caution because many reports from South Asia report effluent As concentrations of a few tens of ppb as a success, whereas in North America and Europe this is the starting point for arsenic removal! Where low standards coincide with high natural As concentrations then only extremely efficient removal systems will be able to achieve compliance (see section 7.8.1). Some methods described later may effectively reduce As concentrations to <50 ppb but not to <10 ppb As.

7.2.2   Source-water quality

Source-water quality plays a key role in selecting treatment systems. Although many parameters can affect performance, potentially confounding parameters can be predicted from the regional hydrogeology and the four basic geochemical mechanisms described in Chapter 2. Table 7.1 summarises the main water quality characteristics that may guide technology selection.

The literature on arsenic removal has generally neglected the geographical variations of groundwater quality, and hence results may not be applicable to all regions. The most important difference is the high iron and manganese concentrations found in RD waters, which may cause clogging of filters or sorption media, but can also aid As removal. Reductive-dissolution-type waters are dominated by As(III), which may require oxidation, and may

Table 7.1   Characteristic source-water quality and potential issues in water treatment

Parameter	Reductive dissolution (RD)	Alkali desorption (AD)	Sulphide oxidation (SO)	Geothermal arsenic (GA)
Oxygen status	Strongly anoxic	Oxic	Oxic	Variable
pH	Neutral	≥ 8	<7	Normally neutral
Dominant As species	As(III)	As(V)	As(V)	Variable
Fe and Mn	Very high Fe normal, and high Mn is common	Low to moderate Fe and Mn	Fe can be high or low	Variable
Possible other toxic elements	Ba	F, Mo, Se, V, Sb	Co, Cr, Ni, Zn	B
Dominant anions	High HCO_3; very low Cl and SO_4	Variable, usually HCO_3, Cl and SO_4 all present. Cl may be high.	High SO_4, with low to moderate HCO_3	High Cl and/or SO_4
Potentially competing anions	PO_4, SiO_2	V, PO_4, SiO_2	PO_4, SO_4, SiO_2	PO_4, SO_4, SiO_2
Dissolved organic matter	High to very high	Low	Low	Low
Exsolving gases	CH_4, CO_2	None	None	Normally absent
Sulphides	Possible	No	No	Possible
Salinity	Fresh	Fresh to brackish	Fresh	Variable
Other				High temperature

also have elevated phosphate concentrations that can interfere with As adsorption. Most RD waters also require removal of iron and/or manganese to produce good quality drinking water. Though not included in Table 7.1, the other critical raw water quality issue is, of course, the As content.

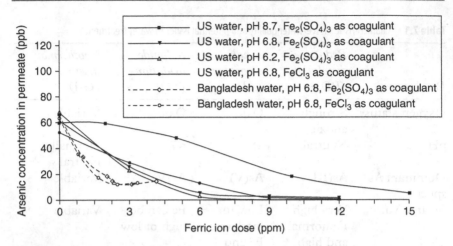

Figure 7.1   Effect of pH and ferric iron dose on arsenic removal by coagulation-filtration. The higher iron dose required for the USA water reflects its low natural Fe-content (0.035 ppm) compared with the Bangladesh water (1.7 ppm). In the USA water, arsenic was present as As(V); the Bangladesh water was pre-oxidised to convert As(III) to As(V).
Source: Wickramasinghe et al. (2004)

For methods such as adsorption, the filter medium is a major cost item that is directly proportional to As concentration. Conversely, other methods such as modified iron removal make use of high natural iron contents to remove arsenic. However, their effectiveness is very sensitive to the Fe:As ratio, and this parameter can vary by several orders of magnitude.

7.2.3   Chemical influences on arsenic removal

The chemical principles controlling inorganic arsenic in water were described in Chapter 2. However, most involve the adsorption of arsenate and/or arsenite onto metal oxides, and the controls most relevant to water treatment are shown in Figures 7.1 and 7.2 and summarised below:

1   In oxic waters, arsenic is readily adsorbed on the common Fe-oxides ferrihydrite and goethite (e.g. Pierce and Moore, 1982), as well as on Al, Mn and Ti oxides and Fe-rich clay minerals.
2   Adsorption of As(V) decreases with increasing pH, especially above pH 7.5–8.0. However, adsorption of As(III) on ferrihydrite and goethite does not decrease until pH 9–10; and adsorption of As(III) on magnetite increases from pH 6 to pH 9.

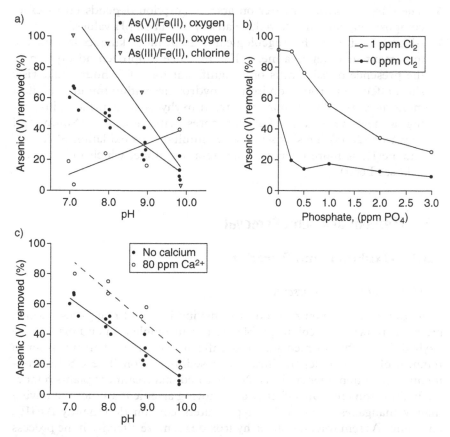

Figure 7.2 Water quality influences of arsenic removal on ferric iron. (a) pH and pre-oxidation. (b) Pre-chlorination and phosphate. (c) pH and calcium. All initial conditions: 1 ppm Fe, 100 ppb As, 10 ppm DIC and saturated with O₂ at 24°C, except (b) constant pH 8.0.
Source: Lytle et al. (2005)

3 Adsorption of both As(III) and As(V) onto iron minerals is stronger than on other minerals. Increasing the Fe:As ratio improves arsenic removal under most conditions.

4 In most situations, As(V) can be adsorbed more rapidly and in greater quantities than As(III). Hence, pre-oxidation of As(III) improves arsenic removal.

5 Phosphate, silicate and dissolved organic matter may reduce arsenic sorption, although sulphate does not. Phosphate significantly reduces adsorption of As(V) at pH > 6, whereas the effect on As(III) reduces with increasing pH.

6   The effect of organic matter on arsenic sorption depends on its exact composition, but tends to reduce adsorption at all pH values.

7   Although of little hydrogeological significance, kinetic factors are important in water treatment. For instance, improved adsorption in the presence of calcium is only significant for a few hours. Likewise, silica affects adsorption on iron oxyhydroxides within minutes as silica monomers and dimers may coat fresh oxyhydroxide surfaces, imparting a negative charge that competes with arsenate (Smith and Edwards, 2005). This explains why simultaneous oxidation of As(III) and Fe(II) is more effective than aeration alone, which only rapidly oxidises Fe(II).

7.3   Methods of Arsenic Removal

7.3.1   Oxidation and filtration

Oxidation of iron and arsenic

Oxidation is a common method of removing iron and manganese, which gives rise to taste and colour problems. The insoluble iron and manganese oxyhydroxides thus formed adsorb significant quantities of arsenic prior to removal of the particles by filtration or sedimentation. The US Environmental Protection Agency (EPA, 2000) noted that treatment plants removing mainly iron are more effective at removing arsenic than those removing mainly manganese. Anoxic RD-type waters contain dominantly As(III), and hence As removal on iron oxyhydroxides is more effective if the process first oxidises As(III) to As(V). In many affected regions, existing iron-removal plants have been successfully adapted to remove arsenic. Iron removal is desirable for its own sake and to prevent clogging of As-removal systems. Many of the methods described below rely on iron to remove arsenic. Whether they utilise the natural iron in groundwater, involve adding ferric salts, or use fixed-bed solid adsorbent, they all rely on the capacity of iron oxyhydroxides to adsorb As(III) and As(V). Earlier evaluations (cited in Lytle et al., 2005) showed that some existing Fe–Mn-removal plants in the USA were already very effective in removing arsenic. Lytle et al. (2005) reviewed theory and practice, to produce the following conclusions and recommendations for optimising iron-removal plants for As removal:

1   As removal is much reduced at pH > 8, and in the presence of high phosphate concentrations;

2   As-removal capacity is always improved by adding extra iron;

3 calcium increases adsorption of arsenate, and tends to counteract the influence of silica;

4 pre-oxidation of arsenic is always desirable because adsorption of As(V) is always more effective than that of As(III);

5 freshly formed (less than a few minutes old) iron particles have a much higher capacity to adsorb arsenic;

6 the formation of iron particles should be simultaneous with oxidation of As(III) to As(V), therefore a strong oxidant such as free chlorine or potassium permanganate should be added before aeration[2];

7 when pH ≥ 8, pH adjustment improves arsenic removal, however, there is a disadvantage because it requires handling hazardous acid on site.

Peyton et al. (2006) examined ways of improving community iron and arsenic removal plants in Illinois (USA) to meet the new 10 ppb standard. Pilot tests were conducted on groundwater from a fluvio-glacial aquifer containing 40 ppb As(III), and elevated iron (1.3 ppm; Fe:As = 33) and DOC (13 ppm) concentrations. They recommended an approach, based on so-called Fenton chemistry, in which hydrogen peroxide reacts with ferrous iron to release the hydroxyl radical. Compliant As concentrations were achieved by adding 0.9 ppm of H_2O_2 (before aeration) and 6 ppm of iron (as $FeCl_3$). Without peroxide, aeration oxidised 25% of As(III) in 30 minutes, but adding H_2O_2 converted 50% of As(III) in less than a minute, and oxidation of As(III) was proportional to the peroxide dose.

Passive oxidation and sedimentation

Passive oxidation is the simplest application of oxidation, which involves storing water in broad-topped containers. The technique requires high iron concentrations in the source water, and needs oxygen from the air to mix with the water during pumping, filling and storage. Iron precipitates adsorb arsenic and sink under gravity. The technique has been applied in Bangladesh by WaterAid, although the results are extremely variable, being dependent on the Fe:As ratio and the rates of oxidation and sedimentation. Microbial contamination can also be a problem. Arsenic removal by oxidation is enhanced by solar radiation, which promotes the oxidation of As(III) to As(V) and therefore eases its removal. Hug et al. (2001) demonstrated a very simple method for disinfection and arsenic removal by pouring tubewell water into UV-A transparent bottles (typical soft drink bottles) to which a few drops of lemon juice are added to promote formation of Fe(III) complexes. The bottles are shaken and left in the sun for 5–6 hours before filtering the water through a cloth. The UV light directly kills bacteria and oxidises As(III) to As(V) which is adsorbed onto the Fe(III) precipitate. Arsenic removal of 50–80% was reported. Although this method has limitations, it is possible that exposure to sunlight during aeration may facilitate other methods of arsenic removal.

Slow sand filtration

Slow sand filtration (SSF) is a widely-used technique in the developing world, mostly for treating surface water (Huisman and Wood, 1974), but is also used for iron removal from groundwater. Generally, water is first cascaded or sprayed into an elevated tank, from where it drains into a bed of graded sand and gravel, which may be aerated to encourage biological activity. Aeration readily accounts for the oxidation of iron, but the precise mechanism of arsenic removal is less clear. As(III) may be adsorbed directly onto fresh iron flocs or, as suggested by Katsoyiannis et al. (2004) and Pokhrel et al. (2005), may first be oxidised to As(V) either inorganically or due to bacteria growing on the media. The method is prone to clogging, and regular backwashing is essential. In Canada, Pokhrel et al. (2005) demonstrated that commercial slow sand filters can remove almost all iron and 95% of arsenic.

Examples of slow and rapid sand filters used for municipal supplies to village and small town supplies (c. 2,500 m³/d) in Bangladesh are shown in Figure 7.3. The urban unit applies chlorination after filtration. M. F. Ahmed (2003) reports that these units remove 40–80% of arsenic, which is currently considered satisfactory when the raw water does not greatly exceed 100 ppb As. However, pre-oxidation of As(III) to As(V) would be required to achieve higher As-removal efficiencies.

In Vietnam, Berg et al. (2006a) reported on the successful use of household (slow) sand filters, achieving an average removal efficiency of 80%. A hand-tubewell pumps into an upper tank, filled with sand, from where water flows under gravity into a lower storage tank at a rate of 0.1–1 L/minute, achieving a contact time of 2–3 minutes. Essential maintenance consists in replacing the sand and brushing the tanks every 1–2 months. Berg et al. (2006a) evaluated 43 filters treating water containing 10–380 ppb As, <0.1–28 ppm Fe, <0.01–3.7 ppm P and 0.05–3.3 ppm Mn. For 90% of the filters, the treated water contained <50 ppb As, and 40% contained <10 ppb As. The sand filters not only removed arsenic, but also 99% of Fe, 90% of P, 71% of Mn, 14% of Si and 39% of Ca. They concluded that the nature of the sand is not critical, and a high Fe:As ratio is the key to efficient arsenic removal, noting that 'adsorption to sand surfaces cannot efficiently remove As without simultaneous precipitation of iron'. They concluded that an Fe:As ratio of >50 is required to achieve <50 ppb As and a ratio of >250 to achieve 10 ppb As, proposing the following equation to predict the efficiency of arsenic removal:

$$\text{As removal (\%)} = 13.6 \ln(\text{Fe, ppm}) + 45$$

a) **Village Unit**   Section X

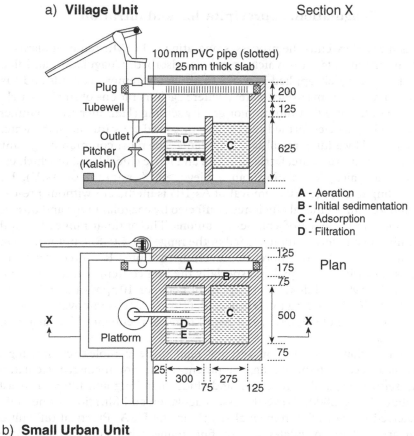

100 mm PVC pipe (slotted)
25 mm thick slab

Plug
Tubewell
Outlet
Pitcher
(Kalshi)

D
C

200
125

625

A - Aeration
B - Initial sedimentation
C - Adsorption
D - Filtration

Plan

A
B

D
E
C

Platform

125
175
75

500

75

25
300   275
75   125

b) **Small Urban Unit**

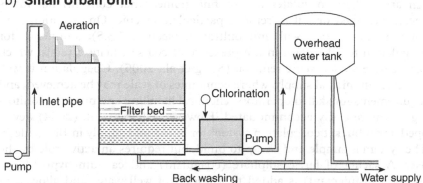

Aeration

Overhead
water tank

Inlet pipe

Chlorination

Filter bed

Pump

Pump

Back washing   Water supply

Figure 7.3 Schematic design of iron and arsenic removal plants used for urban and rural supplies in Bangladesh. (a) Hand-pump operated for rural water supply. (b) A system suitable for supplying a small town via a piped distribution system. All dimensions in millimetres.
Source: M.F. Ahmed (2003)

7.3.2   Coagulation, coprecipitation and filtration

This method extends the processes operating at Fe–Mn-removal plants by adding metal salts onto which arsenic is adsorbed. Coagulation and flocculation are widely applied in water treatment to remove colloids and suspended matter from surface waters, where agglomerations of small particles are separated by either filtration or gravity settling (Hammer and Hammer, 2001). The particles formed can remove dissolved constituents of the water, often aided by adding metal salt coagulants. The most common coagulants are aluminium sulphate, ferric sulphate and ferric chloride, all of which can adsorb arsenic. Coagulation can achieve >90% removal of As(V), but according to EPA (2000) removal of As(III) is inefficient without pre-oxidation. Arsenic-removal efficiency is affected by coagulant type and dosage, pH and the presence of competing anions. The optimal ranges for both aluminium and ferric sulphates fall in the range pH 5.0–8.0, but iron coagulants remove As(III) more effectively than alum. Required coagulant doses vary with water quality, especially the iron content, but according to Edwards (1994) all doses of >20 ppm of $FeCl_3$ or 40 ppm of alum remove >90% As(V). According to Hering et al. (1997), As(III) removal is reduced by the presence of sulphate[3], and As(V) removal is enhanced by calcium at pH >7.0.

Coagulation and filtration systems tend to be complex, comprising a chemical feed system, mixing equipment, basins for mixing, flocculation and settlement, a filter medium, and sludge handling and filter-backwash facilities (EPA, 2000). Nevertheless, coagulation and filtration is one of the preferred methods for municipal supply in the USA. Practical difficulties can arise when coagulates are so fine-grained that conventional filters become clogged or fail to remove particulate arsenic. One solution is to combine coagulation with microfiltration (section 7.3.8); another is for coagulation to take place in the presence of coarse calcite crystals, which can achieve 99% arsenic removal (Song et al., 2005). Coagulation is well suited for municipal supply, where economies of scale may be achieved, and requirements for skilled operators, chemical handling and process monitoring are more easily accommodated. However, Cheng et al. (2004) developed a two-bucket coagulation system for household supply in Bangladesh. The system is simple and cheap to build, but requires an active role by the user. A sachet of ferric sulphate (coagulant) and calcium hypochlorite (oxidant disinfectant) is added to a bucket of well water and allowed to react for 5–10 minutes. The water with iron flocs is then poured into the second bucket containing local sand, retained by a cloth. Groundwater containing 187–753 ppb As was reduced to <50 ppb 95% of the time, and <10 ppb 50% of the time.

7.3.3 Lime softening

Lime softening is used at large treatment plants to reduce excessive hardness caused by high concentrations of calcium and/or magnesium. The process raises the pH by adding sufficient lime (calcium hydroxide) or soda ash (sodium carbonate) to precipitate calcium carbonate at pH 9.0–9.5 or magnesium hydroxide at pH > 10.5. Lime softening may also involve the precipitation of iron hydroxides, formed either from natural iron or iron added as a coagulant. From a survey of operational plants, McNeill and Edwards (1995) showed that plants precipitating only calcium carbonate removed <10% of the As(V), but those precipitating magnesium or ferric hydroxide removed 60–95% of the As(V). The removal of arsenic by lime softening is affected by pH and other dissolved components (McNeill and Edwards, 1997). Optimum removal of As(V) occurs at about pH 10.5, and that of As(III) is at about pH 11.0. However, at lower pH the removal efficiency reduces sharply (EPA, 2000). The removal efficiency of As(V) is much greater than that of As(III), where pre-oxidation is recommended. Arsenic removal is subject to interference by sulphate and carbonate at pH < 11, and by phosphate at pH < 12. After calcium and magnesium have been removed, the pH is neutralised with carbon dioxide gas. Although lime softening can reduce concentrations to below 3 ppb As, EPA (2000) only recommends the method where a reduction in hardness is also desired.

7.3.4 Adsorption processes

A major group of treatment technologies relies on the adsorption of arsenic onto the surfaces of oxides of aluminium, iron, manganese, titanium and cerium and some biological materials. Other adsorbents, including sulphur-modified iron (SMI), iron-modified activated alumina, modified zeolite, and iron-oxide impregnated activated-carbon are also under development (Shevade and Ford, 2004; Payne and Abdel-Fattah, 2005; Westerhoff et al., 2006). In all cases, As(V) is more readily adsorbed than As(III). The adsorbent is normally placed in a tank, or fixed-bed reactor, through which water flows either under gravity or under pressure. The latter is convenient in groundwater treatment where the well pump can be used as a source of power. Adsorption systems are particularly convenient for waters low in iron and manganese, which cause clogging and require regular periodic back-washing.

Adsorbents are often described in terms of their adsorption capacity and a sorption isotherm, which measures the partitioning of the contaminant between solid and liquid. These are important, but the most useful measure is the number of bed-volumes[4] prior to breakthrough (i.e. when the effluent As concentration exceeds a predetermined level). Effluent concentrations increase over time, but the rate at which this happens varies between adsorbents and between waters, and so there is no universal best solution. A related parameter, the empty bed contact time (EBCT), is the time that the water is in contact with the medium, and determines the maximum allowable flow rate. As adsorbents become saturated, they must be replaced or regenerated. They also tend to slump in the reactor vessel, slowing the flow of water, although some recently developed adsorbents have been bonded into a polymer matrix to overcome this problem.

Activated alumina

Activated alumina (AA, or γ-Al_2O_3) is an amorphous aluminium oxide prepared by dehydrating $Al(OH)_3$ at high temperature, so that the surface can exchange contaminants, including arsenic (plus fluoride, selenium, silica and natural organic matter) for hydroxyl groups. Activated alumina is capable of removing >90% of As(V) but, as with many other techniques, removal of As(III) is much less efficient. Arsenic removal on AA is strongly pH-dependent, and is optimal between pH 5.5 and 6.0, which often requires acidification, and subsequent neutralisation to prevent corrosion. Operated under even slightly alkaline conditions, As removal may be reduced by an order of magnitude (EPA, 2000). Activated alumina has a strong affinity for arsenate, but not arsenite, and is affected by competition in the following sequence (EPA, 2000):

$$OH^- > H_2AsO_4^- > Si(OH)_3O^- > F^- > HSeO_3^- > DOC > SO_4^{2-} > H_3AsO_3$$

The sequence differs from that for ion exchange (section 7.3.6), and importantly, AA readily adsorbs fluoride, which ion exchange (IX) does not. Also, sulphate and chloride have little effect on arsenic removal, which gives it a significant advantage over ion-exchange in AD and SO waters. The American Water Works Association (AWWA, 1999) conducted trials on AD-type waters in the southwest USA that show how pH adjustment and pre-chlorination improve arsenic removal on AA, measured in terms of adsorption capacity and the number of bed volumes (BV) to breakthrough at 50 ppb As. The waters had a range of As(V):As(III) ratios, and were run at the natural pH (8.6–9.0) and the optimal pH, with and without pre-chlorination. They also tested synthetic groundwater with 100% As(III) and 100% As(V), both at optimal pH. The results (Table 7.2) demonstrate that both pH adjustment and complete oxidation of As(III) are required to achieve cost-effective and long-lasting removal of arsenic, and can increase the capacity and breakthrough times of AA columns by two orders of magnitudes.

Table 7.2   Influence of speciation, chlorination and pH on arsenic adsorption on activated alumina

Source Water	As (ppb)	As(V) %	pH	Bed volumes to 50 ppb As	Adsorption capacity (g/m³)
Synthetic groundwater	100	0	6	300	20
Synthetic groundwater	100	100	6	23,000	1920
Hanford, California					
Natural groundwater	90	11	8.6	800	61
Chlorination only	98	100	8.8	900	83
pH adjustment only	90	11	6.0	700	60
Chlorination and pH adjustment	98	100	6.0	16,000	1410
Fallon, Nevada					
Chlorination only	110	100	9.0	800	42
Chlorination and pH adjustment	110	100	5.5	13,100	1280

Source: AWWA (1999)

Activated alumina can be regenerated with a few BVs of sodium hydroxide, followed by neutralisation with sulphuric acid, but both pose safety and disposal issues. Regeneration may be repeated, but each cycle reduces the time to breakthrough by about 10–15%. The American Water Works Association (AWWA, 1999) suggested that at very small systems it may be preferred to dispose of the spent medium. Activated alumina columns may be affected by fouling by silica and mica (AWWA, 1999). Over time, as AA dissolves, the medium is prone to becoming 'cemented', although this can be minimised by vigorous backwashing. Operating AA columns in parallel maximises the flow rate, but EPA (2000) recommend operating the columns in series, using the first as a 'roughing' tank and the second as a fail-safe measure to prevent unexpected breakthrough. Each time the 'roughing' tank becomes saturated, it is replaced by the 'polishing' tank, which in turn is replaced by fresh AA.

Synthetic iron oxyhydroxide adsorbents

Granular ferric hydroxide (GFH) and granular ferric oxide (GFO) can remove both As(III) and As(V) without pH adjustment or pre-oxidation, and can also remove phosphate, selenium, antimony, vanadium, molybdenum, copper, lead and chromium. Granular ferric hydroxide and GFO do not produce highly toxic sludges or require dosing with chemicals. These granular media are engineered to be permeable and have large surface areas. Granular ferric hydroxide has a specific surface area of 250–300 m²/g and an adsorption capacity of up to 55 g As/kg (Driehaus et al., 2002). The residue contains of the order of 1–10 g/kg of arsenate, and while regeneration is theoretically possible, direct disposal of the waste is preferred (EPA, 2000). Recently, such media have been incorporated into polymer beads to improve permeability and structural stability, and to make regeneration more practical (DeMarco et al., 2003).

Much of the early experience with GFH came from community supplies (4–160 m³/hour) drawn from sandstone aquifers in Germany that produced groundwater with up to 40 ppb As (Driehaus, 2000; 2002). The GFH became saturated after 50,000 to 200,000 BVs, thus requiring replacement of the media at intervals of 6 months to 2 years. The adsorption capacity (measured in bed volumes) correlated poorly with total As concentration, and was reduced by a factor of four between pH 7 and pH 8, and was also reduced by silica. Because this non-ideal behaviour cannot readily be modelled, Sperlich et al. (2005) recommended the use of rapid small-scale column tests to predict breakthrough behaviour. Backwashing and water quality monitoring were conducted monthly, but routine maintenance requirements were low, no personnel were needed for normal operations, and neither was chemical dosing nor a separate power supply. The method appears well suited for small water utilities with low-Fe sources. No sludge is generated, and it is claimed that spent adsorbent can be sent to landfill without pre-treatment (section 7.5). Synthetic adsorbents have a different cost structure to other treatment systems. Capital investment in pipework and vessels is less, labour expenses are minimal, but the cost of the media is critical and depends strongly on the breakthrough characteristics for the particular water quality.

Iron oxide coated sands

The use of iron-oxide coated sand in fixed-bed reactors was described as a 'rare' process for arsenic removal by EPA (2000), but the use of naturally Fe-rich sands has received attention in India. The process is basically the same as for GFH/GFO and involves adsorption of arsenate, arsenite and other anions onto ferric hydroxide coatings. Depending on cost, the sand may be either replaced or regenerated with sodium hydroxide when exhausted. As(V) is adsorbed more readily than As(III), but adsorption of As(V) decreases as the water becomes more alkaline, especially at pH≥8.5. Although chloride and sulphate are not significant, high concentrations of DOC can reduce As(V) adsorption. Vaishya and Agarwal (1993) showed that Ganges river sand could remove high concentrations of As(III) from groundwater, at the rate of 24 µg/g over a 2-hour period. Joshi and Chaudhuri (1996) showed that iron oxide-coated sand has promise as an adsorbent for household treatment units, and it has since been used in the Family Filter (section 7.5).

Greensand filtration

The geological material known as 'greensand' contains the Fe-rich clay mineral glauconite, which is formed naturally in marine sediments. In water treatment, glauconitic sand is usually pre-treated with $KMnO_4$. The manganese oxide coating promotes oxidation, exchange and adsorption reactions, where arsenic is initially exchanged on the oxide surface, oxidised from As(III) to As(V), and then adsorbed to the sand (Subramanian et al., 1997). The effectiveness of greensand filtration is strongly correlated with the ferrous iron content of the raw water. Both Subramanian et al. (1997) and EPA (2000) report As-removal efficiencies of 80% when the Fe:As ratio exceeds 20. The use of greensand has become increasingly popular for use in pressure filters, of the type shown in Figure 7.4, for community and industrial supplies. The coarse upper layer, which provides rough filtration and retains most of the precipitated iron, is a light material such as coal or anthracite so that it remains on the top during backwashing. Conversely, the garnet filter is denser than the greensand and remains at the bottom during backwashing. Raw water containing a substantial component of As(III) should be pre-oxidised with chlorine or permanganate, and where the Fe:As ratio is <20, it should be dosed with ferric chloride (EPA, 2003a).

Manganese oxides

Manganese oxides can scavenge arsenic from solution, although the adsorption capacity reduces rapidly from $470\,\mu g/g$ at pH 3 to $230\,\mu g/g$ at pH 7,

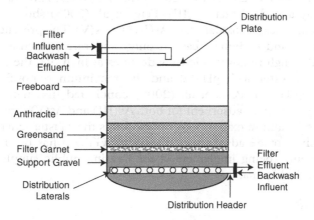

Figure 7.4 Schematic design of a vertical greensand pressure filter.
Source: EPA (2003c)

and only 30 µg/g at pH 10 (Ouvrard et al., 2001, 2002). In practice, pH adjustment would be required. Breakthrough in Mn-oxide filters also depends on the flow rate and should be limited to low-flow systems. Manganese oxides can be regenerated with caustic soda, but this requires acid-neutralisation and produces fine particles that are difficult to remove. Although there are significant constraints to the use of pure Mn oxides, natural materials containing both Fe and Mn oxides show promise, where Mn promotes the oxidation of As(III) to As(V). In India, Chakravarty et al. (2002) used a ferruginous manganese ore, readily available (at \$50–56/t) in Bihar and Orissa, and comprising 77% pyrolusite (MnO_2) and 8% goethite (Fe_2O_3). Under laboratory conditions, it removed almost 100% of arsenic from groundwaters containing 40–180 ppb As, and adsorbed As(III) more strongly than As(V). The material also reduced iron to <0.1 ppm. Similarly, Deschamps et al. (2005) demonstrated that a natural Fe- and Mn-rich material, found in the Iron Quadrangle of Brazil, could remove both As(III) and As(V) without pre-treatment. Manna and Ghosh (2005) conducted trials of a handpump-operated double-column unit, where the first column contained manganese dioxide and the second contained crystalline goethite. Using groundwater containing 4–7 ppm Fe and 70–220 ppb As, breakthrough of arsenic (10 ppb) occurred before that of iron (0.3 ppm) at between 10,000 and 15,000 BV. The waste produced was classified as non-hazardous by the toxicity characteristic and leaching procedure (TCLP; see section 7.5).

Titanium oxide

Nanocrystalline titanium dioxide has been shown to have potential to remove both As(III) and As(V) from drinking water. Although As(V) is more readily adsorbed than As(III), Pena et al. (2005) showed that TiO_2 efficiently catalyses the oxidation of As(III) to As(V). The presence of phosphate, silicate and carbonate caused only moderate reduction in arsenic removal. Although removal efficiency declines at high pH, the effect is not significant in water with pH < 8, and the maximum removal of As(III) occurred at pH 7.5. Pena et al. (2005) concluded that nanocrystalline TiO_2 is a very efficient adsorbent for both As(III) and As(V). The particular advantage of titanium oxides over iron oxides is their faster kinetics. A synthetic titanium oxide adsorbent (Absorbsia™ GTO™) has been marketed, and is currently being implemented for treating public supplies in New Mexico and California.

Cerium oxide

Hydrous cerium oxides have a high selectivity for adsorbing both As(III) and As(V) under a wide range of geochemical conditions, without need for either pre-oxidation or pH-adjustment (M.F. Ahmed, 2003). In the READ-F technology[5], cerium oxide has been combined with an ethylene-vinyl alcohol copolymer to produce beads that are used in a household or community filter. The polymer beads can be regenerated with sodium hydroxide. The filters also include sand filtration to remove iron and prevent clogging of the resin bed. The household units have been certified for use under Bangladesh's Environmental Technology Verification programme (M.F. Ahmed, 2003; section 6.8.4).

Biological adsorptive filtration

Katsoyiannis et al. (2002) and Katsoyiannis and Zouboulis (2004) showed that iron-oxidising bacteria can remove arsenate and arsenite from groundwater rich in ferrous iron, and simultaneously reduce high iron and manganese concentrations. They conducted tests in fixed-bed columns packed with polystyrene beads, using Fe-rich (2.8 ppm) groundwater spiked with up to 200 ppb of As(III) and As(V). The bacteria *Gallionella ferruginea* and *Leptothrix ochracea* were present naturally in the groundwater, and grew to produce an Fe-rich biofilm in the columns. Optimum iron removal occurred at pH 7.2 and 2.7 ppm DO, whereas optimum removal (95%, and residual <5 ppb As) of As(III) occurred when the DO was raised to 3.7 ppm. The advantages of bacterial catalysis are that it (a) reduces the time taken to oxidise As(III) to As(V) to just a few minutes, (b) requires no chemical dosing, and (c) has no breakthrough point because the sorbent (iron) is continuously produced *in situ*. The method is potentially cheap, but may be prone to biofouling, and is yet to be tested in a full-scale application.

Water hyacinth

Use of dried water hyacinth (*Eichhornia crassipes*) offers the win-win zprospect of using an unwanted plant that chokes waterways and ponds to remove an unwanted chemical from water. Al-Rmalli et al. (2005) conducted batch experiments using air-dried and ground hyacinth roots from a pond in Dhaka, and deionised water spiked with 200 ppb of As(III) or As(V), and adjusted to pH 6.0. After a critical mass (30 mg/ml) of root powder was added, the removal of arsenic (93% for arsenite, and 85% for arsenate) occurred at a constant rate for about 40 minutes, and stabilised after about 60 minutes. Arsenic removal was constant between pH 2.0 and 8.0. It was estimated that the hyacinth root has an As-removal capacity of 50 µg/g. Al-Rmalli et al. (2005) suggest that water hyacinth root could be a cheap and effective alternative to iron-based filters. However, significant field testing and development will be required, and it will also be necessary to demonstrate that the treated water meets microbiological standards and does not acquire unpleasant tastes or odours.

The huge quantities of water hyacinth clogging water bodies might have potential in removing arsenic from irrigation water.

7.3.5 Zero-valent iron

The use of low-cost iron filings, also referred to as zero-valent iron (ZVI) or Fe(0), to remove dissolved arsenic has received much attention in recent years. The process appears to work either by coprecipitation and adsorption on iron oxyhydroxides or, when used with sulphate, by forming arsenopyrite. Zero-valent iron has the potential to remediate many organic and inorganic pollutants, and has been used in permeable reactive barriers (PRBs) where iron filings are mixed with sand and placed in trenches or caissons through which groundwater is encouraged to flow (i.e. a buried 'gate'). Lien and Wilkin (2005) used PRB technology to clean up an industrial site where groundwater contained tens of ppm of As(III).

The mechanism of arsenic removal by ZVI is complex, and may vary between different geochemical environments. In theory, ZVI could reduce arsenate and arsenite to elemental arsenic, although Bang et al. (2005) could not detect this in the reacted solids, and concluded that arsenic is adsorbed onto the oxyhydroxides produced by corrosion of the iron. Leupin and Hug (2005) deduced a sequence of reactions whereby oxygen oxidises ZVI to release soluble ferrous and hydroxyl ions, and then oxygen further oxidises the ferrous to ferric ions and As(III) to As(V). Next, hydrolysis of ferric ions precipitates hydrous ferric oxides, followed by a series of surface reactions involving the competitive adsorption of arsenate, arsenite, silica and phosphate.

Leupin et al. (2005) conducted field trials of ZVI filter columns in Bangladesh with an RD-type groundwater containing 441 ppb As, 4.7 ppm Fe, and 6 ppm DOC. In the tests, water flowed under gravity through a stack of inverted plastic funnels (similar to the 3-Kolshi filter), each containing a mixture of sand and iron. Columns with three or four filters of sand and iron lowered As concentrations to a few ppb, although competition from DOC reduced arsenic removal by about 20%. The columns also removed most iron and phosphate, and reduced calcium and silica. An important conclusion, however, and one which will constrain upscaling, is that slow addition of Fe(II) to aerated water is needed to avoid the use of a chemical oxidant. They stress the importance of repeated contact with air, and advocate a high sand:iron ratio to maintain high permeability. Iron filings or nails are also included in household ARPs such as the '3-Kolshi' filter in Bangladesh, and the Kanchan filter in Nepal (Murcott, 2001; M.F. Ahmed, 2003).

7.3.6 Ion exchange

Ion exchange (IX) resins can be weak or strong-base anion exchangers or weak or strong-acid cation exchangers (EPA, 2003b). Generally, strong-base resins are selected to exchange arsenate or arsenite with chloride ions. Exchange is only effective for charged ions, and so only works well for As(V), but pre-oxidation and pH-increase are required to remove As(III). Ion exchange therefore works best for AD-type waters, and least well for RD waters. The selectivity of resins (i.e. their ability to remove a particular ion) is greater for the divalent anions, and so arsenic removal works better at high pH. The preferred order of exchange for most strong-base resins (EPA, 2000) is:

$$CrO_4^{2-} > ClO_4^- > SeO_4^- > SO_4^{2-} > NO_3^- > HAsO_4^{2-} > CN^-$$
$$> Cl^- > H_2AsO_4^- > OH^- > F^-$$

The selectivity for chromate and selenite is not a practical drawback because, if present at significant concentrations, they also require treatment. The selectivity for sulphate is important, and IX is not economic when SO_4 exceeds 150 ppm and TDS exceeds 500 ppm (AWWA, 1999). When the resin is saturated with arsenic, it must be regenerated with a strong solution of HCl or NaCl, which creates a toxic liquid effluent that requires careful disposal, probably involving regulation and significant cost. Korngold et al. (2001) used a strong-base anion resin (Purolite A-505) to remove 99% of As(V) from a water containing 600 ppb As(V), but the process became inefficient when sulphate and chloride were present, and disposal of the regeneration effluent was troublesome. Vaaramaa and Lehto (2003) tested six ion exchangers, both cationic and anionic, of which four were organic and two inorganic, on groundwaters in Finland where arsenic was just one of a range of contaminants (uranium and its breakdown products, various transition metals and fluoride). The most effective exchanger for most metals and arsenic was sodium titanite ('CoTreat'), but none of the exchangers removed fluoride.

7.3.7 Membrane technologies

Membrane filtration relies on synthetic membranes containing billions of microscopic holes that act as selective barriers to the movement of molecules under the influence of a pressure gradient. Membrane technologies are divided into high-pressure (0.3–7 MPa) and low-pressure (5–100 psi; 0.03–0.7 MPa) categories (Shih, 2005). High-pressure systems include reverse osmosis (RO) and nanofiltration (NF), and mainly remove contaminants by chemical diffusion. Low-pressure systems include microfiltration (MF) and ultrafiltration (UF), and remove contaminants by physical sieving.

Reverse osmosis

Reverse osmosis is the oldest established membrane technology, and is best known for its use in desalination. The charged arsenate ion is more easily separated than the uncharged arsenite ion, so increasing the pH and pre-oxidation are recommended (Ning, 2002). Removal efficiency depends on the type of membrane. The older, cellulose-acetate membranes removed 90% of As(V) but only 70% of As(III). More recent polyamide and polyvinyl alcohol membranes can remove 95% of As(V) and 90% of As(III) at pH 10. However, at subneutral pH, removal of As(III) can be as low as 20% (Shih, 2005). High DOC reduces the effectiveness of As(V) and As(III) removal, but RO is advantageous where salinity is also a problem, and is generally more appropriate for AD- and SO-type waters. If the source water contains very high As concentrations, reductions of 90% may achieve a 50 ppb As target, but not a 10 ppb As target.

Nanofiltration

Nanofiltration requires much less energy than RO and removes both arsenate and arsenite because of both the small size of the membrane pores and charged-ion effects that depend on the particular membrane. At pH 6–8 the removal efficiency of arsenite is much less than that of arsenate. The removal efficiency of arsenic increases in water rich in sodium chloride, making NF more favourable for AD- than RD-type waters. Removal of arsenite is only significant at pH ≥ 10, when the As(III) molecule becomes ionised. Oh et al. (2000) field-tested bicycle-powered NF and RO membranes on typical RD-type groundwaters in Manikganj and Sonargaon upazilas of Bangladesh. A common disadvantage of reverse osmosis and other membrane systems for developing countries is the high energy requirement. The bicycle-powered pumping system, which delivered pressures of up to 5.0 MPa, was used with a cellulose triacetate NF membrane and with a hollow-fibre RO membrane. At Sonargaon, the raw water contained 1100 ppb As, 9.2 ppm Fe and 6.4 ppm Mn, and the treated water contained 130–180 ppb As. At Manikganj, where the raw water contained 410 ppb As, 4.7 ppm Fe and 1.1 ppm Mn, the treated water contained 20–40 ppb As. The RO membrane achieved much poorer removal of As(III) than As(V).

Microfiltration and ultrafiltration

Microfiltration removes particles with molecular weights of >50,000 or physical sizes of >0.05 μm, both much greater than either arsenate or arsenite, but MF has potential in combination with coagulation (see below). Ultrafiltration also relies mainly on physical sieving to remove constituents and so has limited application in arsenic removal, although bench tests suggest some potential when combined with electric repulsion (Shih, 2005). As with other membranes, it works better for As(V) than As(III).

7.3.8 Combined coagulation and microfiltration

While coagulation (section 7.3.2) can be effective in removing arsenic from solution, a common practical problem is that the coagulate is so fine that conventional filters either become clogged or simply fail to remove particulate arsenic (Song et al., 2005). Coagulation and microfiltration (CMF) seeks to combine the best features of the membrane and coagulation techniques. CMF entails high capital cost but can achieve low operating costs in large systems (EPA, 2000). Wickramasinghe et al. (2004) compared the use of CMF for an AD-type water from the USA and an RD-type water from Bangladesh. Although only at laboratory scale, these tests demonstrated how source water quality, a systematic geographical variable, affects the selection and design of treatment. The USA water was alkaline (pH 8.7) and oxic, containing 68 ppb As, predominantly as arsenate, and with low Fe and Mn concentrations but a very high silica content (141 ppm). The Bangladesh water contained 138 ppb As, had pH 7.5 and was anoxic, with no sulphate or nitrate but high Fe and Mn concentrations. Note that in the tests, pre-oxidation would have converted the predominantly As(III) in the Bangladesh water to As(V). The coagulant was either ferric chloride or ferric sulphate, and the membrane had 0.22 μm pores. Both combinations removed arsenic, but the efficiency depended on the raw water quality. As shown earlier (Figure 7.1), a much higher dose of ferric iron was required to achieve ≤10 ppb As in the filtered USA water than in the Bangladesh water, which was attributed partly to the higher Fe concentration in the Bangladesh water but mainly to interference from silica in the USA water.

7.3.9 Electrolytic methods

Electrodialysis reversal (EDR) is a complex form of ion exchange controlled by alternating electric currents in which ions migrate from the less to the more concentrated solution. Electrodialysis reversal systems are complex to design but are fully automated, require little operator attention and no addition of chemicals. Routine maintenance consists in changing cartridge filters, calibrating instruments, replacing membranes and electrodes, and maintaining pumps. Electrodialysis reversal typically removes 70–80% of TDS, and EPA (2000) cite removal of both As(III) and As(V) ranging from 28% to 86%.

Electrocoagulation is used mainly in industrial wastewater treatment, but has been used for pilot water-supply applications in Region Lagunera, Mexico (Parga et al., 2005). The removal mechanism involves oxidation, reduction, adsorption, precipitation and flotation. A DC electric current is applied to the water to which some salt is added. Polyvalent cations are produced at a sacrificial anode made of iron or aluminium. As(III) and As(V) react with hydroxyl ions produced at the cathode to form hydroxides that adsorb pollutants. The process is sensitive to the electrical conductivity of the water, but is not pH-dependent in the range pH 6–8 (Kumar et al., 2004). Parga et al. (2005) suggested that magnetite and ferrihydrite produced in the reactor were responsible for arsenic removal. Following bench tests, they constructed a mobile treatment plant with a capacity of 30 L/minute that was tested at wells containing 25–50 ppb As, EC 600–4000 μS/cm, and pH 5.5–7.1. After passing through the electrocoagulation reactor, the residual arsenic was only 2 ppb (99% removal), pH 8.5 and EC 500–2000 μS/cm.

7.3.10   Phytofiltration

Phytofiltration is an emerging technology where plants are used to remove contaminants from water, and has been applied successfully to remove chromium, uranium, caesium and lead (Elless et al., 2005). Recently, various hyperaccumulating ferns, including *Pteris vittata*, have been discovered that can accumulate as much as 22,000 mg/kg of arsenic into its fronds. In hydroponic batch tests, *Pteris* ferns reduced As concentrations from 500 ppb to <2 ppb. A pilot-scale, continuous-flow, phytofiltration system was built at Albuquerque, New Mexico, to treat groundwater with a pH of 7.9 and containing 12 ppb As. *Pteris vittata* ferns were grown in potting mix, wrapped in foam inside slotted plastic pots, and suspended in tanks of water. The tanks were kept in a greenhouse and arranged in series. The volumes and flow velocities were adjusted to ensure the necessary contact time. Initial bench tests showed that water spiked with >50 ppb As of either arsenate or arsenite was reduced to acceptable concentrations in about 50 hours, and was relatively insensitive to the length of daylight, and therefore the period of transpiration and water uptake. The pilot plant was operated for 3 months and consistently produced an effluent with <2 ppb of arsenic. The pH and EC of the effluent was unchanged, dissolved oxygen increased, and no micro-organisms such as protozoa, nematodes, amoeba or ciliates were detected in the effluent. The ferns would normally require disposal to landfill, although in some countries they might be dried and used as straw in brick making.

7.3.11   Removal of organic arsenic species

Organic forms of arsenic are rarely encountered at significant concentrations in natural waters. According to Cullen and Reimer (1989), only MMA and DMA (section 2.1.2) are ever likely to be significant in natural groundwater, and most likely in RD-type waters. Thirunavukkarasu et al. (2002) conducted column studies to examine the removal of organic forms of arsenic with manganese greensand (MGS), two types of iron-oxide-coated sand[6] (IOCS) and a ferric ion-exchange resin (IXR). Canadian tap water (pH 7.6) was spiked with arsenic in the form of DMA. Arsenic-removal efficiencies decreased in the order IXR > IOCS2 >> MGS > IOCS1. Batch studies determined As-removal capacities of $8\,\mu g/g$ for IOCS2, and $5.7\,\mu g/cm^3$ for the ion exchange resin. The results show that, if present, organic As species could be removed by existing technologies.

7.3.12   Arsenic removal *in situ*

Background

The methods described above all involve removal of arsenic from water immediately prior to its distribution, however, it is also possible to remove arsenic prior to its abstraction from the ground. *In situ* arsenic removal works by modifying the redox conditions in an aquifer, although in common with many other methods, it exploits the capacity of iron oxyhydroxides to adsorb arsenic and other trace elements. Here we do not consider permeable reactive barriers that have been used for remediating small sites. The idea of *in situ* groundwater treatment is not new, apparently having been patented in Germany in 1900 (www.aquamedia.at). *In situ* iron removal has been used extensively to reduce high iron concentrations in the Rhine alluvium (van Beek, 1980; Appelo and Postma, 1996). The basic set-up for *in situ* treatment (Figure 7.5) involves cyclically injecting oxygenated water into reducing aquifers, causing precipitation of oxyhydroxides which adsorb arsenic. After each injection cycle, a larger volume of water can be withdrawn before iron returns to its original concentration. Rott and Friedle (1999, 2000) use the term efficiency coefficient (EC_f) for the ratio of the volume of water extracted (meeting the particular quality criterion) to the volume injected. They suggest that the coefficient is normally between 2 and 12 depending on the aquifer and water quality characteristics.

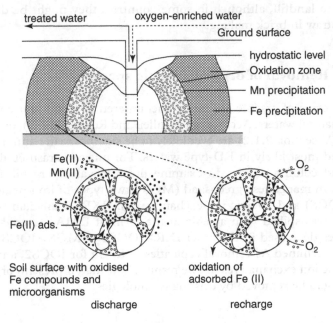

Figure 7.5   Principles of *in situ* iron, manganese and arsenic removal. Note that concentric zones of decreasing oxidation potential gradually expand around the injection well.
Source: Rott and Friedle (1999)

Geochemical processes

During the injection cycle, oxygen reacts with Fe(II) and Mn(II) leading to their precipitation as oxyhydroxides. During the discharge cycle, As(III), Fe(II), Mn(II) and other ions such as NH_4 and DOC are adsorbed onto the oxidised grain surfaces. Appelo and de Vet (2003) have described the geochemical processes occurring in *in situ* iron and arsenic removal, in which the ability of freshly precipitated iron oxyhydroxide to adsorb ferrous iron is critical. To increase removal and minimise clogging, the pH should remain >6, otherwise oxidation of Fe^{2+} is impaired and oxidation of pyrite may acidify the water. Appelo et al. (1999) described the reactions in the first two injection–withdrawal cycles.

- Initially, cations from the outwardly flowing injection water exchange with exchangeable Fe^{2+}. The dissolved Fe^{2+} reacts with oxygen to form Fe^{3+}, which is precipitated as iron oxyhydroxide. Because oxygen is consumed in the reaction, it is retarded relative to the injected water. An inner zone develops where the exchange surfaces are completely depleted in Fe^{2+}, such that eventually oxygen passes through this zone without reaction.

- When injection stops and pumping commences, Fe^{2+} from beyond the oxygen front is drawn towards the well where it is adsorbed onto the depleted oxyhydroxides[7], and so now the iron front lags behind the incoming water front. Provided injection of oxygenated water is resumed before iron concentrations return to their original level, and hence all of the depleted exchange sites have not been refilled by Fe^{2+}, in the next injection cycle oxygenated water will be able to penetrate further into the aquifer. Thus the oxidised zone becomes larger and can adsorb more iron in the following pumping cycle. This sequence of events is repeated indefinitely and so the removal efficiency keeps improving over time.

When operated by alternating injection and abstraction at a single well, it follows that there will always be unused oxygen in the oxidised zone at the end of an injection cycle, and so the system is inherently inefficient. However, if water is injected through separate wells, then all the oxygen can be usefully consumed in oxidising iron. In either case, commencing reinjection before the exchange sites near the well are filled is crucial to ensuring the oxidised zone keeps growing and clogging is avoided. According to Rott and Friedle (1999), the removal process is aided by the autocatalytic effects of Mn oxides in oxidising arsenite, but inhibited by ammonium, common in RD-type waters, which consumes much oxygen when oxidised to nitrate. Although the reaction products are deposited in the aquifer, this does not cause significant clogging because they are deposited in 'dead-end' pores and also because the ageing of oxyhydroxides (e.g. recrystallisation as goethite) is accompanied by a large volume reduction. At an *in situ* treatment plant operating for 10 years in Switzerland, Mettler et al. (2001) found that iron was precipitated as ferric oxides (50–100% goethite, with ferrihydrite as the minor phase), whereas manganese was deposited as Mn(II), probably within carbonates.

7.4 Aquifer Clean-up

Contaminated aquifers contain finite amounts of arsenic, distributed in variable proportions between groundwater and minerals. When water is withdrawn, the partitioning of arsenic between solid and liquid phases readjusts, and eventually the extractable store of arsenic will be depleted. Since arsenic, unlike organic pollutants, cannot be destroyed, the only alternatives are to extract and 'dispose' of it or permanently sequester it beneath the ground, the latter being inherently preferable. Aquifer clean-ups by human action may be deliberate, incidental (by safe disposal of treatment waste) or accidental (such as in pumping for irrigation). The scale of clean-up is very important. It is already practised for industrially contaminated sites using pump-and-treat, electroremediation, phytoremediation and *in situ* reactive barriers (Redwine, 2001; Morrison et al., 2002). The clean-up of entire aquifers is done by nature on a geological timescale, as is evident in the Bengal Basin by the virtual absence of arsenic in aquifers more than about 20,000 years old. Deliberate clean-up of naturally contaminated aquifers is beyond the financial and institutional capacity of less-developed countries, and perhaps most rich countries also. However, it is possible to adopt management strategies to promote the clean-up of shallow aquifers as a long-term public good.

In many affected aquifers, the largest component of abstraction is irrigation. Shallow tubewell irrigation in Bangladesh has often been described as the largest pump-and-treat system in the world, even though, as discussed in Chapters 3 and 4, this may be transferring a problem from drinking water to the food chain. In areas of intensive irrigation, the store of dissolved arsenic in shallow groundwater will be removed in a few decades. What is not known, however, is the rate at which this will be replenished by release from the sediment. Practically, it is difficult to predict how long it will take for As concentrations to decline to acceptable levels. As discussed above, incidental clean-up is accomplished where *in situ* As removal is practised or where contaminated groundwater is withdrawn for treatment. The *in situ* method works best where the Fe:As ratio is high. However, even without stimulation, brown (oxic) sediments can adsorb arsenic as contaminated groundwater flows through them (Stollenwerk et al., 2007). Herein lies a dilemma. On the one hand, while pumping from brown sand risks spreading pollution, on the other hand, it may permanently remove arsenic from exposure pathways. This, in fact, is what is happening where safe wells continue to operate in shallow aquifers. More research is needed to quantify these processes, and develop risk assessment and management methodologies.

The hydrogeochemical processes described above also operate on longer timescales during flow between aquifers. Wells pumping from low-As aquifers that underlie high-As aquifers must place the deeper aquifer at risk. However, the intervening sediments have some (unquantified) capacity to adsorb and immobilise arsenic, perhaps permanently. The conventional view is that deep aquifers should be preserved and protected as sources of potable supply. To advocate exploiting this capacity by deliberately drawing polluted shallow groundwater towards the deeper aquifers would be considered controversial, and yet this is what current practice is doing. Unfortunately, this is neither acknowledged nor is it being monitored. Indeed, it can be argued that if a deep aquifer cannot support potable needs it is not a useful resource, and so its progressive contamination, if it occurred, would be tolerable. Hence, the controversial aspect of increasing interaquifer transfers rests only in allowing or encouraging irrigation pumping from deep aquifers. Such a strategy offers potentially massive benefits both for supplying drinking water and in halting the accumulation of arsenic in irrigated soils. On the other hand, it is untested and risks drawing down arsenic and inducing saline intrusion. The challenge, therefore, is to establish a sufficient knowledge base, both scientifically and institutionally, to manage the process. This can be done through controlled field investigations and by monitoring what is already happening. However, unlike major surface-water schemes that involve massive 'lumpy' investments and once started are difficult to stop, monitored aquifer-transfer and clean-up could be implemented incrementally, halted at any stage, and implemented on a regional basis. For instance, subsidy for deep irrigation wells could be prioritised where As accumulation in irrigated soils is greatest, and there is no practical alternative to maintain food production.

7.5   Disposing of Waste from Treatment Processes

All arsenic removal systems, except *in situ* techniques, generate solid or liquid waste, although there are qualitative differences between spent adsorbents and sludges on the one hand, and toxic liquid wastes (from IX, RO and regeneration of adsorbents) on the other. Liquid wastes are challenging and require a mature waste-management industry and regulatory framework for proper disposal. Spent adsorbents and sludge can be assessed for their stability and leachability using tests developed in the USA to assess the acceptability for disposal to landfill. For solid waste disposal to landfill, attention focuses on whether a waste is legally hazardous, which affects the type of landfill that can accept it, whether additional taxation is incurred, and the need for pre-treatment. The two most widely used tests are the TCLP and California's Waste Extraction Test (WET). The USEPA's TCLP uses a 0.1 M acetate solution, whereas the WET uses a 0.2 M citrate solution.

Leaching test results

Chen et al. (1999) tested sludge from various USA plants and found that only one, from a coagulation plant, would be classified as hazardous by the TCLP. M.F. Ahmed (2003) cites using the TCLP on 18 samples of arsenic removal wastes from Bangladesh, all of which produced a leachate containing <50 ppb As, and mostly <10 ppb As. Recent research shows that the TCLP may significantly underestimate arsenic mobilisation in the strongly reducing conditions that apply in landfills (Hounslow, 1980), and highlights the importance of selecting the test that best approximates the proposed means of disposal. Jing et al. (2005) compared five adsorbents (GFH, GFO,

TiO_2, AA and modified-AA) and found that the WET test predicted As leaching rates up to ten-times higher than the TCLP test. Ghosh et al. (2006a) noted that even though most solid residuals pass the TCLP, As leaching from AA and GFH residuals is sensitive to pH[8], DOC and phosphate (but not bicarbonate, sulphate and silicate). Using a column to simulate the biogeochemical conditions in a mature landfill, Ghosh et al. (2006b) found that both iron and arsenic were readily mobilized from GFH.

Non-landfill disposal

Where well-regulated landfills operate, disposal of residues may be treated as a financial cost, and the risks to health and the environment should be acceptable. Where no such facilities exist, the options include (a) disposal to informal landfill, (b) spreading on land, (c) dilute and disperse disposal to rivers and (d) semi-permanent storage of waste. None of these solutions is entirely satisfactory, although the risks may be acceptable in individual cases. Under these conditions, the ethical responsibility for safe disposal therefore rests with the sponsor of treatment, who should conduct a quantitative risk assessment of disposal options; and since As-removal technologies that produce toxic wastes have alternatives, they should not be promoted unless a credible and verifiable procedure for waste management is in place from the outset. Particularly problematic situations arise in the disposal of waste from domestic and small community ARPs, where no proper facility exists. Yet even here, the risks can be managed. Dipankar Chakraborti has suggested that if the sludge is mixed with cow-dung, arsenic will be lost by methylation, while Sarkar et al. (2005) have demonstrated that the sludge can be practically collected and stored in a small brick-built sand-filter (section 7.6.2). Further, M.F. Ahmed (2003) suggested that sludge and solid waste can be disposed of, immobilising arsenic, by mixing them with clay used to make bricks. However, he warns that this can create a risk of air pollution due to volatilization at high temperature in the brick kiln.

7.6   Examples and Operational Experience of Arsenic Removal Technologies

7.6.1   Household systems

The Family Filter

The Family Filter is a point-of-use (POU), adsorption-based device developed by IHE (Institute for Water Education) in the Netherlands (Petrusevski et al., 2002). It operates by gravity flow through a PVC column (69 mm in diameter and 500 mm high) containing iron-coated sand (ICS), and is intended to supply a family with low-As water for about 6 months. Testing with five ICS samples from Dutch groundwater treatment plants and tap water spiked with 500–1500 ppb As showed that, while As(V) is easily removed, efficient removal of As(III) only occurs if manganese is present in the coating. However, ICS with a thick iron coating effectively reduces As concentrations to <10 ppb As within 15 minutes.

Kanchan Arsenic Filter, Nepal

The Kanchan™ Arsenic Filter was developed in Nepal by the Massachusetts Institute of Technology (MIT) and Environment and Public Health Organization (ENPHO). It combines slow sand filtration with adsorption on iron oxyhydroxides in a large plastic bucket (Figure 7.6). A perforated pipe, with a tap at the end, is set in a layer of gravel and covered with coarse sand and then fine sand. Above this, a perforated plastic tray (diffuser basin), containing brick chips and 5 kg of iron nails, is suspended from the top of the bucket. Water poured into the tray causes rusting of the nails, and the fresh rust adsorbs arsenic. The fine sand below filters the iron particles and also helps to remove bacteria. The filter removes 85–95% of arsenic in waters containing tens to hundreds of ppb As, and can produce 15–20 L of water an hour. To help the private sector to promote the Kanchan Filter, MIT and ENPHO trained and certified entrepreneurs from various districts of Nepal. Including a 10% profit, the Kanchan Filter is sold for less than $20.

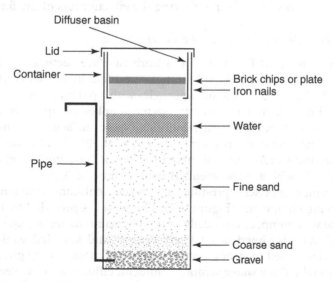

Figure 7.6   Schematic design of the Kanchan household filter from Nepal. Well-water is poured into the diffuser basin, where corrosion of the iron nails forms oxyhydroxides that adsorb arsenic. *Source*: Ngai et al. (2006)

By January 2006, more than 3000 filters had been installed in various parts of the Nepal Terai (Chapter 8), serving more than 25,000 rural people (Ngai et al., 2006). Eventually, the nails need replacing, but the difficulty with this, as with most household devices, is that it is not practical to tell when the medium is exhausted.

The Sono Filter, Bangladesh

The Sono Filter was developed by Abul Hussam in 2001 from the traditional 3-Kolshi filter (Chapter 6), and in January 2007 was awarded the $1 M Grainger Challenge Gold Award[9]. The Sono Filter comprises three vertically-stacked plastic buckets. The top bucket contains coarse sand and a composite iron matrix which removes the arsenic. The second bucket contains coarse sand and charcoal, which removes organic compounds. The third bucket contains brick chips and fine sand to remove any fines. The filter, which is intended to be placed in the household, produces up to 20 L of water an hour, and can last for up to 5 years depending on the raw water quality. The Sono Filter is manufactured in Kushtia (Bangladesh) and retails at less than $40. About 200 devices are manufactured each week, and over 30,000 have been distributed. Schroeder (2006) reported on successful use of Sono Filters over a 3-year period in Kushtia and Rajbari districts, where it consistently reduced As concentrations of hundreds of ppb to below 10 ppb As, and required minimal maintenance. As with the Kanchan Filter, there is no system for monitoring the effectiveness of the filter.

A household adsorption unit in the USA

An application of GFH/GFO type adsorbents (see section 7.3.4) is the ArsenX[np] technology, developed by Solmetex Inc. in the USA. ArsenX[np] combines hydrous iron oxide nanoparticles with a polymer substrate, and is aimed at domestic and community water supplies of up to 60 L/s. The porous beads ensure high permeability and large surface area while being resistant to collapse in the reactor (Sylvester et al., 2007). The media specifications indicate an As-removal capacity of up to 38,000 μg/g of resin in the range pH 4–9, with a recommended contact time of 3 minutes. A typical ArsenX[np] unit comprises a pre-filter, two reactor columns, instrumentation and sampling equipment (Figure 7.7). The power is provided by the pressure of the well pump, and no daily or weekly maintenance is required. This type of product is aimed at relatively wealthy and knowledgeable buyers who are accustomed to strong vendor support. Customers are given a sampling kit to take three water samples (influent, effluent and between tanks) after a fixed period, typically 6 months, to be analysed. The effectiveness of such systems is contingent upon a strong and enforceable warranty and support arrangements.

a) System Front View

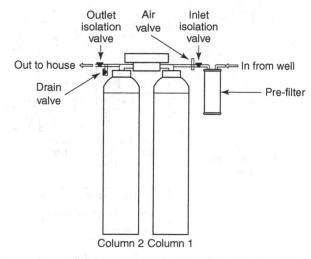

b) System Top View

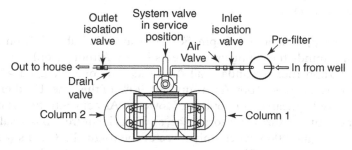

Figure 7.7   Example of a household adsorption system used in the USA: (a) front view; (b) top view. Note: ArsenX^{np} is a product of Solmetex Inc. (USA).

7.6.2   Community arsenic removal plants in West Bengal

The Technology Park Project

In a paper graphically entitled 'Ineffectiveness and unreliability of arsenic removal plants in West Bengal', Hossain, Sengupta et al. (2005) present a bleak picture of the performance of community ARPs, which they monitored for 4 years in a peri-urban area near Kolkata. Under the Technology Park Project[10], 18 ARPs produced by 11 manufacturers with broadly similar designs[11] (Figure 7.8) were installed at highly contaminated sites

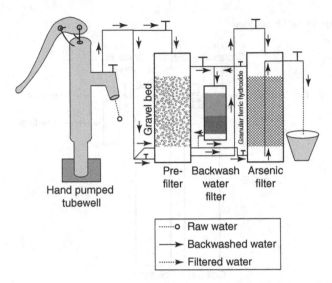

Figure 7.8   Schematic design of the Pal-Trockner arsenic removal plant. This design and similar alternatives have been widely distributed in West Bengal.
Source: Hossain et al. (2006)

(average 320 ppb As and 4.6 ppm Fe). As shown in Table 7.3, on purely chemical grounds their judgement seems harsh. Although only two ARPs met the 50 ppb Indian standard all the time, only one averaged >50 ppb, and most produced <50 ppb As around 80–90% of the time. Further, three units achieved a mean of <10 ppb As. However, As concentration is not the only important measure of performance, as was evident from post-evaluation visits in 2004 and 2005, when only three of the original 18 ARPs were still in use. Of the other 15 ARPs, five no longer worked, three had been removed by the owners, four had been closed down by the local authority and three were simply not used because they were disliked.

Hossain, Sengupta et al. (2005) identified three main causes of poor performance. The first was maintenance: backwashing was not done regularly and its need was not adequately predicted. The second reason was clogging by sand. Even after redrilling, some still did not work reliably. The third cause was a lack of 'user-friendliness': valves became jammed; inadequate packing in the pump-head causes spraying; and injuries occurred due to the handle rebounding. A visit to 12 of the ARPs in January 2006 substantially confirmed these findings, and also identified taste and odour problems. Two ARPs had almost never worked and two were working well; the remaining eight had operated more or less effectively for 3 years, but were abandoned around 2004 when the project stopped paying the operators' salaries. Previously, a local person, usually a poor woman,

Table 7.3   Performance of 18 community arsenic removal plants in West Bengal

Manufacturer	Method or media	Costs ($)		Water quality* (5)		
				As (ppb)		Fe (ppm)
		Capital	Media†	In	Out	
Oxide India	Activated alumina AS–37	1070	326	333	40±10	0.45
				254	8±7	0.1
				–	5±5	0.25
Apyron Tech.	Aqua Bind (AA + metal oxides; pp)	1810	340	366	24±49	0.07
				283	26±32	0.06
PHED	Hematite + quartz + sand + AA	611		843	27±32	0.13
RPM Marketing	Adsorption: AA + AAFS–50 (pp)	1000	453	349	45±37	0.27
				334	19±22	0.06
SOFR, Kolkata	Al-silicate + FH	181	27	466	37±75	0.61
Adhiacon, Kolkata	Catalytic precipitation + IX (pp)	1698		299	94±65	1.37
				148	43±43	0.93
Ionocem	IX (FH)	883		124	15±15	0.27
Pal Trockner	Adsorp As (pp)	1675	566	133	8±17	0.1
				–	13±30	0.73
AIIH and PH	Oxidation-coagulation-filtration	792	‡	227	21±8	110
WSI (USA)	IX: resin + metal oxide (pp)	2088	883	–	33±33	0.38
				–	27±22	0.29
Anir Eng.	Slurry/granular FH	815	192	–	45±54	0.15

AA, activated alumina; FH, ferric hydroxide; IX, ion exchange; pp, patent pending.
*Chemical analyses are the mean and standard deviation averaged from many tens of samples. Multiple rows of analyses indicate multiple units fielded.
†Cost for replacing the adsorbent media.
‡Requires routine expenditure on chemicals.
Source: Hossain, Sengupta et al. (2005)

was paid to carry out backwashing at 15–20-day intervals and routine maintenance. When requested to take over this work, at nine of the ten communities it proved impossible to retrofit a management organisation, although at one site the equipment manufacturer (Pal Trockner) took on this responsibility.

The Technology Park experience demonstrates that the ability to remove arsenic is a necessary but not sufficient condition for a successful water supply. Arsenic-removal plants should only be fitted to good wells with good pumps. Low-cost drilling that suffices for simple hand-pumps may not be adequate for treatment systems that create significant back-pressure. Sand pumping can be reduced by drilling a little deeper and at larger diameter to place a proper gravel pack that will result in better hydraulic performance, and may also result in a lower As concentration. Second, treated water must be palatable as well as potable. Unpleasant tastes and odours make ARPs unpopular and exacerbate any social issues. Bad tastes and odours (due to Fe, Mn or S) should be alleviated by regular backwashing and designs that include effective aeration. Frequent backwashing is also essential to prevent clogging by iron precipitates, and its absence contributed greatly to the abandonment of the ARPs. Sponsors and donors should understand their long-term responsibility to water users. If they do not invest time and money in group formation before construction, they should be prepared to finance the operating and regeneration costs for as long as the ARP is needed. However, a self-sustaining management structure is heavily dependent on community engagement.

Regional surveys of ARPs

Hossain et al. (2006) evaluated 577 out of 1900 ARPs, of similar design to that shown in Figure 7.8, installed in five districts of West Bengal at a cost of around $1500 each. Overall, 25% were not working, 12% contained <50 ppb As in the raw water (i.e. did not require As removal), and 18% did not reduce arsenic to below 50 ppb. Only 45% of the installed ARPs were reducing the As content of water from dangerous levels to <50 ppb As, and 35% to <10 ppb As. While these figures are disturbing in themselves, compliance with the arsenic standard is not sufficient to characterise the performance of the ARPs. Reductive-dissolution-type groundwaters are rich in iron: of 200 samples tested, 93% contained >1 ppm and 22% contained >5 ppm of iron. More importantly, 47% of the treated waters still contained >1 ppm, and only 19% contained less than the desirable level of 0.3 ppm. Thus, it is not surprising that 44% of treated waters became discoloured after standing, and 6% of treated waters had 'bad' odours. Irrespective of As concentration, there were statistically significant differences in willingness to use water that developed colour or odour problems. Clear water was twice as likely to be used, and odour-free water was five times as likely to be used. Interviews with 800 families revealed that 80% of complaints involved poor physical operation and unreliability, leaking connections, water spraying and injuries from the handle 'jumping'. The ARPs had become so unpopular that many people were unwilling to install them, even though some worked well where they were regularly backwashed and the community was involved in their management.

Bengal Engineering College ARPs: a success story

Sarkar et al. (2005) described the performance of 135 well-head ARPs installed by Bengal Engineering College (BEC) in remote villages in Nadia and 24-Parganas North districts[12]. The filter, known as the Amul Filter, is fixed directly to a hand tubewell and removes arsenic in a fixed bed reactor containing 100 kg of activated alumina (Figure 7.9). Each unit serves communities of 100–300 households. Capital costs are met by the donors[13], but villagers pay all operating costs. The design requires no chemical addition, pH adjustment or electricity, and all components are procured in India. At the top of the column, dissolved iron is oxidized by contact with air to precipitate ferrihydrite particles, and both the precipitated iron and the AA are important in removing arsenic. The groundwaters contain 100 to >500 ppb As, but the treated water is consistently <50 ppb, and typically around 20 ppb As. The units have been effective in removing both arsenite and arsenate for as much as 10,000 BV, equivalent to months or years of operation, depending on the water quality.

In addition to the design of the ARP, the BEC programme includes: (a) scheme planning, (b) operational support and (c) health education. When selecting new schemes, initial interest is determined by a field supervisor who tests the water and identifies alternative water sources prior to organising a public meeting. The tubewell cannot be privately owned and there must be 'no objection' from local government. A committee, comprising at least one-third women, is formed and must agree that the ARP can be removed if not used. The committee appoints a treasurer to manage a dedicated bank account. Each family pays Rs10 a month to cover the operator's salary and set aside funds for maintenance and repair. The ARPs are backwashed every day for 10–15 minutes. No users complained of bad smells or taste, which implies that aeration and backwashing is effective. User groups have a strong sense of ownership, regular backwashing is 'enforced' by the users who pay the salary, and the ARP is locked when not in use, so that only members can take water.

The BEC supports the operation, maintenance and monitoring of the ARPs. They analyse raw and treated water every month for arsenic, and periodically for iron and coliforms. They monitor breakthrough of the

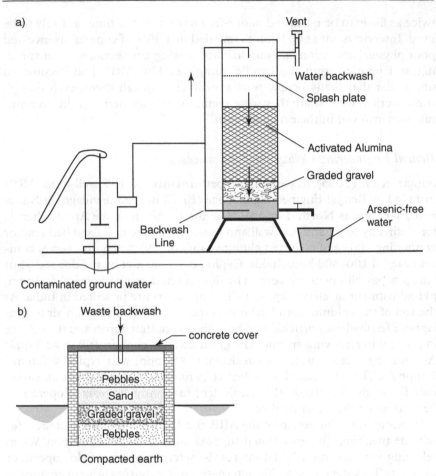

Figure 7.9 Design of the Bengal Engineering College arsenic removal plant: (a) main unit; (b) waste trap. *Source*: Sarkar et al. (2005)

adsorbent and plan for regeneration at a central facility constructed in the project area. Regeneration produces less than 500 g of sludge, which is being stored until proper disposal facilities are available. The third element in BEC's approach is a health education campaign, in which local women are recruited and trained to visit every household to pass on an integrated message on hygiene, sanitation and arsenic. In addition, BEC has pursued an applied technology research programme, which has included (a) dividing the column into two offset lengths to make backwashing more effective, and (b) field testing alternative media such as the Hybrid Ion Exchanger (DeMarco et al., 2003) that is easier to regenerate and less prone to collapse.

It is revealing to contrast the BEC's success[14] with essentially the same technology that has performed poorly elsewhere in West Bengal. Although the design may be somewhat better, the key difference is the attention to both the technical and social sides of operation. BEC also concentrated on a single technology in a restricted geographical area not yet reached by (free-of-cost) government schemes[15].

7.6.3   Comparative evaluations of alternative treatment systems

Evaluation of five conventional arsenic removal plants in the USA

Anticipating a reduction of the drinking water standard, Chen et al. (2002) studied the ability of conventional treatment plants used for community or municipal supply to produce water with <10 ppb As. They monitored two coagulation-filtration plants, two iron-removal plants (IRP) and one lime-softening plant. The coagulation-filtration plants consistently produced water with <10 ppb As, except when one plant temporarily changed the coagulant from alum to polyaluminum chloride. Only one of the IRPs consistently reduced arsenic to acceptable levels, although it was suggested that a coagulant might be added to improve As removal at the other. The lime-softening plant consistently failed to produce water with <10 ppb As, although here it was suggested that raising the pH might improve As-removal efficiency. The study showed that many existing plants would be able to conform to the new standard, and that others could probably conform if modified.

Evaluation of four treatment systems in Canada

Pokhrel et al. (2005) examined the ability of four small commercial technologies to remove arsenic from an RD-type groundwater in a glacial aquifer in Saskatchewan that contained an average of 21 ppb As, 7.4 ppm Fe, 0.96 ppm Mn, and had pH 7.3. The plants each produced about 4.5 L/minute and included a slow and a rapid sand filter, a biological activated-carbon filter (BAC) and a coagulation system. The BAC system comprised a slow sand filter followed by a tank of granulated activated carbon, both of which were aerated. In the slow sand filter, groundwater was sprayed into an elevated tank and then drained into the tank containing 550 mm of filter media. The contact time was 37 minutes, and clogging became significant after about 17 hours, when backwashing was performed. In the rapid sand filter, the media depth was 864 mm but the contact time was only 10 minutes. In the coagulation system, water was mixed with polyaluminium chloride in

Table 7.4   Comparison of four arsenic removal systems in Canada. The numbers in parentheses are the percentages of arsenic removed

Treatment system		Raw water*	Treated water, without ozonation (%)	Treated water, with pre-ozonation (%)
Coagulation	As:	24	7.2 (70)	1.1 (95)
	Fe:	8.3	1.3 (84)	0.6 (93)
BAC	As:	17.4	0.7 (96)	0.2 (99)
	Fe:	7.9	0.0 (100)	0.0 (100)
Slow sand filter	As:	17.4	0.8 (95)	0.7 (96)
	Fe:	7.9	0.0 (100)	0.0 (100)
Rapid sand filter	As:	18.2	8.6 (53)	6.6 (64)
	Fe:	8.3	0.0 (100)	4.2 (49)

BAC, biological activated carbon.
*As in ppb; Fe in ppm.
Source: Pokhrel et al. (2005)

a 450 L settling-tank, and allowed to stand for 3 hours before draining, flushing and repeating the cycle. The performance data (Table 7.4) show that, even without ozonation, both the biological system and the slow sand filter were effective at removing both iron and arsenic. Ozonation further improved the BAC system but not the slow sand filter. Without ozonation, the coagulation system performed poorly, but with ozonation it was highly effective in removing both arsenic and iron. The rapid sand filter was not effective in removing arsenic. The BAC and SSF systems were most attractive because they achieved high As removal without pre-oxidation.

The Stadtoldendorf Waterworks trial, Germany

Jekel and Seith (2000) and Jekel (2002) described full-scale trials of four As-removal technologies at Stadtoldendorf in Lower Saxony. Groundwater drawn from Triassic sandstones (Chapter 9) was oxic with pH 7.9 and contained 21 ppb exclusively of As(V). It was also moderately hard and contained 0.5 ppm of phosphate, 50 ppb of fluoride and 15 ppm of silica. The treatment plant had a capacity of 2450 m³/day and was set up with four parallel pressure filters: F1 – coagulation with Fe(III) chloride; F2 – granulated ferric hydroxide adsorbent; F3 – coagulation with Fe(II) sulphate; and F4 – activated alumina (AA). Each cylinder was 3 m high, with an area of 5.3 m², and equipped for backwashing. Both coagulation systems were set up for washing by air-scouring and required sludge disposal. Filter F2 was filled with 5 m³ of GEH® ferric hydroxide, and F4 with 11 m³ of activated alumina. A control value of 5 ppb As was used to determine media replacement and to guarantee compliance.

All four methods produced water with <10 ppb As, and had particular advantages and disadvantages. Activated alumina was least successful because it developed 'cement-like' properties until it had been thoroughly backwashed, and was later abandoned. Coagulation with Fe(II) salts was superior to ferric iron because oxidation of ferrous iron takes place within the filter bed, leading to better filtration and lower head losses. Both salts required a coagulant dose of 1 g/m³ to achieve 90% As removal. The GFH process was easiest to operate, most reliable and required least labour input. The media achieved compliance for more than 70,000 BV, the crossover point for being economically preferred. On the other hand, GFH lost much of its activity if it dried out, was less stable than AA, and required backwashing after 8000 BV.

Jekel (2002) compared the capital and operating costs of the coagulation systems and GFH systems for breakthrough periods of 70,000 and 100,000 BV. The annualised costs in Table 7.5 (based on a 7% interest rate and 20 year amortisation period) suggest that coagulation using Fe(II) salts has the lowest long-term cost, but GFH is competitive if a long bed life is achieved. Jekel (2002) estimated that at neutral pH, the GFH could operate for more than 200,000 BV. However, as the calculations show, if the bed life is shorter,

Table 7.5 Arsenic treatment costs (DM) at the Stadtoldendorf Waterworks, Germany

Item	Coagulation		GFH	
	Fe(III)	Fe(II)	70,000 bv	100,000 bv
Capital costs:				
treatment plant	0.139	0.139	0.041	0.041
sludge disposal	0.020	0.020	0	0
Total	0.159	0.159	0.041	0.041
Annual operating costs:				
chemicals	0.005	0.005	0.178	0.124
flush water	0.005	0.005	0.002	0.002
maintenance	0.050	0.034	0.010	0.010
sludge disposal	0.073	0.018	0	0
Total	0.136	0.062	0.190	0.136
Annualised cost:	0.151	0.077	0.194	0.140

Note: In 2000–01, DM1 was worth $0.47
Source: Calculated from unit cost data in Jekel (2002)

the cost is very high, emphasising the importance of rapid small-scale column testing (section 7.3.4).

Granular ferric oxide treatment for community supply in the UK

In the English Midlands, Severn Trent Services Ltd (STSL) applied granulated ferric oxide to treat groundwater containing 12–24 ppb As from the Triassic Sherwood Sandstone (Selvin et al., 2002). Following a 20 ML/day prototype that cost €4.6 M, STSL installed 17 plants with capacities of 2–21 ML/day that had been operating for 6–24 months at the time of reporting (Figure 7.10). After passing 10,000 to 76,000 BV, the plants produced water containing <5 ppb As. The plants produced only 0.1% of wastewater, which was disposed to sewer. Replacement media are either injected from a tanker or delivered in 1 m³ bags on flat-bed trucks. Before operation, the media required conditioning by backwashing to remove fines and stratify the bed. Backwashing is conducted monthly to ensure good bacteriological quality, to restratify the bed and to prevent excessive

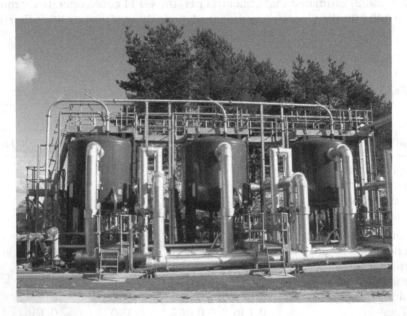

Figure 7.10   Arsenic adsorption plant in the UK. The plant at Chaddesley Corbett in Worcestershire has the capacity to treat 6.4 ML/day of groundwater from the Permo-Triassic sandstone in fixed-bed reactors containing the synthetic granulated ferric oxide adsorbent SORB 33™.
Source: Photograph courtesy of Severn Trent Services Ltd.

differential pressures. Exhausted media are fluidised and removed by tanker for disposal to landfill.

Based on pilot test results, an 8% interest rate and a 20–year life, Selvin et al. (2002) estimated the total life-cycle costs for all 17 new treatment plants using alternative technologies. Membrane technologies were most expensive, ranging from €56–98 M. Various configurations of activated alumina were evaluated, with costs ranging from €70.6 M without either pH control or regeneration, to €52 M for no pH control but with a central regeneration facility. The costs for GFO media[16] were nearly 20% cheaper (€42.8 M) than the next best alternative.

7.6.4 Arsenic and iron removal *in situ*

The concept of *in situ* treatment involves injecting oxygenated water into reducing aquifers to precipitate iron and manganese oxyhydroxides within the aquifer that can also adsorb arsenic (section 7.3.12). The process can be carried out by alternating injection and withdrawal from a single well, or by injection of aerated water through a ring of boreholes surrounding the pumping well.

Germany

In situ iron-removal plants have been operating successfully for 20 years in Germany, and have been shown to remove arsenic. Rott and Friedle (1999) described the performance of three plants at Paderborn. Plant A comprised two wells 115 m deep, screened for 50 m in a fissured (sandstone?) aquifer. Water is pumped from the first well, aerated, and injected into the second. The groundwater contained 0.94 ppm Fe, 0.20 ppm Mn and 15 ppb As (Fe: As 63). Removal of all three elements began within a few treatment cycles; arsenic was first to conform to the water quality objectives and manganese the last (Figure 7.11). To find out whether arsenic might be remobilised, one of the plants was pumped continuously (i.e. no injection) for a month (equivalent to an EC_f of 23), when arsenic remained almost constant at about 5 ppb, and iron rose slightly but remained low (<0.05 ppm). However, manganese rose steadily from about 0.03 to 0.37 ppm. At Plant B, where two wells were operated alternately for production and recharge, groundwater contained 1.97 ppm Fe, 0.35 ppm Mn and 38 ppb As (Fe:As 52). Fe and As concentrations began falling after a few cycles, but it took 20 cycles before As concentrations were consistently <10 ppb. At Plant C (0.94 ppm Fe, 0.15 ppm Mn and 15 ppb As, Fe:As 63), a single well was used. Again, concentrations began falling after a few cycles and reached the 10 ppb standard after 16 cycles.

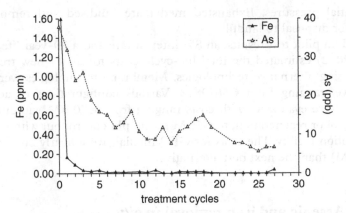

Figure 7.11   Arsenic and iron concentrations at an *in situ* removal plant at Paderborn, Germany. Iron concentrations fall almost immediately, but arsenic requires 10 cycles to reach 10 ppb.
Source: Rott and Friedle (1999)

Bangladesh

In Bangladesh, Sarkar and Rahman (2001) conducted trials at three hand tubewells in Noakhali District, where groundwater was highly contaminated (110, 520 and 1270 ppb As) and contained high iron concentrations[17] (1.0–2.4 ppm). For a month, 500 L of aerated water was fed into the well under gravity every evening, and 3000 L were pumped out every morning, with samples collected after each 500 L. Water withdrawn from the wells had As concentrations of 50, 200 and 520 ppb respectively. In each case, As concentrations were reduced by about 50%. The results are nonetheless encouraging in that they show that arsenic can be removed in highly contaminated aquifers, and hence that large quantities of arsenic might be permanently sequestered below ground. On the other hand, the results should be treated with caution because of the very small volume of water injected, which would have reached less than 0.5 m into the aquifer.

7.7   Costs of Arsenic Removal

7.7.1   Preamble

As may be expected from the above, there is no single best or cheapest treatment method. Costs will vary between countries due to differences in labour costs, financing arrangements, import requirements, and the chemistry of the contaminated water. Availability of low-cost natural materials such as ferruginous or manganiferous sands, zeolites or diatomite could also be important. The basis of cost comparisons differs for the public and private sectors, and for more- and less-developed economies. Public supplies, especially in developed countries, tend to be larger and dominated by a long-term, economic perspective, have access to competitive finance, and consider externalities, opportunity costs and the public good. In the private sector and less-developed country scenarios, such considerations are less prominent.

The greatest benefits of As removal, of course, derive from the cases of arsenicosis and associated mental stress avoided or alleviated. It is common to assess and compare schemes according to cost-effectiveness criteria using discounted cash-flow techniques intended to determine the lowest economic cost option over 10 to 20 years or more. This approach is normally satisfactory, but where a community is suffering from diagnosable arsenic poisoning, the economic benefits of preventing death and disease, distributed over time, should be included in the analysis. Including these benefits is likely to lead to a preference for solutions with rapid implementation.

7.7.2   Cost estimates from the USA

Centralised treatment

The most comprehensive cost data come from the USA[18] (Chen et al., 1999; EPA, 2000), particularly the southwestern states, and so may be biased towards a combination of AD-type water, high labour costs, and a strict and litigious regulatory environment. This does not invalidate the results; but they may need to be recalculated to suit local circumstances. Chen et al. (1999) calculated annualised costs[19], including removing secondary contaminants and waste disposal. They considered four options: (a) modified conventional treatment (optimised lime-softening, coagulation, or Fe–Mn removal); (b) activated alumina; (c) ion-exchange; and (d) reverse osmosis. They considered sizes of plant[20] between 400 and 400,000 m³/day, and concluded that modified conventional treatment is much cheaper than all other options; that AA and IX have similar average costs; and both are cheaper than RO.

The EPA (2000) combined three cost models for different sizes of treatment plant to derive capital, operating and waste disposal costs for nine types of treatment used for centralised supply, as summarised in Table 7.6. There are huge variations in the balance of capital, operation and maintenance and waste costs, and in the variation of each cost-component with increasing design flow. The EPA also concluded that modified conventional systems (coagulation-filtration and lime-softening) have by far the lowest

Table 7.6 US Environmental Protection Agency cost estimates for centralised arsenic treatment

Technology	Capital ($000)	O&M ($000/yr)	Waste Disposal‡ ($000/yr)	Annualised Cost† ($/m³)
Small Systems (4): 100m³/day				
ECF	7.5	0.4	nd	0.03
CAM	210	26	2.2	1.26
ELS	9.0	1.3	nd	0.06
AA (pH 8.0–8.3)	25	17	0.4	0.53
AA (pH 6.0)	56	10	0.09	0.42
IX (SO$_4$ <20 ppm)	28	7.0	0.5	0.26
IX (SO$_4$ 20–50 ppm)	32	11.5	0.2	0.40
GF	28	9.0	0.6	0.32
Medium Systems: 1000 m³/day				
ECF	10.2	2.0	nd	0.01
CAM	800	45	23	0.33
ELS	11.9	8.5	nd	0.03
AA (pH 8.0–8.3)	140	110	4.0	0.34
AA (pH 6.0)	200	50	0.9	0.19
IX (SO$_4$ <20 ppm)	130	21	1.3	0.09
IX (SO$_4$ 20–50 ppm)	170	27	2.0	0.12
GF	200	23	2.4	0.11
Large Systems: 10,000 m³/day				
ECF	160	40	nd	0.02
CAM	3600	83	150	0.12
ELS	260	80	nd	0.03
AA (pH 8.0–8.3)	1200	1000	40	0.31
AA (pH 6.0)	1300	450	9.0	0.16
IX (SO$_4$ <20 ppm)	800	110	9.5	0.05
IX (SO$_4$ 20–50 ppm)	1000	140	20	0.06
GF	1400	160	21	0.08
Very Large Systems: 100,000 m³/day				
ECF	995	330	nd	0.01
CAM	26,000	440	1000	0.08
ELS	1700	700	nd	0.02
AA (pH 8.0–8.3)	12,000	9000	400	0.28
AA (pH 6.0)	13,000	4400	90	0.15
IX (SO$_4$ <20 ppm)	4000	230	95	0.02
IX (SO$_4$ 20–50 ppm)	4000	400	200	0.02
GF	9000	1600	200	0.07

ECF – enhanced coagulation filtration; CAM – coagulation assisted microfiltration; ELS – enhanced lime softening; AA – activated alumina; IX – ion-exchange; GF – greensand filtration; 'nd' – not determined;

* The EPA costs analysis did not include synthetic iron adsorbents due to lack of performance data at that time.

† Annualised cost is the sum of O&M cost plus the capital cost amortised at 7% over 20 years.

‡ Non-mechanical waste disposal on small and medium systems, and mechanical on larger systems.

§ All systems would require piped distribution.

Source: Data from EPA (2000)

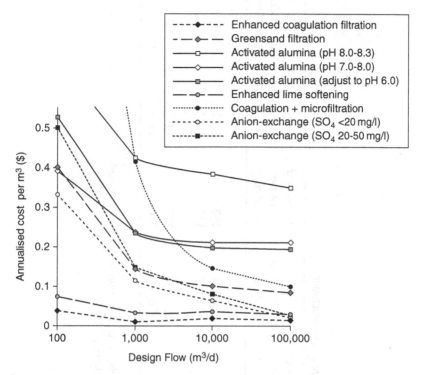

Figure 7.12   US Environmental Protection Agency cost estimates for centralised arsenic treatment. Annualised costs, excluding waste disposal, calculated from EPA (2000) based on a project period of 20 years and 7% interest.
Source: EPA (2000)

operating and capital costs for small and medium systems. By contrast, coagulation-assisted microfiltration is only competitive for large and very large systems. Annualised costs (per m³) were calculated as the sum of operation and maintenance cost and the capital cost amortised at 7% over 20 years, and vary by more than an order of magnitude (Figure 7.12). The unit cost of treated water from modified conventional systems is almost insensitive to design flow, and give least-cost water supply at all flows. Other systems offer major economies of scale. At low flows, the choice between AA and IX will depend on the water chemistry, but at high flows, IX is always preferred. When AA is considered, pH adjustment should be carried out if pH > 8.0, but may be uneconomic for near-neutral waters. Greensand filtration has similar costs to IX over a wide range of flows, but tends to have lower removal efficiency.

Table 7.7 US Environmental Protection Agency (EPA) cost estimates for point-of-use arsenic treatment

Technology	Capital ($)	Operation and maintenance ($/year)	Annualised cost* ($)	Annualised cost ($ per household†)	Water use (m³/day)	Annualised cost ($/m³)
Small systems: 100 households						
LP reverse osmosis	60,000	21,000	26,664	267	1.14	0.64
Activated alumina	22,000	32,000	34,077	341	1.14	0.82
Medium systems: 1000 households						
LP reverse osmosis	500,000	170,000	217,196	217	11.4	0.05
Activated alumina	170,000	260,000	276,047	276	11.4	0.07

LP, low pressure.
*Annualised cost is the sum of operation and maintenance cost plus the capital cost amortised at 7% over 20 years.
†A household was assumed to comprise three persons consuming 3.8 L/day per head.
Source: EPA (2000)

Point-of-use treatment

The EPA (2000) assessed RO, AA and IX systems for POU treatment for communities of 20 to 5000 households, although in the final analysis, IX and high-pressure RO systems were excluded for technical reasons. Despite higher capital costs, the annualised cost per household of AA was about 25% higher than RO for communities of 100 and 1000 households (Table 7.7). Economies of scale from 100 to 1000 households are significant; the unit cost for RO dropping from $267 to $217. Sargent-Michaud et al. (2006) compared RO, AA and bottled water for household water supply in Maine (USA). Ranked in terms of total annual cost, for households of more than one person, the cheapest solution was RO ($411) followed by AA ($518) and lastly bottled water. Only for single-person households was it cheaper to buy water in gallon jars ($321).

7.7.3 Bangladesh costs

The World Bank (2005) has estimated the costs of arsenic treatment in Bangladesh. Notwithstanding the higher interest rate used (12% as opposed to 7%) and the shorter technical life assumed[21], the costs of treatment in Bangladesh (Table 7.8) appear to be significantly higher than USA costs, except for arsenic and iron removal plants (AIRP), which are comparable with USA costs. The high cost of other systems is probably attributable to the cost of imported materials.

Table 7.8 Estimated costs of community arsenic treatment systems in Bangladesh

Technology	Water output (m^3/year)	Technical life	Capital cost ($)	Operation and maintenance cost ($/yr)	Annualised cost ($/$m^3$)
Coagulation-filtration	246	10	250	250	1.21
Granular ferric oxide/granular ferric hydroxide	860	10	2800	475	1.13
Activated alumina	180	10	425	510	3.25
Ion exchange	25	10	280	35	3.40
Reverse osmosis	328	10	2500	780	3.72
As- and Fe-removal plant	730,000	20	240,000	7500	0.05

Source: Modified from World Bank (2005)

World Bank (2005) also estimated the annualised unit cost of water produced by household filters. The least-cost system used iron filings ($0.24/m^3), followed by iron-coated sand ($0.73/m^3), with the most expensive using synthetic media ($1.84/m^3) and activated alumina ($2.39/m^3). The costs of the iron filings and iron-coated sand based systems are comparable with small AA systems used in the USA (Table 7.7). More remarkably, the two least-cost household systems in Bangladesh are cheaper than all the community systems except for AIRP.

7.8   Guidance for Selecting Treatment Methods and Technologies

The following sections offer guidance on the As-removal methods that are appropriate to particular water qualities, and then indicate how they may be applied through specific technologies to different institutional settings.

7.8.1   Raw water and arsenic treatment process

Even in the most affected areas, few As concentrations exceed about 500 ppb. It is generally inappropriate to treat such extreme waters because (a) operational failure may re-expose water users, (b) compliance is more difficult, and (c) operating costs are higher. These high concentrations can often be avoided by resinking wells to a different depth or installing a longer screen, which might reduce the As concentration by 25–75%.

As Chen et al. (1999) showed, if other chemicals (e.g. Fe, Mn, Cl, SO$_4$, NO$_3$, F, B, Se, Mo and V) need to be removed, methods that combine their removal with that of arsenic are likely to be the cheapest overall. Although the list of potential co-contaminants appears long, it becomes simpler when the regional geochemistry is considered (see Table 7.1).

Publications from Europe and North America often address input concentrations (<50 ppb As) that are currently acceptable as outputs in most developing countries. Hence, methods that comply with the 10 ppb level but with low removal efficiencies may fail for raw waters containing hundreds of ppb of arsenic. Table 7.9 shows the maximum achievable removal efficiencies for a variety of technologies; these must be viewed in the context of raw water quality and the applicable drinking water standards.

Wherever iron concentrations are high, this is an opportunity to reduce the cost of treatment by utilising the capacity of freshly precipitated iron hydroxides to adsorb arsenic. Chen et al. (1999) presented a flowchart for cost-based selection of treatment process which, combined with hydrogeochemical

Table 7.9   Maximum achievable arsenic removal

Maximum percentage removal*	Treatment technology	Maximum treatable input concentration to achieve:	
		50 ppb As	10 ppb As
>95	Reverse osmosis	–	–
95	Coagulation-filtration	1000	200
	Enhanced coagulation-filtration		
	Ion exchange (SO$_4$ <50 ppm)		
	Activated alumina		
90	Coagulation-assisted microfiltration	500	100
	Lime-softening		
	Point-of-use activated alumina		
80	Greensand filtration (20:1 Fe:As)	250	50

*The removal efficiencies quoted are indicative, and will vary with the particular technology and raw water quality.
Source: EPA (2000)

insights and Sorg's (2002) technology-screening chart (Figure 7.13), can be reformulated as a set of simple rules, as described below.

Reductive-dissolution-type waters (anoxic, high Fe and Mn)

The designer should try to optimise conventional treatment such as Fe–Mn removal, coagulation or lime-softening, guided by the Fe:As ratio[22] and drinking water quality criteria, as follows.

- If Fe > 0.3 ppm, As > 10 ppb and Fe:As > 20, consider normal iron-removal (oxidation) processes, but optimised for As removal.
- If Fe > 0.3 ppm and As > 10 ppb but Fe:As < 20, consider a modified iron-removal process, adding more iron.
- If either of these fail to meet the required standard, conduct bench tests with AA or GFH/GFO. If that also fails, consider RO.

Alkali-desorption- and sulphide-oxidation-type waters (oxic, low Fe)

If already in place, attempt to optimise conventional treatment. Otherwise, if iron concentrations are low, methods such as RO, IX and synthetic adsorbents should be considered. The presence of other chemicals requiring

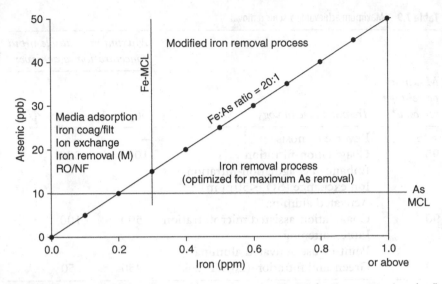

Figure 7.13 Screening tool to select arsenic removal processes. The MCL (maximum contaminant level) values for As and Fe divide the graph into water quality fields that favour specific treatment methods. *Source*: Sorg (2002)

treatment may be critical. Without obviating the need for feasibility studies, the following general points should apply:

- If the total mineralisation, especially chloride concentration, is high, RO may be the preferred option.
- If sulphate exceeds 150 ppm, IX should generally be avoided, and absorbent systems may be preferred. However, if sulphate is low and nitrate also requires treatment, IX may be the preferred solution (Ghurye et al., 1999).
- Where toxic elements such as fluoride or selenium require treatment, an absorbent with a proven ability to remove the specific contaminant should be selected. For example, AA has a successful record in removing fluoride (AWWA, 1999).
- The performance of AA is strongly pH dependent, but can be very efficient with pH-adjustment and, if As(III) is present, pre-oxidation. Regeneration of AA is easier than that of its main alternatives (EPA, 2003a).
- Iron-based adsorbents are less sensitive to pH and the oxidation state of arsenic. Although regeneration is not normally recommended, new polymer-based iron adsorbents may overcome this disadvantage, albeit with higher initial cost. Titanium-based adsorbents are an emerging alternative to iron-based adsorbents.
- Natural adsorbent materials, rich in Fe or Mn, may be preferred where an abundant and cheap local source exists.

Other methods, such as biological techniques, might perform as well or better, but do not have a well-proven record in the field and so can be recommended only for pilot applications. As a general procedure, Lytle et al. (2005) stress the benefit and cost-effectiveness of conducting jar-tests at an early stage in the design process. While not actually contradicting this advice, Smith and Edwards (2005) caution that batch-testing *alone* can result in 'grossly over-optimistic projections of column capacity'. Both Smith and Edwards (2005) and Westerhoff et al. (2006) recommend rapid small-scale column testing (RSSCT) to predict breakthrough curves for granular sorbents. The RSSCT approach gives superior results and can be completed in a few weeks, which is much quicker and cheaper than pilot testing.

In addition to the surface-based methods considered above, *in situ* removal has potential for community and municipal supply, either as a complete treatment or for pre-treatment of highly contaminated groundwater, but requires carefully monitored pilot-studies to optimise the technique for Bangladesh, India and other severely affected countries.

7.8.2   Arsenic treatment technologies and institutional setting

Technologies must be matched to both the system capacity and the nature of the institutions (section 7.1). Household and small community plants that draw water from a handpump or small power-pump generally lack institutional support, and therefore require simple operating procedures and no full-time operator. At centralised treatment plants, strong institutional support for procurement, testing and waste disposal make it possible to employ full-time, skilled operators, and therefore to use methods that are cost-effective but too complex or too demanding of the skilled labour of community systems. Recommendations are summarised in Table 7.10.

Household and small community treatment plants

The selection of technologies for supplies serving between a single and a few hundred households is most influenced by social and operational factors. Based on successful experience with wellhead ARPs in West Bengal (section 7.6.2), Sarkar et al. (2005) proposed the following guidelines for small treatment systems in developing countries:

1 avoid chemical addition, pH adjustment and use of electricity;
2 simple and manual operation;
3 procure all materials indigenously;

Table 7.10   Arsenic removal systems related to raw water quality and demand

Institutional Setting	*Raw water quality type*	
	Reductive dissolution	*Alkali desorption/sulphide oxidation*
Household/ small community	Aeration+AA/GFH adsorbent ZVI with sand filter	AA/GFH adsorbent reverse osmosis
Piped, community system	Aeration+slow sand filter (Fe:As > 20) Pressure filter + ICS/GFH adsorbent (Fe:As < 20)	AA/GFH adsorbent Ion exchange (low (SO$_4$) Reverse osmosis (high TDS)
Centralised treatment and extensive distribution	Modified IRP Coagulation-filtration	Coagulation-filtration with pH adjustment AA with pH adjustment Ion exchange (low SO$_4$)

AA, activated alumina; GFH, granular ferric hydroxide; ICS, iron-coated sand; ZVI, zero-valent iron; IRP, iron-removal plants; TDS, total dissolved solids.

4   units to serve a few hundred households should be within walking distance;
5   management by a village committee;
6   no potential for indiscriminate disposal of contaminated waste.

These six points all appear necessary, but do not give sufficient emphasis to routine maintenance (e.g. backwashing of iron precipitates), the role of a supporting organisation, and understanding the role and involvement of women in the planning process. Smaller systems still, such as the Kanchan Filter in Nepal or the Sono Filter in Bangladesh, rely on gravity flow and reaction with zero-valent iron and are better suited to serving individual households. It is, however, extremely difficult to monitor the effectiveness of very small treatment systems, and they may be unaffordable for the poorest households.

In wealthier societies, pressurised fixed-bed reactors using AA or iron-based media and low-pressure RO systems are likely to be popular, and can be readily supplied by a responsive private sector (e.g. EPA, 2006). High-iron groundwater from glacial aquifers in Illinois has been treated successfully using Mn-greensand filtration and by oxidation plus SSF, although adding additional iron and potassium permanganate (as pre-oxidant) improved As removal (Wilson et al., 2004). Slotnick et al. (2006) examined 261 private wells in Michigan, of which 46% used no treatment and 31% had only water softening. Of the remainder, 7% had RO plants and 16%

Table 7.11 Effectiveness of point-of-use treatment at private wells in southeast Michigan, USA

Treatment system	Number of Wells (%)	Raw water		Treated water	
		Mean As (ppb)	>10ppb As (%)	Mean As (ppb)	>10ppb As (%)
Softening only	81 (31)	8.8	27	9.4	25
Reverse osmosis*	19 (7)	7.2	26	2.3	0
Non-reverse osmosis*	42 (16)	8.3	24	6.7	21
None	119 (46)	–	–	–	–

*Results include wells both with and without water softening.
Source: Slotnick et al. (2006)

had some other kind of filter. Although not all were installed specifically to remove arsenic, the results provide a useful insight (Table 7.11). Water softening was of no benefit with respect to arsenic removal. Although non-RO systems reduced the average As concentration, they had little impact on compliance with the 10ppb standard. By contrast, RO systems were effective in lowering the average As concentration and eliminated exceedances of the drinking water standard.

Large community treatment plants

These installations have a piped distribution system, but limited institutional capability, which favours methods that do not need constant attention, routine laboratory support, chemical dosing, or complex controls. The ability to cope with erratic electricity supplies is an advantage in developing countries. In RD-type waters, high iron content favours use of modified iron-removal plants with a simple filtration system such as a SSF. This approach has been promoted in Bangladesh, where iron removal is achieved by spray or cascading tower aerators. Where the iron content exceeds about 3ppm, a sedimentation tank helps to reduce the rate of clogging of the filter. The method works best where the Fe:As ratio is high, preferably >20. Although pre-oxidation of As(III) greatly improves removal efficiency, it is often preferred to avoid this for operational reasons. However, while this may achieve compliance at 50ppb, it is unlikely to do so at 10ppb. Where the Fe:As ratio is low, it may be necessary either to add iron or to use a pressure tank with aeration and an iron-based adsorbent, as a compromise between minimising cost and maximising As removal. In AD-type or other low-Fe waters, pressurised fixed-bed reactors may be effective. Where As(V) predominates and the pH < 7, activated alumina may be preferred to iron-based adsorbents. However, unless a support agency organises regeneration, disposal of spent iron–based adsorbents may be easier. Although largely untested, *in situ* Fe and As removal may have potential in reducing aquifers.

Centralised treatment plants

Centralised plants, with extensive distribution systems and strong institutional support, can achieve economies of scale that make process-control and monitoring equipment more cost-effective. No methods need be rejected because of complexity or safety considerations, and hence cost will be the main selection criterion. In general, the preferred solution for Fe-rich RD-type waters (Fe:As > 20) will be modified iron-removal with pre-oxidation. Where iron is high but the Fe:As ratio is less favourable, conventional coagulation-flocculation-filtration combined with pre-oxidation will probably be preferred. In low-Fe AD-type waters, where As(V) dominates, there will be more options. It is more practical for centralised plants to benefit from optimisation techniques such as pH adjustment and pre-oxidation and to manage media regeneration and hazardous waste disposal, all of which are troublesome for small plant operators. Consequently, methods such as coagulation with iron-salts and the use of media such as activated alumina become more advantageous, and techniques such as fixed-bed adsorption with synthetic iron-media lose their relative advantage compared with their use in smaller systems.

7.9   Case Study of Water Treatment Requirements in Bangladesh

Surveys in Bangladesh in 1998–99 not only established that 25% of wells exceeded 50 ppb As, and 42% exceeded 10 ppb As, but also produced a baseline of the water quality in all major aquifers (DPHE/BGS, 2001). This section speculates on what treatment methods would be recommended in the hypothetical case that all mitigation was provided by groundwater treatment to conform with present and possible future standards for both arsenic (50 and 10 ppb) and iron (1.0 and 0.3 ppm). Iron is a major issue because 65% of wells exceeded 0.3 ppm. Manganese, although a health issue, is not a major treatment issue in its own right because only 4% of wells require removal of arsenic and manganese but not iron. Groundwaters requiring treatment have near-neutral pH and typically contain 1–2 ppm of phosphate and around 20 ppm of silica but <10 ppm of sulphate. The Fe:As ratio is negatively correlated with As concentration, indicating that the most polluted waters will be the most difficult to treat

Table 7.12   Hypothetical groundwater treatment requirements for Bangladesh*

To remove	Fe:As	Class†	Treatment method	Current treatment standard (%) As: 50ppb Fe: 1.0ppm	Future treatment standard (%) As: 10ppb Fe: 0.3ppm
As and Fe	>20	A	Iron removal plant	14	29
As and Fe	<20	B	Modified iron removal plant	8	11
As only	<20	C	Adsorption/ion exchange/reverse osmosis	3	2
Fe only	>20	–	Iron removal plant	29	25
Neither	–	–	–	46	33

*As and Fe analytical data for 3523 wells from DPHE/BGS (2001).
†The classification and technology screening criteria are from Sorg (2002). Classes A, B and C are shown in Figure 7.14.

by conventional means. In shallow wells with 10–50 ppb As, the Fe:As averaged 390, in wells with 50–250 ppb As it was 60, and in wells with >250 ppb As it was only 14.

Treatment requirements for Bangladesh were estimated using Sorg's (2002) screening criteria (Figure 7.13 and Table 7.12), which suggest that the majority of treatment could be accomplished using conventional iron-removal plants optimised for arsenic removal. A significant proportion (8–11%) of waters would require treatment by iron removal plants (IRPs) that have been modified to include iron addition, while a small proportion (2–3%) would be appropriate for adsorption technologies. However, as noted earlier, Sorg's scheme recommends processes, not specific technologies, and other factors may dictate selection of other methods for household and small community supplies. In practice, treatment will not be applied at all contaminated wells, the majority of which will probably be replaced by deep wells or other sources.

7.10   Future Needs

The performance of As-removal systems in developing countries has often been poor. To improve this, agencies should give much more attention to community organisation, and supporting operation and maintenance when promoting arsenic removal plants. When treating RD-type groundwater, the predominance of As(III) slows down, and to some extent limits, the removal of arsenic, especially compliance with a target of 10 ppb As. It is therefore important to disseminate knowledge of pre-oxidation techniques that are practical for community systems.

Polymer-bound nanocrystalline iron and titanium oxide adsorbents have many technical advantages, but will require further demonstration in the field, especially in developing countries, and appropriate pricing before they are widely implemented. Biological treatment systems appear to have considerable potential, but need thorough field testing before they can be promoted. The other highly promising technique is *in situ* removal of arsenic, and feasibility studies should be undertaken in severely affected aquifers of South Asia.

NOTES

1   MIT's online database of arsenic remediation technologies (http://web.mit.edu/murcott/www/arsenic/database.html) contains information about technologies that have been field-tested.
2   A potential problem in RD-type waters is that free chlorine may react with DOM to create unwanted, and possibly carcinogenic, chlorinated by-products.
3   This is not significant in RD waters, where sulphate is generally absent, and in AD and SO waters, where As(V) dominates, but it may affect some geothermal waters.
4   The term bed-volume (BV) is the volume of vessel packed with adsorbent.
5   Produced by the Shin Nihon Salt Co. Ltd in Japan.
6   Both were prepared from red flint sand, the first by adding $FeCl_3$ for 12 hours, and the second used $Fe(NO_3)_3$ followed by NaOH.
7   Other 'exchanger' minerals such as clays may also adsorb the ferrous iron, enhancing the overall effect, which it has been suggested can be measured in terms of the cation exchange capacity (CEC).
8   pH is unlikely to be critical in most landfills.
9   The US National Academy of Engineering, with financial support of The Grainger Foundation, offered prizes of \$1 m, \$0.2 m and \$0.1 m for a workable, sustainable, economical, point-of-use treatment system for As-contaminated groundwater in developing countries.
10   The Technology Park Project was implemented in 2001 by the School of Fundamental Research (SOFR) with financial assistance from India Canada Environment Facility (ICEF).
11   A similar system, developed by SIDCO, has been deployed in Bangladesh with assistance from UNICEF (M.F. Ahmed, personal communication).
12   The paper by Sarkar et al. (2005) is written by the promoters of the technology, unlike the paper on the Technology Park Project which was written by an

independent group. However, one of the authors (PR) visited the BEC project in January 2006 to verify their findings.

13 Rotary International and Water for People (USA).

14 In January 2007, the BEC team was awarded the Grainger Challenge Silver Award.

15 This is contrary to the approach of large NGOs and donors in Bangladesh who attempt to offer an 'informed choice' of mitigation options. Though intuitively appealing, this approach may be at the cost of quality since no organisations have long experience in delivering arsenic mitigation.

16 The pH and iron content of the groundwater were probably important in determining the best solution here.

17 The Fe:As ratio decreased with increasing As content.

18 These studies did not include synthetic iron media because there was insufficient operation experience at the time (see EPA, 2003a).

19 As annual operating cost plus 10% of capital cost discounted over 20 years at interest rates of 7–8%. This calculation scheme is appropriate for public utilities and large commercial entities.

20 Equivalent to populations of a few thousand to several million people.

21 Because operation and maintenance costs are a significant part of the total cost of treatment, the difference in the discounted unit cost of water that results from the use of a higher interest rate and variable technical life is <13% for all community technologies, except for the As–Fe removal plant which has a 31% higher unit cost. However, the relative ranking of unit costs is not significantly changed by the choice of interest rate, except that RO is marginally preferred to IX at the lower interest rate.

22 Other studies have stressed the benefit of a high Fe:As ratio for efficient As-removal: Leupin and Hug (2005) report 90% As removal when Fe:As > 30; while Meng et al. (2001) recommend Fe:As > 40 for waters rich in P and Si.

Chapter Eight

Arsenic in Asia

8.1 Introduction

More people are affected by As poisoning in Asia than in the rest of the
world combined. It is probable that more than 100 million people drink
water containing >10 ppb As. The main occurrences of contamination in
Asia are summarised in Table 8.1. In terms of population exposed or at
risk, the impacts in Bangladesh and the adjoining regions of India and
Nepal dwarf all other instances. Remarkably similar patterns of contamination extend in a near continuous band (Figure 8.1) from the Indus
River in Pakistan to Taiwan – the South and Southeast Asian Arsenic Belt
(SSAAB). Only in the inland alluvial basins of Inner Mongolia, Shanxi
and Xinjiang in China is As pollution found on a scale comparable to the
SSAAB. Elsewhere, arsenic pollution, although locally severe, is much
less extensive, and mostly associated with a diversity of bedrock aquifers.
South and Southeast Asia includes a large proportion of the world's
poorest people, many of whom now suffer the additional burden of As-
polluted water supplies. Because of poverty, they are more vulnerable to
the effects of arsenic poisoning and economically less well equipped to
respond to the problem. Life on these densely populated alluvial plains
depends on groundwater for drinking water and irrigation, especially of
rice. More than any other region, this area illustrates the complex interplay between exposure from drinking water, food, irrigation, cooking and
nutrition.

Table 8.1 Case histories of arsenic occurrence in Asia

Name	Country/region	Geology, hydrology and climate	Arsenic (ppb)[†] (max./mean/range)	Water chemistry/ processes	Affected population/significance[*]
Indus Valley, Punjab	Pakistan	Alluvium–semi-arid	Max. 972; 20% > 10; 3% > 50	Anoxic, RD	6 M (E10); 2 M (E50)
Indus Valley, Sindh	Pakistan	Alluvium–semi-arid	Max. 906; 23% > 10; 5% > 50	Not known	
Near Colombo	Sri Lanka	?	?	Not known	One death
Chandigarh and surrounding areas	India (Punjab, Haryana, Himachal Pradesh and Union Territories)	Semi-arid	Max. 545; 60% > 50	Not known	One death by non-cirrhotic portal fibrosis
Chhattisgarh	India	Pre-Cambrian metamorphic rocks, semi-arid	Max. 2350; 8% > 50	Anoxic, RD	10,000 'at risk'; 130 (P)
Chenai	India	Alluvium(?); tropical humid	Max. 146	Not known	
Gangetic plains	India (Uttar Pradesh, Bihar and Jarkhand)	Alluvium; tropical humid	Uttar Pradesh (UP): 2.4% > 50 Bihar: 10.8% > 50 Jharkhand: 3.7% > 50	Anoxic, RD	UP: 0.76 M (E50); 4.4 M (E10) Bihar: 2.7 M (E50); 7.2 M (E10) Jharkhand: 0.01 M (E50); 0.02 M (E10)
Bengal Basin	Bangladesh and India (West Bengal)	Alluvium; tropical humid	Bangladesh: 25% > 50; 42% > 10 West Bengal: 25% > 50; 50% > 10	Anoxic, RD	Bangladesh: 27 M (E50) West Bengal: 6.0 M (E50) and 0.3 M (P)
Brahmaputra plains	India (Assam)	Alluvium; tropical humid	Max. 657; 17% > 50	Anoxic, RD	1.5 M (E50); 6.4 M (E10)
Northeast states	India (Manipur, Arunachal Pradesh, Tripura and Nagaland)	Alluvium; tropical humid	Max. 986; 29% > 50	RD(?)	
Terai	Nepal	Alluvium; tropical humid	24% > 10; 3% > 50	Anoxic, RD	0.55 M (E50); 2.5 M (E10). As-patients identified.
Kathmandu Valley	Nepal	Alluvium; tropical humid	13% > 10; 1% > 50	Anoxic, RD	
Irrawaddy delta	Myanmar	Alluvium; tropical humid	21% > 50	Anoxic, RD	As-patients identified 2.5 M (E50)
Chao Phraya plains	Thailand	Alluvium; tropical humid	Max. 100	Anoxic, RD	No As-patients identified

(contd)

Table 8.1 (cont'd)

Name	Country/region	Geology, hydrology and climate	Arsenic (ppb)† (max./mean/range)	Water chemistry/ processes	Affected population/significance*
Hat Yai	Thailand	Alluvium; tropical humid	Max. 1070	Anoxic, RD	0.48 M (E50); 0.58 M (10)
Mekong river	Cambodia	Alluvium; tropical humid	Max. 1700; 48% > 10; 40% > 50;	Anoxic, RD	
Mekong delta	Vietnam	Alluvium; tropical humid	Max. > 500; 13% > 10	Anoxic, RD	No As-patients identified
Red River delta	Vietnam	Alluvium; tropical humid	Max. 3050; 48% > 50	Anoxic, RD	No As-patients identified
Inner Mongolia	China	Holocene alluvium; semi-arid (including Hetao plain and Huhhot basin)	Max. 1480; 11% > 50	Anoxic, RD	1,025,000 (E50); prevalence 16%
Shanxi	China	Quaternary alluvium; semi-arid (including Datong basin)	Max. 2783; 52% > 50;	AD (and RD?)	932,000 (E50); prevalence 13%
Xinjiang	China		Max. 880; 4% > 50	AD and evaporative concentration	143,000 (E50); prevalence 1.4%
Anhui Pr.	China	?	Max. 150	?	87,000 (E50); prevalence 0.8%
Beijing	China	?	Max. 143; 8% > 50	?	60,000 (E50)
Jilin Pr.	China	?	Max. 360; 12% > 50	?	59,000 (E50); prevalence 18%
Ningxia Pr.	China	?	Max. 100; 1.1% > 50	?	25,000 (E50); prevalence 10%
Qinghai	China	?	Max. 318; 8% > 50	?	12,000 (E50); prevalence 9%
Southwest Coast	Taiwan	Alluvium; tropical humid	Max. 1410; 34% > 10	Anoxic, RD	
Northeast Coast	Taiwan	Alluvium; tropical humid	Max. >3000; 59% > 10; 39% > 50;	Anoxic, RD	
Fukoka Prefecture	Japan	?	Max. 293; 43% > 10	AD and RD	
Yumigahama	Japan	Holocene coastal alluvium	Max. 42	Anoxic, RD	
Citarum River, Java	Indonesia	Volcanogenic sulphur-mud	Max. 279	Geothermal	

Region	Country	Geology and climate	Concentration (ppb As)		Health effects
Mindanao	Philippines	Volcanic		Geothermal	
Ghazni city	Afghanistan	Semi-arid	Max. 100 (surface water); 76% > 10		500,000 (E10)
Western Anatolia	Turkey	Boron-rich sediments and limestone; semi-arid	Max. 7,700		Prevalence up to 33%
Kurdistan province	Iran	?	Max. 1480; mean 290		
Siberia: Sakhalin, the Urals, Trans-Baikal, Kamchatka	Russia	?	Max. 10,000 (Kamchatka); Others all >700	Hot and saline	
Middle Caspian Artesian Basin	Russia and Kazakhstan	Cretaceous sediments; semi-arid to arid	Max. 1500		
Mongolia	Mongolia	Semi-arid to arid	10.3% detection (c. 10ppb)	?	Prevalence 16.5%

AD, alkali desorption; RD, reductive dissolution.

*E10 refers to the number of people drinking water with > 10 ppb As, and E50 to drinking more than 50 ppb As. A number followed by the suffix 'P' refers to the number of patients that have been diagnosed. Where exposure has changed over time, the peak figure is quoted.

†Concentrations normally refer to untreated water sources, either wells, streams or lakes, but not piezometers.

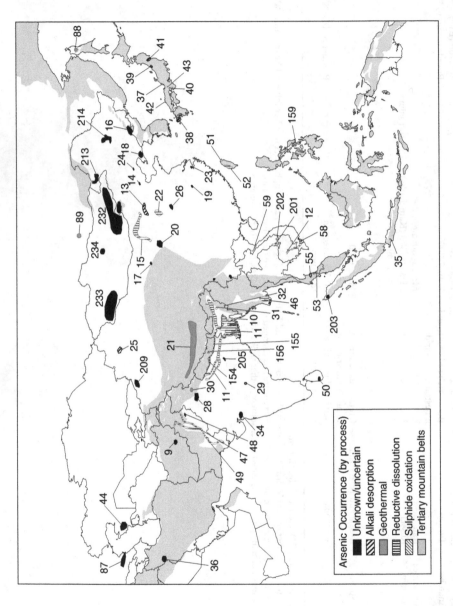

Figure 8.1 Occurrences of arsenic contamination of groundwater in Asia. See Table 1.2 for explanation of numbers. The locations of arsenic pollution compiled by the authors from references cited in the text. Other geographical data from ESRI (1996). Note also that the geographical size of the affected areas bear little relation to the number of people affected.

8.2 South Asia

8.2.1 Regional setting

The Himalayan river systems

Arsenic pollution in the SSAAB occurs predominantly in the alluvial deposits of major rivers flowing south and east from the Himalayas and Tibetan plateau (Figure 8.1). These rivers flow through the highest mountains, with the highest rainfall, and generate the greatest sediment load in the world. The most important Himalayan river system is the Ganges–Brahmaputra–Meghna (GBM). Other major rivers include the Indus which flows into Pakistan, the Yellow (or Huang-He) and Yangtze-Kiang in China, the Red and Mekong in Vietnam and Cambodia, and the Irrawaddy and Salween in Myanmar. All of these have dry and cold upper catchments, steep courses, and hot and humid lower catchments.

The GBM rivers join in central Bangladesh; their combined flow is the third largest in the World and contributes the largest single input of sediment to the oceans. The alluvial plains have tropical monsoonal climates, with 1–3 m of rain a year. Sediments of the Indus, Ganges and Brahmaputra rivers fill alluvial basins along the southern edge of the Himalayas. As the Himalayan front was thrust south, it pressed down the crust in front of it, creating a continuously subsiding foreland basin, now filled with kilometres of sediment, although some of the early sediments have been uplifted to form the Siwalik Hills on the north side of the Ganga plains (Singh, 1996). In the east, the situation is complicated by the east–west squeezing of the Indo-Burman ranges, which created the Bengal Basin (Curray and Moore, 1971).

8.2.2 The discovery of arsenic pollution in South Asia

Initial discoveries in northern India

Arsenic pollution of groundwater was first discovered in north-central India by doctors (Datta, 1976) after a patient who died of liver disease[1] was found to have high levels of arsenic in all internal organs. A survey of wells, boreholes, taps, springs, ponds and canals in Chandigarh and adjoining areas of the surrounding states discovered extensive As contamination, with a maximum of 545 ppb As. The results of the survey are summarised in Table 8.2.

Although some contaminated samples in Himachal Pradesh came from hot springs, no other geological data were presented, except to identify the cause as groundwater. Interestingly, Datta and Kaul (1976) observed that 'Only

Table 8.2   Number of samples containing >50 ppb As in the first survey of arsenic in water supplies in India; the number in parentheses is the total number of samples

State	Wells	Springs	Hand pumps	Ponds	Canals
Punjab	12 (39)	0 (4)	18 (39)	3 (3)	2 (2)
Haryana	1 (24)	2 (5)	1 (5)	–	–
Himachal Pradesh	18 (26)	10 (45)	1 (7)	–	4 (4)
Union Territories	1 (6)	–	2 (12)	1 (1)	–
Uttar Pradesh	0 (4)	–	4 (16)	–	–

Source: Datta and Kaul (1976)

three reports in world literature are available where consumption of arsenic contaminated drinking water has been said to produce some pathologic lesions'. The first was Chile, the second Taiwan and the third was Chandigarh[2]. In the final line of their paper, they added 'Chronic ingestion of arsenic rich water producing a syndrome of 'arsenicosis' ... definitely warrants further study'. Unfortunately their work, published both in an Indian journal and *The Lancet*, was largely ignored (Chakraborti et al., 2003).

West Bengal

Arsenic contamination of groundwater in West Bengal was discovered in 1983 by a dermatologist, Dr K.C. Saha. The results were published not only in Indian medical journals (e.g. Garai et al., 1984) but also the *WHO Bulletin* (Guha Mazumder et al., 1988, 1992). This should have served as a wake-up call to India and surrounding countries, but it did not, and no explanation has ever been offered. Around the same time, As pollution from a pesticide factory was identified in a suburb of Kolkata (Chatterjee et al., 1993), but this turned out to be a red herring in the overall story. By the late 1980s, the arsenic problem was well known to at least six federal or state agencies (e.g. PHED, 1991), but did not lead to the discovery of As pollution in the nearby states of Bihar, Uttar Pradesh and Assam until after 2000 (Chakraborti et al., 2002). Even today, groundwater in many river basins of India appears not to have been tested for arsenic.

Discovery in Bangladesh

Arsenic pollution was apparently discovered in 1993 by the Department of Public Health Engineering (DPHE) in Chapai Nawabganj, close to the West Bengal border. Only after the School of Environmental Sciences

(SOES) organised an International Conference in Kolkata in early 1995 was the possibility of extensive contamination in Bangladesh taken seriously. From 1995, *ad hoc* surveys, particularly by Dhaka Community Hospital (DCH) and SOES, began to map the extent of contamination. Initially, contamination was thought to be restricted to the Ganges delta, but it was soon recognised that the Meghna–Brahmaputra sediments in southeast Bangladesh were even more polluted. Early surveys by UNICEF and DPHE correctly defined the spatial pattern of contamination, but the field kits used missed many exceedances in the range 50–200 ppb. This early period of uncertainty as to the cause, extent and trends of contamination ended with publication of the study by DPHE/MMI/BGS (1999) and the paper by Nickson et al. (1998), which established the cause as natural and not anthropogenic, as had been widely believed.

Other discoveries in South and Southeast Asia

Curiously, neither the publications of the WHO nor the SOES group (e.g. Das et al., 1994, 1996) initiated significant testing outside India. This may have been partly because pollution in India had become associated with anthropogenic causes, and was therefore, implicitly, localised. The first international arsenic conference[3] organised by DCH and SOES in Dhaka in early 1998 played a major role in drawing attention to the problem. Also the obvious geological similarities of the Bengal Basin to other river basins in tropical Asia encouraged governments in the region, often with the assistance of UNICEF, to undertake surveys. These surveys led to the discovery of arsenic contamination in Vietnam (Berg et al., 2001; Stanger et al., 2005), Myanmar (Tun, 2002), Thailand (Kohnhorst et al., 2002), Nepal (Shrestha et al., 2003), Pakistan (Ahmad et al., 2004) and Cambodia (Polya et al., 2005). Some countries, however, remain unsurveyed.

Why was arsenic not discovered earlier?

The reader may wonder why the discoveries in northern India and West Bengal did not trigger investigations across South and Southeast Asia sooner, and led to the question of how long people had been exposed to high levels of arsenic. Some towns and cities had exploited groundwater for many decades, but ironically many of these are sited on As-free aquifers[4], while in rural areas groundwater was tapped by dug-wells which contain low levels of arsenic. In Bangladesh, awareness of arsenic was very low, and most water resource[5] studies gave only cursory attention to water quality. Groundwater was assumed to be safe, except for faecal contamination. Notable exceptions to this complacency were studies of groundwater quality in Bangladesh (Davies and Exley, 1992) and Vietnam (Trafford et al., 1996) by the British Geological Survey (BGS). Unfortunately, although genuinely far-sighted in analysing for trace elements, they did not test for arsenic, which eventually led to a class action in the UK courts as described in Annexe 8.1. In another irony, Matlab, the field study area of the International Centre for Diarrhoeal Disease Research, turned out to be one of the most severely affected upazilas. Matlab had been visited by hundreds, perhaps thousands, of national and international medical researchers, but none of these experts recognised arsenic poisoning, presumably because they were not looking for it. A final irony was that three wells had been tested for arsenic in Dhaka City (DWASA, 1991), but all analyses were (correctly) below the detection limit (10 ppb As), and so gave no impetus to further testing.

The failure to test for arsenic earlier or more widely raises two questions: why was not arsenic tested for on a precautionary basis; and why did it take so long for the news of arsenic in West Bengal to reach Bangladesh? The first question has no good answer, and the testing in Dhaka shows that it could have been done. As for the second, arsenic pollution in West Bengal was well-known in India by 1990 (e.g. PHED, 1991). By the early 1990s, suspected patients were crossing into India for treatment. Chakraborti et al. (2002) state that correspondence was sent to the Government of Bangladesh and UN agencies, but was not acted on. The political climate of the time did not encourage scientific dialogue between India and Bangladesh, but agencies such as UNICEF and WHO worked on both sides of the border. As Chakraborti et al. (2002) ask 'Why is it so hard to admit that mistakes were made?'

8.2.3 Arsenic contamination in the Bengal Basin

Geology and hydrogeology

The Bengal Basin occupies most of Bangladesh and West Bengal and is roughly equivalent to the delta of the GBM rivers (Morgan and McIntire, 1959). Bounded by the Indian craton to the west, the Shillong Plateau to the north, and the Indo-Burman ranges to the east, it is filled by kilometres of alluvial sediment that form one of the most productive aquifers in the world. The Ganges and Brahmaputra carry sediment derived from metamorphic rocks in the Himalayas, but the Ganges alluvium contains more detrital calcite. Meghna sediments are derived partly from the Shillong Plateau, but mainly from the Indo-Burman ranges.

The distribution of arsenic in the Bengal Basin is closely related to its Quaternary history. Table 8.3 shows the general relationships between landforms, stratigraphy, aquifers and arsenic occurrence. The greatest differences in the aquifer properties relate to the age of the sediment, which

Table 8.3 Simplified relationship between landforms, stratigraphy and aquifers in Bangladesh

Age	Landform/ physiographic unit(s)	Equivalent stratigraphic unit(s) and lithology	Hydrogeology and arsenic occurrence
Holocene	Chandina Surface/ Old Meghna Estuarine Floodplain	Chandina Formation; silt and sand	Good yields; severe As pollution
	Ganges River and Tidal Floodplains	Undifferentiated; silt and sand	Good yields; severe As pollution
	Brahmaputra and Jamuna Floodplains	Dhamrai Formation; silt and sand	Good yields; moderate As pollution
	Sylhet Basin	Undifferentiated; silt and sand	Moderate yields; locally severe As pollution
Pleistocene	Madhupur and Barind Tracts	Madhupur Clay	Important aquitard and redox barrier
	Exposed in Sylhet and Chittagong hills. Frequently encountered in boreholes	Dupi Tila Formation; weathered sand and clay	Moderate to good yields, uncontaminated
Pliocene and older	Chittagong Hill Tracts and Sylhet hills	Tertiary sandstones	Minor and localised aquifers, uncontaminated

Source: Modified after Ravenscroft (2003)

was controlled by fluvial incision during the Last Glacial Maximum (LGM; Ravenscroft, 2003), whereby the Holocene channel-fill sequences are separated by Pleistocene terraces known as the Madhupur and Barind Tracts (Figures 8.2 and 8.3). During the LGM, the water table stood many tens of metres below the surface of these interfluves, promoting flushing, oxidation of organic matter, and the formation of iron oxides and clay minerals. These older aquifers are brown, intensely weathered sands, with slightly reduced permeability (20–30 m/day) but contain groundwater of excellent quality, low in iron and total dissolved solids, and with arsenic mostly below detection limits (Ravenscroft, 2003).

After the LGM, the incised channels of the GBM rivers were invaded by long estuaries that were later displaced by prograding deltas and aggrading fluvial sequences (Figure 8.3). In the early Holocene, rising sea level flooded most of the Pleistocene interfluves, but not the present Madhupur and

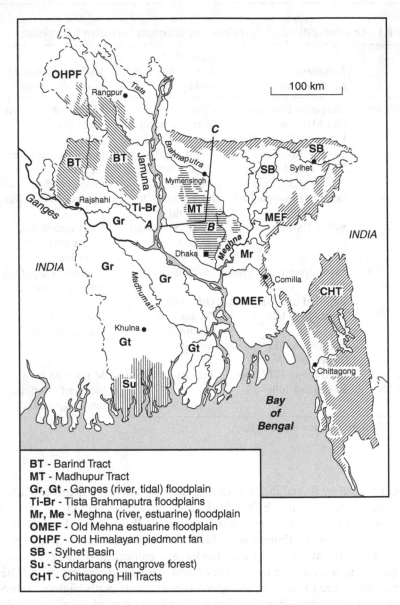

Figure 8.2 Major landforms and rivers in Bangladesh. The Chittagong Hill Tracts are formed of Tertiary sedimentary rocks, the Barind and Madhupur Tracts are of Pleistocene age, while all other units are of Holocene age. ABC is the line of cross-section shown in Fig. 8.3.
Source: Brammer (1996) and Soil Resources Development Institute (SRDI) digital database

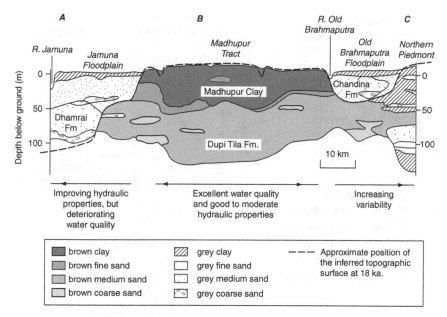

Figure 8.3   Hydrogeological section through Bangladesh. The 18 ka timeline separates the Holocene channel-fill sediments from the As-free Pleistocene deposits, which formed the surface of an elevated terrace surface during the Last Glacial Maximum. Within the plane of section, groundwater flows from the Madhupur Tract towards the major rivers, but at a local scale is strongly influenced by pumping and micro-topographic features.
Source: After Ravenscroft (2003)

Barind Tracts, forming extensive peat basins (Goodbred and Kuehl, 2000a; Goodbred et al., 2003). The Holocene aquifers are grey, high permeability (30–50 m/day) sands containing water of variable quality, characterised by high iron, manganese and arsenic concentrations (Ravenscroft, 2003).

The Holocene and Pleistocene aquifers are extensively pumped for drinking water and for dry-season irrigation, and are fully recharged during the monsoon. Because of the flat topography, regional groundwater flow is sluggish, where vertical flows (pumping and rainfall-recharge) dominate the water balance, and rivers are relatively minor sources of recharge (MPO, 1987). The aquifers in West Bengal are similar to those in Bangladesh (e.g. PHED, 1991; Nath et al., 2005), although the layering of aquifers, which are classified as the first, second and third aquifers (Figure 8.4), is apparently more regular.

In shallow aquifers in Bangladesh and West Bengal, although framboidal pyrite may be present, most sedimentary arsenic is associated with iron oxides (e.g. Nickson et al., 2000, and many others; see below), whereas in deep

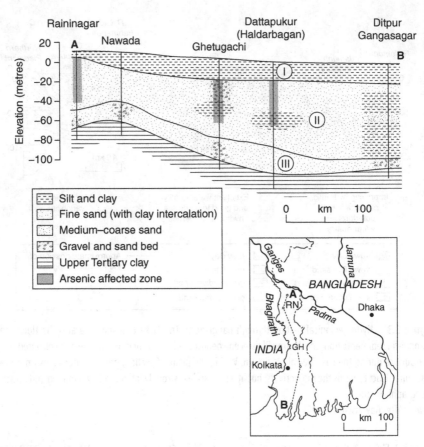

Figure 8.4 Hydrogeological section through West Bengal: I, First Aquifer; II, Second Aquifer; III, Third Aquifer. This generalised sequence does not apply at all locations in West Bengal.
Source: Acharyya et al. (2000)

aquifers in Bangladesh, most sedimentary-As is contained in massive pyrite, with a much smaller component held by iron oxides (Lowers et al., 2007).

Distribution of arsenic in groundwater in West Bengal

Arsenic pollution of groundwater in West Bengal has been mapped less systematically than in Bangladesh, but hundreds of thousands of wells have been tested, both by government and the SOES group (Table 8.4). These data were collected over many years, often with sampling focused where arsenicosis patients were suspected, and so these numbers should be treated as best estimates, and not the outcome of a systematic survey[6]. The distribution of As contamination in West Bengal (Figure 8.5) shows that the

Table 8.4 Status of arsenic contamination in West Bengal

Population (2001)	80 million
Affected districts	9 of 18
Affected villages	3,150
Water samples analysed	115,000
Analyses exceeding 10 ppb	50.3%
Analyses exceeding 50 ppb	25.1%
Population exposed to water with >50 ppb	6.0 million
Estimated population with skin lesions	300,000

Source: Chakraborti et al. (2003)

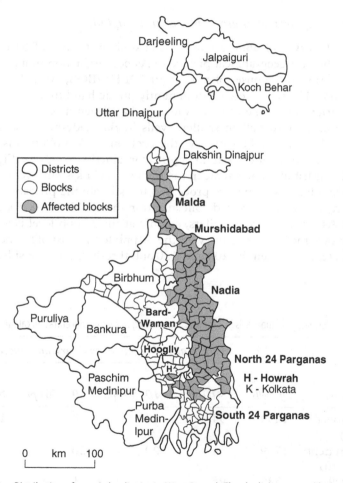

Figure 8.5 Distribution of arsenic by district in West Bengal. The shaded areas are blocks in which a significant proportion of wells produce water containing >50 ppb As.
Source: Nickson et al. (2007)

most severely affected areas are located in a belt between the Bhagirathi river and the Bangladesh border. The vertical distribution of arsenic in West Bengal has been closely correlated with the layering of the first, second and third alluvial units. The first unit is unconfined, occurs within a depth of 30 m, and only slightly contaminated. The second unit, which extends to a maximum of about 70 m, is extensively contaminated. Arsenic is generally absent in the third aquifer (Bhattacharya et al., 1997). Although the GBM rivers derive their sediment mostly from the Himalayas, the headwaters of the As affected Damodar basin, in the west, lie in peninsular India (Acharyya and Shah, 2007).

Distribution of arsenic in groundwater in Bangladesh

A 1998–99 survey of 3500 evenly spaced wells in 61 out of 64 districts[7], provides the best geographical picture of As contamination in aquifers and exposure prior to the onset of mitigation (DPHE/BGS, 2001; Ravenscroft et al., 2005). The wells were predominantly public hand tubewells, selected without prior knowledge of their water quality. When it is considered that there are around 10 million shallow wells in Bangladesh, the statistics in Table 8.5 demonstrate how massive the problem of As pollution is. Nevertheless, the majority of wells at all depths contained <10 ppb As. Figure 8.6 shows the distribution of arsenic in the upper aquifer system (wells < 150 m deep). Data for this map were processed to estimate the probability that a well at any point would exceed concentration thresholds of 10, 50, 200 and 400 ppb As[8]. In the upper aquifers, arsenic at the 10 ppb level is a massive problem over most of the country. At the 50 ppb level, most of the northwest is unaffected, and when the 200 and 400 ppb thresholds are considered, it is

Table 8.5   Percentage of tubewells in Bangladesh according to arsenic concentration category

		Percentage of tubewells with arsenic concentration			
Depth class	Number of wells	<10 ppb	10–50 ppb	50–250 ppb	>250 ppb
Shallow wells (<30 m)	1459	54	16	20	10
Medium depth (30–150 m)	1739	54	20	20	6
Deep wells (>150 m)	325	95	4	1	0

Source: Based on 3523 samples from DPHE/BGS (2001)

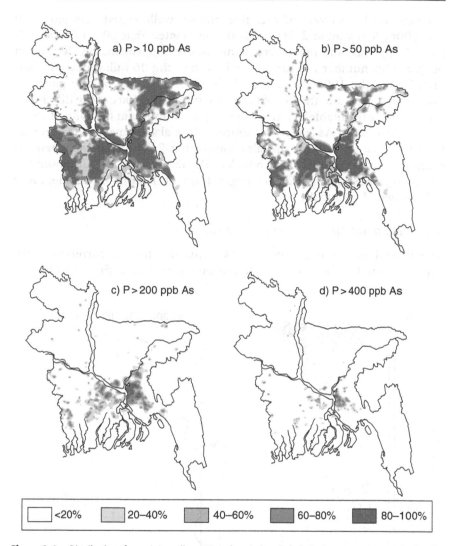

Figure 8.6   Distribution of arsenic in wells <150 m deep in Bangladesh. Each map was prepared using the ArcView Spatial Analyst program with 3500 data points from DPHE/MMI/BGS (1999) and DPHE/BGS (2001). Each point was assigned a probability of 0 or 1 according to whether the threshold was exceeded, and then interpolated using eight nearest neighbours, with the display limited to 3 km of the nearest data point.

seen that extreme As concentrations are strongly concentrated around the Meghna Estuary. Since the health impacts of arsenic are strongly dose-dependent, these maps show the areas that should be targeted for early mitigation (see also Table 6.1).

From blanket surveys of over five million wells tested between 2000 and 2006, Johnston and Sarker (2007) estimated that 20% of tubewells had >50 ppb As, and these were being used by approximately 20 million people. This number is significantly less than the 26 million people estimated from the 1998–99 surveys. This difference may be due partly to sampling density and the use of field kits, but a large part of the difference is probably attributable to well-switching, abandonment of polluted wells, and installation of As-safe water sources. It is also of major concern that follow-up testing in three upazilas found that 24% of the wells painted green (i.e. safe) contained >50 ppb As[9]. Blanket testing also disclosed the horrifying statistic that in 2316 villages, home to 1.2 million people, every well exceeded 50 ppb As.

Statistical trends of arsenic in groundwater

The probability of encountering As contamination is correlated with depth. Figure 8.7 shows the DPHE national survey data, first as a raw plot

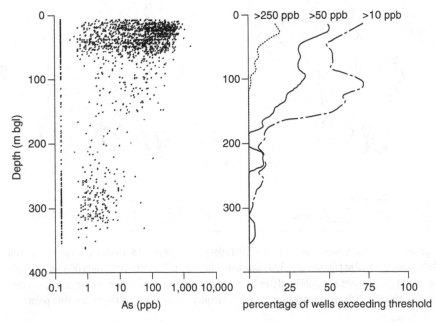

Figure 8.7 Depth distribution of arsenic in wells in Bangladesh. (a) Individual analyses are plotted against the total depth of the well (metres below ground level). (b) The data have been processed to show the probability of exceeding various concentration thresholds in each 10-m band. The plots are based on analyses of more than 2000 hand tubewells by DPHE/MMI/BGS (1999). The wells all have short screen lengths of between 3 and 6 m.

of concentration against depth, and second as the probability of exceeding thresholds of 10, 50 and 250 ppb As. Beyond a very shallow zone exploited by dug wells, at all concentrations the probability of exceeding the threshold decreases steadily with depth. The chance of exceeding 250 ppb As is negligible below 100 m, but the probability of not complying with drinking water standards is significant until depths of 150–200 m. Nevertheless, As-safe wells can be installed at any depth in most areas, albeit with a low probability of success, and perhaps a high risk of failure during operation. Due to local geological variations, the depth at which there is a high probability of obtaining As-safe water varies between regions, and may be as little as 30–50 m where Pleistocene strata are encountered. The cut-off level is primarily due to the depth of fluvial incision at the LGM, and hence the thickness of Holocene sediment (DPHE/MMI/BGS, 1999).

There is a strong tendency for As concentrations to increase with increasing well-age, which indicates that arsenic either migrates within aquifers or is mobilised by organic-rich water draining from adjacent aquitards (Chapter 3). The probability of a well exceeding 50 ppb As increases from around 20% in new wells to about 40% after 10 years of operation. However, these statistical inferences, although based on thousands of analyses, remain to be verified by time-series monitoring.

Relation of arsenic to geomorphology

As implied above, the location of the Holocene channel-fill deposits is expressed in the surface sediments and landforms. Hence, by way of the lithology of the shallow sediments, geomorphological features (Figure 8.2) can be related to the regional distribution of arsenic in groundwater (Figure 8.6). Analysis[10] of the DPHE data (Table 8.6) using GIS showed that the worst contamination occurs beneath the estuarine and river floodplains of the Meghna and Ganges rivers. The main difference is between the aquifers underlying the Holocene floodplains and those beneath older units. A second difference relates to sediment texture. The floodplains and fan deposits in the northwest (i.e. upstream) are less contaminated, due to their coarser grain size and lower organic content (DPHE/MMI/BGS, 1999), which explains the low level of contamination beneath the Brahmaputra floodplains. Arsenic concentrations beneath the Ganges River Floodplain are more variable, which is consistent with deposition in meandering channels, where extreme small-scale differences in continuity between sand and peat horizons can be expected. By contrast, sand bodies underlying the tidal and estuarine floodplains are of greater lateral extent, and therefore have a more uniform distribution of As contamination.

Table 8.6 Arsenic occurrence related to physiographic unit in Bangladesh

Physiographic Unit*	Number of wells	Maximum As (ppb)	Percentage of wells >50 ppb
Meghna River Floodplain	82	744	71
Old Meghna Estuarine Floodplain	380	1086	61
Young Meghna Estuarine Floodplain	51	862	41
Sylhet Basin	297	254	40
Ganges Tidal Floodplain	244	735	39
Ganges River Floodplain	1473	1665	34
Brahmaputra and Jamuna Floodplains	472	270	26
Tista Floodplain	32	66	19
Madhupur and Barind Tracts	90	140	18
Old Himalayan Fan	13	66	8
Northern and Eastern Hills	74	123	4

*See Figure 8.2 for location of physiographic units.
Source: Ravenscroft (2001)

Arsenic in surface waters

While it is commonly assumed that surface waters are free of arsenic, where arsenic is presumed to be adsorbed to iron oxyhydroxides in the suspended load, this is not universally true. In Bangladesh, Islam et al. (2000) compared filtered and unfiltered (always slightly higher As concentrations) samples of surface water to groundwater in the same area. In an uncontaminated area in the southeast (Comilla), they measured 5–6 ppb As. At two contaminated sites in the southwest, they measured between 8 and 15 ppb As, and in a highly impacted part of Chapai Nawabganj, they measured 97 ppb As. Also in Bangladesh, Mazid Miah et al. (2005) reported that surface water from ponds, rivers and canals contained between 2 and 63 ppb As. The highest concentrations were in the northwest, where wells were used to top-up ponds.

Arsenic is also present in the suspended load of the rivers. Stummeyer et al. (2002) found that suspended sediment at the confluence of the Ganges–Brahmaputra contained an average of 15 mg/kg As, three times the global average in rivers. It is also twice that of the bed sediment in the estuary, indicating that arsenic is transported preferentially in the finer fractions. The As content of the suspended load increased from 5.5 mg/kg 'far' from the coast to around 15 mg/kg near the coast and at the river mouth, and then dropped to 4.5 mg/kg in the estuary. Leaching experiments showed that around 90% of arsenic was held in crystalline iron oxides, and that the sum of the exchangeable and reducible[11] arsenic fractions was fairly constant at ≤ 1 mg/kg.

Hydrogeochemistry and causes of arsenic pollution

Initially, arsenic pollution in West Bengal was blamed on oxidation of As-rich pyrite, induced by lowering of the water table by irrigation wells (e.g. Das et al., 1994; Mallick and Rajagopal, 1996). This hypothesis developed in a vacuum of alternatives, and gained support from people who were predisposed to blame 'big development projects' and foreign aid, and advocated banning tubewell irrigation. Between 1995 and 1998, a variety of anthropogenic explanations were put forward including pesticides, contaminated fertilisers, wood preservatives[12], industrial sources, mineral processing and acid mine drainage, construction of river barrages in India, and burning of fossil fuels (DPHE/MMI/BGS, 1999). Although none of these was derived from field data, all implicated sources had caused pollution elsewhere in the world. Alternative explanations came from Bhattacharya et al. (1997) in India and Nickson[13] et al. (1998) in Bangladesh, who attributed contamination to the natural reductive dissolution of iron oxides, now the accepted interpretation (Chapter 2). Importantly, this showed that demands to ban tubewell irrigation lacked scientific support. The key lines of evidence for the new interpretation were the association of dissolved arsenic with anoxic waters rich in iron and bicarbonate, and the correlation of diagenetically available arsenic and iron in the sediments.

After 1999, there was an explosion of interest from national and international organisations to study the geochemistry of arsenic in the Bengal Basin, resulting in voluminous publications, too numerous to review individually here. The majority were conducted in Bangladesh[14], but significant investigations were also conducted in West Bengal[15]. A consensus soon emerged that reductive dissolution (RD) is the dominant mobilisation mechanism, occurring where channel sands with iron-rich coatings are deposited in close juxtaposition to overbank peat and organic-rich mud (McArthur et al., 2001). Decomposition of sedimentary organic carbon (SOC) produces strongly reducing groundwater with high DOC concentrations which, under the influence of natural flow and/or pumping, migrates into adjacent aquifers where it reduces the iron oxide coatings of the sands, releasing adsorbed arsenic. However, other interpretations have been put forward, mostly relating to competitive adsorption and desorption (see section 2.3). Acharyya et al. (1999, 2000) suggested that excess application of phosphate fertilisers[16] might enhance arsenic mobilisation, and Appelo et al. (2002) and Anawar et al. (2004) suggested that carbonate and bicarbonate ions mobilise arsenic

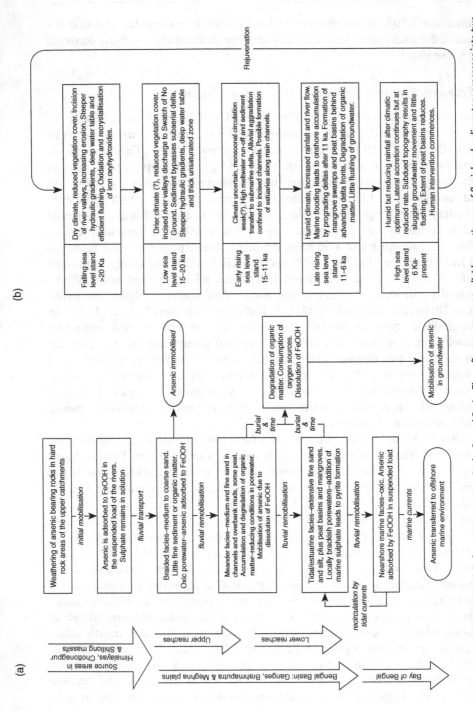

Figure 8.8 Conceptual model of arsenic occurrence in the Bengal Basin. These figures attempt to divide a continuum of fluvial and sedimentary processes into two parts. (a) The progression of events along the long-profile of the rivers. (b) How these events responded to Late Quaternary falling and rising sea levels.

Source: From Ravenscroft et al. (2005).

through formation of complexes and/or desorption. However, neither hypothesis appears consistent with field observations (e.g. Ravenscroft et al., 2001; McArthur et al., 2004).

In a variation of the conventional RD model, Harvey et al. (2002, 2006) suggested that the organic matter driving reduction is derived from the soil zone and surface water bodies, and not SOC. This was strongly disputed by Aggarwal et al. (2003) and van Geen et al. (2003b) amongst others, for various reasons but mainly based on groundwater age dating. Although these models are not mutually exclusive, the question is important because Harvey's suggestion implies that future As mobilisation is not limited by SOC, and hence that all oxide-bound arsenic could be released. Thus isotopic dating of groundwater has a bearing on both whether present pollution is natural or anthropogenic, and how As concentrations will evolve in the future. Dating (^{14}C, ^3H) of groundwater indicates groundwater in contaminated aquifers was mostly recharged a few hundred and a few thousand, but not tens of thousand, years ago (DPHE/MMI/BGS, 1999; Aggarwal et al., 2000; van Geen, Zheng et al., 2003a). However, this does not preclude current arsenic mobilisation, and subsequently $^3H/He$ dating by Klump et al. (2006) at Harvey's site in central Bangladesh showed that most contaminated groundwater was recharged more than 30 years ago (i.e. before tubewell irrigation), but some arsenic has been mobilised more recently. This is important because the store of dissolved arsenic could be depleted in a few decades, but if the sorbed As is still being released, flushing may take centuries (section 3.8).

The geochemical processes described above can be placed in a geological context that explains the three-dimensional distribution of As pollution (Figure 8.8). The key drivers for this model, which apply to all deltas, are first the sedimentary distribution of organic matter and As- and Fe-rich coatings on sands, and second the sedimentary response to Quaternary sea level change (see also section 3.5). The model explains the immobilisation of arsenic in 'older' sediments by oxidation and flushing, and mobilisation of arsenic in 'younger' anoxic sediments by RD.

Health effects

The human dimensions of the 'the largest poisoning of a population in history' (Smith et al., 2000) are awesome. In 1999, 33 million people in Bangladesh and West Bengal were estimated to drink water with >50 ppb As, and roughly double that number to consume water with >10 ppb As (DPHE/BGS, 2001; Chakraborti et al., 2003). Reliable estimates on the number of people who are, or will be, clinically affected by arsenic poisoning are not available, although Chakraborti et al. (2003) reported that 300,000 are afflicted by skin lesions in West Bengal. Estimates of the prevalence of skin lesions in people drinking water with >50 ppb As for long periods are in the range of 21–29% (Rahman et al., 1999, 2006), although Ahsan et al. (2006) showed there is a significant risk of developing skin lesions even when drinking water in the range of 10–50 ppb As. Many non-dermatological effects have also been identified, with significant dose–response relations for hypertension and diabetes, poor lung function in men, and peripheral neuropathy, although Blackfoot disease is almost unknown (Chapter 5). Using Taiwanese dose–response data, Chen and Ahsan (2004) estimated that mortality from liver, bladder and lung cancers will be doubled. In addition, Wassermann et al. (2004) inferred that the intellectual development of children is impaired at concentrations as low as 10 ppb As.

Contrary to earlier opinions, food, especially groundwater-irrigated rice, is now known to be an important source of arsenic exposure, and can easily exceed the FAO/WHO recommended maximum (130 µg/day) without any contribution from drinking water or other foods. In Murshidabad, Uchino et al. (2006) found that for >50% of patients with skin lesions, rice was the principal source of dietary arsenic. Also, in West Bengal, Guha Mazumder et al. (2003) demonstrated the benefits of removing exposure to arsenic in drinking water. Tracking 306 people over 5 years, they showed that the condition of skin lesions improved in 49% of people, while for 48% their conditions were unchanged, and in only 3% of cases did they become worse. On the other hand, 30% of people who did not previously have skin lesions, developed them during the monitoring period.

Social impacts

Poverty and outdoor labour lead to high consumption of well-water and rice relative to meat, vegetables, fruit and processed drinks. This in turn leads to a higher intake of arsenic and reduced ability to resist its effects. Sarkar and Mehrotra (2005) confirmed that poor people are more likely to develop severe clinical manifestations and have a higher mortality rate. Although women are less likely to develop arsenicosis, they face worse social consequences, such as being unable to get married or being forced to divorce (Hassan et al., 2005). Irrespective of gender, to be diagnosed with arsenicosis or to have one's well painted red carries a stigma that can lead to ostracism and social exclusion (Hanchett, 2004). Arsenicosis has economic impacts, both because of medical costs and because adult males, the main wage earners, are most likely to be affected; and if a man cannot work, he may be unable to feed his family, accelerating the downward spiral into poverty.

Impacts on soil and agriculture

The agricultural economy of Bengal is dominated by rice which, as noted above, can be a major source of arsenic exposure. Arsenic uptake in rice depends on its concentration in the soil, and there is evidence to suggest that irrigation with As-rich groundwater is leading to the build-up of arsenic in soil and rice grain sufficient to have significant health effects. Islam, Jahiruddin et al. (2005) found that: (a) irrigated topsoils (0–15 cm) contain more arsenic than non-irrigated soils in the same area; (b) under irrigation, topsoil contains more arsenic than subsoil; and (c) on average, straw contains seven times more arsenic than rice grain and therefore poses a risk to cattle fed on straw.

Arsenic accumulation in rice is especially important in Bengal because dietary intake is very high, around 480 g per person per day (Hossain et al., 2005). The As content of rice in Bangladesh is higher than most other countries, averaging 260 µg/kg in (largely irrigated) *boro* rice (Williams et al., 2006). Rice with the highest As concentrations came from districts where As concentrations in groundwater are also high. A second concern is that As accumulation in soil leads to toxicity to rice and dramatic declines in grain yield, and this has already been reported in some areas (Duxbury and Panaullah, 2007). Given that tubewell irrigation has been so important in achieving food-grain self-sufficiency, these issues raise profound policy implications and require urgent action (Chapter 11).

Mitigation in Bangladesh

The Arsenic Policy Support Unit (APSU, 2005) summarised water-supply interventions for arsenic mitigation up to July 2005. In Table 8.7, the results are summarised by technology, from which it is estimated that up to 22 million people living in As-affected areas obtain drinking water from new installations containing <50 ppb As, and most of this low-As water has been obtained from deep tubewells (i.e. from wells 150 to 300 m deep). This will, however, over-estimate the population who have actually been removed from As exposure because some deep wells will have replaced non-functioning (but As-safe) deep tubewells, and others installed where the shallow aquifer is contaminated by salinity not arsenic. Another issue concerns whether new water supplies are actually 'safe' or only 'arsenic-safe'. Therefore the numbers should be further down-graded because of the proportion of dug-wells (89%), pond sand filters (96%), rainwater systems (53%) and deep tubewells (5%) that fail microbiological standards (Ahmed et al., 2005). Applied rigorously, this would reduce the population that benefited to about 18 million.

While deep tubewells have been the dominant mitigation technology, it has been the routine programmes of the Bangladesh Government that have delivered the bulk of mitigation (Table 8.8). This is surprising, because it does not reflect the publicity given to some agencies and projects. Even in combination, the flagship BAMWSP project, the UNICEF supported programme and five of the largest NGOs, have delivered less than 10% of

Table 8.7 Arsenic mitigation options installed in Bangladesh

Technology	Number	Families per device*	Average operational status† (%)	Arsenic compliance (%)	Persons served‡	Contribution to mitigation (%)
Dug well	6268	50	64	99	1,086,620	4.9
Pond sand filter	3521	50	33	98	315,987	1.4
Rainwater harvesting	13,324	10	95	100	696,179	3.2
Deep tubewell	74,809	50	91	99	18,533,743	84.4
Arsenic removal plant	3771	10	82	80	136,058	0.6
Piped water	33	250	90	95	38,796	0.2
Shallow, shrouded tubewell	5080	50	90	90	1,131,570	5.2
Deep-set handpump	133	50	90	90	29,626	0.1
Total	106,939		79	94	21,968,578	100

*Each device is assumed to serve 50 families except for piped schemes (250) and rainwater harvesting and arsenic removal plant (10).
†Based on data from Kabir et al. (2005) and Ahmed et al. (2005).
‡The beneficiaries estimate assumes 5.5 persons per family, with the population served down-rated by the average proportions that are out of operation or exceed 50ppb As.
Source: Data from APSU (2005); Ahmed et al. (2005); Kabir et al. (2005)

Table 8.8   Arsenic mitigation in Bangladesh by agency; see text for explanation

Agency	Devices installed	Persons served	Contribution to mitigation (%)
Non-government organisations			
AAN	63	11,605	0.1
DCH	112	32,700	0.1
IDE	1072	88,469	0.4
NGO Forum	1486	122,274	0.6
World Vision	2154	138,048	0.6
Others	206	16,507	0.1
Government departments and projects			
BRDB	336	47,785	0.2
BAMWSP	5619	748,537	3.4
DPHE–UNICEF	9957	838,483	3.8
DPHE	85,934	19,924,170	90.7
Total	106,939	21,968,578	100

AAN, Asian Arsenic Network ;BAMWSP, Bangladesh Arsenic Mitigation Water Supply
Project; BRDB, Bangladesh Rural Development Board; DCH, Dhaka Community Hospital;
DPHE, Department of Public Health Engineering (Bangladesh); IDE, International
Development Enterprise.
Source: APSU (2005)

the mitigation services[17]. Mitigation provided by Government was largely in
the form of deep tubewells.

The increased number of deep tubewells has raised concerns about the
sustainability of deep aquifer abstraction. The number of deep wells
increased from about 32,000 in 1993 (UNICEF/DPHE, 1994) to around
150,000 by 2005. Assuming a per capita water use of 10 L/day, and that
abstraction is spread evenly over the 96 upazilas of the coastal zone
(UNICEF/DPHE, 1994), this amounts to an abstraction of about 4 mm/
year. This is small compared with the (1996) national average of 77 mm/
year abstracted for irrigation alone from unconfined aquifers in the centre
and north of the country (Ravenscroft, 2003). Nevertheless, this is a proper
concern because the recharge mechanism is poorly understood, and there is
potential for downward migration of arsenic, and both downward and lateral inflow of brackish groundwater (see Chapter 3).

Mitigation in West Bengal

Mitigation in West Bengal has proceeded more gradually, and has followed
a supply-led path through the Public Health Engineering Department

(PHED) in both urban and rural sectors, and differs fundamentally from the demand-led approach, with up-front financial contributions from villagers, in Bangladesh. Although the latter is conducive to effective operation and maintenance (e.g. Hoque et al., 2004), it has been widely questioned whether this is appropriate to the severity of the hazard, which it has been argued demands an emergency response. In rural West Bengal, the PHED initially installed thousands of handpump-based, arsenic removal plants (ARP), but these have performed poorly (Hossain et al., 2006), while NGO-led schemes have had very variable performance records (section 7.6.2). Partly because of these problems, PHED has since focused on rural piped distribution systems as the basis of long-term mitigation (Bhattacharjee, 2007). The water sources are either high-capacity deep tubewells, or treated and chlorinated river water. Each source serves a cluster of villages, with a cyclic distribution such that water is supplied in turn for about 1–2 hours at a fixed time in the morning and afternoon. Water is drawn from public standpipes, free of cost to users, or through household connections on payment of a fixed charge. Inevitably, NGOs find it difficult to operate where PHED supplies free water, and has led to abandonment of some schemes.

8.2.4 Arsenic contamination on the Ganga Plains and Terai

Geology

The Ganga Plains are taken here to include the Terai (largely in Nepal) and much of the densely populated Indian states of Bihar, Uttar Pradesh (UP), Jarkhand and part of West Bengal. Although generally less severe than in the delta, there is extensive groundwater contamination by arsenic. Investigation of arsenic on the Ganga Plains has lagged behind that of the delta, and hence knowledge of its extent and characteristics is less advanced. The geology and geomorphology of the Ganga Plains were described by Singh (1996) who mapped five major geomorphological surfaces (Table 8.9 and Figure 8.9). Quaternary sea-level change has not had the extreme effect seen in the delta, but neotectonics have had a greater relative effect (Singh, 1996). River incision, which created the accommodation space for young and organic-rich sediments, has been concentrated in narrow belts along the main river channels.

The Terai occupies only 20% of Nepal but is home to 47% of its population and produces 60% of its food grain (Gurung et al., 2005). The Terai runs in an E–W belt, 10–50 km wide, along Nepal's border with India and follows the E–W structural trend created by the suture of the Asian and Indian plates (NASC/ENPHO, 2004), and is filled by about 1500 m of alluvium, which has been accommodated by rapid subsidence. It is divided

Table 8.9 Geomorphological surfaces of the Ganga Plains

Unit		Age (ka)	Description
T0	Active floodplain	<10	Narrow and entrenched floodplains, a few hundred metres to about 2 km wide
PF	Piedmont fan	25–10	10–30 km wide belt of coalescing fans, characterised by shallow, ephemeral channels that form the Bhabar zone and are adjacent to the Terai.
T1	River valley terrace	33–25	This surface stands several metres above the active floodplain, and is not normally flooded by overtopping. It is underlain by coarse sands
F	Megafan surface	74–35	Relict features of the Kosi, Gandak, Sarda and Yamuna-Ganga rivers; typically 100–150 km across
T2	Upland terrace surface	128–74	This complex surface covers a large area north of the Ganga. The streams are incised, sinuous, under-fit channels and not flooded by overtopping.

Source: Singh (1996)

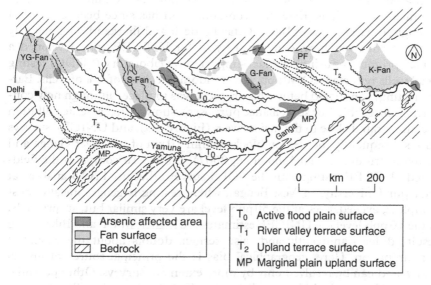

Figure 8.9 Geomorphology and arsenic occurrence on the Ganga Plains. Based on geomorphological mapping from Singh (1996) and arsenic survey data from Nickson et al. (2007). Megafan surfaces: YG, Yamuna-Ganga; S, Sarda; G, Gandak; K, Kosi; PF, piedmont fan. Although the mapping of arsenic is probably incomplete, contamination is concentrated along the most recent (T_0) surface.

into the Inner Terai or 'Bhabar' zone of gravelly sediments near the foothills, and the flat, marshy Terai Plain proper (south of the Churia Hills) formed of finer grained sediments (Singh, 1996). A spring line follows the boundary of the two zones. Only four major rivers cut across the Terai and this influences the composition of alluvium because only these streams carry sediment from the Himalayas. Annual rainfall on the Terai is typically 1800–2000 mm, of which only 10% recharges groundwater, but abstraction is only 10% of potential recharge (Gurung et al., 2005). Terai soils have characteristically organic-rich topsoils (Brammer, 1996). Productive aquifers are found in the top 50–60 m, and flowing artesian wells are common on the Lower Terai. There are 0.5 M shallow tubewells on the Terai supplying 11 M people, 90% of whom rely on groundwater for their drinking water (NASC/ENPHO, 2004). Aquifers and aquitards tend to have lateral continuity from north to south, but not from east to west, demonstrating the effects of incision by rivers that cut across the strike of the Terai.

Arsenic on the Ganga Plains

Although predicted since 1997, arsenic contamination in Bihar was confirmed by Chakraborti et al. (2003). In one village in Bhojpur District they tested 95% of tubewells, finding 82% contained >10 ppb, 57% >50 ppb and 10% >500 ppb As. Of 550 self-selected volunteers examined, 11% had arsenical skin lesions. Extensive contamination has since been confirmed throughout large areas of Bihar, Uttar Pradesh and Jharkhand. The majority of this testing has been conducted by or for UNICEF who developed a survey protocol of using field kits supported by laboratory (SDDC) testing of all wells reported as >40 ppb, plus random checking of 5% of wells. Earlier testing, conducted before this protocol was in place, although now considered unreliable (for surveillance purposes), showed that arsenic pollution is concentrated close to the major rivers (Figure 8.9), and UNICEF surveys have subsequently focused on blocks within 10 km of the River Ganga and its major tributaries (Nickson et al., 2007). Table 8.10 compares the field-based UNICEF testing with the SOES surveys that used AAS analysis at Jadavpur University. In West Bengal, where testing is geographically most complete, exceedances at the 50 ppb level are very similar but, surprisingly, at the 10 ppb level the UNICEF estimates are higher. In UP and Bihar these results differ significantly and raise serious doubts about the extent of contamination. Here, geographical bias is the principal source of uncertainty, and can be resolved only by more extensive surveys. Other potential sources of error include sampling bias (SOES) towards villages where patients were suspected, and inaccuracy of field kits (UNICEF) and consequent underreporting. If the latter is correct, then estimates of contamination in Jharkhand and Assam (see below) may also be low.

Table 8.10 Comparison of arsenic surveys on the Ganga Plains of India

State	Number of samples		Percentage >10ppb As		Percentage >50ppb As	
	UNICEF	SOES	UNICEF	SOES	UNICEF	SOES
West Bengal*	132,262	115,000	57.9	50.3	25.5	25.1
Jharkhand†	9007		7.5	–	3.7	–
Bihar	66,623	19,961	28.9	32.7	10.8	17.8
Uttar Pradesh	20,126	4780	21.5	45.5	2.4	26.5

SOES, School of Environmental Sciences (Jadavpur University)
*Samples are mostly from the delta.
†All data are from Sahebganj District.
Sources: SOES (http://www.soesju.org/arsenic/); Nickson et al. (2007)

Arsenic contamination on the Ganga plains occurs mostly beneath the younger T_0 or T_1 geomorphological surfaces (Figure 8.9). In Bihar and UP, Shah (2007) described the occurrence of contamination in wells installed beneath the most recent floodplains of the Ganga. Compared with the delta, during sea-level lowstands channel incision on the Ganga plains was shallower and more localised, but nonetheless extended for great distances inland (Singh, 1996). Thus, beneath the terraces the water table is, or was, located at considerable depth below ground surface for tens of thousands of years, promoting the removal or immobilisation of arsenic by oxidising organic matter, precipitating and recrystallising iron oxides, and flushing reaction products. Contamination is therefore concentrated close to the main rivers in recent sands that contain more organic matter and have shallow water tables. In the Terai, continuous subsidence has favoured the preservation of organic matter and the maintenance of reducing conditions. Thus the probability of encountering As-safe water in deep wells is uncertain, although more likely in the central plains than in the Terai, and it has been noted that concentrations of >50 ppb As occur mainly in wells <60 m deep, while the few deeper wells rarely contain >10–20 ppb As (R. Nickson, personal communication, 2006).

In the south of Jharkhand, arsenic contamination has been detected along the Son River in Garwha District where 10.4% of 672 wells surveyed exceeded 10 ppb As, and 6.1% exceeded 50 ppb As (R. Nickson, personal communication, 2007). Garwha District is an area of largely crystalline bedrock, where 27% of wells also contained >1.5 ppm of fluoride, and 90% of wells contained elevated nitrate, indicating that different geochemical conditions apply.

Arsenic on the Nepal Terai

The first investigation of As contamination in Nepal was in 1999, and by 2003 >18,000 tests had been conducted, of which 7.5% exceeded 50 ppb (the Nepal interim standard) and 24% exceeded 10 ppb As (Shrestha et al., 2003; NASC/ENPHO, 2004). It was estimated that 2.5 million people were drinking water with >10 ppb As. There was significant variation between the 20 districts on the Terai (Figure 8.10). In Chitwan, no wells exceeded 10 ppb, while in Nawalparasi 26% of wells exceeded 50 ppb, with a maximum of 2,620 ppb As. Shrestha et al. (2003) described a pattern of generally low-level contamination interrupted by hot-spots where a high proportion of wells exceed 500 ppb As.

Arsenical skin manifestations have been identified, mostly melanosis and keratosis of palms, trunk and soles, and had a prevalence of 2.6% in the four most exposed districts. Only 20% of cases were at the moderate stage, and there was one confirmed and several suspected cases of Bowen's disease. In severely affected communities of Nawalparasi the prevalence of skin lesions was 9%. Maharjan et al. (2006) reported similar results: an overall prevalence of arsenicosis of 2.2% (3.0% in men, 1.4% in women) amongst 18,000 people in six districts. The prevalence increased with age, being very low (0.1%) in persons under 15 years, 1.3% in the 15–49 year age group, and increased to 10.3% in persons over 50 years. In four affected villages they found a prevalence of 10.2%, of which 73% were classed as mild, 25% moderate and 2% severe.

The heterogeneous distribution of arsenic contamination along the Terai may be partly explained by the division of the Terai into inner and outer parts where only four major rivers carry sediment from the Himalayas, and hence determine where relatively unweathered sands accumulate. Shrestha et al. (2003) found a poor correlation between As concentration and well age, and also that most contaminated tubewells were <50 m deep, and especially <30 m deep, where as many as 68% contained >10 ppb As. Few wells were deeper than 60 m, and only one >100 m. Thus although most were low in arsenic, the numbers are too small to say whether deeper aquifers are an important mitigation option. Mitigation activities in Nepal have given strong emphasis to household treatment systems, and especially the Kanchan filter (section 7.6.1).

In Nawalparasi, Gurung et al. (2005) found that organic-rich Holocene clays, which separate the fine-sand horizons from which hand tubewells draw water, contained up to 31 mg/kg As. Arsenic concentrations of up to 740 ppb in groundwater were negatively correlated with redox potential, had near-neutral pH, and an average iron concentration of 5.3 ppm. They concluded that arsenic is mobilised under strongly reducing conditions similar to those in the Bengal Basin.

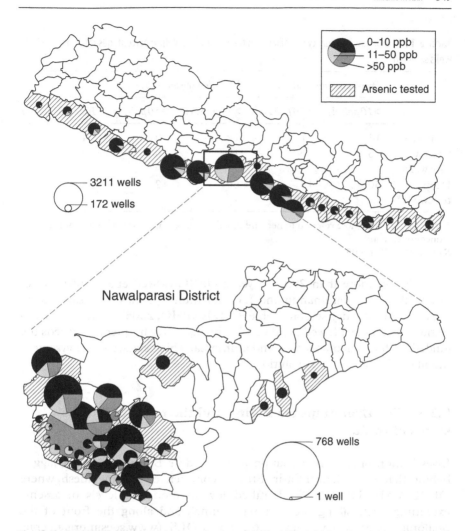

Figure 8.10 Distribution of arsenic contamination on the Nepal Terai. (a) Arsenic concentrations in wells by district. (b) Arsenic concentrations in Nawalparasi District. The Terai is dominated by the E–W structural trend of the Himalayas, such that only four rivers cut across the Terai. Nawalparasi is the most affected district, and even here, contamination is very heterogeneous.
Source: NASC/ENPHO (2004)

Interior Nepal

Arsenic pollution also occurs in fluvio-lacustrine sand and gravel deposited by the Bagmati River in the Kathmandu Valley. The unconfined aquifer is separated by 200 m of clay from a deeper alluvial aquifer that contains

Table 8.11   Groundwater quality surveillance in the Kathmandu Valley; percentages refer to the >300 wells sampled

	Post-monsoon (%)		Late dry season (%)		
	>10 ppb As	>50 ppb As	>10 ppb As	>50 ppb As	Escherichia coli
Dug wells	14	1	12	0	44
Shallow tubewells	6	0	11	0	9
Deep tubewells*	50	13	69	12	34

* It is believed that those referred to here are mostly screened in the deeper parts of the unconfined aquifer.
Source: ENPHO (2005)

groundwater more than 200,000 years old (Cresswell et al., 2001). Over 300 wells in the Kathmandu and Lalitpur municipalities were sampled in the early and late dry season (Table 8.11; ENPHO, 2005). Arsenic concentrations increase with well depth, and drinking water frequently exceeds the guidelines for iron, manganese and ammonia, which suggests that arsenic is mobilised by reductive dissolution.

8.2.5   The Brahmaputra Plains and the northeast states of India

Investigation of As contamination in the middle Brahmaputra has lagged behind that in the Bengal Basin. Studies commenced in Bangladesh, where DPHE/MMI/BGS (1999) identified low to moderate levels of arsenic extending north along the Jamuna channel, and along the front of the Shillong Plateau (see Figure 8.6). The SOES (www.soesju.org/arsenic/misc_crip) reported arsenic in Dhemaji district in the far northeast of Assam, and in Karimganj district, adjacent to Bangladesh on the south of the Shillong Plateau. Of the 241 water samples analysed by SOES, 42% exceeded 10 ppb and 19% exceeded 50 ppb As. More extensive surveys of >2000 boreholes and dug wells in the seven states of northeast India were reported by Singh (2004) and are summarised in Table 8.12, which lists only the districts where 'significant' contamination was found.

Although the samples are widely spaced and much of the terrain is mountainous, it is clear that arsenic pollution is widespread in the middle catchment of the Brahmaputra. The proportions of contaminated wells are comparable to those in Bengal, and extreme concentrations (>400 ppb) were

Table 8.12 Summary of arsenic surveys in northeast India; arsenic was not detected in Meghalaya, Mizoram or Sikkim states

State*	District	Number of samples	Percentage of wells > 50 ppb As	As (ppb)	pH	Fe (ppm)
					Maximum value of	
Assam (1500)	Naogaon	76	13	112	7.9	11.0
	Jorhat	80	21	657	7.6	30.6
	Lakhimpur	76	21	550	7.0	49.4
	Nalbari	72	19	422	6.9	22.3
	Golaghat	60	13	200	8.5	25.3
	Dhubri	52	19	200	8.4	19.4
	Darrang	52	8	200	8.2	20.9
	Dhemaji	44	22	200	6.8	26.8
Manipur (60)	Thoubal	12	50	986	7.6	4.3
Arunachal Pradesh (296)	Papum Pare	24	33	74	6.2	2.0
	West Kameng	20	2	127	7.8	4.9
	East Kameng	20	2	58	8.0	1.1
	Lower Subansiri	28	43	159	7.5	0.1
	Dibang Valley	19	42	618	7.5	0.3
	Tirap	28	14	90	7.4	0.3
Tripura (117)	West Tripura	38	22	191	7.1	11.0
	Dhalai	19	42	444	8.3	8.9
	North Tripura	21	57	283	8.1	1.0
Nagaland (132)	Mokok Chong	21	33	278	7.5	1.9
	Mon	20	25	159	7.4	1.3

*The number in parentheses is the total number of samples collected in the state.
Source: Singh (2004)

found in around a third of districts. However, Singh (2004) noted that there had been no reports of arsenicosis in the region, which may be due to the shorter duration of exposure than in Bengal (R. Nickson, personal communication, 2007). Although no geological data were reported, the high iron concentrations and generally near-neutral pH suggest that RD is the most likely release mechanism. More recent surveys in Assam found that 7.4% of 5700 samples collected from within 25 km of the Brahmaputra contained >50 ppb As (Nickson et al., 2007). An intensive survey of the central Manipur valley has confirmed severe groundwater pollution where 41% of wells exceeded 50 ppb As, and 65% exceeded 10 ppb (Chakraborti et al., 2008). However, to date there have been limited health impacts because well-water has been used only for short time, and many people rely on rainwater collection.

8.2.6 The Indus Plains, Pakistan

Although there are similarities between the geology of the Indus (e.g. Shroder, 1993) and the Ganges–Brahmaputra river systems, there are important differences with regards to the semi-arid to arid climate, and the fact that the sediments are extensively oxidised. Since Mughal times, the Indus Plains have been transformed by canal irrigation, where leakage from unlined canals has caused the water table to rise and has resulted in water-logging and soil salinisation. Information on arsenic pollution comes from surveys by UNICEF and the Pakistan Council for Research in Water Resources who tested about 23,500 samples using field kits and 4000 samples in the laboratory (Ahmad et al., 2004). In the Punjab, 20% of samples exceeded 10 ppb and 3% exceeded 50 ppb As. The most affected districts were Bahawalpur (18% >10 ppb), Rahim Yar Khan (19% >10 ppb) and Multan (38% >10 ppb). Overall, 6% of wells <30 m deep exceeded 50 ppb, and only 4% of those >30 m exceeded 50 ppb.

An epidemiological study of 28,000 people in seven districts of the Punjab found elevated arsenic in finger nails of people drinking >50 ppb As. Arsenicosis was diagnosed, although its prevalence (0.1%) was low. It was estimated that 6 million people in the Punjab drink water with >10 ppb, and 2 million with >50 ppb.

Ahmad et al. (2004) found that pollution was worse further south in Sindh Province, where 36% of samples exceeded 10 ppb and 16% exceeded 50 ppb. No epidemiological data were available for Sindh Province, although there were anecdotal reports of skin ailments. They found the probability of encountering arsenic increases with well depth in Sindh, with a peak at around 30 m, and arsenic being absent below 45 m (Table 8.13). They noted that districts near the Indus River in Sindh and its tributaries in the Punjab were more likely to be contaminated, an association similar to that noted on the Ganga Plains.

Table 8.13   Depth distribution of arsenic in Sindh Province

Depth (m)	Number of samples	>10ppb (%)	>50ppb (%)
3–15	12,398	16	4.0
15–30	9,931	31	7.0
30–45	173	34	7.5
>45	69	0	0.0
Total	22,571	23	5.3

Source: Ahmad et al. (2004)

A geochemical study by Nickson et al. (2005) at Muzaffargarh in the Punjab found that 53% of wells exceeded 10 ppb and 13% exceeded 50 ppb, with a maximum of 906 ppb As. High (>25 ppb) As concentrations were largely restricted to urban areas, which they attributed to RD of iron oxides promoted by leakage of sewage. In wells <10 m deep, almost all dissolved components were extremely variable due to evaporative concentration. Below 10 m, arsenic and phosphorus concentrations increase with depth, whereas sulphate decreased over the same depth range, suggesting reduction of sulphate and dissolution of iron oxides. There was a slight tendency towards enrichment in arsenic at high pH, with no very low As concentrations at >pH 7.8. Farooqi et al. (2007) described a local occurrence in the eastern Punjab where arsenic and fluoride pollution coexist, which is not observed in the Ganges–Brahmaputra system.

8.2.7   Chhattisgarh, central India

Arsenic contamination of groundwater was reported in weathered bedrock in Chhattisgarh in central India by Chakraborti et al. (1999) and Pandey et al. (1999, 2002). In Rajnandagaon District, where 7–8% of wells exceeded 50 ppb (maximum 1010 ppb), 10,000 people were estimated to be 'at-risk'. In the adjacent district of Kanker, the mean concentration in 89 wells was 144 ppb As (Pandey et al., 2006). Exposure to arsenic was confirmed by analysis of nails, hair and urine; and skin lesions (melanosis and keratosis) and suspected Bowen's disease have been identified. In one village alone (Kaurikasa), 130 people had advanced symptoms of arsenicosis. The main river in Rajnandagaon, the Seonath, contained up to 60 ppb As during the monsoon[18], but was below detection limits in the dry season. In Kanker, surface waters contained an average of 74 ppb and a maximum of 900 ppb As.

Geologically, the As-affected areas of Chhattisgarh are restricted to the Early Proterozoic Dongargarh–Kotr rift zone, which comprises acid and basic volcanics, volcaniclastics, intrusive rocks, and sulphide-rich quartz 'reefs' along the shear zones (Acharyya et al., 2005). The area is mineralised, and arsenopyrite-rich zones contain up to 15,000 mg/kg As. The affected area has gently undulating topography, where weathered bedrock extends from the surface to about 20 m. Contaminated groundwater is drawn both from wells drilled into bedrock and from dug-wells that exploit either the over-burden or the weathered zone at the bedrock contact. Two dug wells, near an area of former alluvial gold and uranium mining, contained 520 and 880 ppb As (and <0.1 ppm Fe). Drilled wells are cased to the top of bedrock, and then completed with open-hole construction to depths of 50–75 m. The fractured rhyolite aquifer is moderately permeable, supporting well yields of a few litres per second with drawdowns of the order of 10 m. Groundwater abstraction has been increasing in recent years, but is mainly used for pota-ble purposes. Arsenic-polluted groundwater is strongly correlated with out-crops of porphyritic rhyolite, hydrothermally enriched in arsenic, and to a lesser extent the contemporaneous granite, but is not found in wells overly-ing basic volcanic rocks (Acharyya et al., 2005).

No complete groundwater analyses have been reported, and there are differences between the reported partial analyses. Pandey et al. (1999) reported subneutral pH and consistently low (<0.01 ppm) iron concentra-tions, but high (236–288 ppm) sulphate concentrations. However, Acharyya et al. (2005) reported low sulphate (10–40 ppm) and higher iron (33% >1 ppm) concentrations. Acharyya et al. (2005) concluded that arsenic is mobilised partly by oxidation of sulphides at shallow depth (affecting dug wells), but mainly by reduction of iron oxyhydroxides at greater depth.

In the same area, agricultural soils, used for monsoon rice cultivation, contain up to 252 mg/kg As, and rice grown there contains up to 446 µg/g As and high levels of copper and lead (Patel et al., 2005). There is limited groundwater irrigation, and so the accumulation of As, Cu and Pb is attri-buted to rainwater leaching these elements from a geologically enriched soil. The occurrence of arsenic in Chhattisgarh differs from all others in South Asia. The extent and mobilisation of arsenic and its fate in agriculture are all poorly understood and require further investigation.

8.2.8 Other areas of South Asia

India

Somasundaram et al. (1993) and Ramesh and Ramanthan (cited by Mukherjee et al., 2006) reported As concentrations of up 420 ppb in shal-low wells in Chennai, but both tentatively attributed this mainly to anthro-pogenic pollution. The situation in the remainder of southern India is mostly unknown, but Datta and Kaul (1976) reported that five of nine wells tested from the city of Vapi in Gujarat contained >50 ppb As.

Sri Lanka

The earliest report of As pollution in South Asia was by Senanayake et al. (1972) who reported seven cases of polyneuropathy caused by arsenic in well-water near Colombo. Arsenic poisoning was confirmed by analysis of water, urine and nail clippings. Symptoms included vomiting, facial swelling, 'Mees line' on nails, gastroenteritis, eye irritation, and weakness, numbness and jerky movements of the limbs. A 70-year old man continued drinking this water and died of severe gastroenteritis after 2 weeks.

8.3   Southeast Asia

8.3.1   The Red River of Vietnam

Berg et al. (2001) described As pollution in the Red River Delta (or Bac Bo Plain) of northern Vietnam, which is home to 11 million people. At Hanoi, in the upper part of the delta, groundwater has been exploited for over 90 years, currently at the rate of 500 Mm³/day. In 1999–2000, raw water from the wellfields ranged from 15 to 430 ppb As. Severe contamination was also found in private tubewells around Hanoi (Table 8.14). Despite the high levels of exposure, no symptoms of arsenicosis were identified.

The Red (or Song Hong) River delta has a tropical monsoonal climate, with a mean temperature of 23°C and annual rainfall of 1800 mm. It occupies a NW–SE, fault-bounded basin, 500 km long, 50–60 km wide and >3 km thick, bounded by Precambrian crystalline rocks and Palaeozoic to Mesozoic sediments (Tanabe et al., 2003). The prograding delta contains abundant organic matter, and at Hanoi, where the Quaternary sequence is 50–90 m thick, municipal wells draw water from depths of 30–70 m, and private wells draw water from 12–45 m. According to Berg et al. (2001), the Quaternary sequence can be divided into: (a) a fine-grained upper sequence

Table 8.14   Arsenic in private wells near Hanoi

| District | Number | Percentage of wells with As exceeding | | Maximum As (ppb) |
		10 ppb	*50 ppb*	
Dong Anh	48	50	25	220
Tu Liem	48	70	32	230
Gai Lam	55	77	52	3050
Thanh Tri	45	97	90	3010

Source: Berg et al. (2001)

of clay to fine sand; and (b) a lower sequence of coarse sand and gravel, interbedded with layers of peat up to several metres in thickness. Arsenic concentrations in core samples from 12 to 20 m ranged from 6 to 33 mg/kg in brown to black clays, 2 to 12 mg/kg in grey clay and 0.6 to 5.0 mg/kg in brown to grey sands. The As and Fe contents in sediments are positively correlated (see Figure 2.11). The polluted groundwater is anoxic and contains high concentrations of iron, manganese, alkalinity and ammonium (up to 48 ppm). Tritium dating suggests that the affected waters have residence times of a few decades to more than 50 years. Berg et al. (2001) concluded that the mobilisation processes in the Red River delta are the same as in the Bengal Basin.

Around Hanoi, groundwater arsenic is strongly concentrated to the south and west of the urban area (Figure 8.11), and its distribution has been

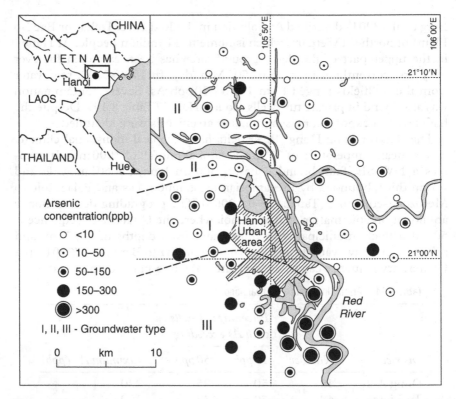

Figure 8.11 Arsenic concentration in groundwater in the Hanoi area, Vietnam. Arsenic pollution is concentrated on the right bank of the Red River, especially to the south of the Hanoi metropolitan area, where it is associated with both Type III groundwater and buried peat.
Source: After Berg et al. (2001) and Duong et al. (2003)

correlated with the three water types defined by Duong et al. (2003): (I) high bromide, (II) low bromide, and (III) high bromide with high ammonia and DOC. High levels of pollution occur mainly in Type III waters. The low-As Type II waters parallel the active channel of the Red River, similar to what has been observed along the Ganges in Bangladesh (Ravenscroft et al., 2005). In both cases, these low-As aquifers are formed by clean fluvial channels that lack a sufficient redox driver, and cut through earlier deltaic sands that are thinner, finer grained and richer in organic-matter.

Information on mitigation in Hanoi is given by Duong et al. (2003) and Berg et al. (2006a). Water from the municipal wellfields is passed through eight treatment plants that employ aeration, sedimentation, sand filtration and chlorination prior to distribution, which is only partially effective, and reduces concentrations to 25–91 ppb As. However, As concentrations in water collected from households are further reduced by around 50%, probably due to adsorption onto iron pipes (Berg et al., 2001). At community level, Berg et al. (2006a) described the use of small arsenic removal plants (ARPs) based on the slow sand filter concept (see section 7.3.1). The filters, which are coupled to hand tubewells, reduce high iron concentrations, and achieved an As removal efficiency of 80%. Berg et al. (2006a) attributed their social acceptability to the simplicity, low cost and use of local materials.

8.3.2   The Mekong River of Vietnam, Cambodia and Laos

Groundwater in the Mekong basin of Vietnam and Cambodia typically contains <10 ppb As, but there are areas of slightly elevated (10–130 ppb) arsenic, and occasional hot spots with up to 600 ppb As. Of 932 samples tested by Stanger et al. (2005), mostly using the Hach field kit, 13% exceeded 10 ppb As. In Cambodia, 22% of over 1000 water samples analysed by Polya et al. (2005) contained >10 ppb, 14% > 50 ppb and 5% > 200 ppb As. Buschmann et al. (2007) demonstrated that the affected area is restricted to the floodplains of the Mekong and Bassac rivers, where 1.2 million people drink untreated well-water, of which 48% is > 10 ppb and 40% > 50 ppb As. There are no reports of widespread arsenicosis from the Mekong delta, but Berg et al. (2006b) noted skin lesions in Cambodia. They suggested that the rarity of symptoms in both countries is due to the short duration (mostly <10 years) of exposure, and fear it will increase rapidly. They also estimated that 13.5% of the 11 million people in Vietnam were exposed to >50 ppb As.

Contamination also occurs higher up the Mekong River in Inchampasak and Saravane provinces of Laos, and also along the Se Kong tributary into Attapeu Province (UNICEF, 2004). Although 16% of the 2000 wells tested exceeded 10 ppb As, only 1% exceeded 50 ppb As.

The Lower Mekong floodplain is divided into three units: the main channel, the Tonle Sap (Great Lake) and the Cuu Long Delta (Stanger, 2005; Stanger et al., 2005). From the Lao border to Phnom Penh (where its major distributary the Bassac divides) the Mekong floodplain is narrow, and runs through hills of Mesozoic volcanics and sediments, probably explaining the (apparent) lack of continuity with contamination in Laos. Annual rainfall ranges from 1000 to 2000 mm. The Mekong Delta has a high tidal range, strong currents and broad tidal plains, but differs from the Ganges–Brahmaputra in that it is underlain by crystalline basement at depths of <200 m (Morgan, 1970). The alluvial valley is about 50 km wide and surrounded by extrusive igneous rocks that supply coarse sediment to the delta. Deposition occurs in levee ridges and basins that terminate in a coastal accretion ridge, which forms a 20 m thick sheet of sand extending over thousands of square kilometres (Morgan, 1970). The maximum Holocene transgression, between 6 and 5 ka, reached up to 4.5 m above present sea level on Late Pleistocene terraces (Nguyen et al., 2000).

According to Stanger et al. (2005), the alluvial stratigraphy of the Lower Mekong comprises a thin cover of recent sands and silt, overlying Holocene fluvial silts and coastal sand dunes up to 20 m thick. Beneath these are Upper to Middle Pleistocene sands, silt and clay, 10–30 m thick, which are widely abstracted from, and at the base are Lower Pleistocene sands that underlie 90% of the delta. Contamination is found in all four units, and high As concentrations are found in both shallow and deeper (100–120 m) aquifers. However, the shallow aquifers are often brackish, so most drinking and irrigation water[19] is pumped from depths of 150–250 m, which is generally arsenic-free (Berg et al., 2006b).

Groundwater is near-neutral (pH 7.0–7.6), and negative redox potentials suggest it is strongly reducing (Stanger et al., 2005). In Cambodia, Polya et al. (2005) inferred a strong geological control, noting that high-As tends to be found in wells 16–80 m deep, in aquifers of Holocene age, and close to major channels of the Mekong and the Bassac (Table 8.15). Buschmann et al. (2007) present strong evidence that arsenic is mobilised by RD.

8.3.3   The Irrawaddy River delta, Myanmar

The limited information (Tun, 2002, 2003) on As pollution in the Irrawaddy Delta suggests that the situation is similar to that in Bangladesh and Vietnam. In one survey, Tun (2002) found that 66% of 99 wells exceeded 50 ppb As, although only 37% of household water samples exceeded 50 ppb As. He identified arsenicosis patients and linked this to drinking water. Nine samples were from dugwells and all contained <50 ppb As. Tun (2003) reported more detailed surveys of 1912 wells in four townships in the Irrawaddy delta using the Merck field-kit backed up by laboratory tests on 25 random samples. The results, summarised in Table 8.16, show levels of

Table 8.15 Relation of arsenic in groundwater to geology in Cambodia

| Geological unit/age | Percentage of area in Cambodia | Number of samples | Percentage of wells with As exceeding | | | Maximum As (ppb) |
			10 ppb	50 ppb	200 ppb	
Holocene, near Mekong and Bassac	3	401	46	32	11	1700
Holocene, other areas	30	346	9	4	1	390
Pleistocene	30	217	8	5	3	270
Pliocene volcanics	6	27	0	0	0	8.7
Neogene–Quaternary sediments	5	13	0	0	0	7.9
Older units	27	68	9	0	0	38

Source: Polya et al. (2005)

Table 8.16 Arsenic survey of four townships in southern Myanmar

Township	Number of wells	>10 ppb As (%)	>50 ppb As (%)	>100 ppb As (%)
Kyonpyaw	701	43	23	3.9
Thabaung	512	65	36	19
Hinthada	371	31	11	4.9
Laymyathna	324	34	4.6	0.6

Source: Tun (2003)

contamination that are comparable to Bangladesh and West Bengal. Depth profiles of arsenic in three townships peak at 40–50 m before declining rapidly below 60 m. Caussy and Than Sein (2006) estimated that 2.5 million people use drinking water containing more than 50 ppb As in Mynamar.

8.3.4 Thailand

Chao Phraya delta, central Thailand

Kohnhorst et al. (2002) detected low-level As contamination in Nakorn Chaisi District, 20 km northwest of Bangkok. They sampled wells with depths of 80–200 m in the Bangkok and Phrapadaeng alluvial aquifers, analysing arsenic on site with a locally developed field kit. All surface waters and most wells contained ≤10ppb As, and only one well, in the Phrapadaeng aquifer, contained >100ppb As. Human exposure is minimal because most people use municipal supply or bottled water for drinking. Nevertheless, Kohnhorst et al. (2002) recognised that the depth (i.e. >80m) of the wells may have resulted in few detections of arsenic. The Holocene sequence of the Chao Phraya delta is thin, and at Bangkok much of it is marine (AIT, 1981). Hence, regional experience suggests further contamination may be found at shallower depth and/or further inland, where water is drawn from Holocene fluvial sediment.

Hat Yai, southern Thailand

In an investigation of the impact of urbanisation on groundwater quality at the city of Hat Yai, Lawrence et al. (2000) discovered severe contamination (>1000ppb As) in strongly reducing waters that also contained high Fe, NH_4 and DOC concentrations. Hat Yai obtains about 50% of its water supply from the semi-confined Hat Yai (25–40 m), Khu-Tao (45–80 m) and Kho-Hong (>100 m) alluvial aquifers. The aquifers are separated by fine sand, silt and clay, and are recharged by rainfall and leakage from water mains, canals and sewage. Arsenic occurs in two associations. In the first, extreme arsenic values are found in water with tens of ppm of iron and near-neutral pH. The second is in water containing a few tens of ppb of As and a few tens of ppm of SO_4, with pH 5–6. Lawrence et al. (2000) proposed that a descending plume of sewage creates reducing conditions, mobilising arsenic from iron oxyhydroxides (Figure 8.12) and inferred that the plume had taken 30–35 years to migrate into the Hat Yai aquifer.

Ron Phibun Tin Belt, southern Thailand

Arsenic contamination of surface and groundwaters (up to 5000ppb As) in Ron Phibun District has been widely cited (e.g. Williams et al., 1996; World Bank, 2005). The problem occurs in an area where tin is mined from both bedrock and alluvium. Contamination of shallow groundwater was attributed to oxidation of mining waste, which is rich in arsenopyrite and its alteration products, and finely disseminated arsenopyrite in the alluvium. Over 1000 people have been diagnosed with arsenical skin conditions (World Bank, 2005).

8.3.5 Other parts of Southeast Asia

Java, Indonesia

Sriwana et al. (1998) reported concentrations of arsenic, aluminium, boron, iron and manganese, all exceeding drinking water standards, along the Upper

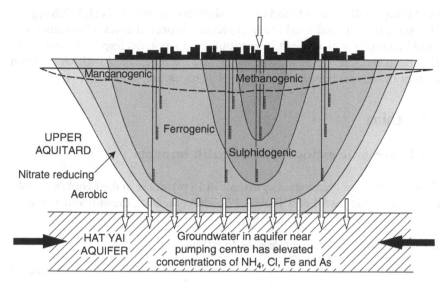

Figure 8.12   Evolution of contaminated groundwater at Hat Yai, Thailand. Under the influence of municipal abstraction from the Hat Yai, a zoned plume of increasingly reducing water, originating from urban wastes, has gradually been drawn into the aquifer, mobilising arsenic from iron-rich coatings on the sediments. *Source*: Lawrence et al. (2000)

Citarum River in West Java. Water is drawn for irrigation and 'other' purposes. The Citarum catchment contains active and recently extinct volcanoes, and hydrothermal features that are the probable sources of the contaminants. The volcanogenic pollutants drop to baseline levels within 30 km of the source.

Western Malaysia

Chow (1986) recorded the presence of 'excessive' arsenic and fluoride in well-water in Kampong Sekolah on the western coast of Malaysia. No details of the geology or chemistry were given, although it was noted that both As and F concentrations in soil correlated well with those in groundwater, and both fluorite and limonite were abundant in the soil, which might be sources of fluoride and arsenic respectively.

Philippines

Near the Mount Apo geothermal power plant on Mindanao Island, Webster (1999) reported that the Marbel and Matingao rivers contain up to 140 and 260 ppb As respectively, along with elevated concentrations of boron, lithium and antimony. Arsenic in the rivers is attributed to leakage from hot springs that contained between 3100 and 6200 ppb As. Villagers living near the Matingao River were found to have slightly elevated levels (1.5–2.8 mg/kg) of arsenic in hair, and local medical records reported cases of anaemia and 'skin irritations' which might be attributable to arsenic. Exposure had probably been reduced because river water had been replaced with water from springs of normal temperature about 8 years earlier.

8.4   China

8.4.1   Arsenic exposure and health impacts

Groundwater is contaminated by arsenic in 19 provinces of the People's Republic of China (Figure 8.1 and Table 8.17). Unfortunately, the available mapping

Table 8.17   Arsenic contamination of groundwater in China

Province	Wells tested*	Percentage of wells >50ppb*	Maximum As (ppb)[†]	Exposed population[†]	Prevalence of arsenicosis (%)[†]
Shanxi	3079	52.4	1932	932,000	13.1
Inner Mongolia	5885	11.3	1860	1,025,000	15.5
Xinjiang	14,050	4.8	880	143,000	1.4
Jilin	8200	12.2	360	59,000	17.7
Ningxia	8276	1.1	100	25,000	9.5
Qinghai	24	8.3	318	12,000	8.6
Anhui	ND	ND	150	87,000	0.8
Beijing	ND	8.0	143	60,000	0.0
Heibei[‡]	525	0.0	48	ND	ND
Sichuan[§¶]	3870	9.3	>600	860	ND
Zhejiang	293	ND	70	ND	ND
Zhengzhou**	622	ND	186	ND	0.0
Liaoning[¶††]	3500	0	<50	ND	0.0
Gansu[¶]	5016	2.7	>250	22,954	ND
Henan[¶]	28,068	0.7	>500	7855	ND
Heilongjiang[¶]	43,344	0.5	>100	ND	ND
Yunnan[¶]	9535	0.3	>200	6839	
Shandong[¶]	19,899	0.2	>50	31,799	–
Hunan[¶]	10,000	0.1	>50	348	0.0

ND, no data.

*Sun (2004); [†]Xia and Liu (2004); [‡]Lu et al. (2004); [§]Bin et al. (2004); [¶]Yu et al. (2007); **Wei et al. (2005); [††]Liu et al. (2003).

is either site-specific or aggregated at provincial level, such that it is difficult to portray the spatial patterns in a geologically meaningful way. Sun et al. (2001) estimated that 14.7, 5.6 and 2.3 million people, respectively, were drinking water with >10 ppb, >50 ppb and >100 ppb As. Most identified areas are in the arid north of the country. In addition, there is widespread arsenic poisoning in Guizhou Province due to burning of high-As coal (Ding et al., 2001).

Xia and Liu (2004) reported that the prevalence of arsenicosis in Inner Mongolia increases with age, especially between 20 and 40 years. They also reported no gender difference in prevalence, but Luo et al. (1997) reported that skin lesions were more frequent in males. Xia and Liu also presented summary data showing a strong dose–response function, as summarised in Table 8.18. The results not only demonstrate how rapidly the risk of arsenicosis increases at higher concentrations, but also provide some justification for not reducing the 50 ppb standard due to the absence of symptoms in persons exposed to lower concentrations. The correlation with cumulative arsenic intake was an even stronger relationship ($r^2 = 0.98$).

The prevalence of skin lesions in Xinjiang and Inner Mongolia both followed well-defined dose–response trends (Figure 5.5), with most studies finding thresholds of between 50 and 200 ppb As (Yang et al., 2002). Xia and Liu (2004) reported associations of arsenic with peripheral vascular disease, polyneuropathy, hypertension and cancer. Fujino et al. (2004) showed that arsenic adversely affects mental health, and Li et al. (2006) and Otto et al. (2006) showed that arsenic affects neurological function at concentrations below the threshold reported by NRC (1999). Removing exposure to arsenic in drinking water has been only modestly successful in alleviating dermatological symptoms (section 5.14).

8.4.2 The Yellow River Basin, Inner Mongolia

The As-affected areas of Inner Mongolia, the worst affected and most intensely studied province of China, mainly follow the semi-arid middle

Table 8.18 Prevalence of arsenicosis in China related to arsenic dose in drinking water

Arsenic (ppb)	Persons examined	Patients identified	Prevalence (%)
<50	624	0	0
50–200	641	29	4.5
200–400	321	39	12.1
400–650	1021	278	23.1
>650	1179	581	49.3

Source: Xia and Liu (2004)

reaches of the Yellow (or Huang He) River. Although its discharge is seven times less than the Yangtze-Kiang, it carries by far the largest sediment load (34 kg/m³) of any major river. Arsenic pollution occurs mainly along the first two arms of the Great Bend, where the river heads north towards the arid realms of Mongolia before turning south to enclose the loess plateau. The eastern side of the Great Bend receives much more rain and a massive input of loess, increasing both sediment load and discharge, and influencing the quality of the alluvial groundwater. On the western side of the Great Bend, the Hetao Plain receives 130–220 mm of rain, and potential evaporation is >2000 mm (Lin et al., 2002). This is one of the oldest irrigation districts in China, and 45% of the irrigated soils have been salinised. Aquifers are recharged by the Yellow River and the irrigation canals contain fresh groundwater, but otherwise shallow groundwater is saline.

The Great Bend occupies a fault-bounded basin filled with 2000 m of post-Jurassic lacustrine sandstone and shale (Lin et al., 2002). Quaternary deposits range from 200 m thick in the southeast to 1500 m in the northwest, but thin to a few tens of metres at the foot of the mountains. The lower Pleistocene comprises muds with sand and peat. The present Yellow River migrated into the area in the late Pleistocene or early Holocene. As a result of channel avulsion, there are many oxbow lakes filled with organic-rich muds, although due to the dry climate, there was also evaporative concentration and salt accumulation. In the upper 200 m, there are three to five aquifers with variable water quality. On the Hetao Plain, arsenic occurs in both deep (50–200 m) and shallow aquifers (Luo et al., 1997), and Lin et al. (2002) reported that 40% of 161 wells exceeded 50 ppb and 7% exceeded 500 ppb As. Groundwater is anoxic, with iron concentrations of >0.3 ppm in 20% of deep wells and 6% of shallow wells. High As concentrations are associated with organic–rich sediments, methane gas and abundant humic acids (0.2–17 ppm), and the water is often brownish-yellow or yellowish-green. Arsenic mobilisation was attributed to the reducing conditions, and it was suggested that arsenicosis is worsened by the humic acids. Groundwater is also contaminated by fluoride, which exceeded 1 ppm in 14% of wells. Zhang et al. (2002) and Zhang (2004) proposed a causal link to As–Sb–Cd and Cu–Pb–Zn mineralisation in the Yin Mountains to the north of the basin.

The Huhhot Basin is an important sub-basin that joins the Yellow River where it turns to the south. This lacustrine basin has an area of 4800 km² and is bounded by mountains on both sides. Smedley et al. (2003) found lower median As concentrations (2.9 ppb; maximum 1480 ppb) in 59 shallow wells than in deep (>100 m) wells (128 ppb and 308 ppb As). Groundwater also contains up to 6.8 ppm of fluoride, dominantly in shallow wells. These As statistics are skewed by their spatial distribution, because deep wells are concentrated in the centre of the basin, whereas many of the less contaminated shallow wells are located along the basin margins. Shallow

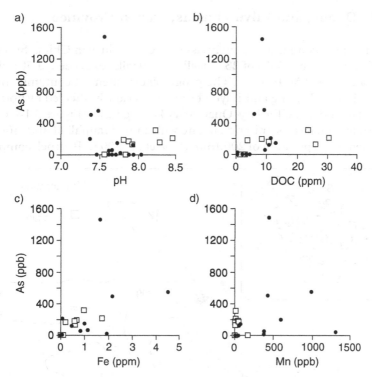

Figure 8.13   Hydrochemistry of groundwater in the Huhhot Basin, Inner Mongolia, China. The plots show the relation of arsenic in groundwater to pH, DOC, iron and manganese. Solid circles represent shallow (<100 m) wells, and open squares represent deep (>100 m) wells.
Source: Smedley et al. (2003)

groundwater quality is also affected by evaporative concentration. High As concentrations are found in anaerobic groundwater with elevated concentrations of iron, ammonium, phosphate and DOC, and low sulphate concentrations (Figure 8.13). Manganese is only enriched in the shallow aquifer. Smedley et al. (2003) concluded that As mobilisation is caused by 'desorption coupled with reductive dissolution of Fe oxide minerals', although this appears to conflate processes operating in different parts of the aquifer. All samples with high Fe (>0.3 ppm) and NH_4 (>1 ppm) have elevated arsenic, but some high As concentrations are associated with low Fe and NH_4. In shallow groundwater, arsenic is negatively correlated with pH, but a few deep waters have pH 8.2–8.5 and are enriched in phosphate and DOC (11–31 ppm). It appears that RD, enhanced by evapoconcentration, is the dominant process in the shallow aquifer, but desorption may be significant in the deeper aquifers.

8.4.3   Datong and Taiyun basins, Shanxi Province

Shanxi is the second most severely As-affected province in China. Sun et al. (2001) reported that 35% of 2373 wells in 129 villages exceeded 50 ppb As, and 5% exceeded 500 ppb As. The geographical extent of contamination is unclear, but the Datong and Taiyun basins are seriously affected by both arsenic and fluoride. The Tertiary–Quaternary Datong Basin (Figure 8.14) covers 60,000 km^2 and has a semi-arid climate with annual rainfall of 300–400 mm and potential evaporation of 2000 mm (Guo et al., 2003). Bedrock comprises

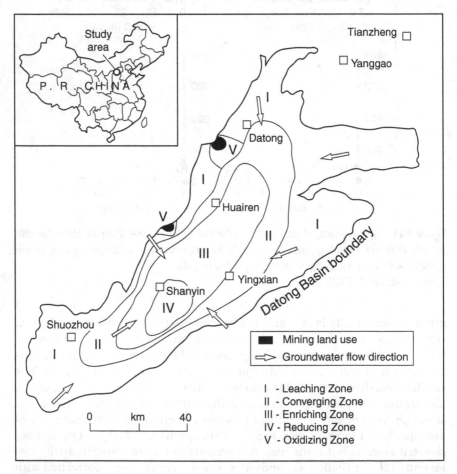

Figure 8.14   Hydrogeology and chemical zoning of groundwater in the Datong Basin, Shanxi Province, China. Groundwater is recharged at the basin margins by surface water from the adjacent mountains, and is partly discharged by evaporation in the basin centre.
Source: Guo and Wang (2005)

Precambrian gneiss and basalt in the west, and Palaeozoic limestone, sandstone and shale in the east. At Shanyin City, alluvial and lacustrine sediments are up to 3 km thick, with fluvial sediment dominating the Holocene sequence. The aquifers are alluvial sands, gravelly at the margins, but passing into lacustrine fine sand and organic-rich mud towards the centre of the basin (Guo and Wang, 2005). The sediments typically contain 1–10 mg/kg As and up to 1% by weight of organic carbon. Of 30 wells 10–50 m deep, sampled in 1999 and 2001, 50% exceeded 10 ppb and 40% exceeded 50 ppb As. Although samples were not preserved in the field, As(III) was still the dominant arsenic species when tested in the laboratory.

The average composition of groundwater at Shanyin in the Datong Basin is given in Table 8.19. High As (maximum 1932 ppb) is associated with elevated phosphate and DOC, and low concentrations of sulphate and nitrate. High As is positively correlated with pH. Maximum enrichment in arsenic occurs at pH 8.5, and arsenic is virtually absent below pH 7.7 (Figure 8.15). While iron is generally present in solution, high-Fe and high-As tend to be mutually exclusive. Guo et al. (2003) deduced that arsenic is positively correlated with organic compounds (measured as naphthenic acid) in water at concentrations of <400 ppb As, but the correlation breaks down at higher concentrations. All four wells with >400 ppb As had pH > 8.0, suggesting that the data include two superimposed trends, reflecting the operation of different processes.

Groundwater flow converges on the centre of the Datong Basin, producing concentrically zoned chemical water-types in shallow (<80 m) groundwater (Figure 8.14). These are characterised by Guo and Wang (2005) as follows.

1   A leaching zone in the recharge areas, with Ca–HCO_3 water, nitrate and <5 ppb As.
2   A 'converging' zone with low As, carbonate dissolution and cation-exchange.

Table 8.19   Average groundwater chemistry at Shanyin, Shanxi Province, China

Parameter	Unit	Average	Parameter	Unit	Average
T	°C	12.4	As	ppb	64
pH		7.7	Ca	ppm	62
HCO_3	ppm	476	Mg	ppm	62
SO_4	ppm	287	Na	ppm	244
NO_3	ppm	72	Fe	ppb	90
Cl	ppm	170	Mn	ppb	50
F	ppm	3.2	PO_4	ppm	0.24

Source: Guo et al. (2003)

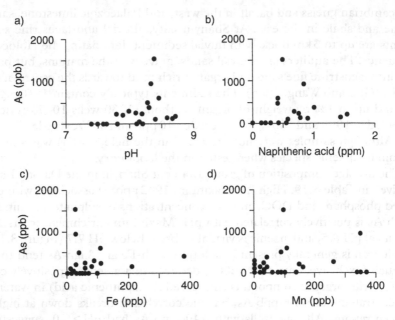

Figure 8.15 Hydrochemistry of groundwater in the Datong Basin, Shanxi Province, China. The plots show the relation of arsenic in groundwater to (a) pH; (b) naphthenic acid, a product of organic decomposition; (c) iron; and (d) manganese.
Source: Guo et al. (2003)

3 An 'enriching' zone of relatively stagnant groundwater, concentrated by evaporation, enriched in sulphate and nitrate, and modified by ion-exchange to produce Na–HCO$_3$ water with high pH that promotes desorption of fluoride (mean 7.2 ppm) and arsenic (mean 13 ppb; maximum 197 ppb).

4 An anoxic 'reducing' zone, also Na–HCO$_3$ type, where sulphate and nitrate are reduced, which has the highest As concentrations (mean 366 ppb; maximum 1530 ppb). Fluoride remains high (mean 3.7 ppm), and phosphate, iron and manganese are slightly elevated.

5 An oxidising zone (within Zone 1) in coal-mining areas. Pyrite oxidation generates high sulphate concentrations, but arsenic is very low (maximum 1.2 ppb).

In the Taiyuan Basin, De et al. (2006) reported the co-occurrence of arsenic and fluoride at Wusu City, where 59% of 1069 wells contained >50 ppb As and 41% contained >1 ppm F. In wells 30–60 m deep, the mean As concentration is only 10 ppb As, but concentrations below 60 m increase to 150–200 ppb As. Fluoride concentrations are more uniform with depth.

8.4.4 Xinjiang Province

Xinjiang is the third most As-affected province and, at Kuitin in 1980, it was the source of the first report of extensive arsenicosis in China (Sun, 2004). Arsenic-polluted groundwater is found in the Dzungaria Basin, north of the Tian Shan mountains. This relic back-arc basin has been subsiding since the Mesozoic, and is bordered by ophiolitic rocks on three sides. It is probable that groundwater is withdrawn from both Quaternary and Tertiary strata (Zheng, 2007). The climate is hyperarid. At Urumchi, annual rainfall is only 99 mm, and is even lower to the north. Monthly temperatures range between −15°C and +23°C, and the area is subject to red and black (evil) dust storms that last for 2–3 days. Lianfang and Jianzhang (1994) sampled groundwater and surface waters (average 10 ppb As) along the Kuntun valley that leads 250 km to the saline Lake Aibi (175 ppb As) at the bottom of the catchment. Arsenic concentrations in groundwater increase with distance along the flow path, and with increasing well depth (Table 8.20). Wang et al. (1997) reported that arsenic co-occurs with fluoride, and that 50,000 people use water containing high As and F from wells that were installed in the 1960s. Although separate data for arsenic were not reported, 16.5% of 619 wells contained both >1.0 ppm F and >100 ppb As. The highest As concentration was 880 ppb, and the highest F-concentration was 21.5 ppm. Based on these limited data, it appears possible that arsenic is mobilised by AD and concentrated by evaporation.

8.4.5 Qinghai–Tibet Plateau

Sun (2004) reported that 8% of wells in Qinghai province contain >50 ppb As. Mianpiang (1997) described the occurrence of arsenic in saline alkaline

Table 8.20 Arsenic concentration and well depth in Xinjiang Province

Well depth (m)	Number	As (ppb)
2–10	11	7 ± 5
76–156	7	95 ± 50
156–236	12	157 ± 20
236–316	37	217 ± 28
316–400	5	251 ± 77

Source: Lianfang and Jianzhang (1994)

lakes and hot springs on the extremely arid Qinghai–Tibet plateau, on the north side of the Himalayas. Many lakes are centres of internal drainage, and are so highly concentrated by evaporation that some are several times more saline than seawater. Many, but not all, lakes are alkaline. Twenty-two lakes that contained arsenic had an average concentration of 9900 ppb As and chloride concentration of 25,000 ppm. The highest As concentrations were found in carbonate-type lakes.

The Qinghai–Tibet plateau is also one of the world's most active geothermal areas, containing more than 600 groups of hot springs and mud volcanoes (Mianpiang, 1997). The main occurrences of arsenic in hot springs are in the Shiquanhe–Yarlung–Zangbo geothermal zone, where waters are also enriched in B, Li, Cs, Cl and in some cases F. Extreme As concentrations occur around Moincer in the west of this zone, and include the world's highest recorded natural concentrations of arsenic: 126 ppm at the Sogdoi hot-spring and 31 ppm at the Semi hot spring. The Sogdoi hot-spring also contains an astonishing 1917 ppm of boron. However, the human impact of arsenic in these lakes and hot-springs is apparently small.

8.4.6   Other provinces of China

There are reports of As contamination from many other parts of China (Table 8.17), but few details are available concerning the hydrochemistry, health impacts or geographical extent. In Zhejiang Province, Zhou et al. (2004a,b) identified a few arsenicosis patients and concentrations of 50–70 ppb As around Tong Xiang City, Zhouquan and seven other cities. Li, Zhou et al., (2006) reported that 20% of wells exceeded 10 ppb, and 3% exceeded 50 ppb As in Wuhe County of Anhui Province, and found five persons with mild arsenicosis. The reports from Zhejiang and Anhui provinces are potentially significant because they are both located in the lower catchment of the Yangtze-Kiang. Similarly, the report from Zhengzhou Province, where Wei et al. (2005) identified arsenic in wells 20–40 m deep in Zhongmou County (but no patients), is significant because it is the only case of As contamination in the Yellow River catchment downstream of the Loess Plateau. Some additional information is given for Sichuan by Bin et al. (2004), for Hebei by Lu et al. (2004), for Jilin by Zhemming et al. (2000) and for Beijing by Dou et al. (2006). Mitigation of contaminated water supplies is being implemented by government through construction of piped distribution systems based on either deep groundwater or treated surface water (Yan Zheng, personal communication, 2007).

8.5 East Asia

8.5.1 Taiwan

Epidemiological studies

Arsenic pollution on the southwest and northeast coasts of the island of Taiwan has been well known since the 1960s, and Taiwan has a special place in the history of epidemiological studies of arsenic ingestion. Boreholes have been used as a source of water supply since the 1910s, although groundwater usage reduced after a reservoir was constructed in 1956, which served about 50% of the population. However, many villagers were still drinking from wells containing hundreds of ppb of arsenic through the 1960s and 1970s (WHO, 2001). In addition to skin lesions, arsenic ingestion was linked to cancers of the skin, lung, bladder, liver and kidney, as well as cardiovascular disease and a particular form of peripheral vascular disease known as Blackfoot Disease (BFD), which can lead to gangrenous amputation of the extremities (Lamm et al., 2006a). The disease had been known since the 1930s, although a connection to arsenic was not made until the late 1960s. A curious feature of arsenic in Taiwan is that BFD is endemic in the southwest but not on the northeast coast. Blackfoot Disease was first recorded in southwest Taiwan in the 1930s and peaked between 1956 and 1960 with between 6.5 and 19 persons per 1000 contracting BFD in the affected villages (Tseng, 2005).

Some workers have questioned whether Blackfoot Disease, which is almost unknown in other As-affected areas, has a causal link to arsenic (e.g. Lu, 1990). Although there are increased incidences of cardiovascular disease (CVD) in both the affected areas, a significant dose–response relationship has been identified only in the non-BFD endemic northeast (WHO, 2001). Lamm et al. (2006a) identified distinct thresholds for both lung and bladder cancer (Figure 5.6), with no increased cancer risk thresholds ranging from 117 ppb (lung cancer in men) to 217 ppb (lung cancer in women), but were not able to 'disentangle' the BFD dose-relationships, and consider that the cause of BFD remains in some doubt.

Hydrogeochemical studies

In Taiwan, which has a monsoonal climate with annual rainfall of 1400 mm, hydrogeochemical investigations of arsenic have lagged behind epidemiological studies. In northeastern Taiwan, Hsu et al. (1997) reported that 59% of 377 wells exceeded 10 ppb and 39% exceeded 50 ppb As, and Chiou et al. (2005) reported concentrations in excess of 3000 ppb As in the Lanyang

Table 8.21   Average well-age and depth as a function of arsenic concentration in northeastern Taiwan

As (ppb)	Number (%)	Well depth (m)	Well age (years)
<10	154 (41)	16	15
10–50	75 (20)	30	14
50–300	110 (29)	34	17
300–600	19 (5)	41	16
>600	19 (5)	36	13
Total/average	377 (100)	26	15

Source: Hsu et al. (1997)

Basin. These data (Table 8.21) suggest no strong relationship between As concentration and either the age or depth of wells, although the shallowest wells are less affected. Earlier reports that As contamination was associated with black shales were incorrect and, as described by Yen et al. (1980), Liu et al. (2004) and Liu, Wang et al. (2006), contamination actually occurs in a Late Quaternary fluvio-deltaic aquifer sequence, similar to the situation in the Bengal Basin and Vietnam. Three aquifers, located at depths above 50 m, between 100 and 180 m, and below 200 m are separated by fine-grained, partially marine aquitards.

The first geological model of arsenic occurrence in Taiwan by Yen et al. (1980) associated arsenic with the Quaternary evolution of the coastal plain, and contained key elements of current thinking. The black shales, noted above, were identified as sources of sedimentary input to the alluvium. The accumulation of arsenic was linked to regressive phases of the Pleistocene, but no mobilisation mechanism was identified. More recent hydrogeochemical investigations of the Choushui alluvial fan (a non-BFD endemic area) by Liu, Wang et al. (2006) found concentrations of up to 590 mg/kg As in marine aquitards deposited between 9000 and 3000 ka. They also showed that, although the depth of peak As concentration differs between areas (20–70 m in the Choushui fan, and 70–250 m in the BFD endemic Chianan Plain), the age of the sediments is the same. Liu, Wang et al. (2006) concluded that arsenic originated in the marine aquitards, and was mobilised by RD processes, in the same way as described in Bangladesh by Nickson et al. (2000).

8.5.2   Japan

The volcanic chain of the Japanese islands is rich in arsenic, which occurs at high concentrations (up to 25.7 ppm As) in geothermal waters

(WHO, 2001) and also in Quaternary alluvium. Arsenic-contaminated hot springs discharge into sedimentary aquifers on the Niigata Plain in central Japan (10 ppb As and up to 40°C) and the Shinji Lowland (up to 114 ppb As and 85°C) in western Japan (Kubota et al., 2003). Shimada (1996) recorded As contamination of alluvial aquifers at four locations in southern Japan. The most affected, and best investigated, area was the South Chikugo alluvial plain in Fukuoka Prefecture, where groundwater has been exploited for drinking and irrigation since 1910. Although 23% of the 12,000 wells exceeded 10 ppb As, and had a maximum of 370 ppb, no arsenicosis patients were reported (Kondo et al., 1999). Wells ranged from 15 to 60 m deep, and high-As was found mainly at depths of 30–50 m. While low-As groundwater had a wide range of compositions, high-As water was a sodium-bicarbonate type with pH 7.2–8.0, and was moderately reducing (Eh −100 to +100 mV). At the most polluted site, Shimada (1996) identified six aquifer horizons within a depth of 55 m. High-As concentrations were detected in Pleistocene brownish-grey, clayey gravel in the fourth, fifth and sixth aquifers. Two pyroclastic flow deposits, separated by a red palaeosol horizon, overlie the fourth aquifer. The upper (Aso–4) pyroclastic layer was dated at 80 ka. The sediments contained 2 to >30 mg/kg As, associated with goethite and amorphous iron hydroxides. Kondo et al. (1999) proposed that both anionic exchange at high pH and RD mobilise arsenic in different areas, but that anion exchange was more important.

On the Kumamoto Plain, 50 km south of Chikugo, Shimada (1996) reported contamination (10–66 ppb As) in wells 5–110 m deep, but strongly concentrated at 30–50 m. Arsenic occurs in Pleistocene marine silt and sand (Shimbara Formation) filling a buried valley, and overlies the Aso–4 pyroclastic layer. Compared with uncontaminated waters (Table 8.22),

Table 8.22 Comparison of high- and low-arsenic groundwater from Kumamoto, Japan

	As-rich water		As-poor water	
	Average	Maximum	Average	Maximum
pH	8.2	9.1	7.1	8.2
As (ppb)	32	66	1	<5
Fe (ppm)	0.58	1.3	0.07	0.57
PO_4 (ppm)	5.5	11	0.5	11
NO_3 (ppm)	1	16	10	52
NH_4 (ppm)	0.12	1.1	0.03	0.28

Source: Shimada (1996)

the high-As groundwater is a more reducing and alkaline, Na–HCO$_3$-type water containing more phosphate, ammonium and iron. Superficially, there are similarities between arsenic occurrences described by Shimada (1996) and those in the Bengal Basin and in parts of China. However, there are also distinct differences: first the interbedded pyroclastic flow deposits might contain easily weatherable volcanic glass; and second, arsenic is not encountered in the shallowest aquifers, and not even in the Holocene sequence.

At Fukui, in the extreme south of Fukuoka Prefecture, a shallow coastal aquifer, comprising fluvial sand and gravel and dune sand interbedded with peat, contains 10–50 ppb As (Shimada, 1996). Concentrations of up to 60 ppb As were found in municipal wells 50–70 m deep at Takatsuki, where both shallower and deeper wells were free of arsenic.

In the south of Osaka Prefecture, Oono et al. (2002) reported As concentration of up to 10.6 ppb in a Quaternary alluvial aquifer, containing high iron (2.4–8.0 ppm) and ammonium (>1 ppm) concentrations, which they attributed to reductive dissolution of iron hydroxides. At Yumigahama in western Japan, Torres and Ishiga (2003) described contamination (up to 42 ppb As) in Holocene coastal sands containing subneutral (pH 6.1–7.1) and slightly oxic (DO 1.5–4.0 ppm) groundwater.

8.6   Western, Central and Northern Asia

8.6.1   Western Anatolia, Turkey

Kütahya

There are unusual occurrences of arsenic pollution of groundwater in Western Anatolia. Çöl et al. (1999) described an arsenic patient who worked at the Emet-Hisarcik borax mine in Kütahya Province who had been exposed to both airborne arsenic at work and arsenic in drinking water at home (405 ppb As). The 35-year-old man, who had worked at the mine for 15 years without using gloves or a mask, was diagnosed with keratosis on his palm which developed into squamous-cell carcinoma, and Bowen's disease on his thigh. Dogan et al. (2005) conducted clinical investigations in two villages, and identified widespread skin lesions, with an apparent dose–response relationship. At Dulkadir village, water ranged from 300 to 500 ppb As, and three of the 56 people examined had skin lesions. At Igdekoy village, the water contained around 9000 ppb As, and 33 of the 99 people examined had skin disorders including keratosis, hyperkeratosis, hyperpigmentation, basal-cell carcinoma and Bowen's disease.

In the semi-arid Kütahya area (annual rainfall 490 mm), As-rich groundwater is associated with boron-rich sediments laid down in an E–W-trending graben (Colak et al., 2003; Meltem, 2004). The Emet-Kütahya graben contains alternating lacustrine, volcanic and volcaniclastic deposits of Cretaceous to Quaternary age, underlain by Palaeozoic schists and marble. The Neogene fill comprises limestone, marl, lignite, marl and tuff overlain by borate-bearing clay of Pliocene age. The ore, which has been mined since 1956, is colemanite ($CaB_3O_4(OH)_3$–H_2O) containing 51% B_2O_3 and 1000 mg/kg As in the form of realgar (AsS) and orpiment (As_2S_3). The borate-enriched zone is up to 450 m thick and is overlain by an upper limestone unit. The sedimentary boron and arsenic were probably both derived from volcanic geothermal waters.

Colak et al. (2003) identified two distinct aquifers: a lower, karstified marble containing geothermal water with concentrations of 10–20 ppb As; and a more important, Upper Limestone aquifer containing up to 7700 ppb As. The borate-enriched zone forms an aquitard between the two aquifers. In the Upper Limestone, water is frequently drawn from springs located at the contact with the underlying aquitard, and these have the highest As concentrations. High-As groundwater is generally Ca–HCO_3 or Ca–HCO_3–SO_4 type, weakly alkaline (pH 7.4–8.4) and has negative redox potentials. Concentrations of iron (mostly <0.2 ppm) and manganese (<0.01 ppm) are very low. Boron concentrations are very high, up to 4.4 ppm, but do not correlate with arsenic. Colak et al. (2003) attributed arsenic mobilisation to dissolution (oxidation) of realgar and orpiment by groundwater flowing along the base of the limestone.

Nearby, on the Kütahya plain, Kavaf and Nalbantcilar (2007) have described more extensive contamination of river water (up to 37 ppb As) and groundwater from springs and wells (up to 136 ppb As) drawn both from recent alluvium and the underlying Kütahya Formation which consists of lavas and interbedded sediments.

Afyon

Gemicic and Tarcan (2004) described As- and B-rich groundwaters from around the Heybeli Spa at Afyon, where geothermal waters (up to 48°C) have been used since Roman times for bathing and drinking. This is of some concern because they contain up to 1240 ppb As and 5.7 ppm of boron. The main geothermal reservoir lies in Palaeozoic to Mesozoic schists and marbles, and discharges upward through Tertiary limestone, sandstone, tuff and finally into Quaternary alluvium. The waters are subneutral (pH 6.3–7.0) and slightly brackish (EC 3370–4410 μS/cm), with high alkalinity and sulphate. Iron concentrations are mostly <0.5 ppm and manganese is low (<0.06 ppm). Chloride and arsenic are well correlated, a common characteristic in geothermal waters.

Izmir

Arsenic is mobilised by sulphide-oxidation at concentrations of up to 463 ppb in a karstic limestone aquifer in the Nif Mountain area southeast of Izmir (Simsek et al., 2008).

8.6.2   Kurdistan Province, Iran

Bijar County (580 km^2) in western Iran, at 1750 m a.s.l. near the border with Iraq, has a semi-arid climate with 500 mm rainfall and a mean annual temperature of 12.5°C. The water supply is drawn from deep wells, dug wells, springs and qanats (i.e. a subterranean channel dug at a near-horizontal angle to intersect the water table, and hence carry water to the land surface). In a survey of 18 villages, Mosaferi et al. (2003) found a mean As concentration of 290 ppb with a maximum of 1480 ppb. Springs, some of which are piped for drinking, contain the highest As concentrations. They estimated that the exposure has been ongoing for at least 30 years and has produced widespread keratosis and hyperpigmentation in the exposed population, and has even required amputation of gangrenous limbs. Neither the nature of the aquifers nor the water chemistry were specified, although it was reported that the source of arsenic is geological.

8.6.3   Middle Caspian Artesian Basin, Russia and Kazakhstan

Kortsenshteyn et al. (1973) detected high-As groundwater during hydro-carbon investigations in Cretaceous rocks in the East Caucasus foothills in Russia and Jurassic rocks of the South Mangyshlak zone in Kazakhstan (on opposite coasts of the Caspian Sea). They reported As concentrations of up to 1500 ppb from 50 boreholes, although it must be emphasised that many of the waters were highly saline and could not be considered for potable use without desalination. Many of the wells were thousands of metres deep, and had open or screened sections tens of metres long. The mechanism of arsenic mobilisation is not known, although Kortsenshteyn et al. (1973) noted that arsenic appears to be associated with mineralisation of the High Caucasus. Arsenic concentrations decrease with increasing chloride content, which is contrary to the normal trend in geothermal water (e.g. Webster and Nordstrom, 2003). However, their plots suggest that the waters may belong to distinct groups rather than defining a general trend. In the East

Caucasus foothills, As concentrations of up to 1.5 ppm are found in methane-bearing waters[20] and/or saline waters rich in Br, I, B and NH_4.

8.6.4 Afghanistan

Reconnaissance surveys by Saltori (2004) identified As contamination in eastern Afghanistan. The western province was surveyed but no arsenic was detected, while other regions could not be surveyed. A total of 647 wells, between 15 and 65 m deep, were tested. In most districts, no arsenic was detected, but eight wells in Logar Province exceeded 10 ppb As, and in the Ghazni metropolitan area, 76% of 74 wells exceeded 10 ppb. A follow-up survey of three mining regions found three mountain villages where people were seriously exposed to arsenic in drinking water. Here the source of arsenic was presumed to be oxidation of arsenopyrite associated with copper mineralisation. This interpretation appears reasonable for the mountain villages, but may not apply to Ghazni.

8.6.5 Mongolia

The Public Health Institute in Ulan Bator conducted extensive well-water surveys and clinical examinations (MOH, 2004). Results are quoted only in terms of the presence of arsenic in the water, as determined by a semi-quantitative Gutzeit-type field kit, with a reported detection limit close to the WHO guideline. Experience (Chapter 6) suggests that such kits are not reliable in the range 10–50 ppb (the Mongolian standard); nevertheless, the percentage of wells in which arsenic was detected is likely to be close to the percentage exceeding 10 ppb, and the results clearly indicate the existence of a significant arsenic problem that requires further investigation and mitigation. Overall, 10.3% of 867 samples from 21 aimags (provinces) and Ulan Bator contained arsenic. The highest levels of contamination were observed in the southeastern provinces (Dornogobi, 54%; Dundgobi, 31%; Sukhbaatar, 27%; Dornod, 14%) and in the southwest (Gobi-Altai, 24%; Hovd, 19%), but in most of the north and centre (except Arkhangai, 19%) of the country levels were low. The exposed population is probably of the order of 100,000. Analyses of urine and nails confirmed uptake of arsenic in the exposed population[21], and clinical examinations found evidence of arsenicosis in 16.5% of persons. The Ministry of Health (MOH, 2004) found that well depth had a significant influence, with the highest proportion of contaminated samples drawn from wells either less than 10 m deep or more than 40 m deep. They also found a weak positive correlation between the arsenic content and age of wells, but did not identify an anticipated relationship between arsenic content and proximity to As-rich coal deposits.

8.6.6 Russia

In an account of mineral waters in Russia, Voronov (2000) described several occurrences of high-As groundwater. Within the Russian classification, As-rich mineral waters are defined as having >700 ppb As, and are very rare. It is thought their formation requires As ores, high temperature and alkaline conditions. They have been recorded in Sakhalin, the Urals and Trans-Baikal. The largest body of As-rich water, at Nalachenskoye in Kamchatka, contains 10 ppm As and is very hot (77°C) and saline (4 ppt).

8.7 Suspect Terrain and Research Needs

This section applies the model of four geochemical processes operating in geological and climatic contexts to predict where else As-contaminated groundwater might be located. What follows is not a comprehensive list, but is indicative, and could be elaborated at different scales in individual countries.

8.7.1 Bengal Basin, India and Bangladesh

No major new discoveries are expected, but research is needed to (a) understand the migration of dissolved arsenic, (b) to predict the sustainability of presently As-safe wells in shallow and deeper aquifers, and (c) to predict the accumulation of arsenic in irrigated soils and its transfer to crops. The first two issues require monitoring of piezometer nests for periods of years to a few decades in order to provide the basis for robust modelling. These issues are urgent and important because present practice is drawing polluted water towards safe wells, and it is not known to what extent the arsenic will be attenuated in the subsurface. The fate of arsenic in irrigation water requires monitoring soil and water concentrations, quantification of 'available-As' in the aquifer sediments, and surveys of water quality at all irrigation wells in As-affected areas. Research is also needed to find ways of reducing the uptake of arsenic by plants (Chapter 4), and reducing the intake and impact of arsenic in food by modified cooking methods and dietary supplements (Chapter 3).

8.7.2 Peninsular India and Pakistan

Arsenic contamination in the Precambrian rocks of Chhattisgarh appears unique in Asia, but is probably not. There are large areas of broadly similar geology, where reconnaissance surveys, focused on down-faulted rift blocks with sulphide mineralisation, ought to be conducted. Most As-affected areas are located along the main channels and Himalayan tributaries of the Indus, Ganges and Brahmaputra rivers. However, occurrences of arsenic in the Damodar fan-delta and the Son River demonstrate that a Himalayan provenance is not an absolute prerequisite. The areas of Haryana, Punjab and Himachal where Datta and Kaul (1976) identified arsenic three decades ago, but which have been ignored since, should be investigated urgently. Saxena (2004) estimated that India contains about 10% of the world's hot springs, which often contain high levels of F, Cs and Li. However, these have not been analysed for arsenic (V.K. Saxena, personal communication, 2007), and the presence of arsenic in at least some of these springs is likely.

8.7.3 Southeast Asia

Mapping of As contamination is probably significantly incomplete in Vietnam, Laos, Cambodia, Thailand and Myanmar. It appears that groundwater in some of the smaller rivers, and tributaries of the Red, Mekong, Irrawaddy and Salween rivers, has not been tested. The continuity of contamination in the Mekong should be investigated. Hydrogeological conditions in the region are similar to those in the Bengal Basin, where groundwater has been developed more intensively, and so there is much scope for learning lessons.

Conditions may be favourable for As mobilisation in the Chiang Mai Basin, Northern Thailand, as described by Asnachinda (1997), although no arsenic analyses were presented. The Late Tertiary Chiang Mai graben is surrounded by metasediments and Permo-Triassic volcanics and granite. The Quaternary alluvial fill contains abundant peat and organic matter. The groundwater was classified into 'normal' (near-neutral pH; high Fe and Mn) that could mobilise arsenic by reductive dissolution; and 'high F' types that could favour alkali-desorption.

8.7.4 Indonesia, Malaysia and the Philippines

These countries have many geological similarities. The basic risk factors are the volcanic sources of arsenic, both directly as geothermal arsenic and also input to alluvium that could be mobilised by RD. Although there are no arsenic data, volcaniclastic alluvial aquifers on Java (Indonesia) are strongly reducing, with high concentrations of iron, manganese, bicarbonate and ammonium, and discharges of methane gas are common (IWACO, 1994). Geothermal sources of arsenic are likely to be more widespread in the region than has been reported to date, but their geological setting or temperature should make them easy to identify, except perhaps where deep sources seep into the base of alluvial deposits. Arsenic has also been detected by UNICEF in water wells in Aceh Province of Sumatra (Indonesia), but no details are available. The report from Malaysia by Chow (1986) may be indicative of more extensive contamination.

8.7.5 China

Although well documented in Shanxi and Inner Mongolia, and to a lesser extent in Xinjiang Province, little is known about the occurrence of arsenic in the other affected provinces. In Shanxi and Inner Mongolia, pollution occurs mainly in inland subsiding basins where there has been insufficient base-level lowering to oxidise and/or flush out organic matter. However, there are no unambiguous reports[22] of As contamination from either the Yellow River delta or the whole of the Yangtze-Kiang and Zhujiang rivers and their tributaries. It also seems anomalous that arsenic has not been reported from river basins closest to the Red River of Vietnam.

The sedimentology of the Yellow and Yangtze deltas, as described by Saito et al. (2001) and Li et al. (2002), offers a perspective on the likelihood of encountering arsenic in groundwater. The Yellow River delta is characterised by high sediment discharge, thin Holocene deltaic sediments and a steep longitudinal profile. By contrast, the Yangtze delta is characterised by high water discharge, large seasonal water-level range, a tide-dominated coast, thick Holocene sediments filling a deep incised channel formed during glacial periods, and continuous seaward progradation with isolated river-mouth sand bodies. Marine sediment underlies the coastal parts of both deltas, but there was greater accommodation space for Holocene sands in the Yangtze delta. The enormous silt load of the Yellow River probably reduced the accumulation of channel sands and organic-rich mud. The Yangtze sediments show much more evidence of weathering of Na- and Ca-silicate minerals (Yang et al., 2004). In general, the Yangtze-Kiang shows greater similarity to the Ganges–Brahmaputra delta, and therefore perhaps a greater likelihood of As contamination of groundwater. However, the lower slope and greater weathering of the sediment may have acted to reduce the availability of arsenic.

8.7.6   Northeastern Russia

No information of arsenic is available, but alluvial and glacial basins adjacent to the extensive Tertiary mountain chains should be considered suspect (Chapter 11).

8.7.7   Korea

Numerous reports relate anthropogenic As pollution to mining (e.g. Lee et al., 2004, 2005). Although there are no reports of natural contamination, it would not be surprising if shallow groundwaters were affected in highly mineralised regions.

8.7.8   The Alpine–Himalayan belt of southwest Asia

Arsenic may be present in various settings. The Shiquanhe–Yarlung–Zangbo geothermal zone, which forms an As-rich province in the Qinghai–Tibet area of China, extends westwards into Afghanistan, Iran and Turkey, and eastward in Thailand and Myanmar (Mianpiang, 1997). It is anticipated that high As concentrations will be found in geothermal waters in these countries too. In the same general areas, there may be occurrences of arsenic in bedrock aquifers, mobilised by SO, similar to those noted earlier in Turkey and Iran. Although there is no direct evidence, it is suspected that alluvial groundwater in semi-arid basins draining areas of Tertiary volcanic activity may mobilise arsenic by alkali-desorption.

8.7.9   The Arabian Peninsula

Apart from one report by Sadiq and Alam (1996) of minor contamination (11 ppb As) from a shallow aquifer at the city of Jubail in Saudi Arabia, very few arsenic determinations[23] have been reported from the Arabian peninsula but, as in the Alpine–Himalayan belt, it is suspected that arsenic may be mobilised by AD in alluvial basins draining areas of Tertiary volcanic activity in the west and southwest of the Arabian Peninsula.

Annexe 8.1   The British Geological Survey Court Case

A8.1.1   Background

In 1992 the British Geological Survey (BGS) conducted a survey of ground-water quality in central and northeastern Bangladesh (Davies and Exley, 1992; hereafter 'the BGS report') that explicitly considered potential toxicity to humans but did not analyse for arsenic. If it had, it would, beyond any reasonable doubt, have found it. In August 2002, lawyers in London, acting on behalf of 400 Bangladeshi villagers, issued a claim for compensation against the National Environmental Research Council (NERC); a British Government agency of which BGS is a part. A summary[24] of the case and its implications is given by the Open University (OU, 2006). The basis of the claim in 'Sutradhar vs the NERC', in which Mr Sutradhar belonged to a class of people 'affected' by the BGS report, was that:

1 the Bangladesh Government was not properly equipped to do this type of testing;
2 the survey was financed as 'aid' and was intended for use by the Bangladesh Government;
3 the BGS report included an assessment of 'toxicity to humans', knowing the water would be used for drinking;
4 BGS should have known that arsenic might be present in groundwater;
5 readers would rely on the BGS judgement as to which trace elements to analyse for.

These points appear reasonable to the scientific eye, although they involve value judgements about what might be expected from a prestigious organisation such as the BGS, and whether there should be a distinction between a priori knowledge and application of the precautionary principle[25]. However, this was a legal case and not a judgement on the quality of BGS' work. From a legal perspective, the claim may be summarised by saying that the BGS owed Mr Sutradhar a 'duty of care'. Legally, the duty of care is subject to three tests: proximity, foreseeability and fairness (OU, 2006). The existence of a duty of care depended on there being a chain of reliance between the BGS and Mr Sutradhar, and also on the length of that chain, which is referred to by the legal term 'proximity'. It was not disputed that the pollution was natural, nor was it suggested that BGS was responsible for the existence of the pollution. The grounds for compensation were that, if BGS had tested for arsenic in 1992, they would have found it, and a mitigation programme would have commenced 5 years earlier. Therefore it was alleged that the BGS bore responsibility for the incremental health impacts. This Dickensian nightmare eventually went to the highest court in the land, the House of Lords, and it took 4 years to decide whether or not a trial should take place. The following is summarised principally from the account given by OU (2006).

A8.1.2 The Court Case

In March 2003, the case of 'Sutradhar vs the NERC' came before the High Court of Justice, where NERC's lawyers moved to strike out Mr Sutradhar's claim on the grounds that there was no prospect that the claim could succeed at trial by jury. The NERC disputed the duty of care because (a) the study was made under contract to the British and not the Bangladeshi Government, (b) BGS did not specify how the report should be used, and (c) neither BGS nor Mr Sutradhar knew of the other's existence. The judge, Mr Justice Simon, without attempting to reach a conclusion, said that the decision on whether or not to test for arsenic was part of the definition of a competent hydrogeological survey. Regarding proximity, he considered there was a chain of reliance from the claimant to the BGS. The judge dismissed NERC's application, concluding that it raised a 'novel point in a developing area of law', and was not bound to fail at trial, and observed that it is very difficult to separate proximity from foreseeability and fairness.

In January 2004, NERC's case came before three Law Lords in the Court of Appeal and returned to the issue of proximity (OU, 2006). The NERC raised the issue of 'construction', referring to limitations on how the findings should have been used, although the Claimant countered by pointing out the reference to 'possible toxicity to fish and humans' in the report's title and text. Lord Justice Kennedy rejected the construction argument, but took a different view on proximity, stating that to extend reliance on a 'short term pilot project' to Mr Sutradhar would be 'a mighty leap which would render the concept of proximity almost meaningless'. On the other hand, Lord Justice Clarke, citing expert evidence, was satisfied that the Government of Bangladesh relied heavily on donor's reports, and hence the claim of proximity could be reasonably argued. The decisive judgement thus came from Lord Justice Wall, who decided that there was insufficient proximity between BGS and Mr Sutradhar. So, by a 2:1 majority, the claim was struck out, but the claimant was given permission to appeal to the House of Lords.

Finally, in May 2006, the case went to the House of Lords, which in July 2006 ruled that the BGS did not owe a duty of care to the Bangladeshis. The rationale for the decision appears to be that (despite the reference in the title to toxicity to humans) the 1992 report did not specify that the BGS should test the water to ascertain whether it was suitable to drink. As the lawyers representing the Bangladeshi villagers comment 'It is simply unimaginable that such an omission could have occurred in the developed world leading to such a human tragedy.' (http://www.leighday.co.uk/doc.asp?doc=885).

A8.1.3   The Wider Picture

The BGS case, which through Legal Aid, the British Government paid to bring against itself, has implications for all scientists conducting research in the developing world. Some western scientists argued that the case would, for fear of prosecution, inhibit research in poor countries, and therefore be to the detriment of those countries. Attaran (2006) reflected on the broader implications for foreign aid, citing examples[26] where international aid had done positive harm or was given in a form (e.g. contaminated food aid) that would have been illegal in the donor country but was accepted through diplomatic coercion. No-one was held legally accountable for those activities, and so Attaran's interest in the BGS case is that it is the first foreign aid case to be pleaded as negligence in common law jurisdiction anywhere in the world. His view is that those responsible for foreign aid should be as accountable as those plying any other trade, and focuses on whether the BGS ought to stand trial and not on the chances of conviction.

Attaran (2006) considers that negligence law must be seen in the broader context of foreign aid. He stressed the newness of foreign aid and takes issue with the 'daisy chain of reliance' argument put forward by counsel for NERC. He suggests rather that technical assistance[27] is a norm in foreign aid. It is normal and necessary because the scientific support required is not available in the recipient country, and lies outside the capability of the donor agency. He takes the view that liability for the quality of advice should not depend on whether it is paid for as aid, alleging blatant double standards by donor countries. He argues that the Appeal Court confused lack of proximity with the length of the supply chain, the latter being built on natural 'partnerships' necessary to the functioning of foreign aid. Finally, he rejected the view that trial could reduce the quantity of aid given, arguing that any reduction in quantity would be more than compensated for by an improvement in quality, citing the British Government's response to the Pergau Dam scandal[28] as evidence.

Two perspectives on the BGS Court Case are important. The original claim was based on the proposition that the BGS had been negligent in not testing for arsenic, an issue that would have been tested if a trial had taken place. However, the decision not to go to trial was based on the legal criterion of proximity, and so the question of whether there was negligence has not and, without a change in the law, will not be tested. The second question is why the BGS, who did not actually install drinking water tube-wells, were singled out for legal action. United Nations' agencies such as WHO, who advise governments on drinking water standards, and UNICEF, who financed the installation of tubewells, have not been subject to such action. In fact, an attempt was made to bring a case against UNICEF in a Bangladesh court, but was rapidly abandoned because all UN agencies have immunity from prosecution, leaving the BGS an easier target for those seeking to assign legal blame for the oversight of many agencies, over many years, and in many countries.

In retrospect, it is also worth questioning whether the courts are the best means by which to judge such cases. An absolute judgement of guilt or innocence regarding the quality of scientific advice underpinning aid programmes is not appropriate or fair. It may be argued that the BGS Court Case delayed the delivery of mitigation to Bangladesh, and a successful outcome for the claimants could only have resulted in an increase in Britain's aid programme in Bangladesh. This could, and should, have been done without an expensive court case, with questions of responsibility and lessons to be learned left to an independent enquiry. However, if donor agencies or governments do not initiate such responses, the courts may offer the only line of redress to those who feel wronged.

NOTES

1   Non-cirrhotic portal fibrosis.
2   A better search might have discovered Argentina, but no more.
3   International Conference on Arsenic Pollution in Groundwater in Bangladesh: Causes, Effects and Remedies. Dhaka Community Hospital, 8–12 February 1998.
4   This is not really ironic because, to avoid flooding, most large settlements (e.g. Dhaka) developed on terraces that are underlain by the Pleistocene Dupi Tila Formation, which is free of As contamination.
5   Rahman and Ravenscroft (2003) summarise studies in Bangladesh.
6   This is because exposure patterns change as soon as people are aware of As pollution.
7   The survey excluded the Chittagong Hill Tracts.
8   Wells > 150 m deep are predominantly located in the coastal area and almost all contain < 10 ppb As.
9   Unfortunately, it appears that neither survey included laboratory quality control, so it cannot be said with certainty which is correct and therefore it reduces confidence in the blanket testing.
10 The analysis used national-scale mapping of landforms, which introduces some error close to the boundaries of mapping units, but the overall patterns are clear.
11 The exchangeable As was defined as the acetic acid soluble fraction, and the reducible As was that extracted by 0.04 m hydroxylamine hydrochloride.
12 This idea was treated with sufficient seriousness that a study (NRECA, 1997) was conducted virtually in secret because of the fear that arsenic pollution might have been caused by copper chromatic arsenic compounds in electricity pylons financed by American aid.
13 Initially a 1997 MSc thesis at London University, and presented at the DCH Conference in February 1998.
14 Notable investigations on Bangladesh include AAN (2000), Aggarwal et al. (2000), K.M. Ahmed (2003), Anawar et al. (2002, 2004), Appelo et al. (2002), Bhattacharya et al. (2001b), Breit (2000), Breit et al. (2005), Dowling et al. (2003), DPHE/BGS (20001), DPHE/MMI/BGS (1999), Harvey et al. (2002, 2006), Horneman et al. (2004), Islam, Bootham et al. (2004, 2005), Klump

et al. (2006), McArthur et al. (2001), Nickson et al. (1998, 2000), Ravenscroft et al. (2001, 2005), Stollenwerk et al. (2007), Swartz et al. (2004), van Geen et al. (2003a, 2004) and Zheng et al. (2004, 2005).

15 Notable studies in India include Acharyya et al. (2000, 2005), Bhattacharya et al. (1997, 2001b), Chakraborti et al. (2001), McArthur et al. (2004), Nath et al. (2005), PHED (1991), Sengupta, Mukherjee et al. (2004), Shivanna et al. (2000) and Stüben et al. (2003).

16 Higher fertiliser applications and irrigation are required by modern high-yielding varieties of rice, and hence impacts on groundwater should be correlated with the intensity of tubewell irrigation.

17 The Bangladesh Arsenic Mitigation Water Supply Project (BAMWSP), in addition to mitigation, undertook a huge tubewell testing programme. UNICEF and some NGOs have also been very active in both testing and awareness raising (Davis, 2003; Lokuge et al., 2004).

18 The data of Pandey et al. (2002, 2006) were derived from acidified and unfiltered samples, and may therefore exaggerate the dissolved arsenic load.

19 No information has been found concerning the use of As-rich irrigation water in Vietnam or Cambodia.

20 This suggests the possibility of degradation of organic matter, although the methane might be lithogenic gas that has migrated from deeper strata.

21 Thought to be of the order of 100,000.

22 There are As occurrences in Anhui, Zhejiang and Zhenzhou provinces, but it is not known if these are located on the alluvial plains.

23 There is also indirect and dubious evidence of As-contamination in Saudi Arabia. The BBC reported that bottled water being sold in London, purporting to come from the Zam Zam well in Mecca, contained >30 ppb As (http://news.bbc.co. uk/2/hi/uk_news/england/london/5405348.stm). Westminster City Council (WCC) pointed out that Zam Zam water cannot legally be exported and hence the water being sold was 'unlikely to be authentic'. If WCC are correct, it still leaves open the question as to the source of arsenic, which could not be local tap water. The Zam Zam is a hand-excavated well, about 30 m deep, that taps groundwater from wadi alluvium overlying diorite (http://www.sgs.org.sa/index.cfm).

24 The OU S250 course text includes full transcripts of the hearings in the supporting material.

25 Arsenic might have been anticipated on the basis of comparable hydrogeological conditions in West Bengal, Hungary or Taiwan. Alternatively, it might have been tested for because it was a well-known and highly toxic groundwater pollutant and there were almost no data from Bangladesh.

26 Attaran (2006) cited examples of the European Union sending butter oil containing faeces to Tunisia and mouldy wheat flour to Djibouti, and the WHO's anti-bilharzia programme in Egypt.

27 Whereby a chain of reliance runs from the expert, by way of the donor and recipient government, to the intended beneficiaries.

28 The Pergau Dam in Malaysia was opposed by the British Overseas Development Administration as 'uneconomic' and 'an abuse of the aid programme', but was forced through by the Foreign Ministry, reputedly as a sweetener for an arms deal (Attaran, 2006).

Chapter Nine

Arsenic in North America and Europe

9.1 Introduction

North America and Europe are included in one chapter because of their broadly similar geological and socio-economic conditions. Also, baseline hydrogeochemical studies are more extensive than elsewhere, and so it is likely that a higher proportion of occurrences of As contamination have already been discovered. In terms of geographical extent, though not of exposed population, the USA and Mexico form the most extensively contaminated region of the world. The USA contains the greatest geochemical diversity of As contamination, including all the mobilisation mechanisms described in Chapter 2. Europe also includes a great diversity of As contamination but, with the notable exception of the Great Hungarian Plain, the occurrences are of rather limited extent and/or human impact. Elsewhere in Europe, contamination is reported mainly from bedrock aquifers, and in Europe and North America the overall pattern of contamination has surprisingly little in common with the polluted river basins of Asia[1].

9.2 United States of America and Canada

9.2.1 National data for the United States of America

The main occurrences of natural arsenic contamination in North America are listed in Table 9.1, and their locations are shown in Figure 9.1. Occurrences of arsenic in Canada (Wang and Mulligan, 2006) are less common than, but are often contiguous with, those in the USA. Overviews of arsenic occurrence in the USA by Welch et al. (2000), Focazio et al. (2000) and Ryker (2003) estimated that 8% of public water supplies and 10% of all

Table 9.1 Case histories of arsenic occurrence in North America

Country/region	Name	Arsenic (ppb)† (mean/ range, Max.)	Geology, hydrology, climate	Water chemistry	Affected population/ significance*
Canada	Nova Scotia	13% > 50; Max. 1050	Crystalline bedrock; temperate	AD and SO	As-patients identified
USA	New England	30% > 10; Max. 408	Crystalline bedrock; temperate	AD	103,000 (E10)
USA	Illinois	19% > 10; Max. 266	Buried Valley Aquifer; temperate	RD	130,000 (E10)
USA	Michigan	70% > 10 Max. 220	Fluvio-glacial sediment; temperate	RD	Circulatory, cerebro-vascular diseases and kidney diseases; diabetes
USA	Minnesota, Iowa and the Dakotas	26% > 10; Max. 145	Fluvio-glacial sediment; temperate	RD	
Canada	Saskatchewan	23% > 10; Max. 117	Fluvio-glacial sediment; temperate	RD	
USA	Wisconsin	20% > 10; 4% > 50 Max. 12,000	Mineralised, Palaeozoic sandstone; temperate	SO	Lung and cardiovascular disease
USA	Oklahoma	Max. 232	Permian, red-bed sandstone; temperate	AD	Norman City, municipal wellfield
Canada	Ontario	Max 3780	Sulphide-rich Ordovician limestone; temperate	SO	1–4 deaths in 1937
Southwest USA	Basin-and-Range Province	Max. 1300	Alluvium; semi-arid	AD	
Oregon, USA	Willamette Basin	22% > 10; 8% > 50; Max. 2150	Alluvium and volcaniclastic rocks; temperate	AD	Skin diseases
Washington State, USA	Granite Falls	18% > 50; Max. 33,000	Mineralised granite; temperate	SO	

Region	Location	Concentration†	Geology; climate	Process	Number affected*
British Columbia, Canada	Bowen Island	40% > 10	Jurassic metasediments and metavolcanics; temperate	AD	
Alaska, USA	Fairbanks	40% > 10; 28% > 50 Max. 1370	Quaternary fluvio-glacial sediment and complex bedrock; sub-arctic	Various, including RD and SO.	
Alaska, USA	Cook Inlet	8% > 50; Max. 110	Quaternary fluvio-glacial sediment; sub-arctic	RD	
Northern Mexico	Sonora	9% > 10; Max. 305	Alluvium; semi-arid	AD?	
Northern Mexico	Baja California	Max. 410	semi-arid	SO?	
Central Mexico	Rio Verde	Max. 54	Alluvium over limestone and volcanics; semi-arid	?	
Central Mexico	Región Lagunera	50% > 50; Max. 624	Volcanic(?); semi-arid	?	400,000 (E50) 2,000,000 (R)
Central Mexico	Zimapán Valley	50% > 50; Max. 1100	Alluvium over limestone; semi-arid	SO	

AD, alkali desorption; RD, reductive dissolution; SO, sulphide oxidation.

*E10 refers to the number of people drinking water with >10 ppb As, and E50 to drinking more than 50 ppb As. A number followed by the suffix 'P' refers to the number of patients that have been diagnosed. Where exposure has changed over time, the peak figure is quoted. R indicates at risk.

†Concentrations normally refer to untreated water sources, either wells, streams or lakes, but not piezometers.

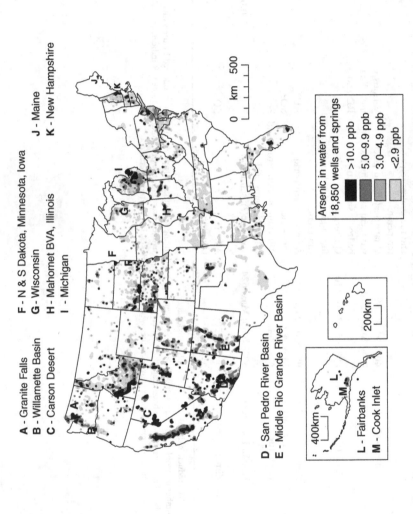

A - Granite Falls
B - Willamette Basin
C - Carson Desert

F - N & S Dakota, Minnesota, Iowa
G - Wisconsin
H - Mahomet BVA, Illinois
I - Michigan

J - Maine
K - New Hampshire

D - San Pedro River Basin
E - Middle Rio Grande River Basin

L - Fairbanks
M - Cook Inlet

Arsenic in water from
18,850 wells and springs

>10.0 ppb
5.0–9.9 ppb
3.0–4.9 ppb
<2.9 ppb

Figure 9.1 Distribution of arsenic in groundwater in the USA. The map illustrates the wide extent of arsenic in diverse geological settings across the USA. The named locations, indicated by letters on the map, are referred to in the text. BVA, Buried Valley Aquifer.

drinking water sources contain >10ppb As, although only 1.0% of public water supplies exceeded 50ppb As[2]. Many polluted supplies have presumably been abandoned in recent years because earlier estimates, cited by Smith et al. (1992), suggested that 350,000 people drank water with >50ppb As, and 2.5 million drank water with >25ppb As. The statistics are complicated by a trade-off between growing awareness, new discoveries and progressive abandonment of polluted wells. The extension of the 50ppb drinking water standard until 2006 led to there being a large stock of operational wells producing water with 10–50ppb As, but very few wells with >50ppb As. Historically, there was probably widespread exposure to higher As concentrations. In their landmark *Geochemistry of Arsenic* paper, Onishi and Sandell (1955) noted the common occurrence of arsenic in hot springs and volcanic exhalations, but did not mention other occurrences in groundwater. Ferguson and Gavis (1972) noted that in a 1969 survey of nearly 1000 water supplies, only 0.5% exceeded 10ppb, and 0.2% exceeded 50ppb As, and represented 'no current threat to public health in the US'. Apparently the scale of the problem in the USA was not recognised until the 1990s.

Much of the early USA literature on arsenic focused on the oxidation of pyrite or arsenopyrite, and many of the current explanations for As contamination were only recognised after 1990. In some cases this remains the preferred explanation, but in others the explanation has been revised. The diverse forms of arsenic contamination in the USA include the following associations:

1 widespread contamination of glacial and fluvio-glacial deposits in the temperate mid-west and northeast, mobilised by reductive dissolution (RD) of iron oxides;
2 contamination of fractured bedrock in the temperate New England, Nova Scotia and the northern Pacific Coast, where arsenic is mobilised by either sulphide oxidation (SO) or alkali desorption (AD);
3 contamination of 'basin-fill' alluvial aquifers in the semi-arid southwest, mobilised by alkali-desorption;
4 geothermal arsenic in areas of recent volcanic activity, mostly, but not exclusively, in the Rockies;
5 evaporative concentration in the arid southwest, increasing concentrations of arsenic mobilised by other processes;
6 anthropogenic pollution related to mining activities.

9.2.2 Health impacts

Compared with the rest of the world, arsenic in drinking water appears to have less effect on health in North America than in most other affected regions. Remarkably, of the hundreds of publications on groundwater arsenic in the USA, very few make explicit reference to the presence or absence of health impacts. There are, however, exceptions that have demonstrated symptoms of As poisoning in Ontario (Wylie, 1937), Nova Scotia (Grantham and Jones (1977) and Washington State (Frost et al., 1993). Reviewing data from Lassen County, California, Goldsmith et al. (1972) noted that people drinking water with above 50 ± 30 ppb As had elevated As concentrations in their hair, but showed 'no evidence of any specific illness associated with elevated arsenic'. Attempting to explain the low prevalence and intensity of arsenical symptoms in the USA compared with Taiwan, Argentina and Chile, Pershagen (1983) suggested that this could be explained by the better health[3] and nutrition of the American population, and in some cases lower intake of water and shorter duration of exposure.

The limited recognition of a link between an As hazard and clinical effects in the western USA may account for what Walker et al. (2006) call a 'paradox of awareness'. Their surveys found that 66% of persons who were 'not at all concerned' about the possible health effects were actually consuming water with >10 ppb As, whereas only 38% of persons who were 'highly concerned' about the possible health effects used water with comparable arsenic contents. While Pershagen's findings may be essentially valid, there is evidence that the American population is affected by As poisoning. Tollestrup et al. (2005) identified arsenical skin conditions (including hyperpigmentation and hyperkeratosis) in New Mexico, Arizona, and western Texas by sending questionnaires to dermatology practices. However, no causal link to drinking water could be determined.

Attributing non-dermatological symptoms of arsenic poisoning is more difficult. Engel and Smith (1994) found statistically significant[4] higher incidences of heart disease[5] in counties where the mean As concentration in public supplies (ranging from 5 to 92 ppb) exceeded 20 ppb As. In Wisconsin, Zierold et al. (2004) used self-reported questionnaires[6] to look for a connection between As exposure and cardiovascular disease in a population that had been consuming the well-water for an average of 30 years. They concluded that people drinking > 10 ppb As were statistically more likely to suffer from high blood pressure, heart attack and circulatory problems or to have had bypass surgery than those drinking < 2 ppb As. Reanalysing the same data set, Knobeloch et al. (2006) concluded that 'of residents aged over 35 years, those who had consumed arsenic-contaminated water for at least 10 years were significantly more likely to report a history of skin cancer than others'.

The risk of bladder cancer has received particular attention. Based on seven counties with long-term exposure to concentrations of around 100 ppb, Steinmaus et al. (2003) found no increased risk of bladder cancer at As intakes of over 80 μg/day, but did find an increased risk in smokers who drank contaminated water. Similarly, Lamm et al. (2004), examining 30 years of records from 133 counties, found no increased risk of bladder cancer in the exposure range of 3–60 ppb As. These studies suggest a higher cancer threshold for the USA population than inferred from earlier studies in Taiwan. On the other hand, Siegel et al. (2002) inferred a small, but significant, increased risk of bladder cancer at concentrations of >10 ppb As in some parts of New Mexico, while Ayotte et al. (2006a) presented evidence to suggest a possible link between bladder cancer and elevated As concentrations in New England.

Studies in the USA have focused on arsenic in drinking water and so direct comparison with studies in Asia must be qualified by the generally greater per capita consumption of water and As intake from food in the latter studies, and differences in general nutrition that must be taken account of before any possible role of genetic factors can be identified.

9.2.3   An early case of arsenic poisoning from well-water in Ontario, Canada

An early case of As poisoning from well-water was reported by Wyllie (1937) from Halifax County, Ontario. The study is particularly interesting because of its then innovative, interdisciplinary nature. One man died and his whole family were affected, and the almost immediate deaths of three out of four live births may have been caused by arsenic. In 1932, a 29-year-old farmer suffered from weakness, inability to walk, keratosis of the palms and soles, liver disease and hypertension. He was diagnosed with advanced liver disease and died 2 months later. After his death, his younger brother took over the farm and soon felt unwell. By 1935, the widow and daughter, and the brother all showed signs of skin pigmentation and hyperkeratosis. The brother was also suffering from gastrointestinal disturbance, swelling of the ankles, numbness of fingers and toes, dryness of hair and an irritated bladder. The brother had an appendectomy to relieve gastrointestinal symptoms, but when he went home, the symptoms returned. At this point, the farm's well came under suspicion, and was found to contain 3780 ppb As.

Wyllie (1937) conducted investigations around the farm based on three hypotheses: use of arsenical insecticides; leaching and percolation of urine from the new piggery; and naturally occurring arsenic in local rocks. The family denied ever using arsenical insecticides. Dr Wyllie established that the well had been drilled in 1922 to a depth of 29 m. The previous owner informed him that the well had been drilled into 'red rock' (limestone), and also that he had felt unwell for the last 12 years. On examination he was found to have hyperkeratosis of the palms which he had previously attributed to 'hard work'. This indicated that the pollution was not a recent phenomenon, and he recognised the now well-known phenomenon of latency in developing arsenicosis, in this case 2–3 years.

Dr Wyllie sampled four other wells in the area. None contained detectable arsenic, but all were much shallower. From the literature, he established that a gold mine at Deloro, 15 km away, was an internationally important source of arsenopyrite. A piece of limestone, dug out from a depth of 1 m during excavation of the piggery, contained 11.5 mg/kg As, further pointing to a geological source. Lime-scale in the farm's kettle contained 0.4% arsenic, and through filtering experiments he inferred that the arsenic was probably present as a fine suspension. The association of arsenic at the farm and the gold mine may have been fortuitous[7], because the gold and arsenic at Deloro occur in Precambrian basement, whereas the limestone found at the farm is probably of Ordovician age. Bredberg (2004) reports that the Ordovician limestone contains commercial deposits of sphalerite (ZnS) and galena (PbS). These deposits would almost certainly contain pyrite, and all three minerals could release arsenic if exposed to a fluctuating water table.

9.2.4   The Basin-and-Range Province, southwest USA

Regional data

Arsenic contamination affects dozens of alluvial basins in the Basin-and-Range Province, of Arizona, New Mexico, Nevada and California, where many cities and small communities depend on groundwater for their water supply. The area is tectonically active, has a semi-arid to arid climate, and was not directly affected by Pleistocene glaciation. Welch et al. (1988) documented 28 occurrences of groundwater As in the western USA, of which 14 were in basin-fill aquifers. In 10 basins, the source of arsenic was 'unknown', whereas 12 years later, Welch et al. (2000) identified Fe oxides as the predominant source and a combination of evaporative concentration and 'limited adsorption' as the likely cause.

Robertson (1989) presented data from 24 basins in Arizona with As concentrations > 50 ppb, and a maximum of 1300 ppb (Figure 9.2). The Basin-and-Range Province comprises N–S-trending fault blocks, where basin-fill alluvium is separated by linear ranges of Precambrian to Tertiary igneous and metamorphic rocks, and where geothermal activity is common. The basins have been greatly affected by subsidence, and are filled by Late Tertiary to recent fanglomerate deposits at the margins that pass laterally into silt, clay and sometimes evaporites in the basin centres. The alluvial sediments contain 2–88 mg/kg As, and are locally interbedded with volcanic layers.

The aquifers are recharged from three sources: by direct infiltration; by runoff from the adjacent ranges; and by leakage from regional rivers. Many

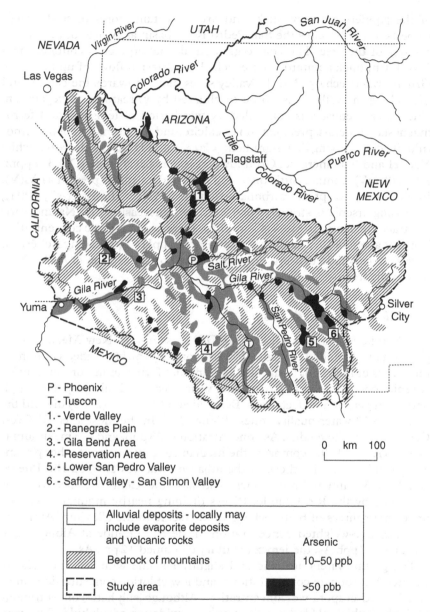

P - Phoenix
T - Tuscon
1. - Verde Valley
2. - Ranegras Plain
3. - Gila Bend Area
4. - Reservation Area
5. - Lower San Pedro Valley
6. - Safford Valley - San Simon Valley

0   km   100

	Alluvial deposits - locally may include evaporite deposits and volcanic rocks
	Bedrock of mountains
	Study area

Arsenic

| | 10–50 ppb |
| | >50 pbb |

Figure 9.2   Arsenic in the Basin-and-Range Province, Arizona. Arsenic is concentrated in fault-bounded basin-fill alluvial deposits, but locally also from springs in bedrock.
Source: Robertson (1989)

of the aquifers are very thick, and are important stores of fresh water. Robertson (1989) cites the San Pedro River basin as typical of the hydrogeology of the area. The coarse-grained alluvial aquifer is confined by a 100–400 m thick aquitard, where wells have artesian flows of up to 30 L/s. Groundwater recharged at the valley sides moves towards the centre, and then along the valley axis, to be discharged by phreatophytic vegetation. The water chemistry is controlled by weathering of feldspars and ferromagnesian minerals, precipitation of calcite, and the formation of montmorillonite clay. Moving down-gradient, Ca, Mg and HCO_3 all decrease, while Na, pH and F all increase. Groundwater is pervasively oxic (DO 3–7 ppm; Eh > 200 mV), contains little dissolved iron, and arsenic is present as As(V). In all basins, except the carbonate-rich Verde Valley (Foust et al., 2004), increasing arsenic is strongly correlated with increasing pH, Na and various trace elements (F, Mo, V, U and Pb). Increases in arsenic concentration began at about pH 7.5, and were pronounced at pH > 8.0, leading Robertson (1989) to conclude that arsenic was released by desorption of As(V) from iron oxyhydroxides.

The Middle Rio Grande Basin

The Middle Rio Grande Basin (MRGB) in semi-arid New Mexico occupies a fault-bounded trough, 150 km long by 50 km wide, containing thousands of metres of basin-fill alluvium that forms an important aquifer. Arsenic concentrations of >20 ppb are widespread, and values up to 600 ppb have been detected in deep wells. Bexfield and Plummer (2003) divided the basin into 13 water-quality zones (Figure 9.3). In the most affected (West Central) zone, the median As concentration is 23 ppb, and the maximum is 264 ppb As. Table 9.2 compares the median concentrations of other parameters in this zone with those in the adjacent, but less-affected Rio Puerco and East Mountain Front zones, and also the Central Zone, which is recharged by the Rio Grande. Rivers draining nearby mountains can be important sources of both recharge and arsenic to the alluvium. Although the discharge-weighted concentration in the Rio Grande at Albuquerque was only 1.7 ppb As, the Jemez tributary contained 12 ppb As.

The groundwaters are oxic and slightly alkaline with only moderately elevated bicarbonate concentrations, and low chloride concentrations indicate limited evaporative concentration. Although sulphate concentrations are high, the high pH is not consistent with oxidation of sulphides. The zone with the highest pH also had the highest Na:Ca ratio, suggesting a link with ion-exchange reactions. Most high As concentrations occur at pH > 8.4. Indeed, above pH 8.4, As concentrations of <20 ppb are rare (Figure 9.4), which led Bexfield and Plummer (2003) to attribute elevated arsenic to desorption from iron oxides. However, they also concluded that desorption

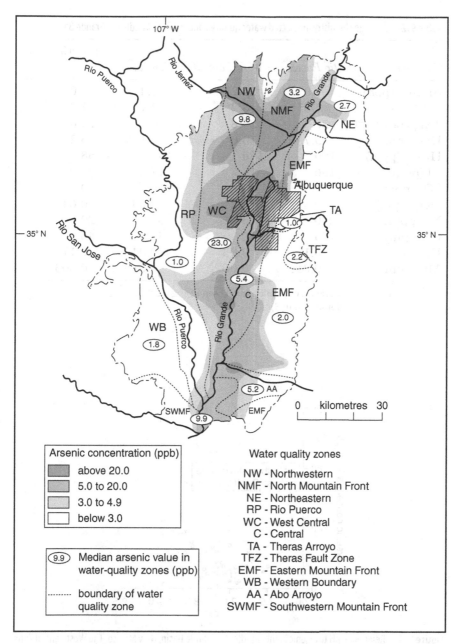

Figure 9.3 Water quality zones and arsenic distribution in the Middle Rio Grande Basin, New Mexico. *Source*: After Bexfield and Plummer (2003)

Table 9.2 Average chemistry in selected water quality zones* of the Middle Rio Grande Basin

Parameter	Rio Puerco	West Central	Central	East Mountain Front
Arsenic (ppb)	1.0	23.2	5.4	2.0
pH	7.5	8.2	7.7	7.7
Temperature (°C)	20.0	23.8	18.1	22.0
DO (ppm)	3.7	3.0	0.1	5.2
HCO_3 (ppm)	190	174	158	158
Cl (ppm)	186	13	17	23
SO_4 (ppm)	1080	92	66	390
NO_3 (ppm)	0.88	1.2	0.08	0.64
Na (ppm)	290	103	31	29
Ca (ppm)	135	12	43	45
Fe (ppm)	0.13	0.03	0.04	0.17
Mn (ppm)	0.015	0.002	0.015	0.003

*The locations of the water quality zones are shown in Figure 9.3.
Source: Bexfield and Plummer (2003)

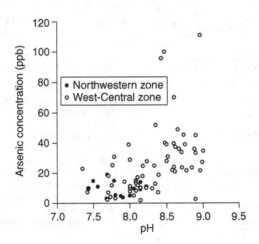

Figure 9.4 Relation of pH to arsenic in the Middle Rio Grande Basin, New Mexico. The West Central Zone is the most As-affected zone in the Rio Grande Basin. Note that although As concentrations are most elevated above pH 8.4, many wells produce water with >10 ppb at lower pH.
Source: Bexfield and Plummer (2003)

does not account for the widespread low-level arsenic in near-neutral water, which they attribute to the reaction of water infiltrating through geothermally altered rocks in the Jemez Mountains, and not mixing with geothermal water[8].

The Carson Desert

Shallow aquifers in the Carson Desert of Nevada contain high arsenic and uranium concentrations that impact on domestic supplies and a wildlife management area (Welch and Lico, 1998). During the Pleistocene, the area was covered by Lake Lahontan, which deposited thick silt that is overlain by permeable fluvial–deltaic sands, and finally by aeolian sands with interbedded volcanic ash beds (Figure 9.5). Sediments deposited in the distal part of the basin are finer grained and rich in organic matter. The sediments are derived from granitic and acid-volcanic rocks. Before the advent of irrigation, groundwater was recharged mainly by leakage from the Carson River, which contains 11 ppb As. In the west, groundwater flow is dominantly horizontal, but in the east flow is upward and discharges by evapotranspiration or leakage into lakes. Where flow is horizontal, total dissolved solids (TDS) range from 200 to 1000 ppm, but in the discharge zone TDS increase from 2000 to nearly 100,000 ppm. Groundwater contains little or no dissolved oxygen, and high DOC (10–100 ppm) but also hundreds of ppm of sulphate. Ferrous iron is mostly < 0.5 ppm, but manganese concentrations are often high. Arsenic, mainly present as As(V), increases from < 100 ppb to around 1000 ppb As in the saline zone, where uranium concentrations reach several hundred ppb. Evaporative concentration profoundly influences both the bulk chemistry and concentrations of arsenic (and uranium) but does not account for its initial presence. Welch and Lico (1998) used a mixing model (Figure 9.5) to deduce that at low chloride concentrations (<100 ppm) there is 'excess arsenic' due to RD of Fe(III) oxyhydroxides. However, at high chloride concentrations (>1,000 ppm) there is a 'deficiency' of arsenic that they attributed to increased adsorption at high salinity.

Owens Lake, California

Owens Lake area has not been a surface water body since the early 20th century, when diversion of stream flows to the Los Angeles aqueduct completely dried up the lake, and turned the former lake bed into a sink for the evaporative discharge of groundwater. The surrounding mountains are formed of marine and continental sediments, and intrusive and extrusive igneous rocks (Levy et al., 1999). Artesian wells are common, and produce groundwater that is slightly alkaline (pH 7.5–8.8), relatively fresh (EC 1300–3300 µS/cm), strongly enriched in sodium relative to calcium, and that contains significant sulphate. The artesian waters

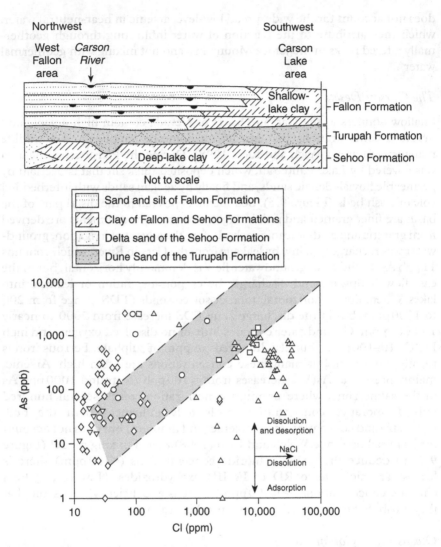

Figure 9.5 Relation between chloride and arsenic in groundwater in the southern Carson Desert, Nevada. (a) Cross-section through the Fallon–Carson Lake area. (b) Relationship between As and Cl. Upward pointing triangles represent upward-flowing water (in discharge areas); downward pointing triangles represent the Carson River; and diamonds the lateral-flow area. The shaded area shows the trends of evaporative concentration from two of the freshest waters. Because most plot below this range, it indicates that other reactions, such as adsorption or halite dissolution, must operate.
Source: Redrawn after Welch and Lico (1998)

contain up to a few hundred ppb of arsenic. Due to evaporation, shallow groundwater has evolved into high-alkalinity, high-pH brines that contain tens of ppm of fluoride and between a few ppm and 163 ppm As. Locally, saline waters contain > 130,000 ppm of chloride[9] and pH 9.1–9.8. Low calcium concentrations ensured that fluoride remained undersaturated with respect to the mineral fluorite, and the high pH inhibited adsorption of arsenic, and so both elements were concentrated by evaporation (Levy et al., 1999).

Albuquerque Water Supply

Albuquerque, the main city in the MRGB, pumps about 370 ML of groundwater a day, and has seen itself as at 'the forefront of the fight against the national arsenic standard' (NRDC, 2003). In 2005, water in the city supply had a mean concentration of 13 ppb As, but because it is drawn from many individual wells, concentrations in the distribution network vary widely (Figure 9.6). Although the US EPA 10 ppb standard came into effect in early 2006, the New Mexico Environmental Department granted Albuquerque an exemption until the end of 2008 to implement an Arsenic

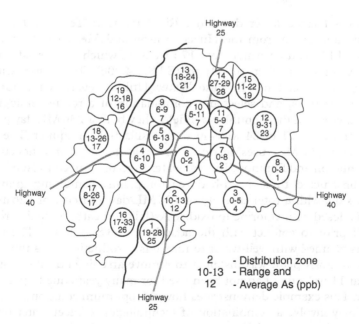

Figure 9.6   Distribution of arsenic in the Albuquerque water distribution system in 2005. The variability of arsenic in the distribution system reflects the distribution of arsenic in wells.
Source: CABQ (2005)

Compliance Strategy (ACS). Their reluctance to implement the lower standard appears to be a reaction to both the cost and the perceived (low) health impact[10] (NRDC, 2003). Indeed, the Water Utility Department only acknowledges ongoing research on the risks of low-level exposure (CABQ, 2005). Due to the characteristics of the aquifer, the cost implications were sensitive to the standard adopted. At 50 ppb, all city wells were compliant, and at 20 ppb, 79% would be in compliance, but this drops to 58% at 10 ppb and 31% at 5 ppb. CABQ (2005) estimated that complying with a 5 ppb standard would cost $190–380 m, and require doubling the water rate, although NRDC (2003) estimated the cost at $40–60 m. To comply with the new standard, Albuquerque is constructing an 11 ML/day arsenic removal plant, using coagulation and flocculation with ferric chloride followed by microfiltration, which was scheduled for completion in 2007 (CABQ, 2005). In addition, Albuquerque will receive an allocation of river water through the San Juan–Chama Diversion Project, which brings water from the Colorado River across the continental divide through 26 miles of tunnel, a solution far removed from what might be considered in most affected countries.

El Paso water supply

El Paso is located lower down the Rio Grande in Texas and relies on groundwater drawn from the Hueco Bolson and Mesilla Bolson alluvial aquifers. El Paso drew water from 175 wells, of which 46 were affected by As concentrations of up to 30 ppb (STSL, 2006). To comply with the January 2006 deadline, El Paso Water Utilities evaluated a range of treatment options, and selected a combination of three technologies for different areas. In the Canutillo wellfield, they built a 230 ML/day plant to treat water from 21 of 24 wells in the Mesilla Bolson aquifer. The plant, which cost $50 M[11], uses ferric chloride as a coagulant, flocculation, sedimentation and filtration. To treat water from the Hueco Bolson aquifer, they constructed three fixed-bed reactor plants, containing granulated ferric oxide, with a total capacity of 190 ML/day and cost of $26 m. Raw water is dosed with chlorine to oxidise As(III) and carbon dioxide reduces the pH prior to contact with the adsorbent (STSL, 2006). The treated water is blended with well-water to maximise production. At a third site, a reverse osmosis plant was installed to remove arsenic and other contaminants at 11 wells that had not been used for many years due to poor water quality. This example demonstrates how the optimum solution for a water utility may involve a combination of technologies to meet water demand that varies in space and time, to balance future and present costs, and to take account of different source-water qualities. Arsenic treatment at El Paso resulted in a 19% increase in the water rate, but was apparently accepted by rate-payers following an effective information campaign to gain support for the scheme (STSL, 2006).

9.2.5   Fluvio-glacial aquifers in mid-west USA and Canada

Regional data

Arsenic contamination is widespread in the glacial and fluvio-glacial aquifers that formed beneath and around the margins of the great ice sheets that built up over the present Hudson Bay–Great Lakes region. The sands and gravels that formed as glacial outwash often occupy deep buried valleys that form major aquifers. The outwash deposits may cut through, or be overlain by, thick tills that form aquitards[12]. The mid-west USA differs qualitatively from New England (section 9.2.6) in that the glacial deposits are thicker and more continuous, and confine the bedrock aquifers. Similar patterns of contamination extend into adjoining areas of Canada, such as Saskatchewan, where Thompson et al. (1999) found that 36% of 25 private wells contained > 10 ppb, and 8% > 50 ppb, with a recorded maximum of 117 ppb As. However, only 14% of public wells exceeded 10 ppb and none exceeded 50 ppb As. They estimated that several thousand private wells exceeded Canada's interim standard of 25 ppb As. In Michigan, Meliker et al. (2007) have inferred links between As exposure and heart, cerebrovascular and kidney diseases, and diabetes mellitus.

In the mid-west USA, contaminated wells mostly contain <100 ppb As, but occasionally >1000 ppb As. Matisoff et al. (1982) and Korte (1991) were the first to recognise that arsenic was derived from iron oxides under reducing conditions, though others (e.g. Kim et al., 2002; Kolker et al., 2003; Warner, 2001) have continued to emphasise the role of bedrock and oxidation of pyrite. Erickson and Barnes (2005a) demonstrated the influence of the glacial history advance on the occurrence of arsenic in groundwater by highlighting the difference in contamination between wells inside and outside the 'footprint' of the late Wisconsinan Drift (Table 9.3). Overall, wells inside the footprint are nearly five times more likely to be contaminated (see Figure 6.2). They also found a difference, albeit less dramatic, between the proportion of bedrock wells containing >10 ppb As inside (7%) and outside (3.5%) the Wisconsinan footprint. The Late Wisconsinan Drift is characterised by a fine-grained matrix, carbonate and shale clasts, and entrained organic carbon (Erickson and Barnes, 2005b). The abundance of organic matter is thought to be due to the incorporation of Pleistocene coniferous forests, soils and lake-sediments into the Des Moines lobe. The activity of organic matter is demonstrated by the presence of methane in

Table 9.3   Arsenic occurrence in glacial drift in relation to provenance in mid-west USA

	Public water supply wells			*Other wells*		
Wisconsinan Glaciation	*Number of wells*	*Average depth (m)*	*>10ppb (%)*	*Number of wells*	*Average depth (m)*	*>10ppb (%)*
Inside footprint	551	44	16.3	3724	27	33.1
Outside footprint	219	26	0.5	842	14	8.7

Source: Data from Erickson and Barnes (2005a)

water wells, and the greater degree of As contamination within the Wisconsinan footprint probably results from the higher organic matter content, a pattern comparable with pre- and post-LGM sediments in the Bengal Basin (Chapter 8). Erickson and Barnes (2005b) also drew attention to the frequently overlooked conclusion that 'high-arsenic sediment is not necessary to cause arsenic-impacted ground water'.

The Mahomet Buried Valley Aquifer

The development of the current explanation, a variation on the Bengal Basin model where alluvial sources are replaced by glacial ones, is illustrated by the different accounts of the Mahomet Buried Valley Aquifer (MBVA) in Illinois, where Warner et al. (2003) reported that 19% of 886 wells contained > 10 ppb As. The MBVA (Figure 9.7) comprises outwash deposits, tills and palaeosols with a complex geological history (Kelly et al., 2005). The main aquifer unit, the Illinoian-age Banner Formation, consists of up to 50 m of outwash sands resting directly on bedrock, and supplies 320 ML/day to 800,000 people (Warner, 2001). At the top of the Banner Formation is a discontinuous palaeosol which is overlain by the Illinoian Glasford Formation, comprising two tills with discontinuous sands near the base that support domestic wells and some community supplies. The Glasford Aquifer is thinner but more extensive than the Mahomet Aquifer, and has an organic-rich palaeosol at the top. The uppermost unit is the Wisconsinan Wedron Till. In the Mahomet Aquifer, groundwater flows from east to west and discharges into various rivers. In the east, the MBVA is underlain by Silurian dolomite and Devonian sediments, and in the west by Carboniferous sandstones, dark limestones and coal (Kelly et al., 2005).

Although Warner (2001) inferred a primary lithological control, noting median concentrations of 7.9 mg/kg in clay, 4 mg/kg in sand and gravel, and 21 mg/kg As in shale, this was challenged by Kirk et al. (2004) and

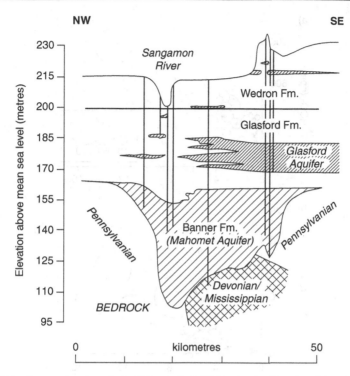

Figure 9.7   Cross-section through the Mahomet Buried Valley Aquifer. Note that although the surface formation (the Wedron Till) dates from the most recent (Wisconsinan) glaciation, the main affected aquifer (the Banner Formation) is of Illinoian age.
Source: Kelly et al. (2005)

Kelly et al. (2005). Arsenic is present predominantly as As(III), and As-affected groundwater has near-neutral pH with very low DO and sulphate concentrations (Figure 9.8). The mutual exclusivity of arsenic and sulphate is cited as reason to reject sulphide oxidation, and the pH suggests that desorption of arsenate would be insignificant. Groundwater also contains high concentrations of bicarbonate (500–750 ppm), iron (1–3 ppm) and DOC (0.5–16 ppm). Tritium dating indicates that the waters were recharged more than 50 years ago. Strong correlations of DOC with both ammonia and bicarbonate indicate microbial degradation of organic matter (Figure 9.8). Significant sulphate is only found when DOC is < 2 ppm, whereas significant methane concentrations are found only when DOC > 2 ppm (Kirk et al., 2004). High As concentrations are mainly confined to areas of less than 1 km in diameter. Thus, it appears that arsenic is mobilised by reductive dissolution of oxyhydroxides where the aquifer is in good vertical continuity with overlying palaeosols containing organic matter.

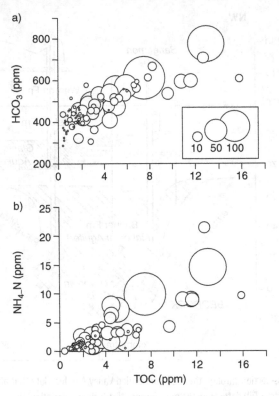

Figure 9.8   Relationships between As, total organic carbon (TOC), NH₄ and HCO₃ in the Mahomet Buried Valley Aquifer. The positive correlations between dissolved organic carbon (DOC), bicarbonate and ammonium characterise the decay of organic matter. The diameter of the circles represents arsenic concentration in ppb. *Source*: Kelly et al. (2005)

Sedimentary controls

The complexity of the MBVA is a warning against simplistic generalisations about glacial aquifers. Although the MBVA lies beneath the Wisconsinan footprint, neither the aquifer nor the palaeosols are of Wisconsinan age. Figure 9.9 illustrates the complexity of glacial drift aquifers using four scenarios from Michigan described by Szramek et al. (2004). In the Manistee and Kalamazoo areas, where coarse-grained outwash is in hydraulic continuity with the bedrock, no wells exceeded 10 ppb As. Conversely, in the Thumb Area, where there are extensive (organic-rich?) lake bed deposits, 70% of wells exceed 10 ppb As. In an intermediate condition at Huron there is a complex interlayering of outwash and till, and 10% of wells exceed 10 ppb As. In summary, the complex interplay of glacial and interglacial processes

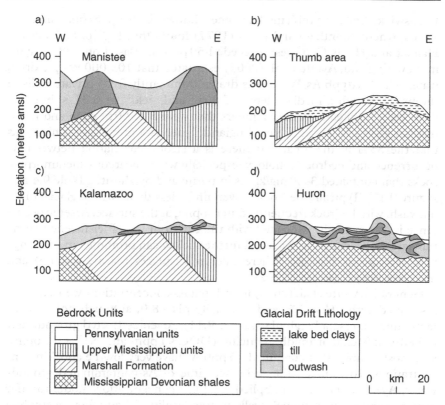

Figure 9.9 Hydrogeological cross-sections through drift deposits in Michigan. (a) At Manistee, where the drift is thickest and most permeable, no wells exceed 10 ppb As. (b) In the 'Thumb' area, bedrock is covered by thin and organic-rich low-permeability lake deposits where 70% of wells > 50 ppb. (c) At Kalamazoo, the drift is thin, permeable and uncontaminated. (d) In interbedded outwash and till at Huron, 10% of wells exceed 10 ppb.
Source: Szramek et al. (2004)

creates widespread reducing conditions in both drift and bedrock aquifers that provide a model for predicting As occurrence in other glaciated regions.

9.2.6 Bedrock aquifers in New England and Nova Scotia

Regional data

Arsenic-contaminated groundwater, at low to moderate concentrations, is widespread in crystalline bedrock in New England, Nova Scotia and New

Brunswick. Arsenic problems have been known in Nova Scotia since the 1970s, where Grantham and Jones (1977) found that 13% of 825 wells in Halifax and Hants Counties[13] exceeded 50 ppb As. Based on 888 analyses in New England, Ayotte et al. (2003) estimated that 103,000 people drink water with > 10 ppb As. Water was drawn dominantly from private wells in the bedrock with a median depth of 80 m and yield[14] of 0.3 L/s, but also from wells in unconsolidated aquifers that were 8 to 50 m deep and had a median yield of 19 L/s. In New England, igneous and metamorphic rocks underlie 85% of the area, and there is a strong correlation between As occurrence and bedrock lithology, especially with calcareous metamorphic rocks that contained 3–40 mg/kg As in pyrite and pyrrhotite (Table 9.4 and Figure 9.10). Typically, bedrock is overlain by less than 10 m of glacial till or outwash, with bedrock frequently outcropping at the surface. Arsenic occurrence is also spatially associated with the extent of Late Pleistocene marine transgressions, which as discussed further below can promote ion-exchange reactions during flushing (where calcium displaces marine sodium) and increases the pH (section 2.6.2).

Generally, Ayotte et al. (2003) found that As concentrations were strongly associated with pH > 7.5, and especially pH > 8.0, although not all contaminated waters had high pH (Figure 9.11). Arsenic-affected groundwater in bedrock is oxic or mildly reducing (DOC < 1 ppm and NH_4 < 0.1 ppm), and most samples that contained > 5 ppb As have very low Fe and Mn concentrations. To estimate the residence time of As-contaminated groundwater, Ayotte et al. (2003) applied a CFC[15] concentration model to infer ages of 3–50 years. Although wells in unconsolidated aquifers mostly had relatively high yields of low-As water, two wells were contaminated (10 and 48 ppb), and contained low DO and high DOC, Fe, Mn, NH_4 and CH_4 concentrations, strongly suggesting RD of iron oxides. In addition to the regional data of Ayotte et al. (2003), smaller scale studies found the following, broadly similar, characteristics.

Table 9.4   Relation of arsenic concentrations to lithology in New England

Aquifer type	Number of wells	Percentage of wells exceeding		
		10 ppb	20 ppb	50 ppb
Unconsolidated aquifers	175	3	3	1
Calcareous metamorphic rocks	215	21	9	2
Other metamorphic and igneous rocks	488	7	3	1

Source: Ayotte et al. (2003)

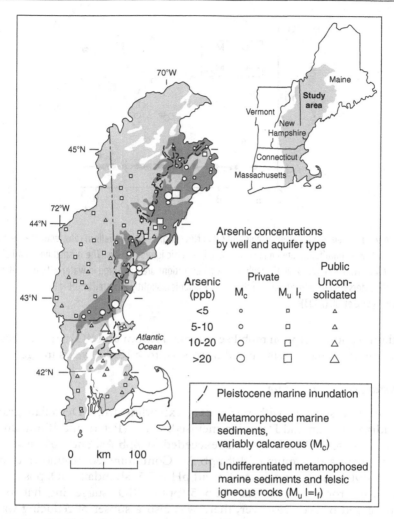

Figure 9.10 Distribution of arsenic concentrations in wells in eastern New England. The relation of this distribution should be compared with the As-risk map in Figure 6.3.
Source: Ayotte et al. (2003)

Nova Scotia and New Brunswick

In New Brunswick, arsenic is associated with iron oxide aggregations in a Carboniferous tuff, and in Nova Scotia with arsenopyrite in Lower Palaeozoic metasediments (Bottomley, 1984). In both areas, well yields were low, consistent with the estimated regional transmissivity of 2.5 m²/day (Nova Scotia). Most groundwaters were both alkaline and oxic, with pH≥8.0 accompanied by low DO and iron. Bottomley (1984) suggested that both

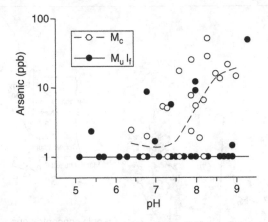

Figure 9.11   Relation between arsenic and pH in New England. M_c – wells in calcareous marine meta-sediments; M_u – undifferentiated metasediments; I_f – felsic igneous rocks. The dashed line is a LOWESS best-fit line. Note that although the highest As concentrations are measured in water with pH > 8, many high-pH waters contain low-As, and in other waters arsenic is slightly elevated at pH < 8.
Source: Ayotte et al. (2003)

oxidation and desorption mobilise arsenic. Tritium and ^{14}C dating indicated that contaminated waters ranged from < 10 to > 10,000 years in age.

Central New Hampshire

Arsenic is associated with pegmatites extending from Devonian granite intruding Silurian and Devonian metasediments (Peters and Blum, 2004). Here, 62% of 127 bedrock wells exceeded 10 ppb As, and 20% exceeded 50 ppb, with a maximum of 408 ppb As. Contaminated groundwater contained > 90% As(V) and generally had pH > 7.5, abundant DO, positive Eh values, low iron concentrations and 5–50 ppm of SO_4, suggesting that arsenic is mobilised by AD. However, there was also a subset of reducing waters that contained high iron concentrations with pH < 7, low DO, negative Eh and dominantly As(III), where arsenic is mobilised by RD.

Goose River Basin, Maine

Here, arsenic is associated with garnet-bearing granite and adjacent migmatites, pyritic schists and pegmatite veins (Sidle et al., 2001). Again, well yields are low, the highest being 2.5 L/s (Sidle, 2002). As in the other areas, the affected waters are generally oxic with positive Eh values and high DO (median 8.1 ppm), but the pH ranges widely (pH 6.2–8.2) and sulphate is much more abundant, typically 50–100 ppm. By measuring the ^{34}S contents of sulphate in groundwater and in arsenical pyrite, Sidle et al. (2001)

deduced that both the sulphate and arsenic were derived from oxidation of pyrite in the bedrock. Using tritium and krypton–85[16] isotopes, Sidle and Fischer (2003) inferred that the contaminated groundwater had been recharged since 1950.

Conclusion

In New England and Nova Scotia, bedrock lithology has an important influence on arsenic distribution, but multiple mobilisation mechanisms operate. The principal cause appears to be desorption from iron oxides at high pH, supplemented by the geochemical effects of pleistocene marine inundations. However, SO is also important, and locally RD mobilises arsenic in the drift. The thin or absent drift cover, the absence of organic carbon, and the stores of arsenic in sulphide and/or iron oxides provide an environment favourable for mobilising arsenic by either oxidation or desorption, depending on the local conditions.

Ayotte et al. (2003) showed that high As concentrations occur mainly at depths of between 50 and 120 m. Although drilling deeper is an option, it would be expensive, likely to be accompanied by lower yield, and with only a modest probability of success. Relocating wells might be an option for municipal supplies, but it is unlikely to be practical for private well owners. Hence point-of-use treatment may be the most economic solution for many private water supplies, especially where Fe and Mn concentrations are low.

9.2.7 Sandstone aquifers, eastern Wisconsin

Occurrence

Schreiber et al. (2000, 2003) presented a classic demonstration of arsenic mobilisation due to oxidation of sulphide minerals in the vicinity of a fluctuating water table. Although the area lies in the mid-west USA, As mobilisation is not controlled by the glacial history. In the Fox River valley, As concentrations up to 12 ppm have been recorded from a sequence of Cambrian to Ordovician sandstones and limestones. The critical element in this sequence is a mineralised zone called the Sulphide Cemented Horizon (SCH) that occurs at the contact between the St Peter Sandstone and the Sinnipee Group (Figure 9.12). The SCH is a layer of nodular sulphides, 20–60 cm thick, containing As-rich material bound to pyrite and marcasite (but not arsenopyrite), as well as in colloidal iron oxides. Sulphide mineralisation also occurs throughout the St Peter Sandstone, on average with < 10 mg/kg in the pink sandstone, around 90 mg/kg in the grey sandstone, and up to 585 mg/kg in the SCH. Contamination is not restricted to the

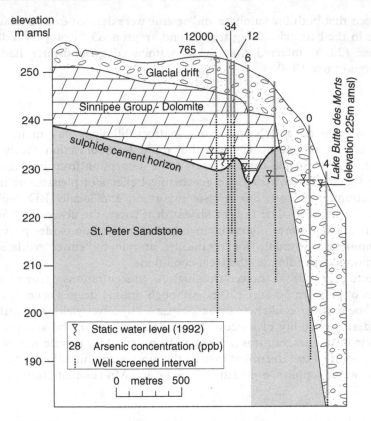

Figure 9.12   Hydrogeological section through Algoma Township, Wisconsin. Note that the open sections of the polluted wells are intersected by both the sulphide cemented horizon and the water table. *Source*: Redrawn after Schreiber et al. (2000)

small area described by Schreiber et al. (2003), as Zierold et al. (2004) reported that water from 20% of the more than 20,000 wells overlying the outcrop and subcrop of the St Peter Sandstone exceeded 10 ppb As.

Groundwater that is not impacted by arsenic is typically a Ca–Mg–HCO$_3$-type water with pH 7–8. Schreiber et al. (2000) showed that arsenic is mobilised where the open sections of wells, the SCH, and the zone of water table fluctuation all coincide (Figures 9.12 and 9.13). Conversely, where the SCH has been eroded, where it is permanently saturated or where the open sections of wells are tens of metres below the water table, high As concentrations are not encountered. They concluded that direct passage of air along the borehole is the most important pathway by which oxygen reaches the SCH. The Fox River study is a convincing example of how pyrite oxidation can cause high As concentrations due to a combination of natural and

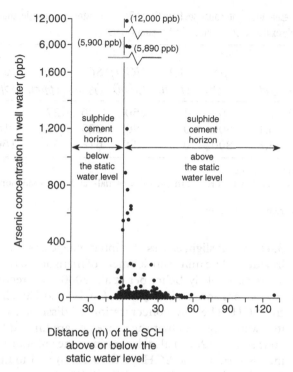

Figure 9.13 Relation between arsenic concentration, the sulphide cemented horizon (SCH) and the water table in eastern Wisconsin. Note that the extreme As concentrations are strongly concentrated in wells where the SCH lies within a few metres of the static water table.
Source: Redrawn after Schreiber et al. (2000)

pumping-induced water-table fluctuations, and yet the special conditions and distinct chemical signatures suggest that it is exceptional. In a later paper, Schreiber et al. (2003) identified low-level As contamination in low-SO_4, neutral-reducing waters in the confined section of the St Peter Sandstone that they attributed to RD.

Oxidation of the SCH produces a distinctive geochemical effect. The three water analyses in Table 9.5 approximate the 'before' (RW2), 'partial' (RW3) and 'after oxidation' (RW1) conditions. Despite the loss of bicarbonate, the total mineralisation is doubled, and can be accounted for by the increases in sulphate and iron. Although gypsum is present in overlying strata, this is discounted as a source of sulphate because of the small increase in calcium. The characteristic signatures are the massive iron concentration and the very low pH, both of which are rare in natural waters. After deducting the background sulphate concentration, the mass ratio of SO_4:Fe (3.7) is very close to

Table 9.5   Representative water analyses from the St Peter Sandstone, Wisconsin, showing the inferred impacts of sulphide oxidation on arsenic and other parameters

Well	As (ppb)	pH	EC (μS/ cm)	DO (ppm)	HCO₃ (ppm)	SO₄ (ppm)	Ca (ppm)	Fe (ppm)	Mn (ppm)
RW2	0.3	7.2	400	4	250	26	27	0.20	BDL
RW3	23	6.1	500	0.4	80	223	58	18	0.7
RW1	166	3.8	800	0	BDL	618	59	160	0.9

BDL, below detection limit
*Wells RW2, RW3 and RW1 represent the before-, partial-, and after-oxidation conditions respectively.
Source: After Schreiber et al. (2000)

that of pyrite (3.4); and the slight excess of sulphate suggests some precipitation of iron oxyhydroxides[17]. The minor enrichment of manganese further suggests that an oxide source is unlikely. Schreiber et al. (2000) also recorded that the contaminated waters are enriched in Zn, Cr, Co, Ni and Cu, all of which are abundant in the SCH. The low concentration of dissolved oxygen in the As-contaminated water suggests that the processes are limited by the supply of oxygen. Schreiber et al. (2003) also determined the sulphur isotope signature of the minerals forming the SCH ($\delta^{34}S$ –6.15‰) and found it was very close to that of sulphate in groundwater ($\delta^{34}S$ –6.48‰).

Health effects

As described in section 9.2.2, Zierold et al. (2004) and Knobeloch et al. (2006) investigated the possible health effects of arsenic in the St Peter Sandstone aquifer, finding that people drinking > 10 ppb As were significantly more likely to report a history of high blood pressure, heart attack, circulatory problems and bypass surgery than those people drinking < 2 ppb As. Dermatological symptoms and cancer were not assessed.

Mitigation

This type of As contamination requires hydrogeological expertise in constructing new wells, or possibly modifying existing wells[18]. Historical water-level fluctuations, plus a safety factor, should be used to define the depth of seasonal aeration. Wells should be redrilled and cased to below this depth, and the annular space grouted to the surface. Due to the highly aggressive groundwater close to the water table, the casing should be resistant to corrosion, and the grout should be based on bentonite or sulphate-resisting cement. From a regional perspective, water resource managers should try to ensure that, where possible, the SCH remains permanently saturated, and where not possible, the appropriate authorities, drillers and house owners should be informed.

9.2.8 Sandstone aquifers in Oklahoma and Pennsylvania

Central Oklahoma

Arsenic in the Central Oklahoma Aquifer is mobilised by desorption during flushing of Permian red-bed sandstones that contain up to 232 ppb As and elevated concentrations of chromium, selenium and uranium, all in the deeper and confined parts of the aquifer (Schlottman et al., 1998; Smith, 2005). Solid phase arsenic is concentrated in goethite-cemented sandstones. The groundwater is oxic, and arsenic > 10 ppb coincides with pH > 8.5. Arsenic pollution is strongly depth related. Most domestic and agricultural wells, which are < 100 m deep, are not affected, but arsenic is a common problem in municipal wells that are typically 180–250 m deep. A more detailed description of the hydrogeological controls of arsenic in the Central Oklahoma Aquifer is given in section 3.7.2.

Newark Basin, Pennsylvania

A similar occurrence of arsenic was reported by Senior and Sloto (2006) from Mesozoic sandstones in the Newark Basin in southeastern Pennsylvania, where As concentrations of up to 70 ppb As coexist with elevated concentrations of boron, fluoride, molybdenum, selenium, uranium, lithium and strontium. Arsenic was associated with pH≥8.0. It was found that arsenic and other trace elements were spatially associated with diabase (dolerite) intrusions, where there was a 20% probability of arsenic exceeding 10 ppb, compared with 10% in the basin as a whole. It was suggested that magmatic fluids associated with the intrusions had enriched the surrounding rocks in arsenic and other elements, from where they were subsequently mobilised by circulating groundwater.

9.2.9 The Willamette Basin, Oregon

The Willamette Basin occupies 31,000 km^2 of northwest Oregon between the Coastal and Cascade mountain ranges, and is home to 69% of the state's population. A 1962–63 survey of 174 wells found that in Lane County 30% of wells contained > 10 ppb, and 16% > 50 ppb As (Whanger et al., 1977).

More recently, Hinkle and Polette (1999) reported that 22% of 728 wells contained >10 ppb, and 8% > 50 ppb As. The maximum concentration was 2000 ppb, with six wells containing >1000 ppb As. Whanger et al. (1977) found elevated arsenic levels in blood, hair, nails and urine to confirm the uptake of arsenic. They found little evidence of acute toxicity, but did find evidence of chronic poisoning in the form of anaemia, and vascular and dermatological ailments. However, there was no relationship with skin cancer. The diagnosis was supported by the relief of symptoms when the source of drinking water was changed.

The Coastal Range is formed of marine sediments and volcanics, while the Cascade Range is predominantly volcanic. Conlon et al. (2005) described the hydrogeology of the alluvial Willamette Basin, as summarised in Table 9.6.

Table 9.6   Hydrostratigraphy of the Willamette Basin, Oregon

Hydrostratigraphic Unit	Age	Hydrogeology
HCU, High Cascade Unit	Holocene	unconfined aquifer on summits of Cascade Range; discharges to mountain streams (K = 30–300 m/day).
USU, Upper Sedimentary Unit	Late Pleistocene – Holocene	unconfined sand and gravel aquifer in lowlands; ≤15 m thick in valley centre (K = 60 m/day).
WSU, Willamette Silt	Pleistocene	Aquitard; separates the USU and MSU
MSU, Middle Sedimentary Unit	Pleistocene	Confined, weakly cemented, sand and gravel aquifer (K = 0.01–100 m/day).
LSU, Lower Sedimentary Unit	Plio-Pleistocene	mudstone and cemented sand and gravel aquifer (K = <10 m/day).
CRBU, Columbia River Basalt Unit	Miocene	Aquifer, basalt lavas with permeable interflow horizons (K = 0.001–100 m/day).
BCU, Basal Confining Unit	Eocene	marine sediments; volcanics and volcaniclastics (Fischer and Eugene formations) (K = <0.01 m/day).

Source: Conlon et al. (2005)

Most abstraction, of which 81% is used for irrigation, is drawn from the USU and MSU in the lowlands (Conlon et al., 2005). The USU and MSU, however, cover only a small proportion of the area of the Willamette Basin, although they are found close to the main centres of population.

Whanger et al. (1977) and Hinkle and Polette (1999) both reported that high As concentrations were spatially associated with outcrops of both the Fischer and Eugene Formations. Comparing the As-mapping of Hinkle and Polette (1999) with the As mapping of Conlon et al. (2005), it is observed that many of the most contaminated wells are located where the Upper Sedimentary Unit (USU) and/or Middle Sedimentary Unit (MSU) are present, but are also close to the outcrops of the Fischer and Eugene Formations. Further research is required to determine the relative importance of bedrock and alluvium as sources of arsenic.

Arsenic-rich groundwater is characterised by a high ratio of Na to Ca+Mg, high pH, and by high concentrations of boron and phosphate. However, the concentrations of TDS, sulphate and chloride were highly variable. Hinkle and Polette (1999) found that arsenic was poorly correlated with well depth, and also ruled out anthropogenic sources. Speciation measurements in five samples ranged between 68% and 100% of As(III), implying reducing conditions. Hinkle (1997) reported that four samples with As > 50 ppb had low DO and variable concentrations of phosphate (0.36–2.0 ppm) and iron (0.16–1.9 ppm). Arsenic in hot-springs further complicates interpretation of the data. In summary, the chemical associations suggest the possibility of AD similar to volcanic-loessal aquifers in South Dakota[19] and Argentina, but it is unclear how important this process is compared to reductive-dissolution and geothermal activity.

9.2.10   Mineralised granitic rocks, Washington State, USA

Frost et al. (1993) reported As poisoning from well-water around Granite Falls, in an area mined for gold, silver, lead and arsenic until the early 20th century. In 1985, a patient was diagnosed with arsenic poisoning that was traced to a dug well containing 7 ppm As. A survey of 400 wells found that 70 (18%) contained >50 ppb, with As concentrations as high as 25 and 33 ppm As. Monthly sampling of 26 wells for a year showed that concentrations varied by factors of between 1 and 19, and four of the wells fluctuated about the 50 ppb standard. Although the cause, which is probably SO, cannot be determined from this evidence alone, the observations have two general implications. First, in bedrock aquifers, very shallow dug wells may pose a higher risk than drilled wells (the opposite of what is observed in alluvial aquifers). Second, single measurements of shallow wells in bedrock may be insufficient, because of seasonal fluctuations, to characterise the As risk.

9.2.11   Metamorphic bedrock, British Columbia, Canada

Bowen Island, northwest of Vancouver, is formed of Jurassic metasediments and metavolcanics, intruded by Late Jurassic granodiorite and monzonite plutons. Boyle et al. (1998) found that 60% of wells drilled into bedrock exceeded 10 ppb As, and 44% exceeded 50 ppb, with a maximum of 580 ppb As. Within the As-affected area, bedrock is cut by veins containing pyrite, arsenopyrite and copper. Where mineralisation is located near the surface, bedrock has been weathered to limonite and clay by percolating ground-waters. During the Pleistocene, the area was covered by about 1500 m of ice, which depressed the land so much that when the ice first melted 13,000 years ago, the island was inundated by the sea. It is estimated that the land that is now Bowen Island was submerged by as much as 150 m, but due to isostatic rebound the area has been land for about 9000 years.

The chemistry of groundwater on Bowen Island is controlled by the hydrolysis of silicate minerals, generating sodium-bicarbonate waters with elevated pH (7.4–8.9) and silica. The dominance of sodium is partly due to ion-exchange, where calcium and magnesium exchange with sodium that was adsorbed onto clays when the island was submerged by the sea. Most waters contain 10–200 ppm of sulphate, low iron (<0.3 ppm) with arsenic predominantly present as As(V), indicating that the water is either oxic or mildly reducing. Increasing concentrations of arsenic are broadly correlated with increasing pH and concentrations of alkalinity, sodium and silica. Lithium, boron and fluoride are also positively correlated with arsenic, but calcium is inversely related to arsenic. For these reasons, Boyle et al. (1998) concluded that desorption from iron oxides was the most likely explanation for As contamination on Bowen Island. However, RD may account for a small subset of samples with high Fe and Mn concentrations, and where As(III) is dominant.

Northwest of Bowen Island, Hall (2005) reported contamination on the Sunshine Coast (52% of 258 samples >10 ppb As) and at Powell River (20% of 199 wells >10 ppb). In both areas, a few wells exceeded 1000 ppb As, and contaminated waters also contained high levels of fluoride and boron. Again, arsenic was associated with granitic bedrock and past volcanic activity. Wells >20 m deep had higher As concentrations, mainly present as As(V). Hall (2005) indicated that, depending on the pH, SO_4, Fe and Mn concentrations, treatment would be the most appropriate mitigation, but did not specify which methods.

9.2.12 Alaska

Fairbanks

Fairbanks is located in the valley of the River Tanana, a tributary of the Yukon, which has long been associated with mining, and as Welch et al. (2000) commented 'oxidation of arsenopyrite associated with gold ore is an obvious source'. While this is one cause of pollution, a re-examination of the data of Mueller et al. (2002) indicates a more complicated pattern, where arsenic is present in at least five geochemical associations. Their 1999–2000 survey showed that 38% of well-waters exceeded 10 ppb As. This is a serious problem in itself, but the statistical distribution of results (Table 9.7) is unusual in that it is bimodal, where well-water tends to be either very good or very bad. However, no clinical symptoms of As poisoning have been reported (Pershagen, 1983).

Fairbanks is located in the 'Yukon–Tanana Terrane' of multiply deformed and metamorphosed Palaeozoic and Precambrian rocks. The main unit, the Fairbanks Schists Group, consists of quartzite and garnet-mica schists, and is succeeded by Devonian volcanics and intruded by Carboniferous gneisses. These units are locally intruded by Cretaceous granites, and subsequently covered by Tertiary basalts. The area is intensely mineralised, most importantly by Au–Sb–As ore in quartz veins associated with Cretaceous granites. The gold also occurs as placer deposits in the alluvium. Bedrock is exposed only intermittently, being extensively covered by Quaternary loess and fluvio-glacial deposits. The main aquifers are formed of lowland alluvium consisting of interlayered gravel and loess. However, fractured bedrock

Table 9.7 Arsenic concentrations in groundwater around Fairbanks, Alaska

As (ppb)	Number of samples	Percentage of samples
<1	65	56.0
1–10	7	6.0
10–50	7	6.0
50–200	4	3.4
200–500	16	13.8
>500	17	14.7

Source: Mueller et al. (2002)

controls groundwater flow in the upper valleys and highland areas. Fractured-rock aquifers also discharge to the alluvium in the valley bottoms, and may be partly geothermal (Mueller et al., 2001), but there is little direct evidence for an association between arsenic and geothermal waters. High-As waters have temperatures in the range 3–7°C and, with a single exception, the warmer waters (up to 21°C) contain low As concentrations. At Fairbanks, five groups of high-As groundwaters can be identified[20].

1   High chloride waters, with Cl of 90 ppm against a background of < 10 ppm. Arsenic concentrations are very high (1376 ppb As) and fluoride (1.1 ppm F) concentrations are also slightly elevated. The water is near-neutral (pH 7.1–7.4) and anoxic, having no nitrate or sulphate but very high Fe concentrations (10.7 ppm) and high alkalinity (400 ppm).
2   High manganese waters, averaging 5 ppm, as against a background of <1 ppm, very high As (1080 ppb) but low Fe (0.06 ppm) concentrations. Groundwater is subneutral (pH 6.3–6.6) and has a trace of dissolved oxygen but high nitrate (170 ppm N) and sulphate (90 ppm SO_4).
3   High antimony waters, with 50–60 ppb Sb, and high (274 ppb) As concentrations. Groundwater is near-neutral (pH 7.1–7.5) and oxic, with high DO (14 ppm) and significant nitrate (4 ppm). Fe and Mn concentrations, however, are very low. Alkalinity is relatively low (142 ppm) and chloride negligible (1 ppm).
4   High sulphate (700 ppm) waters, with >200 ppb As. Groundwater is near-neutral (pH 6.7–7.1) and oxic, with significant DO (2 ppm) and nitrate (9 ppm). Fe concentrations are high (1.7 ppm) but variable, while Mn is low (0.1 ppm).
5   Type 5 waters have distinct groupings on many graphs, and are characterised by high As (300–400 ppb), alkalinity (628 ppm) and EC (1040 μS/cm). Groundwater is near-neutral (pH 6.7–7.3) with negligible DO and nitrate but significant sulphate (40 ppm) concentrations. Iron is very variable (0.4–18 ppm), and manganese is only slightly elevated (0.22 ppm).

The diversity of water types, shown in Figure 9.14, illustrates the complexity that can arise in some geological settings. Each type probably has a distinct origin or geological association. It is difficult to identify all the processes responsible, but it appears that desorption (maximum pH 7.8; 96% <pH 7.5) plays little or no role. The high-antimony and high-sulphate groups (Types III and IV) probably involve SO. Although elevated chloride is often associated with geothermal arsenic (Webster and Nordstrom, 2003), it appears that arsenic in both Type I and Type V waters is released by RD The high-manganese group (Type II) is particularly unusual, not least because the waters have both high bicarbonate and sulphate concentrations[21]. Nordstrom et al. (2006) confirmed the strong influence of shear zones rich

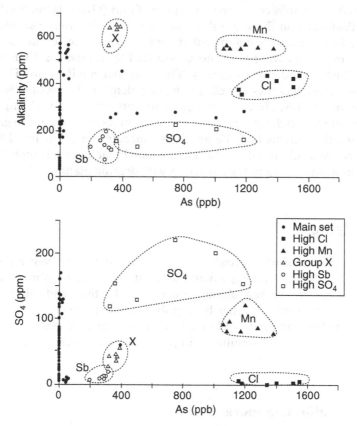

Figure 9.14   Relation of arsenic to sulphate, and bicarbonate in Fairbanks, Alaska. Groundwater conditions in the Fairbanks are highly complex, with at least six water types present and multiple mobilisation processes operating.
Source: Data from Mueller et al. (2002)

in arsenopyrite and scorodite on aqueous arsenic. The major ion chemistry is dominated by increases in bicarbonate up to the saturation concentrations of calcite and dolomite, as a result of rock weathering. High As concentrations are found mainly in waters with high bicarbonate. Although Nordstrom et al. (2006) concluded that reducing conditions, organic decomposition and high HCO_3 are important in mobilising arsenic, other factors including anthropogenic sources of nitrate (fertiliser) mobilise arsenic locally.

Cook Inlet

More than half the population of Alaska live around the Cook Inlet. On the Kenai Peninsula, 8% of 312 wells exceeded 50 ppb, with a maximum of

150 ppb As, and 46% contained > 0.3 ppm of iron (Glass, 1996, 2001). The Kenai Peninsula, on the south shore of Cook Inlet, is a major sedimentary basin and source of oil, gas and coal. It contains 6000 m of Tertiary sediment and 200 m of Quaternary sediment, bounded by Jurassic and Cretaceous metasediments and metavolcanics. The principal aquifers are Holocene alluvium in which domestic wells can be completed at depths of < 30 m and yield up to > 60 L/s. Here, streambed sediments contain 5 to 44 mg/kg As. Peat and organic-rich soils contribute colour and organic matter to ground-water, which contains high Fe and Mn concentrations, but low DO and nitrate concentrations. Glass (2001) concluded that arsenic is mobilised by RD of iron oxides due to their reaction with organic matter.

9.3   Mexico

Arsenic pollution is widespread in Mexico (Figure 9.1). However, there are few descriptions concerning either the distribution or environmental asso-ciations of arsenic. There is abundant geothermal activity and sulphide min-eralisation, and from what has been published, it is recognised that pollu-tion occurs both naturally and as a result of centuries of mining activities, and that it has caused significant impacts on groundwater, surface water and air quality.

9.3.1   Región Lagunera

Del Razo et al. (1990) estimated that 400,000 people were exposed to >50 ppb As in the Región Lagunera of Durango and Coahuila States in northern Mexico, while Parga et al. (2005) suggested that two million people were 'at risk' of As poisoning. Del Razo et al. (1990) reported that 50% of 129 wells exceeded > 50 ppb As, with a maximum of 624 ppb As. Del Razo et al. (1993) also showed that 19% of wells contained > 1.5 ppm of fluoride, with a maximum of 3.7 ppm F, and that fluoride and As concen-trations were positively correlated. Symptoms of arsenicosis were identified in 21% of the exposed population of Región Lagunera, the main effects being skin pigmentation, keratosis, Bowen's disease (5.1%), skin cancer (1.4%), peripheral vascular disease (4%) including Blackfoot Disease (0.7%), and gastrointestinal illness (Cerbrián et al., 1983). Examining arsenic levels in food and water, Del Razo et al. (1990) concluded that food makes an equal contribution of arsenic to adult dietary intake (see Chapter 5). Región Lagunera is also an important area for dairy cattle, and Armienta (2003) reported that cow's milk contained up to 27.4 µg/kg, with 10% of samples exceeding the recommended limit[22] of 10 μg/kg As. Although local alfalfa contained up to 316 μg/kg As, it was considered that water was the main source of arsenic in milk.

Few geological details are available, though Ortega-Guerrero (2004) reported that groundwater is oxic, and that elevated arsenic is found mainly in granular aquifers, but is also found in the underlying carbonate aquifer. Discussing the origin of high As concentrations, he indicated that contamination is associated with pyrite in the recharge area, but that evaporation increases the As concentrations. Little information is available on mitigation, but Armienta (2003) reported that, since 1988, 70% of the population of the region have been provided with better quality water. Parga et al. (2005) described an innovative approach to arsenic removal using electrocoagulation, which removed more than 99% of the As(III) and As(V) present (Chapter 7).

9.3.2   Zimapán Valley, central Mexico

The Zimapán Valley, an important mining region in Hidalgo State, is the best-documented case of arsenic pollution in Mexico (Armienta et al., 1997, 2001; Morse, 2001). Pollution was first detected in 1992 during a survey to find the source of a cholera outbreak, when it was found that more than half the wells contained > 50 ppb As. Armienta (2003) estimated that most of the 12,000 people were still exposed to concentrations of up to 250 ppb As, and had been drinking this water for at least 15 years. Arsenic uptake by humans was confirmed by analysis of hair samples. Of 120 exposed persons examined, only 19% showed no arsenical skin manifestations. Of the remainder, 20% displayed hypopigmentation, 13% hyperpigmentation, 21% both hypo- and hyperpigmentation, and 26% had hyperkeratosis.

The Zimapán Valley is underlain by Mesozoic limestones and Quaternary volcanics, covered by the Zimapán fanglomerate and Quaternary alluvium (Figure 9.15). Mineralisation is related to a quartz-monzonite[23] intrusion, and is concentrated at its margins and along dykes emanating from it. The ore bodies are massive sulphide deposits containing pyrite, pyrrhotite, sphalerite, galena, chalcopyrite, arsenopyrite and other lead, antimony and bismuth minerals. Deeper wells generally penetrate the limestone, while shallow drilled wells and dug wells draw water from the unconfined fanglomerate aquifer. Armienta et al. (2001) analysed water from 60 shallow and deep wells and springs, of which 45% exceeded 50 ppb As, and the highest (in limestone) contained 1100 ppb As. The analyses in Table 9.8 show that alluvial groundwater is dominated by sodium, while the fanglomerate

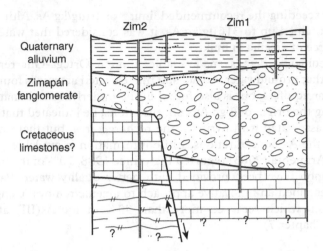

Figure 9.15 Hydrostratigraphic section through the Zimapán aquifer system, Mexico. The dashed line represents the water table or piezometric surface. Elevated arsenic is found in all the units, but tends to be higher in deeper wells and in the limestone.
Source: After Armienta et al. (2001)

and limestone aquifers are dominated by calcium. Both chloride and sulphate concentrations are highest in the alluvium, which suggests that (locally) it does not act as a conduit for recharging the limestone. Although water in the limestone has lower redox potential than the other units, the low iron concentrations and persistence of sulphate confirm that it is not strongly reducing.

The highest As concentrations are generally in oxic groundwater in deep wells. Waters that contain > 1 ppm Fe also have low As contents. Groundwater has moderate to very high sulphate concentrations, although the correlation between arsenic and sulphate is weak. Armienta et al. (1997) identified three sources of arsenic: natural oxidation of As-bearing minerals; leaching of tailings; and percolation through dry deposition of smelter fumes. As regards mobilisation, RD can be ruled out because of the oxic conditions, and the absence of a correlation with either temperature or chloride makes a geothermal source unlikely. Although arsenic is not strongly correlated to either elevated pH[24] or sodium enrichment, two of the five samples with pH > 8.0 contain > 100 ppb As. Hence, the principal mobilisation mechanism appears to be SO, where the characteristic acidity has been buffered by the carbonate aquifer. Rodriguez et al. (2004) suggested that sulphides are oxidised when the water table falls in the dry season, and mobilised when it rises again in the rainy season[25]. Based on batch experiments, Romero et al. (2004) suggested that migration of As(V) is limited

Table 9.8 Chemical analyses of selected wells in the Zimapán aquifer system

Aquifer	Sample	As (ppb)	Eh (mV)	T (°C)	pH	HCO₃ (ppm)	SO₄ (ppm)	Cl (ppm)	F (ppm)	Na (ppm)	K (ppm)	Ca (ppm)	Mg (ppm)	Fe (ppm)
Alluvium	Tule Manan	19	ND	21.0	6.96	385	111	20	–	41	3.7	97	38	1.2
	SAN	54	ND	23.8	7.17	345	257	48	0.56	122	5.6	175	52	0.1
Fanglomerate	SJ02	BDL	582	29.8	7.53	385	18	7	0.78	30	1.1	60	30	0.92
	T. Col	36	454	22.6	6.88	304	31	6	0.34	14	1.7	78	9	0.05
	Zim3	57	408	21.5	7.06	404	20	10	0.36	14	1.5	115	13	BDL
Tamaulipas (limestone)	Zim1	BDL	376	20.0	7.55	280	32	3	0.3	30	2.3	54	14	BDL
	Zim2	526	147	29.0	7.82	271	62	4	0.66	10	1.7	87	13	0.45
	Muhi	1000	154	29.8	7.37	265	87	4	2.1	35	4.2	70	14	0.22

ND, not determined; BDL, below detection limit.
Source: Armienta et al. (2001)

by adsorption onto hydrous ferric oxides, coprecipitation of complex Ca-arsenates and adsorption onto calcite.

9.3.3   Other regions

Wyatt et al. (1998) described extensive pollution of public water supplies by arsenic and heavy metals in the state of Sonora in northwest Mexico, reporting average As concentrations at 29 townships across the state. The water supply to three towns or cities exceeded 50 ppb (the maximum being at Magdalena, with 117 ppb As), and in 19 (66%) townships the supply exceeded 10 ppb As. Many of the supplies contained elevated concentrations of fluoride, which was positively correlated with arsenic. Mercury (> 1 ppb Hg) was also detected in supplies to 13 towns. The association with fluoride, together with its proximity to the Basin-and-Range Province (section 9.1.4), suggest that AD may be responsible, however, further investigations are required.

In the Rio Verde river basin in San Luis Potosi of central Mexico, Planer-Friedrich et al. (2001) reported As concentrations of up to 54 ppb in Tertiary–Quaternary basin-fill deposits, bounded by carbonate and acid-volcanic rocks. Arsenic is present dominantly as As(V), and groundwater is subneutral (pH 6.7–7.2). Positive correlations of arsenic with, *inter alia*, Ca, Mg, Na, K, Cl, F and SO_4 point to evaporative concentration, although the original mobilisation mechanism was not identified.

Cano-Aguillera et al. (2004) reported natural occurrence of arsenic in groundwater in the Guanajuato Mining District, once one of the major silver producers in the world. Both here, and in the San Antonio–El Triunfo mining district, the millions of tonnes of low-grade ore and mine waste, accumulated over hundreds of years, threaten important aquifers (Carrillo-Chávez et al., 2000; Romero et al., 2006).

9.4   Europe

9.4.1   Introduction

The distribution of arsenic in groundwater in Europe (Table 9.9 and Figure 9.16) is complex, and there is no characteristic pattern as observed in Asia or South America. The greater diversity of As contamination recognised in Europe is probably a reflection of the intensity of testing, and the number of research organisations. By far the most important occurrence is beneath the Great Hungarian Plain, but many are at a very low level and might have

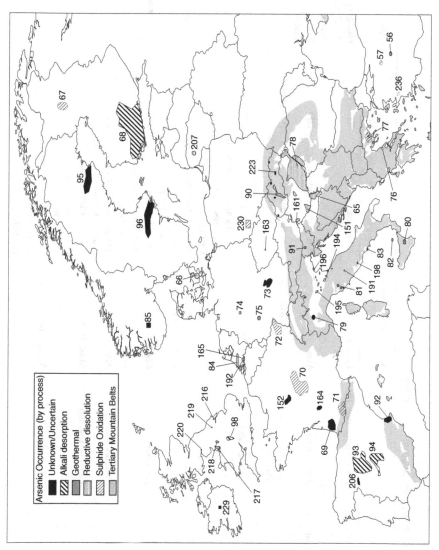

Figure 9.16 Locations of arsenic in groundwater in Europe. See Table 1.2 for explanation of map numbers.

Table 9.9 Case histories of arsenic occurrence in Europe

Country/region	Name	Arsenic (ppb)[†] (mean/range/max.)	Geology, hydrology, climate	Water chemistry	Affected population/significance[*]
Hungary, Romania, Croatia	Great Hungarian Plain	17% > 50; Max. 4000	Alluvium; temperate	RD	Hungary: 500,000 (E50); Croatia: 200,000 (E10)
Belgium, Germany and Netherlands	Rhine delta	Max. 38	Alluvium; temperate	RD	None known (water treated)
Finland	Southwest Finland (Pirkanmaa)	17% > 10; Max. 2230	Precambrian igneous and metamorphic rock; temperate	AD (+SO?)	
N. Finland	Finnish Lapland	Max. 35	Precambrian igneous and metamorphic rock; sub-arctic	AD	
Sweden	Uppsala	4% > 10; Max. < 300	Crystalline bedrock; temperate	?	
Norway		1% > 10; Max. 19	Crystalline bedrock; temperate	?	
Denmark	Fensmark	Max. 30	Glacial outwash over limestone; temperate	RD?	None known (water treated)
Lithuania		Max. 33	Temperate	?	
Poland	Sudetes Mts	Max. 140	Temperate, Palaeozoic mudstone and sandstone	SO	
Czech Republic	Celina-Mokrsko	Max. 1500	Precambrian volcano-sedimentary rocks; temperate	SO	
Germany	Wiesbaden	Max. >100	Geothermal, Palaeozoic metamorphic rocks; temperate	GT	

Country	Region	Concentration	Geology; climate	Mechanism	Exposure
Germany	Bavaria	Max. 150	Triassic red-bed sandstones; temperate	?	None known (water treated at 60 public sources)
England	Midlands	15% > 10; 0% > 50	Triassic red-bed sandstones; temperate	?	None known (water treated at 17 public sources)
England	Northwest	11.5% > 10; 1.6% > 50; Max. 263	Triassic red-bed sandstones; temperate	AD?	None known
France	Massif Central, Vosges and Pyrenees	Max. 100	Crystalline and granitic rocks; temperate	GT and SO	200,000 (E10); 17,000 (E50)
Spain	Duero Basin	Max. 290	Tertiary sediments; Mediterranean	AD	
Spain	Madrid Basin	Mean 25; Max. 91	Tertiary sediments; Mediterranean	AD	
Southern Italy	Active volcanic regions	Max. 6,390	Geothermal; Mediterranean	GT	
Central Italy	Tiber valley	Max. 52	Alluvium; Mediterranean	AD?	
Northern Italy	Siena	8% > 10; Max. 14	Geothermal; Mediterranean	GT	
Northern Italy	Po Delta	21% > 10; 3% > 50 Max. 1340	Alluvium; temperate	RD	
Switzerland	Malcantone watershed	Max. 300ppb	Fluvio-glacial alluvium; temperate	RD and SO	Total population 5000
Slovenia	Tertiary basin	Max. 589 Mean 12;	Geothermal; temperate	GT	
Greece	Thessalonika	Max. 125	Hydrothermally altered metamorphic rocks	SO	5000

AD, alkali desorption; RD, reductive dissolution; SO, sulphide oxidation; GT, geothermal.

*E10 refers to the number of people drinking water with >10ppb As, and E50 to drinking more than 50ppb As. Where exposure has changed over time, the peak figure is quoted.

†Concentrations normally refer to untreated water sources, either wells, streams or lakes, but not piezometers.

gone unreported in other parts of the world. The earliest report of arsenic poisoning from well-water, and one that produced skin cancer, came from Poland in 1898 (Mandal and Suzuki, 2002), while an even earlier determination was made at Wiesbaden Spa by Fresenius in 1885 (Schwenzer et al., 2001), although apparently this water did not cause illness.

9.4.2   Danube Basin: Hungary, Romania, Slovakia and Croatia

Exposure and health impacts

Hungary and the adjoining areas of Romania, Slovakia and Croatia constitute the most severely As-affected region in Europe. Exposure estimates differ, but Csalagovitis (1996) suggested that, at its peak, As affected 0.5 M people in Hungary, while Habuda-Stanić et al. (2007) report that 200,000 are still exposed to >10 ppb in Croatia[26]. He reported that, in the 1800 communities for which data were available, arsenic (>50 ppb As) affected 295 communities in a semi-continuous area in the Bekes Basin, Sarret, and the southern part of the Danube–Tisza interfluve (see Figures 9.19 and 9.20). He also noted that there were no data for 36% of Hungary. It is not known when exposure started, but most public supplies have been in operation since before 1940. Older wells, some in use for over 100 years, have similar As concentrations to modern wells, but some hydrogeologists suggest that concentrations have increased over time (Csanady et al., 2005). However, the working assumption is that the present population has been exposed to similar arsenic levels since birth. Until 1983, some wells had concentrations as high as 4000 ppb As (Mandal and Suzuki, 2002).

Varsányi et al. (1991) examined mortality due to all causes and deaths due to cardiovascular disease and cancer, in two groups of 16,000 people from six high-As (>50 ppb) and six low-As villages. The results (Table 9.10), which they considered controversial, did not show a statistically significant difference in overall mortality between the high- and low-As groups. However, the deaths due to cardiovascular disease were significantly higher in males, although significantly lower in females. For deaths due to cancer, there was no difference in men, but a significantly higher death rate in women.

Between 1971 and 1987, Börzsönyl et al. (1992) conducted epidemiological studies on 25,648 people in southeast Hungary who had drunk contaminated well-water throughout their lives, and compared them with 20,836 people from a nearby area who had drunk low-As water. Arsenic concentrations in hair were correlated with arsenic in water, confirming long-term exposure. Many cases of hyperkeratosis and hyperpigmentation

Table 9.10   Analysis of mortality in the arsenic-affected area of Hungary

As (ppb)		SMR: all causes of death		SMR: cardio-vascular disease		SMR: cancer	
Class	Range	Male	Female	Male	Female	Male	Female
>50	55–137	131	79	129	77	120	109
<50	4–38	124	76	108	94	118	61

SMR, standardised mortality ratio.
Source: Varsányi et al. (1991)

were found in both adults and children in the contaminated area. Serious vascular diseases such as Blackfoot Disease were not identified, and there were no significant differences between the exposed and control populations with respect to cancer, peripheral neuropathy or peripheral vascular disorders. However, they did find significantly higher incidences of spontaneous abortions and stillbirths in the exposed population. Expressed in terms of each 10,000 live births, the rate of spontaneous abortions was 696 as against 511, and the rate of stillbirths was 77 compared with 28 in the low-As area.

Geology

The affected area lies on the Great Hungarian (or Central Danubian) Plain, which forms part of the Pannonian Basin, and covers 100,000 km² with an average elevation of about 100 m a.s.l. The geology of the Great Hungarian Plain (GHP) has been described by various authors including Ronai (1985), Embleton (1984) and Liebe (2002). The main river of the GHP is, in fact, the Tisza and not the Danube, which flows along the western edge. The soils are marshy–peaty soils, chernozems, forest soils and red clays. The Quaternary deposits of the GHP are typically 600–700 m thick and contain abundant organic matter, degradation of which gives rise to methane discharges in water wells. During the Pleistocene, the Danube channel was excavated to depths of up to 200 m. Although subsidence rates increased in the Upper Pleistocene, Holocene sand and gravel rarely exceeds 2–4 m in thickness, but thick peat is developed locally. The Pleistocene sequence comprises 50–70% of high permeability sand (Csanady et al., 2005).

Hydrogeochemistry

A landmark study by Varsányi et al. (1991) sampled 85 wells, 80–560 m deep, and identified a strong correlation between arsenic and humic substances in

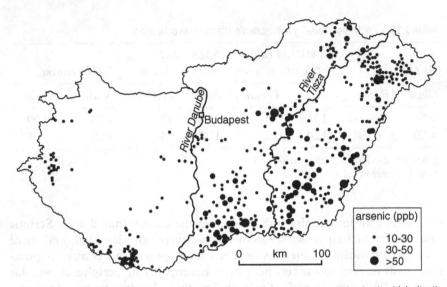

Figure 9.17   Distribution of arsenic in groundwater in Hungary. Arsenic contamination is widely distributed in the alluvium of the Great Hungarian Plain, especially along the Duna–Tisza and Maros tributaries of the Danube.
Source: From Biacs (2005)

groundwater. They distinguished two discrete areas of pollution: one to the west of the Tisza and a more extensive area to the east where the aquifers are finer grained (Figure 9.17). The chemistry of groundwater in the two areas is distinctly different (Table 9.11), and this allowed them to distinguish three water types based on the chemical oxygen demand (COD[27]):

1   waters with < 25 ppb As and high to very high COD (6–12 ppm) are found in the fine-grained aquifers of the southeast;
2   waters with uniformly low COD (*c.* 2 ppm) and moderate to high arsenic (50–150 ppb);
3   waters found in most of the As-affected areas follow a trend that bisects the other two groups, where arsenic is positively correlated with COD, Na, Cl and humic acid, and negatively correlated with Fe.

High As concentrations are most commonly encountered at depths of 100–200 m (Csanady et al., 2005), and are associated with high concentrations of NH_4, Mn, Fe, humic acids and CH_4, and temperatures as high as 30°C (Hlavay, 1997). Csalagovitis (1996) concluded that the origin of arsenic in groundwater is linked to the 'early diagenesis of fluvial, swamp and floodplain formations during the Quaternary', and inferred that arsenic is mobilised by bacterial reduction of iron hydroxides in organic-rich

Table 9.11 Average groundwater quality on the Great Hungarian Plain

Parameter (ppm)	West (coarser sediment)	East (finer sediment)
Na	26	220
Cl	3	11
As (ppb)	25	38
COD	1.8	5.9
Fe	0.4	0.2
NH$_4$	0.93	1.86
Hardness (as CaCO$_3$)	122	37
Humic acid	0.5	8.5

Source: Varsányi et al. (1991)

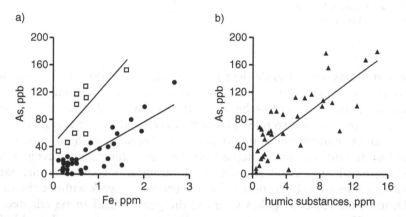

Figure 9.18 Relations of arsenic, iron and humic acids in groundwater in the Duna–Tisza interfluve, Hungary. (a) Arsenic and iron in the recharge area; open squares are from the south of the interfluve, and circles from other areas. (b) Arsenic and humic substances in the discharge area.
Source: Varsányi and Kovács (2006)

sediments. Varsányi and Kovács (2006) elaborated the relationship between arsenic, iron and humic acids (Figure 9.18), also concluding that arsenic is mobilised by RD driven by the degradation of peat, as in the Bengal Basin.

Remediation

In Hungary, remedial action started in 1981, and a centrally funded project ran from 1983 to 1995 to reduce the As concentrations at municipal water works to < 50 ppb, which was achieved in 1997 (Csanady et al., 2005). Initially, improvements were made by blending water from different wells, where the worst wells were either taken out of operation or used only for emergencies, while low-As wells were used continuously. This reduced As

Table 9.12   Arsenic concentrations in arsenic-affected regions of Hungary, Romania and Slovakia

	Hungary				*Romania*		*Slovakia*	
							Banska Bystica	*Nitra*
	Bacs	*Bekes*	*Csongrad*	*JNS*	*Bihor*	*Arad*		
Number of samples	99	23	60	64	54	98	67	65
Median As (ppb)	7.7	17	28	16	0.48	0.70	0.69	0.95
Maximum As (ppb)	39	31	40	88	24	95	37	39

JNS, Jazs-Nagykun-Szolnok.
Source: Lindberg et al. (2005)

concentrations to tolerable levels at about one-third of the affected settlements. In parallel with these measures, a new groundwater source was located 30 km from Bekescsaba, and piped in to blend with existing supplies. Arsenic removal technologies were developed to suit regional differences in As concentrations and interfering substances such as ammonium and humic acid. The main method involved pre-chlorination, coagulation and coprecipitation with ferric salts, and filtration. In some cases the natural iron content was high enough for this process to work without chemical additions. However, in Bekes County, the process had to be adapted to include pH correction, use of permanganate as an oxidant and double filtration (Csanady et al., 2005).

Although the interventions reported by Csanady et al. (2005) have been successful in reducing As exposure at the 50 ppb level, none met the current 10 ppb EU standard, and additional treatment is required. Nevertheless, recent reports by Lindberg et al. (2005) suggest that mitigation has been effective in reducing exposure (Table 9.12). The large majority of 200 water samples from Hungary were < 10 ppb and none exceeded 100 ppb As. In 2005, the Hungarian daily newspaper *Magyar Hirlap* reported that Hungary will spend €4 M between 2006 and 2009 to implement the new standard.

Adjoining areas of Romania, Croatia and Slovakia

Gurzau and Gurzau (2001) reported As concentrations up to 176 ppb in groundwater in Bihor and Arad counties of Transylvania, near the Hungarian border (Lindberg et al. (2005). Elevated As concentrations were also reported from parts of Slovakia (Table 9.12), and Rapant and Krčmová

(2007) showed that arsenic pollution is widely distributed, but is concentrated in the southwest, with 1.2% of groundwater sources exceeding 10 ppb As, and 0.3% exceeding 50 ppb As. However, the main cause of As pollution in Slovakia is oxidation of sulphides in mineralised areas (S. Rapant, personal communication, 2007).

In eastern Croatia, close to the Hungarian border, Cavar et al. (2005) and Habuda-Stanić et al. (2007) recorded high arsenic concentrations in drinking water in and around the towns of Osijek (population 100,000; 38 ppb As), Cepin (population 13,000; 172 ppb As) and Andrijasevci (population of 4000; 612 ppb As). Exposure was confirmed by analysis of hair samples (up to 5 μg/g), which correlate well with arsenic in drinking water. Osijek and Cepin lie in the Drava Depression, and Andrijasevci is located in the Slavonia–Srijem Depression. Andrijasevci is underlain by an aquifer containing between two and 11 layers of sand in the upper 200 m. In the Drava Depression there are three to eight sand and gravel horizons in the top 120 m. The groundwater also contains high concentrations of iron, manganese, ammonium and DOC, which strongly suggests operation of the same geochemical processes as in Hungary. Testing of 18 wells, 100–177 m deep, in Osijek in 1987, 1996 and 2001 indicated large increases in As concentration in most of the wells. In Osijek and Vinkovci, groundwater is treated by coagulation-filtration which reduces As concentrations from around 250 to 40 ppb. Other municipal systems use rapid sand filtration, but this is no more effective. Overall, Cavar et al. (2005) estimated that 3% of the population of Croatia may be exposed to a serious health risk from arsenic in drinking water, and Habuda-Stanić et al. (2007) estimate the currently exposed population at 200,000.

9.4.3 Suomi Finland

In Finland, arsenic predominantly affects rural water supplies drawn from wells drilled into bedrock, where concentrations reach 2230 ppb As, but occasionally affects springs and dugwells in the overburden (Backman et al., 1994; Karro and Lahermo, 1999; Backman and Lahermo, 2004). Finnish bedrock aquifers are also affected by fluoride, uranium and radon. The difference between bedrock and overburden aquifers (Table 9.13) is similar to that noted in New England (section 9.1.6), which has broadly similar bedrock and glacial history. The 'One Thousand Wells' survey showed that, nationwide, only 3% exceeded 10 ppb As, but the proportions were much higher in southwest Finland and parts of Lapland (Figure 9.19).

Hakala and Hallikainen (2004) reported limited health effects in the Finnish population, and did not identify dermatological effects, perhaps because the relatively high exposure in the 1970s was reduced during the

Table 9.13   Arsenic in drift and bedrock wells in Finland

Aquifer	Number	Median As (ppb)	Maximum As (ppb)
Overburden	1197	0.22	138
Bedrock	472	0.65	1040

Source: Data after Karro and Lahermo (1999)

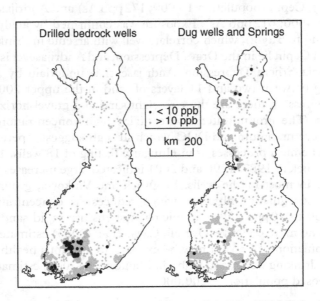

Figure 9.19   Distribution of arsenic-contaminated water wells in Finland. (a) Drilled wells in bedrock. (b) Dug wells and springs.
Source: After Backman and Lahermo (2004)

1980s and 1990s. Analysis of urine and hair as biomarkers by Kurttio et al. (1998) confirmed significant human uptake of arsenic, and they also inferred that arsenic exposure was associated with complaints of muscle cramps, mainly in the legs. Within about 3 months of removing exposure, concentrations in urine of former users (17 ppb) dropped to only three times that in the control group (5 ppb), much less than in those still exposed (58 ppb As). Kurttio et al. (1999) found an increased risk of bladder cancer, but not kidney cancer, associated with elevated As concentrations in drinking water.

Most of Finland is underlain by Archaean granitoids, gneisses and migmatites, and Proterozoic mafic-layered intrusions and greenstone belts.

Bedrock has an extensive cover of glacial sediment, but this is normally only a few metres thick, and in much of the coastal and northern regions the till is discontinuous. At the end of the Pleistocene glaciations, low-lying coastal areas were inundated by seawater, which also left behind a layer of clay and silt. Water in the drift tends to be subneutral and less mineralised than in bedrock (Karro and Lahermo, 1999). Bedrock is fractured to depths of 50–200 m and supports household water supplies for about 20% of the population, but the yields are generally too low to support community supplies. Though covering only 3–4% of the area, eskers[28] are important, high-yielding aquifers.

Although concentrations of >1,000 ppb As are known, contamination is mostly low-level. In southwest Finland, bedrock consists mainly of volcanic-sedimentary rocks, and contaminated wells are mostly found where the rocks have been hydrothermally altered and where arsenopyrite coats fracture surfaces (Karro and Lahermo, 1999). They also noted that concentrations tend to be higher in confined aquifers, and that As-rich groundwater is spatially correlated with the As content of the silt and clay fraction of glacial till (Figure 9.20). Elsewhere, Tarvainen et al. (2001) associated groundwater containing >10 ppb As with black schists, metavolcanics, amphibolite and gabbro.

In the Pirkanmaa As hotspot in southwest Finland, where 17% of wells exceeded 10 ppb As, bedrock consists of granodiorite, mica-schist, gneiss and metavolcanics, and As-contaminated groundwater coincides with high As concentrations in soil. However, Juntunen et al. (2004) concluded that arsenic in groundwater is not related to rock type, but is tectonically controlled, following 'broken, ribbon-like lenses tens of kilometres long'. Compared with the national baseline, groundwater in Pirkanmaa is more alkaline and mineralised, and locally exceeds drinking water standards for Fe, Mn, F, Cl and Ni. As shown in Figure 9.21, arsenic is often associated with elevated pH, suggesting that desorption from iron oxides is significant, but this offers a far from complete explanation.

In central Lapland, Tanskanen et al. (2004) reported two pristine springs containing 24 and 35 ppb As, associated with As-rich (median 40, maximum 929 mg/kg) organic sediments[29] and pH > 8. In the Haukipudas area of northern Finland, Roman and Peuraniemi (1999) described groundwater containing up to 43 ppb As at a site underlain by mica-schists that were so rich in arsenical pyrite, pyrrhotite and arsenopyrite that the authors described it as an 'arsenic geochemical province'. The area was covered by 2–3 m of brown, iron-hydroxide cemented till containing up to 112 mg/kg As. The groundwater was slightly acidic (pH 5.74) and apparently oxic, with high concentrations of iron (4.2 ppm) and sulphate (92 ppm). Arsenic mobilisation was attributed to oxidation of arsenopyrite.

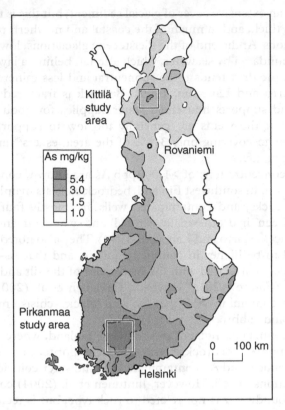

Figure 9.20   Distribution of arsenic in glacial till in Finland. Chemical analyses were performed on the fine fraction (< 0.06 mm) of the till. Note that high As concentrations in till are spatially correlated with high As concentrations in well-waters shown in Figure 9.19.
Source: Redrawn after Tanskanen et al. (2004)

9.4.4   Germany

Triassic Sandstones, Saxony and Bavaria

According to Jekel (1996), the occurrence of arsenic in the Frankonia district of Bavaria and the Solling region of Lower Saxony is typical of certain sandstones, such as the 'Buntsandstein' (Goldberg et al., 1995). Kevekordes et al. (1998) reported that in Saxony only 2% of 150 wells exceeded the 1986 standard of 40 ppb As, but 40% exceeded 10 ppb As. Driehaus (2002) reported that about 300 drinking water supplies were affected by introduction of the 10 ppb standard, of which 60 have been equipped with treatment systems, and the rest have been either withdrawn or are blended with low-As water. Heinrichs and Udluft (1999) described natural As

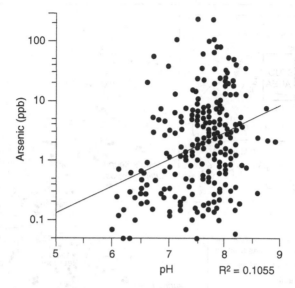

Figure 9.21   Relationship between arsenic and pH in groundwater in Finland. All water samples are from bedrock in the most-affected region around Pirkanmaa (Figure 9.20). Although most of the high As concentrations are associated with high pH, alkali desorption can only explain part of the observed contamination. *Source*: Redrawn after Juntunen et al. (2004)

contamination, mostly at the tens of ppb level, in the Upper Triassic Keuper sandstones of northern Bavaria (Figure 9.22). The sequence comprises 200–500 m of interbedded sandstones and mudstones, which undergo a facies change from shallow marine in the northwest to terrestrial in the southeast. A gypsiferous unit occurs at the base, and deep-seated saline groundwater that contains up to 550 ppb As. They investigated municipal wells, mostly 100–150 m deep, completed with long open sections, and having concentrations ranging from 10 to 150 ppb As. Groundwater is near-neutral (pH 6.7–7.8), mildly reducing, lacking nitrate (< 0.2 ppm) but with significant sulphate (10–100 ppm). Bicarbonate is slightly elevated (150–400 ppm) but Fe and Mn are generally < 0.5 ppm. Heinrichs and Udluft (1999) concluded that As mobilisation is controlled by the sediment chemistry, but did not identify a mobilisation mechanism. It may be that mixing of waters within the long open-sections of the wells disguises the signatures of mobilisation.

Wiesbaden Spa

The famous spa at Wiesbaden, which comprises 40 hot springs, has been known to contain > 100 ppb As since 1886 (Schwenzer et al., 2001). Wiesbaden

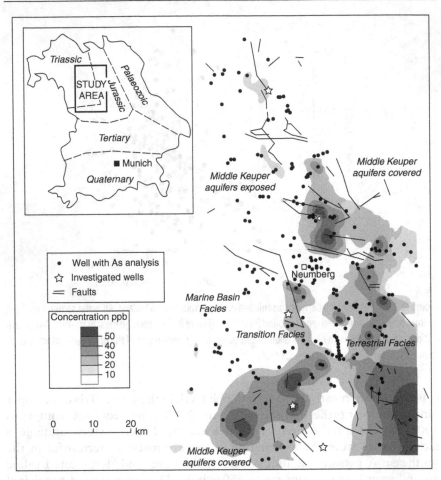

Figure 9.22 Distribution of arsenic in the Upper Triassic sandstone aquifer of northern Bavaria, Germany. High-As in groundwater is associated with particular lithologies that were deposited only in fluvial and terrestrial environments.
Source: After Heinrichs and Udluft (1999)

is built on Ordovician to Devonian metavolcanics and metasediments. The springs lie about 100 m south of a major thrust fault that separates phyllites to the north from crystalline rocks to the south. Groundwater is an anoxic Na–Cl type, where arsenic is present mainly as As(III). The famous 'Kochbrunnen' well has had a virtually constant chemical composition for the past 150 years. Its temperature is 66°C, and it contains 2520 ppm of Na, 4380 ppm of Cl, 557 ppm of HCO_3, 2.9 ppm of Fe and 0.6 ppm of Mn. The pH is 6.0 and the Eh −60 mV. Sulphate reduction is indicated by the odour of H_2S. Schwenzer et al. (2001) observed that hydrous ferric oxide is precipitated around the wells and springs, but only scavenges the trace of arsenate. Through a series of experiments they showed that, at the *in situ* temperature (66°C), oxidation of As(III) takes several hours, too slow to retard As(III) at the wellhead, but fast enough to prevent its migration through surrounding aquifers.

Rhine alluvium

Rott and Friedle (1999), describing *in situ* removal of iron and manganese at Paderborn, near the head of the Rhine Delta, reported arsenic in three wells (15–38 ppb As) drawing water from the Rhine alluvium. The wells contained 0.94–1.94 ppm Fe and 0.15–0.35 ppm Mn. Arsenic is present mainly as As(III) and ammonium is also present, suggesting RD, probably under similar conditions to those found in the Danube and Ganges–Brahmaputra systems.

9.4.5   United Kingdom

England and Wales

A nationwide survey of trace elements found that 10–15% of waters from sandstone aquifers contained 10–50 ppb As, although none exceeded 50 ppb (Edmunds et al., 1989), and there are no associated reports of adverse health effects. Recent baseline surveys by the Environment Agency provide a picture of arsenic occurrence in some bedrock aquifers. The most affected aquifer is the Triassic Sherwood Sandstone (equivalent to the 'Buntsandstein' in Germany), which is a major water resource in the Midlands and northwest England. Arsenic contamination is most common in the northwest region, where monitoring found that 11.5% of 672 water sources exceeded 10 ppb As, and 1.6% exceeded 50 ppb. The highest concentrations were recorded in Liverpool (355 ppb), the Carlisle Basin (233 ppb), Manchester (215 ppb), Cheshire (57 ppb) and the Vale of York (Shand et al., 1999; Griffiths et al., 2003, 2005). In the Midlands, As concentrations of up to 26 ppb are associated with oxic waters. In Nottinghamshire, elevated As occurs where the Sherwood Sandstone dips beneath the Mercia Mudstone, and where the groundwater is aerobic and slightly alkaline, with pH≥8.0, but As concentrations decrease down-gradient in the anaerobic zone (Smedley and Edmunds, 2002). In the Midlands, contaminated water wells operated by Severn Trent Water Services have been equipped with fixed-bed reactors containing a synthetic iron oxide adsorbent (section 7.6.3).

Other sandstone aquifers also contain traces of arsenic. In the Lower Greensand, 11% of samples exceeded 10 ppb, with a maximum of 20 ppb As in reducing waters (Shand et al., 2003). There was a single exceedance

(13 ppb As) in the Devonian Old Red Sandstone of the Welsh borders, and none in either the Millstone Grit of northern England or the Tertiary sands of the Wessex Basin.

The most important aquifer in the UK is the Upper Cretaceous Chalk. In four regional baseline surveys, all samples contained < 5 ppb. In the confined Chalk of North Humberside, however, Smedley et al. (2004) found that 30% of reducing groundwaters exceeded 10 ppb, with a maximum of 63 ppb As. A local As occurrence (25 ppb As) was noted in the Lincolnshire Limestone (Griffiths et al., 2006), but in the other UK limestone aquifers (the Magnesian, the Corralian, the Carboniferous and the Greater and Inferior Oolite), plus the granites of southwest England and Palaeozoic metasediments of Wales, all samples were below 10 ppb, and generally below 5 ppb As.

Few data are available for alluvial or glacial aquifers in the UK, which are generally thin, and exploited mainly for domestic supplies. Estuarine alluvium in Somerset contains several tens of ppb of both arsenic and selenium, accompanied by high concentrations of NH_4, Fe and DOC, indicating reductive dissolution (AGMI, 2004). The Environment Agency has recorded elevated arsenic in private supplies in mid-Wales (R. Ward; personal communication, 2007).

Scotland and Northern Ireland

The Drinking Water Quality Regulator (DWQR, 2006) reported no exceedances for arsenic in piped water supplies, but no data were available for private supplies. In Northern Ireland, two sources (14 and 35 ppb) exceeded the drinking water standard; both were associated with areas of dispersed and vein-hosted As mineralisation (Doe and McConvey, 2005).

9.4.6   France

Grossier and Ledrans (1999) found that 200,000 people in 45 administrative areas were drinking water containing >10 ppb As, and 17,000 people drinking water with >50 ppb As. The most contaminated sources (As > 50 ppb) were located around the Massif Central, the Vosges and the Pyrenees mountains, while waters with 10–50 ppb As were also located in sedimentary basins in the Aquitaine and Centre regions. Based on this survey, Grossier and Ledrans (1999) identified As-risk zones related to the regional geology, which included not only active geothermal and recent volcanic regions, but also granitic rocks. Bonnemaison (2005) reported that most pollution occurrences were associated with arsenopyrite that had been oxidised due to lowering of the water table, and that contaminated groundwater is spatially correlated with arsenic anomalies in soil, which closely reflect the underlying rock type. He also noted that 20% of thermal waters in France contain >50 ppb As, and that, on average, surface waters contained 0.73 ppb As.

In preparation for lowering the drinking water standard to 10 ppb As, Chery et al. (1998) sought to correlate arsenic and other trace elements with the regional geology and geochemical baselines in the 30% of France underlain by crystalline rocks. Geochemical As anomalies were found along the margins of granite intrusions where soil concentrations attain 300–1000 mg/kg As and groundwater often reaches 30 ppb As. They estimated that 20% of water sources in the geochemically anomalous zones would exceed 10 ppb As, although outside the anomalies groundwater sources are expected to contain < 10 ppb As. They predicted that where soil-As exceeds 60 mg/kg there is a significant risk of groundwater exceeding 10 ppb As, and that where soil exceeds 300 mg/kg As there is a significant risk of exceeding 50 ppb As.

9.4.7   Spain

Madrid and Duero Basins

Arsenic contamination in the Madrid and Duero basins was detected during routine drinking water surveillance. The Madrid Basin is an intermontane tectonic depression filled with Tertiary continental deposits, and bounded by mountains formed mainly of Hercynian granitic rocks and schists (Hernández-García and Custodio, 2004). The basin has a complex zoning (Figure 9.23), with detrital arkosic sands, silts and clays near the mountains, and evaporites and carbonates in the basin centre. The aquifers are arkoses interbedded with silts and clays. The Duero Basin comprises Tertiary carbonate and gypsiferous sediments overlain by Quaternary aeolian sands (5–15 m thick), all cut by channels of sand and gravel that contain < 0.2–16 mg/kg As (Garcia-Sanchez et al., 2005). The two basins are geologically similar, but differ in detail and scale. There are also at least nine mining sites associated with As mineralisation on the margins of the Duero Basin.

In the Madrid Basin, wells 50–476 m deep contained an average of 25 ppb As and a maximum of 91 ppb As (Hernández-García and Custodio, 2004). The highest concentrations are found in detrital sediments to the north of Madrid (Figure 9.23). Arsenic concentrations were not correlated with well depth but, as shown in Figure 9.24, are positively correlated with pH, Na + K:Ca + Mg ratio[30], and vanadium. Similar associations have been noted in southwest USA and Argentina, and have been cited as evidence supporting AD, although other factors are probably involved. The presence of nitrate indicates that groundwater is oxic or only mildly reducing.

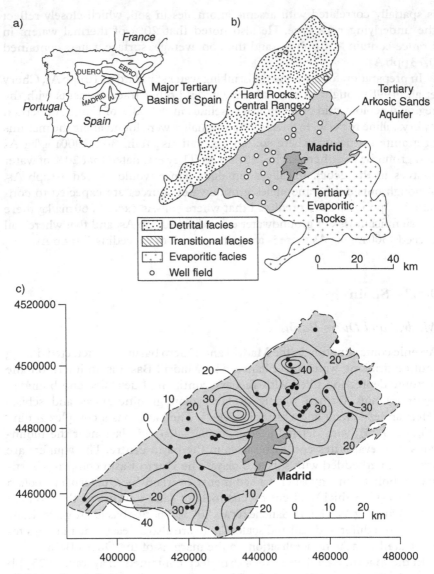

Figure 9.23 Hydrogeological map and distribution of arsenic in the Madrid Basin, Spain. (a) location of the Madrid and Duero basins; (b) geology of the Madrid basin; (c) distribution of arsenic in groundwater. *Source*: Redrawn after Hernández-García and Custodio (2004)

Garcia-Sanchez et al. (2005) reported higher As concentrations (20–260 ppb) from 28 wells, 3–300 m deep, in the Duero Basin. Although there is no overall trend with well depth, As concentrations tend to be lower in shallow wells. A more intensive survey (514 wells) by Gómez et al. (2006)

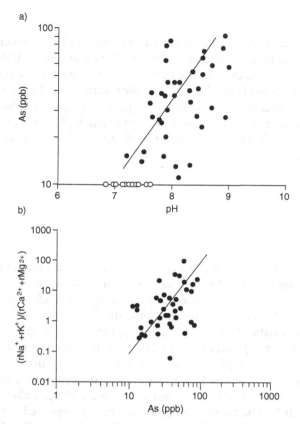

Figure 9.24   Arsenic, pH and ion-exchange in groundwater from the Madrid Basin, Spain. Despite the apparent correlation between As and pH, it is noted that many high-As concentrations occur at pH values of <8.0. *Source*: After Hernández-García and Custodio (2004)

reported a mean of 41 ppb As, and maximum of 613 ppb. Groundwater is oxic, and arsenic was correlated with HCO_3 and pH, but not with SO_4. High As concentrations were also associated with long residence times. Hernández-García and Custodio (2004) suggested that arsenic is released by desorption from clay minerals and/or Fe and Al oxyhydroxides. In the Duero Basin, Garcia-Sanchez et al. (2005) suggested that under oxic conditions, HCO_3 competes with arsenate sorbed to oxyhydroxides. They also suggested that biomolecules called 'siderophores', which bind strongly to Fe, promote dissolution of oxyhydroxides, and hence liberate arsenic. Gómez et al. (2006) noted that high-As in groundwater was closely associated with particular stratigraphic horizons, such as the Middle Miocene organic-rich Zaratan facies. They also proposed that arsenic is mobilised by desorption from Fe and Mn oxyhydroxides under oxidising and alkaline conditions.

Other areas

Garcia-Sanchez and Alvarez-Ayuso (2003) reported As concentrations of up to 52 ppb As in groundwater in the middle reaches of the Duero River in Salamanca Province, close to the border with Portugal, although most pollution in this region is attributed to mining activities. Morell et al. (2006) reported As concentrations of up to 14 ppb in Triassic sandstones in the Mediterranean provinces of Castellon and Valencia, in Ca–Mg–HCO$_3$ type groundwater with Fe concentrations of up to 0.83 ppm and low Mn concentrations.

9.4.8   Italy

Po Basin

Giuliano (1995) reported the presence of arsenic accompanied by high concentrations of NH$_4$, Fe and Mn in an alluvial aquifer in the central-southern Po River Plain. Subsequent investigations identified extensive pollution of alluvial groundwater along the Po, Adda, Adige and Reno rivers in Lombardia (Castelli et al., 2005), Emilia-Romagna (Farina et al., 2005) and Veneto (Boscolo et al., 2005). Groundwater is an important source of potable supply and is also used for irrigation and livestock. Arsenic occurs in confined aquifers down to depths of 150–200 m. In Veneto, 21% of 1303 wells surveyed contained >10 ppb, 3% > 50 ppb and 2% > 100 ppb As. The maximum As concentrations reported were > 400 ppb in Lombardia, 480 ppb in Veneto, and 1300 ppb in Emilia-Romagna. In Emilia-Romagna, groundwaters are near-neutral (pH 6.7–7.8) and have negative redox potentials, and elevated As concentrations are spatially correlated with high Fe concentrations. Fine-grained sediments forming aquitards have high As concentrations: 2–45 mg/kg As in Emilia-Romagna, and 2–45 mg/kg in Lombardia. The aquifer sediments, however, contained < 10 mg/kg. Arsenic is adsorbed onto ferric hydroxides, and contaminated zones are associated with layers of peat and organic-rich clay. Arsenic mobilisation was attributed to RD in Emilia-Romagna (Marcaccio et al., 2005), and the same processes probably operate in all three provinces.

Tuscany

Tamasi and Cini (2004) described concentrations of up to 14.4 ppb As in springs originating from volcanic rocks at altitudes of 600–900 m a.s.l. in the Mount Amiata region of Siena. The spring with the highest concentration, the Santa Fiora, also had a discharge of 650 L/s, and supplies water to the city of Siena. Although the area is geothermally active, the affected waters are neither hot (7.0–15.5°C) nor significantly mineralised (EC 76–804 μS/cm; with only one sample >110 μS/cm). The waters are near-neutral (pH 6.3–7.3) and contain only a few ppm of sulphate. Despite historic mining in the region, Tamasi and Cini (2004) rejected any anthropogenic cause, attributing arsenic to 'mineral deposits in the aquifer'.

Mantelli et al. (2005) reported very high As concentrations from hydrothermally altered volcanic rocks in southeastern Tuscany, which were attributed mainly to geothermal activity, but also to oxidation of sulphide minerals. Although most contaminated wells contained only a few tens of ppb of arsenic, one potable source contained 579 ppb, and one non-potable source contained 13,000 ppb.

Lazio

Vivona et al. (2005) reported As concentrations of 4–52 ppb and fluoride concentrations of 0.2–2.3 ppm in the Tiber River valley in a volcanic-alluvial aquifer formed of sands and carbonate gravel interbedded with Pleistocene alkali-potassic volcanic rocks. Arsenic and fluoride were positively correlated, although water from wells in sedimentary layers had lower As:F ratios. The fluoride is thought to be derived from fluorite and fluorapatite in the aquifer, and it is believed that arsenic is derived from percolation of rainwater through volcanic units that overlie, or feed water laterally into, the Tiber gravels (Vivona et al., 2005). Elsewhere, Giulano et al. (2005) recorded thick alkali-potassic volcanic aquifers containing up to >50 ppb As, and where 10% of wells exceeded 10 ppb As. Again, arsenic and fluoride were positively correlated.

Volcanic arsenic in southern Italy

Although not known to be of health significance, geothermal arsenic is common around the volcanic centres of southern Italy, including Vesuvius, Etna and Vulcano (Aiuppa et al., 2003). Arsenic ranges from below detection to 6390 ppb and is dominantly present as As(III). The highest concentrations are found where active hydrothermal circulation takes place at shallow level. Temperatures range from 38 to 73°C, and chloride concentrations from 30 to 9300 ppm. Groundwater containing > 100 ppb As also has high Cl and SO_4 (320–2300 ppm) concentrations, and variable Fe concentrations of up to 122 ppm (Figure 9.25). However, pH (1.7–7.0) is not systematically related to As concentration. The positive correlation of As and SO_4 was attributed to the dissolution of sulphides, enhanced by the high temperature. The highest arsenic concentrations are associated with intermediate redox conditions, because under hot and reducing conditions arsenic is precipitated in realgar, and under oxidising

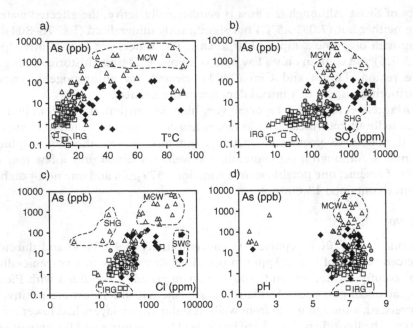

Figure 9.25   Relationships between arsenic, temperature, chloride, sulphate and pH in volcanic groundwaters in southern Italy. MCW, mature chloride waters; SHG, steam-heated groundwater; IRG, Fe-rich groundwater; SWC, seawater contaminated.
Source: Aiuppa et al. (2003)

conditions it is adsorbed by iron oxides. At Etna and Vesuvius, where hydrothermal activity is least, groundwaters have relatively low As concentrations with low temperature and high bicarbonate concentrations. Unlike around the other volcanoes, increasing arsenic is associated with increasing pH, in the range pH 6–8. Although hot springs are not normally used for water supply, volcanic rock can form important aquifers such as the Etnean aquifer which supplies a million people in eastern Sicily. In Campania, Cocozziello et al. (2005) recorded high As concentrations on the isle of Ischia, near Naples, and lower levels of contamination (*c.* 30 ppb As) beneath the Volturno Plain.

9.4.9   Greece

In anticipation of the new EU drinking water standard, Mitrakas (2001) conducted reconnaissance surveys of water sources across Greece. While samples from 24 major cities were all <10 ppb As, 13.6% of 125 tap water samples from smaller cities and communities, mainly from northern Greece, exceeded 10 ppb As. The proportion of irrigation wells with >10 ppb was higher (26.4%), and most thermal mineral waters contained > 10 ppb As. In Thessaloniki Prefecture in northern Greece, Fytianos and Christophoridis (2004) reported that 13.5% of drinking water samples from 52 villages exceeded 10 ppb As. In eastern Thessaly, the mean As concentration in 26 wells, boreholes and springs was 12 ppb, and the maximum 125 ppb As (Kelepertsis et al., 2006). Many of these waters were also contaminated by antimony, and were estimated to affect 5000 people in the Melivoia, Sotiritsa and Ano Polydendri areas. The area comprises rolling hills and small mountains, mostly covered by forest or intensive fruit orchards. The geology consists of Palaeozoic schist, amphibolite and marble overlain by a thrust sheet of Triassic and Cretaceous ophiolite and limestone, and all covered by unconsolidated Quaternary deposits. Arsenic contamination occurred only in hydrothermally altered metamorphic rocks, but in both boreholes and springs, indicating that pollution occurs at shallow and intermediate depths. Groundwater is subneutral (pH 6.0–6.6) and oxidising (Eh > 570 mV), while iron concentrations are low. Kelepertsis et al. (2006) attributed the arsenic and antimony contamination to arsenopyrite and stibnite mineralisation in the affected area.

9.4.10   Other parts of Europe

Czech Republic

Drahota et al. (2006) reported As pollution of shallow wells, containing up to 1500 ppb As, in two small watersheds in the Celina–Mokrsko gold district, where arsenicosis had been identified in the local population. Groundwater in the Mokrsko catchment had an average As concentration of 761 ppb. However, the deposits in the study area had never been mined, and arsenic was mobilised by natural oxidation of arsenopyrite and pyrrhotite associated with Late Precambrian volcano-sedimentary rocks and granodiorite.

Denmark

A paper on water treatment in Fensmark in eastern Denmark by Jessen et al. (2005) reported As concentrations of 10–30 ppb in groundwater from the top 10–20 m of a 'fractured limestone' (Chalk?) aquifer that was overlain by 20–60 m of fluvial sand and clayey till. The water was anoxic, of a Ca–HCO_3 type, and contained 2 ppm of iron and 0.1 ppm of manganese.

Ireland

No details are available, but summary data presented by Toner et al. (2004) indicate the presence of arsenic concentrations in groundwater of up to 28 ppb As.

Lithuania

The Eastern Baltic Lowlands (EBL) occupy a downwarp between the Fennoscandian Shield and the Russian Platform, and are covered by up to 300 m of Quaternary morainic and glacial lake deposits (Embleton, 1984). The lake and bog deposits are assumed to be rich in organic matter and to interdigitate with fluvio-glacial sand and gravel. High ammonium concentrations (mapped as 0.5–16 ppm) are widespread in shallow and deep wells in both Quaternary and pre-Quaternary aquifers (Carl Bro, 2004). In addition, iron concentrations reach up to 15 ppm (UNESCO, 1974), indicating strongly reducing groundwater conditions. Combined with the geological setting, this suggests the operation of RD. To date, only a handful of arsenic analyses have been performed in Lithuania, but concentrations of up to 33 ppb As have been detected (Dr K. Kestutis[31], personal communication, 2006).

Netherlands and Belgium

In the Schuwacht bank filtration scheme at Gouda in The Netherlands, wells 70–200 m from the River Rhine contained 2–14 ppb As (Appelo and de Vet, 2003). The wells were screened in coarse sands at a depth of 20–30 m. Almost all of the abstracted water is drawn from the river, and its chemistry is modified by flow through the alluvium, acquiring increased concentrations of Ca, Fe, Mn, NH_4 and alkalinity, as well as dissolved methane, suggesting reaction with natural organic matter in the sediment. Stuyfzand (1991) described the occurrence of trace elements in groundwater along two cross-sections in southern Netherlands. Shallow groundwater is anoxic, with pH 7.6–7.7, and contains 15–22 ppb As, which is assumed to have been mobilised by RD. However, a deeper well (c. 150 m) in the Brabantian aquifer, recharged in Pleistocene hills to the south, contained 44 ppb As in an acidic (pH 5.2) groundwater containing 226 ppm of sulphate, and was attributed to oxidation of pyrite. To the south, in northern Belgium, Coetsiers and Walraevens (2006) reported As concentrations of up to 60 ppb at depths of between 20 and 300 m in the Neogene alluvial aquifer, where arsenic is thought to be mobilised above 80 m by reduction of iron oxyhydroxides.

Norway

In Norway Frengstad et al. (2000) identified just 1% of 476 groundwater samples exceeding 10 ppb As, with a maximum of only 19 ppb As. Associations with both high pH, and outcrops of 'Caledonian granites, mafic and ultramafic' rocks were noted.

Poland

Dobrzynski (2007) recorded As concentrations of up to 140 ppb in fractured Carboniferous–Permian mudstones and sandstones in the Sudetes mountains of southwest Poland. The sediments were deposited in alluvial and lacustrine environments, and contain carbonate minerals, gypsum, pyrite and organic matter. The As-rich waters have pH 7.5–7.7, quite low Fe (<0.7 ppm) and Mn (<0.13 ppm) concentrations, but contain high levels of B, Sr, Zn and SO_4, with much of the latter attributed to gypsum dissolution. Arsenic was attributed to oxidation of pyrite and arsenopyrite.

Slovenia

Kralj (2004) reported low-temperature (<40°C) thermal springs containing up to 589 ppb As at the margins of small Tertiary basins near to Ljubljiana in west-central Slovenia.

Sweden

The Sveriges Geologiska Undersokning (SGU, 2005) have shown that low-level As contamination is found in many regions of Sweden, with 3.9% of 738 wells surveyed exceeding 10 ppb As. None of the 106 dug wells sampled, and only two of the 101 wells in drift, exceeded 10 ppb As. Arsenic contamination was predominantly found in wells drilled into bedrock (4.3% > 10 ppb), and the most affected region is around Uppsala in east-central Sweden. Only four out of 531 wells exceeded 100 ppb, and none exceeded 300 ppb As.

Switzerland

Pfeifer et al. (2004) traced the movement of arsenic through a small watershed, the Malcantone catchment, in southern Switzerland. Here, arsenic is mobilised (up to 91 ppb, all arsenate) by sulphide oxidation in the upper catchment, transported by streams adsorbed to iron oxyhydroxides, and remobilised (up to 368 ppb, all arsenite) by reductive dissolution in swampy alluvial sediments in the lower catchment (section 3.7.3).

9.5   Suspect Terrain and Research Needs

9.5.1   North America

Alluvial basins

A surprising feature of the occurrence of arsenic in groundwater in the USA is the apparent absence of contamination in the Holocene deltas of the southern and eastern states. Based on the superficial similarities with deltas of South and Southeast Asia, it might be suspected that arsenic would be mobilised by RD in shallow groundwater, especially in the Mississippi Delta. It is not clear whether this apparent absence is due to the particular characteristics of the American rivers or because shallow aquifers are rarely exploited, and thus their water quality has not been examined in detail. However, the former explanation appears more likely (section 3.5.2).

Mexico

Mexico is perhaps one of the most extensively As-contaminated countries on Earth, but to date there appears to have been no nationwide compilation of information of the extent and severity of pollution and, apart from the Zimapán area, few process studies. Both process studies and extensive data compilations are required.

9.5.2 Europe

Alluvial basins of Europe

The occurrences of arsenic in the Danube and Po Basins have many similarities with the As-affected alluvial basins of South and Southeast Asia. It is surprising that As contamination has not been reported more widely from alluvial basins in Europe. Indeed, arsenic pollution has not been reported from the Danube Delta, although description of wellfields at Bucharest, where groundwater contains elevated NH_4 and pH 7.8–8.4, suggest that these aquifers might be affected by arsenic (Zamfirescu et al., 1999). There are, however, minor reports of arsenic from the Rhine alluvium.

As noted in Chapter 3, there appears to be an association between the mineralogy of river sands and the occurrence of arsenic, which led us to identify reports of As contamination in the Tiber and Po basins. This pattern may well be repeated in other rivers draining the Alps, Carpathians and other young mountains, and deserves examination.

Glaciated terrain

In North America, aquifers formed by glacial outwash at the end of the Pleistocene are widely contaminated by arsenic, and have a characteristic chemistry: near-neutral pH, an absence of nitrate and sulphate, and high concentrations of iron, bicarbonate, ammonium, DOC and methane (e.g. Erickson and Barnes, 2005b; Kelly et al., 2005). Similar sediments were deposited around the margins of the north European ice sheets, and groundwater extracted from them might also be contaminated by arsenic, especially in confined aquifers developed in sands and gravel layers at the base of tunnel-valleys in parts of England, northern Germany and Poland. Although As contamination of the overburden was noted in Finland, there is little published evidence of contamination in other countries. However, information on the iron and ammonium contents of groundwaters led us to identify unpublished reports of As contamination in Lithuania, and it is suspected that As contamination may be more extensive across the Baltic Plains from northern Germany to Byelorus, and as well as perhaps also in parts of the UK and Ireland.

NOTES

1   Notable exceptions are the Danube and Po basins.
2   It is presumed these supplies have now been brought into compliance, certainly with 50 ppb, and probably with the 10 ppb standard that became effective in 2006.
3   As expressed by the Body Mass Index.
4   Odds ratios of 1.9 (90% CI: 1.7–2.1) for men and 1.6 (90% CI: 1.5–1.8) for women.
5   Disease of arteries, arterioles and capillaries.
6   Although diagnosis relied on self-reporting, and was not independently confirmed, the forms were completed before the As-test results were made known. The studied population consumed well-water that ranged from below detection to 2389 ppb As, with a median concentration of 2 ppb As.
7   As pollution, partly natural, has also been recorded around the mining town of Cobalt, Ontario (Percival et al., 2004).
8   Due to the absence of a good correlation between As and Cl.
9   Seawater contains 19,000 ppm Cl.
10 The apparent absence of symptoms may be explained by the low exceedances, a diet rich in meat, fruit and vegetables, and low per-capita consumption of tap water.
11 Including additional distribution pipes and pumping stations.
12 River deposits in cold climates are commonly interbedded with appreciable thicknesses of organic-rich mud, fine-sand and peat (Kasse, 1998). Under postglacial, temperate climates, these layers provide the redox driver to mobilise arsenic from adjacent sand and gravel horizons.
13 Although some of the affected parts of Halifax and Hants Counties were designated as 'gold districts', Grantham and Jones (1977) found negligible difference between As occurrences in these and non-designated areas.
14 In fractured-rock aquifers, even where the transmissivity is low, flow that occurs in a few thin, but permeable, fissures can carry contaminants quickly and to considerable depth.
15 Anthropogenic chlorofluorocarbon compounds.
16 ^{85}Kr is an inert tracer that has been increasing in the atmosphere since the start of nuclear fuel reprocessing.

17 High sulphate concentrations may also result from dissolution of gypsum, but this is accompanied by increasing concentrations of calcium, and not iron.

18 Depending on the diameter of the existing well casing, it may be possible to install and seal a smaller diameter casing inside it, but this is technically difficult and in most cases probably not practical.

19 As (< 115 ppb) accompanied by elevated Mo, V, Se and U concentrations is associated with Miocene–Oligocene volcanic ash at Grass Mountain, South Dakota, and is attributed to desorption at pH > 8.0 (Carter et al., 1998).

20 All concentrations are arithmetic means unless stated otherwise.

21 The high-Mn waters may result from nitrogen-rich sludge applied to remediate gold-mining tailings rich in arsenopyrite (D.K. Nordstrom, personal communication, 2007).

22 Virtually the same as the 10 ppb guideline for water.

23 Quartz-monzonite is a coarse-grained intermediate igneous rock containing roughly equal proportions of alkali and plagioclase feldspar, and 5–20% quartz.

24 The most alkaline sample has a pH of 8.97 and arsenic below detection limits.

25 The monthly As concentrations analysed by Rodriguez et al. (2004) are from different years and hence the correlation must be treated as suspect until more time-series data are collected.

26 They also indicate the presence of arsenic in Serbia and Montenegro, but no details are given.

27 COD (chemical oxygen demand) was considered a proxy for DOC, and correlates well with humic acid.

28 Long narrow ridges of sand and gravel deposited by sub-glacial streams.

29 Large areas of Finland are covered by shallow lakes and meres underlain by peat, which often contain more >10 ppm As bound to iron oxides (Virtanen, 2004). The highest As contents are found in the lowest peat layers and are derived from the underlying bedrock or mineral soil.

30 This parameter suggests ion-exchange reactions such as occur where a marine sediment, or a previously inundated aquifer, is being flushed by fresh water.

31 Head of Department of Hydrogeology, Geological Survey of Lithuania.

Chapter Ten

Arsenic in South and Central America, Africa, Australasia and Oceania

10.1 Introduction

The continents of the southern hemisphere have been grouped in one chapter because of their broad geological[1] and climatic similarities, and also because reported occurrences of natural arsenic contamination are relatively rare. The two most notable are both in South America, but neither have true equivalents elsewhere, and both have resulted in severe health impacts. The first is on the Chaco-Pampean plains in Argentina, where arsenic is associated with deposits of volcanic loess. The second arises where geothermal groundwater seeps into Andean rivers that are exploited for water supply on the coastal plains of Chile. In Africa, arsenic contamination is most remarkable for its general absence. To date, no globally important instance has been reported, but overall there is a dearth of information on arsenic in groundwater. However, if the occurrences do not reflect only the lack of data, they are significant for predicting where As contamination will not be found. In Australasia, two minor occurrences have been identified in coastal basins in Australia, but alluvial and geothermal-arsenic in New Zealand are more widespread, although none has resulted in significant human impact.

10.2 South and Central America

The main occurrences of arsenic in South America are listed in Table 10.1, and their distribution (Figure 10.1) can be considered in terms of four main regions: the high volcanic mountains of the Andes; the arid Pacific coastal plains; the tropical river basins of Amazonia; and the semi-arid Chaco–Pampean plains. The western side of South America is rich in arsenic both

Table 10.1 Occurrences of arsenic contamination in South and Central America, Africa and Australasia

Country/region	Name	Arsenic (ppb)[†] (mean/range/Max.)	Geology, hydrology, climate	Water chemistry	Affected population/significance*
South and Central America[‡]					
Nicaragua	Sebaco-Matagalpa Valley	37% >10; Max. 1320	Hydrothermally altered bedrock	Geothermal, Ca-HCO$_3$	1200 (E10)
El Salvador	Ilopanga lake catchment	Max. 770	Geothermal	GT	
Argentina, Chaco-Pampean plains	Cordoba	82% >50	Loess-rich alluvial deposits; semi-arid	AD; pH>8, high Na:Ca; high F, V and Mo	811,000 (E50)
	La Pampa	96% >10; 73% >50			
	Santiago del Estero	98% >10; 53% >50			
	Tucuman	100% >10; 87% >50			
	Buenos Aires	84% >10; 56% >50			
Bolivia	Altiplano	Max. >1000	Geothermal; arid to semi-arid.	GT	
Peru		Max. c. 500	Geothermal	GT	
Ecuador	North-central region	Max. 5080	Geothermal	GT	400,000 (E50)
Chile, Region II	Rio Loa	2000	Geothermal hot-springs discharging into rivers; arid to semi-arid.	GT	
	Rio Elqui	110			
	R. Camarones	1252			
Brazil	Iron Quadrangle	Max. 350	Precambrian basement, ironstone and sulphide mineralisation	SO	
Africa					
Ghana	southwest Ghana	10% >10; Max. >2000	Precambrian basement; tropical	SO	4000 (E50)
Ethiopia	Rift Valley	7% >10; Max. 96	Rift valley; semi-arid	?	

Country	Location	Concentration	Geology/Environment	Source	Notes
Botswana	Okavango delta	30% >10ppb; Max. 117	Alluvial–lacustrine; semi-arid	RD. High DOC, Fe; pH 8.0–8.6	
Burkina Faso	Yatenga	Median 15; Max. 1630	Precambrian basement; semi-arid	?	
Nigeria	Warri–Port Harcourt	Max. 750	Deltaic alluvium; humid-tropical	SO?	Conflicting data – requires confirmation
Nigeria	National survey	1000 water sources sampled by UNICEF all <10ppb	Humid-tropical to semi-arid	None	
Nigeria	Cross State	Median 16; Max. 35	Surface water; humid-tropical	?	
Nigeria	Ogun State	Average 76; Max. 200	Limestone; humid-tropical	?	
Cameroon	Ekondo Titi	Max. 2000	Alluvium	RD	4000 (E50)
Australasia					
Australia	New South Wales	Max. 337	Coastal alluvium over sandstone and granite	SO?	None
Australia	Perth	Max. 800	Coastal alluvium	SO and RD	Livestock affected
New Zealand	Waiotapu Valley, North Island	Max. '>50'	Central volcanic plateau	GT	
New Zealand	Waikato River, North Island	Average 32; Max. 150	River	GT	
New Zealand	Canterbury, South Island	Max. 43	Coastal alluvium	RD?	

*E10 refers to the number of people drinking water with >10ppm As, and E50 to drinking more than 50 ppm As. Where exposure has changed over time, the peak figure is quoted. 'E', now reduced due to mitigation measures.

†Concentrations normally refer to untreated water sources, either wells, streams or lakes, but not piezometers.

‡Arsenic has also been noted in Costa Rica and Guatemala.

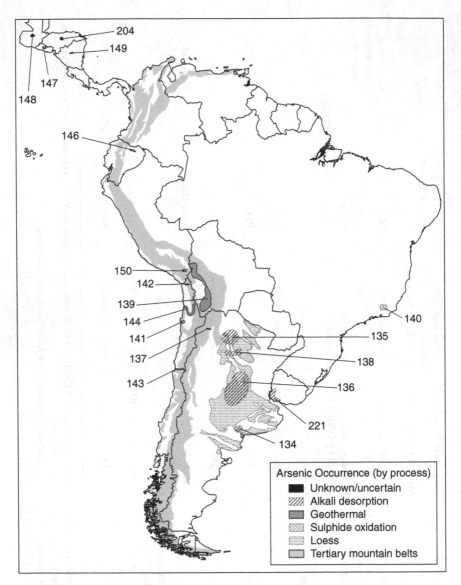

Figure 10.1 Occurrences of arsenic in Central and South America. See text and Table 1.2 for explanation of map numbers. The locations of Tertiary mountain belts and the distribution of loess are from ESRI (1996).

directly, due to volcanic activity, and indirectly because of the contribution of volcanic material to alluvial and aeolian deposits.

10.2.1   The Chaco–Pampean plains

Regional Setting

The Chaco–Pampean plains of Argentina, Paraguay, Uruguay and Bolivia lie between the Andes and the Rio Paraña, and extend up to 1500 km N–S and 500 km E–W. Here 1.2 million, mainly rural, inhabitants depend on groundwater as their only source of drinking water (Bundschuh et al., 2004). The Pampean Plains have a subhumid to semi–arid climate, with rainfall of 532 mm (Santiago del Estero) to 800 mm (Cordoba) and average temperature of 16.5°C. They have hot-wet summers and cold-dry winters. The vegetation is characterised by tall grass with an absence of trees (Clapperton, 1993). The population live mostly in small agricultural settlements, are heavily dependent on irrigation, and tend to be poorer than elsewhere in Argentina. In much of the area, groundwater is the only practically accessible source of water and is used for drinking, livestock and irrigation. On the Chaco Plains in the north, annual rainfall ranges from 400 mm in the west to 1200 mm in the east, and mean summer temperatures range between 24 and 30°C (Iriondo, 1993). Vegetation is characterised by diverse forests and large swamps with floating plant masses in the east, passing to sparse trees, cactus and 'hard' grass in the west.

Arsenic exposure and health impacts

An endemic disease caused by arsenic in drinking water has been known in Cordoba Province since the early part of the 20th century, and is known by the abbreviation HACRE[2] (Nicolli et al., 1989). It is associated with a type of skin cancer known as Bel Ville disease, named after the main town of the affected region. Despite the long history of arsenic poisoning, no systematic geological investigations took place until 1985. Surveys have been conducted in various provinces of Argentina (Table 10.2), and overall 95% of shallow groundwater samples exceeded 10 ppb and 67% exceeded 50 ppb As. Sancha and Castro (2001) estimated that two million people consume water containing >50 ppb As in Argentina, and the pollution extends into Uruguay (Manganelli et al. 2007).

Examining 15 years of mortality data from Cordoba, Hopenhayn-Rich et al. (1996, 1998) identified statistically significant relationships between As exposure and deaths from lung, kidney and bladder cancers. The exposure history was difficult to assess because water is drawn from so many private and public wells. Consequently, the 26 counties ('*Departmentos*')

Table 10.2   Summary of arsenic surveys on the Chaco–Pampean Plains of Argentina

Province	As (ppb) in water samples					
	Number	Average	Maximum	>10 (%)	>50 (%)	Ref.
Buenos Aires	–	–	–	84	56	(1)
Cordoba	60	164	3810	–	82	(2)
Cordoba	66	108	593	–	50	(3)
La Pampa	103	414	5300	95	73	(4)
Santiago del Estero	40	743	14,969	98	53	(5)
Tucuman	31	279	758	100	87	(6)

'–' not reported.
Sources: 1. Paoloni et al. (2005); 2. Nicolli et al. (1989); 3. Farias et al. (2003);
4. Smedley et al. (2002); 5. Bhattacharya et al. (2006); 6. Warren et al. (2005)

of Cordoba were grouped into low, medium and high As-exposure categories, using all available well data and also reports of arsenical skin manifestations. The two counties with the highest number of clinical reports were placed in the high exposure group, and assigned an average As concentration of 178 ppb. The six counties assigned to the medium exposure group also had reports of elevated arsenic concentrations and skin diseases. This classification was refined using data from a national survey that identified towns where water with >120 ppb As had been recorded. The remaining 16 counties were classified as low exposure. Provincial mortality data for 1986–91 were compared with the 1991 national census to calculate standardised mortality ratios (SMR). The results, as shown earlier in Table 5.12, indicate major increases in mortality from all three cancers resulting from arsenic exposure; well-defined dose–response relations are apparent for all three cancers. They also found a small positive trend for liver cancer and that skin cancer mortality was elevated for women in the high exposure group, but considered that associations between arsenic and mortality for these cancers were unclear, and found no relation with stomach cancer.

Although contaminated groundwater is used for irrigation, little is known about its implications for human exposure. Apart from arsenic, groundwater beneath the Pampean plains is extensively polluted by other naturally occurring contaminants, as illustrated by the exceedances of WHO guidelines in Table 10.3, based on a survey of over 100 wells in the northern part

Table 10.3   Exceedances of toxic trace elements in groundwater of La Pampa Province, Argentina

Parameter	Guideline value (ppb)	Exceeding	Maximum (ppb)	Parameter	Guideline value (ppb)	Exceeding	Maximum (ppm)
As	10	95%	5,300	B	0.5	99%	13.8
Mo	70	39%	990	F	1.5	83%	29.2
Se	10	32%	40	NO$_3$-N	11.3	47%	140
U	2	100%	250				

Source: Smedley et al. (2002)

of La Pampa province, and from which it is clear that arsenic pollution here cannot be addressed as an isolated problem.

Geology of the Chaco–Pampean plains

In terms of As pollution, the most important deposit underlying the Chaco–Pampean plains is the Pampean Loess Formation, which comprises 1100 km^2 of surficial sand and loess with an average thickness of 30–40 m deposited over the past 2.5 million years (Clapperton, 1993; Zarate, 2003). The loess is aeolian or reworked aeolian fine sand and silt of Andean volcaniclastic origin. The Pampean Loess is partly true air-fall silt-sized loess (*loess volcaniclasticos*) and partly wind-blown sand (*loess arenosos*), typically forming 1–2 m thick beds separated by erosional discontinuities or palaeosols. Intervening dune sands may have formed in glacial maxima. The southern Pampas is a huge sand sea, with longitudinal dunes up to 200 km long, but only 5–15 m thick, formed of feldspar (50%), volcanic glass and quartz (Nicolli et al., 1989). The loess[3] in Cordoba is a poorly sorted, clayey silt containing 45–70% feldspar, 25–50% volcanic glass and 4.8–12% heavy minerals, mainly pyroxenes and amphiboles[4]. The western Chaco is dominated by rivers draining the *Sierras Subandinas* that flow through deep transverse canyons and carry well-sorted sand (Iriondo, 1993). These subparallel streams terminate in the eastern Chaco where they meet the Paraguay–Paraña belt. Infiltration is limited by 12–20 m of silty clay and peat that accumulate in either permanent (*esteros*) or temporary (*bañados*) swamps. The Paraguay–Paraña belt is formed of clean fluvial sands derived from Cretaceous sandstones in Brazil.

Hydrogeology

Although Smedley et al. (2002) suggested that the Pampean Aquifer consists of (silt size) loess, it is more likely that the aquifer is formed of either dune sands or fluvial material interbedded with loess. In the north of Santiago del Estero, Bhattacharya et al. (2006) described a 100 m sequence of loess interbedded with three to six fluvial horizons that pass from gravel in the west to fine sand in the east. Warren et al. (2002) reported similar profiles in Tucuman province, where unconfined sand, a few tens of metres thick, is separated from a confined alluvial aquifer by variable thicknesses of clay. Wells in the shallow aquifer are commonly of large diameter, from which water is drawn *via* buckets or handpumps. The aquifers described by Warren et al. (2002, 2005) and Bhattacharya et al. (2006) suggest that the chemistry of percolating water is conditioned by reaction with loess and collected by a basal drainage layer of high permeability sand. In La Pampa Province, the saturated thickness of the aquifer increases from about 25 m (with an unsaturated zone up to 120 m thick) in the west, to about 80 m in the east where the water table approaches the ground surface (Smedley et al., 2002). The anomalous water balance estimates[5] are best explained if vertical movements dominate flow in the aquifer, and where most recharge is discharged through local flow cells as baseflow and/or evapotranspiration. The aquifers are recharged from three sources: direct infiltration on the plains; seepage from the Sali River; and infiltration on the piedmont followed by lateral flow through deeper strata (Garcia et al., 2006). The spatial relationship between loess, fluvial deposits and groundwater recharge in the Sali River basin of southwest Tucuman is illustrated in Figure 10.2.

In Santiago del Estero, the advent of irrigation caused the water table to rise from about 4 m to only 1.5 m below the surface, at which depth capillary rise to the surface is significant. In Cordoba, the water table lies mostly between 3 and 8 m below ground, and in Tucuman it ranges from a few metres to 20 m below ground. Thick silty soils have large water-holding capacities, and capillary rise can deposit salts near the surface that are redissolved during major recharge events. This interpretation is supported by Smedley et al. (2002), who used stable isotope measurements to infer a weak evaporative tendency in La Pampa. They also used tritium and radiocarbon dating to infer residence times of a few decades to a few centuries in both shallow and deep (>100 m) wells, and that suggest moderately rapid flow through the unsaturated zone.

Geochemistry

The landmark study by Nicolli et al. (1989), substantially confirmed by later investigations, identified associations of arsenic with volcanic glass in the loess, and with high pH. Arsenic-contaminated groundwater is oxic, slightly alkaline and sometimes saline, with tens to hundreds of ppm of sulphate. Groundwater is either of the Na–HCO$_3$ or Na-mixed anion type. Total mineralisation can be high, with ECs of 10–15,000 μS/cm, and

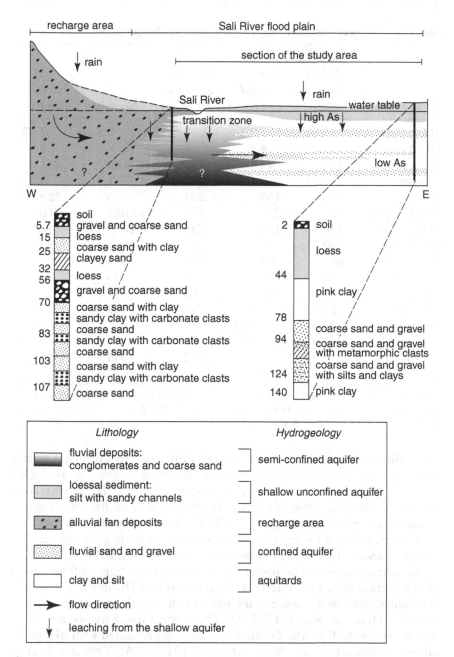

Figure 10.2 Hydrogeological section through the Sali River basin, southwest Tucuman. Note how the three different sources of recharge interact differently with the As-rich loessal sediments.
Source: Garcia et al. (2006)

Table 10.4   Average composition of groundwater from the Chaco–Pampean plains

Parameter	Tucuman shallow 'loess' aquifer'	Tucuman deeper alluvial aquifer	Rio Dulce Fan. San del Estero	Cordoba	La Pampa
pH	7.78	7.12	7.57	7.8	7.82
DO (ppm)	4.6	4.6	–	–	5.9
As (ppb)	279	14	743	164	414
F (ppm)	1.62	<0.05	2.6	1.2	5.2
Cl (ppm)	343	185	221	676	458
HCO$_3$ (ppm)	707	208	581	625	716
SO$_4$ (ppm)	550	160	235	1083	430
NO$_3$ (ppm)	100	7.6	13	–	84
Na (ppm)	680	205	427	1034	667
K (ppm)	32	9.4	22	36	15
Ca (ppm)	65	49	90	51	45
Mg (ppm)	24	8.5	18	39	45
Fe (ppm)	0.057	0.031	4.6		0.13
Mn (ppm)	0.020	0.007	0.57		0.005
EC (μS/cm)*		–	2422	4044	3340

*In Tucuman, where no EC measurements were reported, these may be approximated as 1.5 times TDS, giving 3300 μS/cm for the loess aquifer, and 1100 μS/cm for the deeper aquifer.
Sources: Data from Bhattacharya et al. (2006); Garcia et al. (2006); Nicolli et al. (1989); Smedley et al. (2002); Warren et al. (2005)

although evapoconcentration is important, high salinity correlates poorly with extreme arsenic values. Arsenic is dominantly present as As(V), although in Santiago del Estero, higher proportions of As(III) are correlated with DOC (median 8.6 ppm), and were attributed to infiltration of excess irrigation water (Bhattacharya et al., 2006). In some areas, infiltration of river water, polluted by organic wastes, generates anoxic groundwater that mobilises arsenic by reductive-dissolution (Garcia et al., 2006).

The average chemical composition of groundwater from different parts of Argentina is shown in Table 10.4. High nitrate and DO indicate that both the shallow and deep aquifers are oxic. High arsenic is associated with elevated pH, in the range pH 7.5–9.0. The contaminated waters are rich in Na+K relative to Ca+Mg. Sodium is positively correlated with pH, while calcium is negatively correlated with both pH and As. This is indicative of hydrolysis of silicate minerals and dissolution of carbonates (O. Sracek, personal communication, 2007), which consume carbon dioxide and account for the rise in pH and Si, and the correlation between arsenic and

a) Arsenic and pH

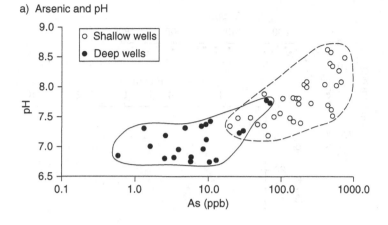

b) Arsenic and fluoride

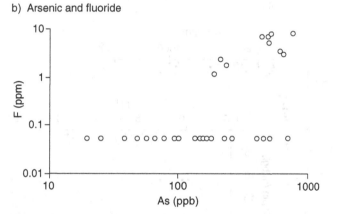

Figure 10.3   Correlation of arsenic with pH and fluoride in Tucuman Province, Argentina. (a) Arsenic and pH. (b) Arsenic and fluoride.
Source: Warren et al. (2002)

bicarbonate. Figure 10.3 shows the correlations between arsenic, pH and fluoride in groundwater in Tucuman Province. Deep groundwater consistently has pH < 7.5 and < 20 ppb As. However, even in the shallow aquifer, a significant minority of waters with high As concentrations have pH < 7.5, where desorption would not normally be expected. While most high F concentrations occur at pH > 8.0, Warren et al. (2002) showed that there are two distinct sources of arsenic, one accompanied by fluoride and one not (Figure 10.3).

In Tucuman, As, F, pH and salinity vary systematically with depth (Figure 10.4). In the shallow aquifer, As concentrations range from 20 to 760 ppb, and fluoride reaches 8.3 ppm. However, very high concentrations are restricted to the uppermost few tens of metres of the saturated zone, and

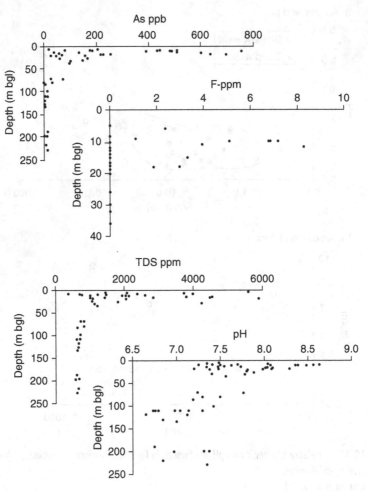

Figure 10.4   Depth distribution (below ground level) of arsenic, fluoride, total dissolved solids (TDS) and pH in Tucuman Province, Argentina. Note the different depth range for the fluoride graph.
Source: Warren et al. (2002)

fluoride is effectively absent below about 20 m. Further, the deeper ground-water cannot realistically evolve from that in the shallow aquifer, and it follows therefore that either this water was recharged before deposition of the upper loess or it was recharged on the mountain piedmont and has reached its present position by lateral flow. This supports the interpretation of stratigraphic control, whereby the occurrence of both arsenic and fluoride is fundamentally linked to the distribution of recent loess

(Warren et al., 2005). The low As concentrations in the deep aquifer may be due to local mobilisation, but may also be the result of leakage from the shallow aquifer.

Arsenic is often associated with elevated concentrations of other toxic trace elements (Table 10.3). In Cordoba, arsenic is positively correlated with F, V and U, but not with Se and Sb. In Santiago del Estero, arsenic is correlated with F, Na, B and V, and in La Pampa with F, B, V, Mo and less strongly with Be and U. Fluoride is a major problem on the Chaco–Pampean plains: 83% of samples in La Pampa, 42% in Cordoba, 40% in Santiago del Estero and 33% in Tucuman exceeded 1.5 ppm. Selenium is a problem in some areas but is not correlated with arsenic or pH. Although most of the trace elements pose an additional health burden, the coincidence of selenium and arsenic can reduce the toxicity of both (Chapter 5).

Nicolli et al. (1989) and later investigators found that the same elemental correlations observed in groundwater were also found in the loess, and this led them to propose a direct lithological control, where arsenic is released directly by weathering of volcanic glass. Differences in the trace element composition of the glass and the loess (Table 10.5) show that the loess is significantly enriched in As and Sb compared with the pure volcanic glass. The low calcium and high silica contents (Chapter 2) of the Pampean loess could promote desorption of As(V) at marginal pH conditions. Sediment analyses by Bhattacharya et al. (2006) indicate that arsenic is mainly bound to Fe and Mn oxides, and led them to invoke a two-step process where silicate minerals react with soil moisture to form iron oxides that subsequently adsorb arsenic released during weathering.

Palaeoclimates have influenced the distribution of arsenic. During drier phases, a higher proportion of rainfall would have been retained in the capillary fringe, to be discharged by evaporation, thus concentrating reactions and soluble minerals at the top of the unsaturated zone. Periodically this was supplemented by falls of loess and volcanic ash, building up a store of oxide-hosted arsenic. Nicolli et al. (1989) reported that the pH values of sediment[6] samples were in the range 8.5–9.5, easily sufficient to desorb

Table 10.5   Trace elements in loess and volcanic glass in Cordoba Province, Argentina

Element	Loess	Glass
As	16.7	>>8.71
Se	1.53	<1.79
U	2.99	<<4.20
Sb	0.545	>>0.314
Mo	3.4	≈3.65

Source: Nicolli et al. (1989)

As(V) under oxic conditions. Arsenic mobilisation above the water table could explain why the pH of some contaminated shallow groundwaters appears too low for desorption of As(V) to operate, and might also explain the less frequent contamination of the eastern plains where the water table approaches the ground surface. However, based on present information, the distribution of the Pampean loess (Figure 10.1) is a risk factor for, but not a unique determinant of, arsenic contamination.

Mitigation

For a problem known for 80 years, mitigation of arsenic pollution on the Pampean Plains appears to have been modest[7]. Hopenhayn-Rich et al. (1998) noted that As exposure has reduced in Cordoba due to construction of aqueducts to bring water from low-arsenic river sources, and also in rural areas where well-water is used in combination with rainwater stored in large outdoor containers ('*aljibes*'). Smedley et al. (2002) noted that some urban supplies have now been equipped with reverse osmosis (RO), although it is not known how successfully, but RO would be advantageous where salinity is also an issue. Experiments have been carried out using local laterite (unsuccessful) and a 'tropical' laterite (successful) from near the Paraguay and Brazil borders (Claesson and Fagerberg, 2003). Rivero et al. (2000) reported that coagulation-filtration systems are being installed in rural communities which use activated clay with alum or ferric chloride as the coagulant and calcium hypochlorite as an oxidant. Results from 16 plants showed that only five removed >75%, while nine removed <40% of the arsenic. Ten plants produced water containing 10–50 ppb As, only two <10 ppb, and four exceeded 50 ppb As.

Hydrogeological solutions appear to have received less attention, but the vertical distribution of arsenic and fluoride in Tucuman and La Pampa suggest that deep groundwater could be a cost-effective means of mitigation. However, this must be accompanied by long-term monitoring to ensure that As and F do not migrate downward from the shallow aquifer.

10.2.2   The Altiplano, Bolivia

In Bolivia, where around 25,000 people are exposed (Sancha and Castro, 2001), numerous rivers on the high-altitude Altiplano are contaminated by arsenic of both natural and anthropogenic origin. Natural arsenic is believed to seep into rivers from geothermal sources. The Altiplano is formed of Late Tertiary to Quaternary volcanic and volcaniclastic rocks overlying Mesozoic and Palaeozoic sediments. Young, active volcanoes of the Cordillera Occidental form its western margin. The region is noted for extensive sulphide mineralisation and supergene[8] enrichment. Active volcanoes, fumaroles depositing native sulphur, and both saline and thermal springs are common. The hydrology of the region is characterised by precipitation on the mountains of the Cordillera Occidental that is discharged by evaporation on the salars (salt flats) of Coipasa and Uyuni. Gross measures of salinity (Cl, TDS, SO_4) increase by three or four orders of magnitude along the flow direction of the streams due to evapo-concentration, and most other elements increase sympathetically. Banks et al. (2004) summarised the occurrence of arsenic and other elements in rivers on the Altiplano, reporting a median concentration of 34 ppb and a maximum of more than 1 ppm As. The rivers have a high median pH of 8.3, which increases downstream and is strongly correlated with arsenic concentration. The relatively uniform Cl: As ratio suggests that there is little attenuation of arsenic within the rivers. According to Banks et al. (2004), the primary sources of arsenic are fumaroles and hot springs, which are concentrated by evaporation, while the high pH and oxic conditions inhibit adsorption or precipitation of arsenic.

10.2.3   The Pacific plains of Chile, Peru and Ecuador

Both natural and anthropogenic (especially from copper and gold mining) arsenic pollution are present in Region II of northern Chile, mainly in rivers draining the Andes, but also in groundwater and soil. The adverse health impacts of arsenic have long been recognised, and the continued development of excess cancers after removal of exposure to arsenic was identified here (Smith et al., 1998). The greatest impacts have been at the regional capital of Antofagasta, but municipal water sources are contaminated at the coastal towns of Tocopilla, Iquique and Arica, and inland at Calama on the Rio Loa. Sancha and Frenz (1998) estimated that, in 1994–96, 11% of the population of Region II drank water containing >50 ppb, and 39% with >10 ppb As. Judging the success of water-supply mitigation since 1998 depends on the criterion applied. Sancha (2006a) reported that currently <0.1% of the Chilean population is exposed to >50 ppb As, but 47% access water supplies containing >10 ppb As. According to Sancha (2006b) arsenic remains a serious health problem, where exposure fluctuates between 81 and 174 µg/day. She indicates that water is the main source of exposure in northern and central Chile, but food is the main source in southern Chile. Sancha and Frenz (1998) highlighted differences between exposure in urban populations, where water supplies are treated to remove arsenic, and in largely aboriginal rural communities, where water is not treated and people consume locally produced food that may have been grown on As-contaminated soils. By contrast, the urban population of northern Chile tends to consume food imported from the uncontaminated south of the country.

Antofagasta, Chile

The most serious pollution has occurred around Antofagasta[9], the capital of Region II (population 400,000). Water supplies were drawn from the Rio Toconce and Rio Holajar that drain a 3000 m high section of the Andes some 300 km to the east (Borgono et al., 1977). The Rio Toconce contains around 800 ppb As, derived from a natural geological source in the upper catchment (Smith et al., 1998). Arsenic (400–600 ppb, dominantly arsenate) is also found in groundwater in sediments derived from Quaternary volcanics (Sancha, 1999). Arsenic concentrations in water supplies in Region II have fluctuated over time (Table 10.6). In all three locations, there were sudden increases and decreases in the As content, presumably corresponding to commissioning of new supplies and treatment plants.

At Antofagasta, the first reports of arsenical skin lesions and respiratory illness came only 2 years after the increase in arsenic concentration in the city supply (Ferreccio and Sancha, 2006). Shortly after peak exposure, there were large increases in the prevalence of peripheral vascular diseases such as Raynaud's symptom and ischaemia of the tongue. At its worst, 35% of the population of Antofagasta displayed arsenical skin lesions. During the period of peak exposure, infant mortality increased, and it was estimated that 18–24% of infant deaths between 1958 and 1965 were attributable to arsenic (Ferreccio and Sancha, 2006). In the 1970s, the commonest symptoms associated with arsenic in drinking water were respiratory and cardiovascular disease. In Antofagasta, 10% of cardiac infarction cases were aged under 41 (compared with 1.5% in Santiago), and of these, 53% had skin lesions. Twenty years after concentrations peaked, 12% of school children had skin lesions and 28% had chronic bronchitis, compared with 4% outside the city (Borgono et al., 1977). Pershagen (1983) suggested that malnutrition

Table 10.6   Average concentration of arsenic in water supplies in three cities of Region II, Chile

Years	Antofagasta (population 258,000)	Tocopilla (population 44,000)	Calama (population 141,000)
1950–1957	90	250	150
1958–1970	860	250	150
1971–1977	110	636	287
1978–1979	110	110	110
1980–1987	70	110	110
1988–2003	40	40	40
2004–2005	10	10	10

Source: Ferreccio and Sancha (2006)

may have contributed to the development of symptoms. Greatly increased risks of cancer (see below) persisted 20–30 years after the water treatment plants were commissioned. However, only in the 1990s was it established that the high prevalence of respiratory diseases and lung cancer was caused by arsenic in drinking water, and not airborne arsenic from mining activities.

Ecological studies by Smith et al. (1998) demonstrated increased cancer mortality in the exposed population. After 1970, the Salar del Carmen treatment plant slowly reduced As exposure, initially only to 260 ppb, but following improvements, to around 40 ppb. Having reconstructed the history of As concentrations in public supplies, they separately estimated the exposure history of men and women in each 10-year age band. They then calculated SMRs by comparing mortality records in Region II for the period 1989–93 with national mortality data for 1991. Their survey data also allowed them to eliminate smoking as a confounding factor for cancer mortality. As shown earlier (Table 5.12), they deduced large increases in mortality from bladder, lung, kidney and skin cancers, both during and after the period of peak exposure, and concluded that 'arsenic might account for 7% of all deaths among those aged 30 years and over'. A later analysis by Yuan et al. (2007) concluded that excess deaths from heart attacks, lung and bladder cancer attributable to arsenic poisoning were four times greater in the period 1971–2000 than in the period of peak exposure from 1958 to 1970 (section 5.14).

Sancha (1999, 2006b) described the use of coagulation to remove arsenic from surface and groundwater at Antofagasta. The river water contained 400–600 ppb As, dominantly arsenate, and is alkaline (pH 8.0–8.4) but not saline (TDS 700–800 ppm). It also contains moderate concentrations of sulphate (80–100 ppm) and silica (30–30 ppm), but negligible DOC (Karcher et al., 1999; Sancha, 2006b). At first, the Salar del Carmen plant was not particularly effective, but it was improved by pH adjustment with sulphuric acid, and pre-oxidation with chlorine, prior to adding $FeCl_3$ as the coagulant. This is followed by sedimentation, filtration and chlorination. By the late 1990s, the plant produced water with 40 ppb As residual. A new plant, with a capacity of 520 L/s was completed in 1978 at a cost of $20 M. Sancha (1999) reported that the operating cost was $0.04/m^3, and suggested that the system would not achieve a standard of 10 ppb As; however, by further improving the pH adjustment and oxidation, it subsequently proved possible to produce an output of 10 ppb As (Ferreccio and Sancha, 2006).

For contaminated groundwater, a coagulation-filtration plant, with a capacity of 32 L/s, is used to treat water containing 70 ppb As at Taltal. However, in this case, sedimentation and post-chlorination are omitted. Initially sludge was disposed of by dumping in the desert, but is now placed in an engineered landfill with a geotextile base and a capping system

Table 10.7   Comparison of three coagulation-filtration plants in Chile

Operational characteristic	Salar del Carmen (New)	Cerro Topater (Calama)	Taltal
Capacity (L/s)	520	500	32
Influent As (ppb)	400	400	70
Effluent As (ppb)	10	10	10
Cl_2 dose (ppm)	1.0	1.0	1.0
$FeCl_3$ dose (ppm)	56	41	8.0
Decantation rate (m/day)	70–75	70–75	–
Filtration rate (m/day)	143	143	150
Sludge generation (kg/day)	25–30	20–30	–

Source: Sancha (2006b)

(Sancha, 2006b). A comparison of the operating characteristics of three plants is given in Table 10.7.

Rio Loa, Chile

The Rio Loa in Region II of Chile is severely polluted by arsenic, with an average concentration of 1400 ppb As (Romero et al., 2003). The Rio Loa rises in the Cordillera Occidental, from where annual rainfall decreases from 3000 mm to almost nothing on the hyperarid Pacific plains. Its source is on the volcano Miño, and it cuts through rhyolitic volcanics and limestones before it is joined by the Rio Salado, a river is fed by geothermal springs including the El Tatio hot spring (84°C), which is saline (TDS 9600 ppm) and contains massive quantities of As (27 ppm), B (130 ppm) and Li (27 ppm), but low SO_4, and affects the lower reaches of the Rio Loa. Downstream, the river runs through Late Tertiary to Holocene alluvium with evaporite beds. There are three major porphyry copper (plus gold, silver and molybdenum) deposits in the basin.

The waters of the Rio Loa are highly saline (Figure 10.5), and also strongly enriched in boron (average 21 ppm), lithium and sulphate. Above the Salado, the Rio Loa is alkaline (pH 8.2), slightly mineralised with TDS of around 2000 ppm, several hundred ppm of sulphate, and 200–300 ppb As. From the confluence with the Salado to the ocean, the salinity steadily increases from around 3000 to 11,000 ppm, while arsenic increases more slowly from 1000 ppb to around 2000 ppb at the mouth. However, the Cl:As ratio remains fairly constant (1.6–1.7), which suggests concentration by evaporation. Under these oxic, alkaline conditions there is little tendency for Fe and Mn oxyhydroxides to adsorb arsenic, so arsenic remains at dangerous levels even though, below the Salado, it is also too saline for direct consumption.

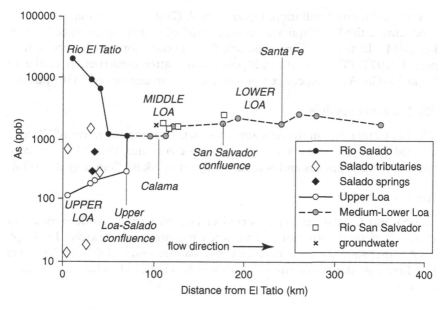

Figure 10.5   Profile of arsenic concentrations along the Rio Loa, Chile. Note that the dashed lines symbolically represent the course of the Rio Loa and its tributaries. In the middle reaches, groundwater and surface water contain approximately the same concentrations of arsenic.
Source: Romero et al. (2003)

Rio Elqui, Chile

The Rio Elqui, 400 km north of Santiago, which supplies water to some 200,000 people, lies at the transition between the Atacama Desert and steppe, with annual rainfall of 100 mm (Dittmar, 2004). River water is derived from snow melt on the Andes, and flow decreases from a maximum at the mountain front due to combination of evaporation and leakage into the ground. The Rio Elqui is both less saline and less polluted by arsenic than the Rio Loa. In its upper and middle reaches, EC decreases from around 1000 to about 650 µS/cm, while in the lower reaches (below the confluence with the Rio Claro) it ranges from 450 to 550 µS/cm. The water is consistently alkaline (pH 8.0–8.5), and contains up to 110 ppb As in the upper catchment, and with even higher concentrations in some tributaries, but below the Rio Claro, concentrations fluctuate in the range 10–18 ppb As.

Oyarzun et al. (2006) attributed contamination primarily to Miocene hydrothermal copper and As mineralisation, which has been exposed to erosion for about 10,000 years. The arsenic is mobilised by oxidation of sulphide minerals in fracture zones, where they are so abundant as to exceed the buffering capacity of surrounding rocks. Mining in the upper catchment of the Rio Elqui, which contains the largest gold mine in Chile (El Indio), has exacerbated natural pollution. Oyarzun et al. (2007) showed that streambed sediments in the Rio Elqui are strongly enriched in arsenic (average 206 mg/kg, $n=14$). In the Rio Toro tributary, As concentrations in the pre-mining period (1975–77) were 360–520 ppb As, but after construction of the El Indio Au–Cu–As mine, concentrations rose to a maximum of 1510 ppb As.

Rio Camarones, Chile

The Rio Camarones in the Atacama Desert, in the extreme north of Chile, is affected by geothermal arsenic and evaporitic concentration. The river contains up to 1252 ppb As and is used locally for drinking (Yanez et al., 2006).

Rio Locumba, Peru

Sancha and Castro (2001) reported arsenic in various Andean rivers of Peru, especially the Rio Locumba where concentrations are around 500 ppb As. Another significant occurrence is at Lake Aricota, which is fed by rivers that flow past the Yucamane volcano, which is believed to be the source of the arsenic.

Rio Tambo, Ecuador

Cumbal et al. (2006) report that arsenic from geothermal sources, in the range 970 to 5080 ppb As, affects springs, a lake, a reservoir and some rural water supplies used for drinking in the Rio Tambo watershed of the north-central Andean region of Ecuador.

10.2.4 Other arsenic-affected areas in South and Central America

The Iron Quadrangle, Brazil

The Iron Quadrangle, in the state of Minas Gerais in southeast Brazil, is one of the richest mining areas in the world. Apart from massive iron deposits, there are important sulphidic hydrothermal gold deposits with associated pyrite, pyrrhotite and arsenopyrite. Borba et al. (2003) estimated that over 300 years nearly 400,000 t of arsenic were discharged to the rivers. Matschullat et al. (2000) sampled 18 rivers and measured a mean of 31 ppb As and a maximum 350 ppb As. Contamination was considered to be mainly anthropogenic, but also partly natural.

São Paulo, Brazil

Campos (2002) identified arsenic contamination (130–170 ppb As) in shallow (12 m) domestic wells, which he attributed to excessive use of phosphatic fertilisers containing traces of arsenic.

Isle of Youth, Cuba

Leon (2004) reported arsenic contamination of surface waters and a bedrock aquifer in a former mining area with gold, arsenic and sulphide mineralization. However, it is not clear to what extent this is natural pollution.

El Salvador

Sancha and Castro (2001) reported arsenic contamination from Ilopango Lake, a large caldera with an area of 185 km² and 240 m deep. It is used as a source of water for 300,000 people (Lopez et al., 2006). The lake is seasonally stratified, and consequently As concentrations vary between 150 and 770 ppb, and boron between 1500 and 8700 ppb. Two sources of arsenic were identified. The first was the sediment of the Chaguite River, and the second was ash deposited when the caldera last exploded, about 2000 years ago. Lopez et al. (2006) suggested that this ash layer may be a regional source of pollution in El Salvador and surrounding countries. Arnórsson (2004) noted high As in geothermal waters at Achuapan.

Nicaragua

Espinoza (2005, 2006) reported concentrations of <10 to 122 ppb As in the Sebaco-Matagalpa Valley of eastern Nicaragua, affecting a community of 3200 where 37% of wells exceeded 10 ppb As. The aquifer is Quaternary alluvium, but the arsenic is derived from hydrothermally altered rocks associated with faults that run parallel to the highly mineralised Nicaragua graben. Most groundwater is of a calcium-bicarbonate type. In 1996, arsenicosis was reported from persons exposed for 6–24 months to groundwater containing 1320 ppb As, and even the dug wells that replaced this supply contained up to 122 ppb As. Soils in the affected area contained up to 95 mg/kg As.

Other countries

Bundschuh et al. (2006) noted the presence of As contamination in water supplies in Costa Rica and Guatemala, but no details were given.

10.3 Africa

What is most notable about known occurrences of natural arsenic contamination in Africa (Table 10.1, Figure 10.6) is their paucity, however, in most countries there is no *evidence* of presence or absence. The only detailed descriptions of As contamination come from Ghana, while there are single references, dating from 2006, for Botswana, Cameroon and Burkina Faso. Incidental detections of arsenic have been noted in Ethiopia and Uganda,

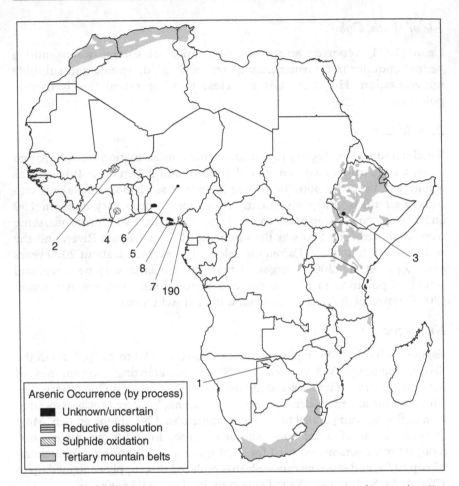

Figure 10.6   Occurrences of arsenic in Africa. See text and Table 1.2 for explanation of map numbers. Note that no information regarding the presence or absence of arsenic could be found for most African countries.

and there are contradictory reports of arsenic from Nigeria. Arsenic concentrations of 5–9 ppb As have also been recorded from wells in weathered and fractured bedrock in the Aroca region of north-central Uganda (Taylor and Howard, 1994).

10.3.1   Botswana

Huntsman-Mapila et al. (2006) documented the occurrence of arsenic in the inland delta of the Okavango River in the semi-arid northwest of Botswana. The Okavango Delta occupies a Quaternary half-graben within the Kalahari Basin, a shallow intracontinental basin covered by sand dunes and lacustrine deposits. Thick alluvial sands were deposited during wet phases of the Pleistocene, derived from late Precambrian granitic, mafic and ultramafic rocks. Groundwater is recharged by seasonal floodwaters, and flows at shallow depths from the floodplains to 'islands' where it is discharged by phreatophytic[10] vegetation. As a result of evapotranspiration, groundwater becomes concentrated in the discharge zones. Traditionally, water supplies were drawn from surface water, but due to the expanding population, groundwater has been increasingly exploited since 1986.

Water in the Okavango River is typically coloured brown by organic acids, and contains 1–3 ppb As. Groundwater from 30% of 20 new boreholes exceeded 10 ppb As, and the highest concentration was 117 ppb As. Arsenic was dominantly present as As(III) and positively correlated with both pH, DOC and bicarbonate. Groundwater containing >20 ppb As mostly has pH 8.0–8.6, which suggests the possibility of alkali-desorption. There is also an association between elevated arsenic and EC, which suggests that evapoconcentration increases arsenic concentrations. The aquifer sands contained 0.2–7.0 mg/kg As, which correlated with iron, organic content, clay content and cobalt concentration. Huntsman–Mapila et al. (2006) concluded that RD of oxyhydroxides is the most likely release mechanism.

10.3.2 Burkina Faso

Appelo and Postma (1996) noted that Blackfoot Disease, a characteristic symptom of arsenic poisoning in Taiwan, was present in Burkina Faso, but gave no details. Following reports of abnormal skin diseases (see http://www.irc.nl/page/32211; accessed 11 January 2007), investigations by UNICEF in 2006 detected arsenic in boreholes and wells in the northern district of Yatenga and Lorum, near the border with Mali. A survey of 36 boreholes revealed a median concentration of 15.1 ppb As and a maximum of 1630 ppb As. The equivalent concentrations in nine dug wells were only 1.5 and 6.1 ppb As, suggesting that arsenic concentrations increase with depth and are not associated with near-surface oxidation processes. The exact locations of affected wells were not reported, but Yatenga lies on the northern edge of the Precambrian Birimian granitic rocks where gold and molybdenum mineralisation occurs, although the northern border region is covered by younger sedimentary rocks (Sattran and Wenmenga, 2002). The soils of the region are described as 'soils of erosion, poorly developed, on gravel material'. The region has an average annual rainfall of around 700 mm, and it is reported that the groundwater is obtained from fissured basement aquifers that are vulnerable to drought (Sattran and Wenmenga, 2002).

10.3.3 Cameroon

Mbotake (2006) reported As concentrations of up to 2000 ppb As in wells in coastal alluvium from the Ekondo Titi region of southwest Cameroon. The Lobe plain is surrounded by hills up to 1500 m high, formed of Cretaceous to Tertiary sandstones and shales and Tertiary to Quaternary basalt. The plain, which receives about 2400 mm of rainfall, has been drained and exploited for agriculture, and passes into mangrove swamp and saltwater creeks in the southwest. It is underlain by thick alluvium, which is interbedded with basalt lavas, and exploited to depths of about 100 m, although most wells are about 30 m deep. Mbotake (2006) estimated that about 4000 people were exposed to high-As concentrations and, because the highest concentrations occur in strongly reducing groundwater, concluded that arsenic is mobilised by reductive dissolution. To date, there are no reports of adverse health effects (I.T. Mbotake, personal communication, 2007).

10.3.4 Ethiopia

In a survey of deep and shallow wells, springs and rivers along the Ethiopian section of the East African Rift Valley, Reimann et al. (2003) found pervasive water quality problems, with 86% of samples failing at least one WHO guideline value. The greatest problems were fluoride[11], which exceeded 1.5 ppm in 33% of samples, and uranium, which exceeded the WHO guideline (2 ppb) in 47% of well-waters. Arsenic, although of lesser significance, exceeded 10 ppb in 7% of samples, and had a maximum of 96 ppb. Arsenic is enriched in hot springs that may impact upon surface waters. The hot springs containing high arsenic also had undesirably high concentrations of B, Be, F, Ge, Li, Mo and Na. Reimann et al. (2003) also noted clusters of deep wells with elevated arsenic in the centre of the Rift Valley which they attributed to hydrothermal sources.

10.3.5 Ghana

The first published report of arsenic pollution was at the Ashanti Gold Mine in southwest Ghana, where soil concentrations of 189–1025 mg/kg and groundwater concentrations of 86–557 ppb As were recorded (Bowell, 1994). The Birimian metasediments and metavolcanics contain more than ten times the crustal average concentrations of both gold and arsenic, and have been mined for gold since the late 19th century. The release of arsenic to the environment was attributed to oxidation of arsenopyrite, either through lateritic weathering or the effects of mineral processing. A geochemical assessment of the Obuasi gold mining area by Smedley et al. (1996) reported concentrations of up to 175 ppb in surface water and up to 64 ppb As in groundwater. The water table is encountered at between 2.5 and 7.5 m b.g.l., and groundwater flow is largely restricted to fractures, especially quartz veins. Smedley et al. (1996) also attributed arsenic pollution to a combination of mining and natural oxidation of sulphides, but also noted that the highest concentrations were in wells 40–70 m deep that contained reducing groundwater. Although they recorded elevated As concentrations in urine, no clinical symptoms could be unequivocally attributed to intake of arsenic.

Norman et al. (2001) tested 127 drilled and 76 dug wells in a 6500 km^2 area of southwest Ghana using the Arsenator™ field kit, and found that water from 18% of drilled wells and 3% of dug wells exceeded 5 ppb As. The maximum As concentration was 2000 ppb, and a higher proportion (41%) of drilled wells than dug wells (20%) contained >0.5 ppm of iron. They detected a strong correlation between skin problems and As concentration in drinking water. They confirmed the association of arsenic with rocks of the Upper Birimian Formation, and speculated that arsenic might be found in groundwater in the other 10 belts of gold mineralisation that cross Ghana. Contaminated groundwater was not only more mineralised, but also, as indicated by negative redox potentials and very low SO_4 concentrations, strongly reducing. Combined with the observation that drilled (i.e. deeper) wells were more often polluted than dug wells, this suggests that arsenic might be mobilised by RD. Norman et al. (2001) estimated that 10% of rural water wells in Ghana may contain >10 ppb[12]. Siabi (2004) indicated that 'high' levels of arsenic have been detected in the Ashanti, Western, Brong Ahafo, Northern, Upper West and Upper East regions. In southwest Ghana, 5% and 19% of boreholes exceed 10 ppb As in the Ankobra and Lower Offin basins (Kortatsi, 2007; Kortatsi et al., 2007), where arsenic was attributed to oxidation of locally abundant arsenopyrite; however, it was also reported that many high iron concentrations were due to reductive dissolution of iron oxides. Obiri (2007) reported concentrations of up to 4500 ppb As at Dumasi in Wassa West District.

10.3.6   Nigeria

There is limited information concerning arsenic in Nigeria, and much of it is confusing. By analogy with Asia, it has often been speculated that groundwater might be contaminated in the Niger Delta, and this finds some support in observations of strongly reducing groundwater (Amadi et al., 1989). However, a survey by UNICEF of 1608 samples from boreholes, dug wells and water vendors in all eight hydrological regions found that all complied with the 10 ppb WHO guideline (Othniel Habila, personal communication,

2006). On the other hand, unpublished analyses (W. Gbadebo, personal communication, 2006) from dug wells and boreholes along the Warri–Port Harcourt axis indicate concentrations of 280–750 ppb As in water that is slightly acidic (pH 4.0–6.0) and contains significant sulphate (48–83 ppm) and modest iron (1.0–1.8 ppm) concentrations. To the east of the delta, Edet and Offiong (2003) measured concentrations of 10–35 ppb As in surface waters from the Lower Cross River basin.

Outside the Niger Delta, Gbadebo and Mohammed (2004) detected concentrations of up to 200 ppb As (average 76 ppb As) in dug wells in the limestone areas of Ogun State in southwestern Nigeria. In an environmental impact assessment at Kaduna in north-central Nigeria, Oke (2003) reported high As concentrations in surface waters and dug wells drawing water from laterite. Oke (2003) reported that groundwater was oxidising and that 'a natural source is strongly suspected for Pb, Fe, Cr and As contamination', however, these results require independent confirmation.

10.4 Australasia

The occurrences of arsenic in groundwater in Australasia are listed in Table 10.1 and their distribution is shown in Figure 10.7, although no human health impacts have been reported. There are also widespread reports of soil

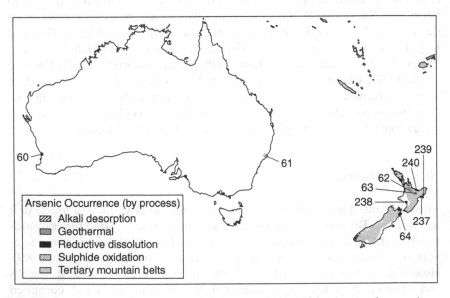

Figure 10.7 Occurrences of arsenic in Australasia. See text and Table 1.2 for explanation of map numbers.

contamination in Australia related to both the disposal of mine waste and the use of arsenical pesticides (Naidu et al., 2006).

10.4.1   Australia

Perth, Western Australia

Groundwater beneath the Swan Coast Plain, near Perth, is affected by arsenic mobilised by sulphide oxidation at shallow depth, and by RD in deeper aquifers (Appleyard et al., 2006). The Swan Coast Plain has a Mediterranean climate (rainfall 860 mm) and is underlain by up to 110 m of Quaternary alluvial and aeolian sands with calcrete layers. Surface soils are permeable and there is little runoff, but water accumulates in surface depressions, forming wetlands that are underlain by peat rich in arsenical pyrite. The underlying sands contain 100–400 mg/kg As. The first and most intensely abstracted (550,000 m³/day) aquifer is formed of unconfined Quaternary sands up to 70 m thick, and includes layers of black, humic peat. The piezometric surface intersects peat layers in the wetlands, which are in partial hydraulic continuity. Above the water table, the peat is weathered, mottled, and contains gypsum and jarosite. The deeper aquifers are confined Jurassic and Cretaceous sediments.

Figure 10.8 shows a conceptual model of groundwater flow and arsenic mobilisation on the Swan Coastal Plain, as discussed below. Perth draws half its drinking water from four aquifers, and has experienced a long-term drought. The water table around the Gwelup wetlands has been falling since the 1970s, triggering oxidation of pyritic sediments. Appleyard et al. (2006) surveyed 800 private wells, which mostly contained arsenic at the tens of ppb level, although some contained a few hundreds of ppb. Many wells produced acidic water (pH 2.5–4.0), with a few hundred to a few thousand ppm of SO_4 and tens to hundreds of ppm of iron – classic signatures of pyrite oxidation. The 2004 survey demonstrated a major decline in water quality compared with a 1976 survey, 1 year after the public wellfield was commissioned, when arsenic was generally below detection limits. Porewater profiling to 15 m confirmed that pH was at a minimum just below the water table, and was accompanied by hundreds of ppb of arsenic, which dropped to a few tens of ppb by 10 m.

The response of municipal production wells, which are screened in the lower half of the unconfined aquifer, was quite different. Iron concentrations rose steadily through the period, whereas calcium and sulphate rose until about 1990 and then stabilised. On the other hand, nitrate, an indicator of oxic conditions, fell after 1990, whereas ammonium rose steadily. In stark contrast to shallow oxidation, the production well data indicate the

a) Pre-development

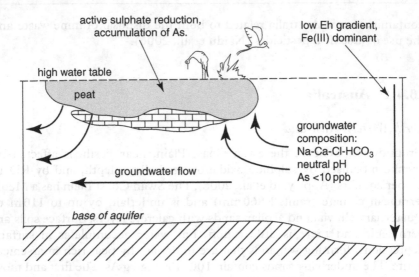

active sulphate reduction,
accumulation of As.

low Eh gradient,
Fe(III) dominant

high water table

peat

groundwater
composition:
Na-Ca-Cl-HCO$_3$
neutral pH
As <10 ppb

groundwater flow

base of aquifer

b) During urban development

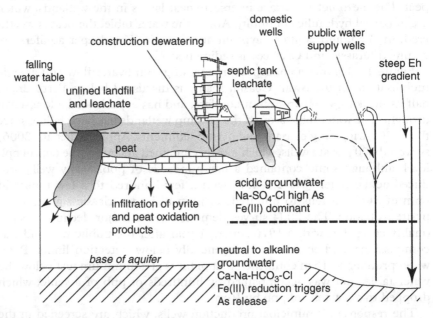

domestic
wells

construction dewatering

public water
supply wells

falling
water table

septic tank
leachate

steep Eh
gradient

unlined landfill
and leachate

peat

acidic groundwater
Na-SO$_4$-Cl high As
Fe(III) dominant

infiltration of pyrite
and peat oxidation
products

neutral to alkaline
groundwater
Ca-Na-HCO$_3$-Cl
Fe(III) reduction triggers
As release

base of aquifer

Figure 10.8 Conceptual model of arsenic mobilisation on the Swan Coastal Plain, Perth, Australia. The two figures compare (a) the presumed natural flow regime with (b) the post-development scenario. Oxidation and reduction processes operate simultaneously at the upper and lower surfaces of the peat. Natural reduction is enhanced locally by leakage from unlined landfills.
Source: Appleyard et al. (2006)

migration of a reducing front into the deeper parts of the unconfined aquifer. For the first 5–15 years, arsenic was not detected in the Gwelup wellfield, but thereafter fluctuated in the range of 5–15 ppb As. The increasingly reducing nature of the deep aquifer is demonstrated by the drop in redox potential of 100–200 mV, and a change in sediment colour from brown to grey, as recorded during drilling. The change was interpreted as a gleying phenomenon, where ferric iron is reduced to ferrous iron. Appleyard et al. (2006) concluded that the fall in the water table caused the products of peat and pyrite oxidation to percolate into the aquifer, promoting reductive dissolution of iron coatings on the sands. Percolation from an unlined landfill constructed in the wetland exacerbated this process. Continued drought threatens the long-term quality of the public water supply to Perth.

Stuarts Point, New South Wales

Smith et al. (2003) reported natural arsenic in Holocene coastal barrier sands in the Stuarts Point coastal sands aquifer (SPCSA) and the underlying Yarrahapinni fractured rock aquifer (YFRA). The SPCSA comprises (a) alluvial swamp deposits overlying (b) Holocene and Pleistocene estuarine clay and sandy clay, and (c) Pleistocene barrier and Holocene marine sands deposited during a period of marine submergence. Sandy horizons have permeabilities of up to 36 m/day. The Holocene clays were classified as having high acid-sulphate soil risk[13]. Rocks of the upper catchment, that form the YFRA, comprise Permian sandstones and granitoids with Ag–Pb and Ag–As mineralisation. Groundwater flow follows the topography towards the coastal wetlands. The maximum As concentration in the SPCSA is 70 ppb, and in the YFRA is 337 ppb. There was no simple correlation between As and SO_4, S, or HCO_3; and As and Fe were also poorly correlated. Recharge water is oxygen-rich and acidic. Two peaks were observed in profiles measured in piezometer nests. The first, at about 10–12 m, was oxic and slightly acidic (pH 5.6) with low Cl and HCO_3. The second peak, at 25 m, is dominantly As(III) and associated with elevated Na and Cl. Smith et al. (2003) concluded that the shallow As(V) peak in fresh acidic water was due to either hydrolysis of Al-hydroxides or pH-controlled desorption from iron oxyhydroxides, while they attributed the deeper As(III) peak to alkaline-desorption[14].

10.4.2   New Zealand

North Island

In the Central Volcanic Plateau (CVP), geothermal waters contain up to 8500 ppb As (Webster and Nordstrom, 2003; Mandal and Suzuki, 2002). An early case of arsenic poisoning from well-water was described by

Grimmett and McIntosh (1939) in the Waiotapu Valley in the CVP. Cattle kept on swampy ground with signs of geothermal activity (hot springs and mud volcanoes) suffered from a form of 'paralysis'. Springs and drains in the area contained up to 2000 ppb As, and some drinking water wells also contained up to 50 ppb As, although no cases of arsenicosis were reported (Grimmett and McIntosh, 1939). The affected area was small, being less than 1000 ha with about 30 farms.

The Waikato River, at 425 km, is the longest river in New Zealand and contains geothermal arsenic originating from the CVP. It is the source of water supply to the city of Hamilton (population 100,000) and about 30 community supplies, some of which are untreated and contain up to 150 ppb (McLaren and Kim, 1995). Hamilton relies on coagulation with alum and filtration to render its water fit for drinking. The Hamilton source shows regular fluctuations in As concentration that do not follow a simple relationship to discharge. Arsenic monitored in treated and untreated water at Hamilton for a year had an average concentration of 32.1 ± 3.7 ppb As. Arsenic concentrations are about 10–25 ppb higher in the summer than winter, but are hardly affected by changes in discharge. McLaren and Kim (1995) suggested that the changes in arsenic concentrations result from microbiological activity that alters the partitioning of arsenic between particulate and soluble forms. Similarly, Mroczek (2005) reported geothermal-arsenic contributing to a background of 21 ppb As in the Tarawera River.

Although there is little published information, arsenic concentrations of 1–5 ppb occur widely in reduced groundwaters in alluvial aquifers in many parts of New Zealand including North Hawkes Bay, the Bay of Plenty, Wanganui and Gisborne. The groundwater is used for various purposes including drinking water, irrigation and livestock. Approximately 10% of 157 monitoring sites have concentrations of >10 ppb, with a maximum 260 ppb As (C. Daughney[15], personal communication, 2007).

South Island

Wilkinson (2005) described arsenic pollution in the Rarangi area, near Marlborough, on the Wairu River plain, an area of glacial outwash overlain by marine and lagoonal sediments and beach ridges. The Wairu plains are underlain by 500 m of glacial and fluvial sediment. The upper unit, the Dillons Point Formation (DPF), is 25–30 m thick in the affected area. The plain is surrounded by hills of Palaeozoic schists that rise to >100 m. Beach ridges separate the plains from wetlands. Post-glacial fluvial aggradation was choked by rising sea level and caused Wairu River to 'disappear' into the swamp. The main source of groundwater is gravel in the Rarangi Shallow Aquifer (RSA), which was deposited after 14 ka, is found in the upper 5 m, and contains layers of peat. The RSA is a highly transmissive

($450\,m^2$/day) unconfined (storage coefficient 0.1) aquifer (Wilkinson, 2005). The underlying Wairu Aquifer is $<20\,m$ thick, confined by marine silts of the DPF, and is of minor importance but contains 2–21 ppb As. Shallow (5–8 m) wells in the RSA, which are used for drinking, dairy farming and irrigation, contain between <1 and 43 ppb As. Groundwater quality in the RSA is highly variable, ranging from slightly acid (pH 6.3) to weakly alkaline (pH 8.2). The wide range of concentrations of redox sensitive species such as SO_4 (0.2–191 ppm), NO_3 (0.002–10.7 ppm), Fe (0.002–5.6 ppm) and Mn (0.001–1.0 ppm) indicates that oxidation and reduction reactions operate in close juxtaposition.

10.5   Arsenic in the Ocean Basins

No major reports of As contamination on oceanic islands have been identified, although Vuki et al. (2006) measured a trace of arsenic in springs on the Pacific island state of Guam. Webster and Nordstrom (2003) reported concentrations of up to 48 ppb As in hot springs on Iceland, and up to 70 ppb in geothermal wells on Hawaii. These concentrations are low compared with continental geothermal systems. It appears that geothermal sources acquire little arsenic from flow through oceanic crust, whereas continental systems acquire arsenic more from sedimentary rocks such as shales than from their magmatic host (Nordstrom and Webster, 2003).

10.6   Suspect Terrain and Research Needs

10.6.1   South America

South America provides numerous examples of arsenic mobilisation through AD and from geothermal sources, but only one case of SO and none of RD. This stands in sharp contrast with Asia, where arsenic is mobilised principally by RD in humid areas and alluvial sediments. There is considered to be a particular risk in three regions of South America: parts of the Chaco–Pampean plains; alluvial basins on the Pacific Plains; and the Amazonian foreland basin.

The Chaco–Pampean plains

The severe arsenic pollution beneath the Chaco-Pampean plains is attributed to the high volcanic content of the Pampean loess. The extent of arsenic pollution appears to have been incompletely mapped. Geomorphological mapping by Zarate (2003) shows that the loess extends into Paraguay,

Brazil, Uruguay and Bolivia. A regional hydrogeochemical study including Argentina and adjoining countries should be conducted to determine the full extent of pollution and/or the factors that limit it.

South American river systems

As discussed in Chapter 3, the quartz:feldspar:rock fragment (QFR) ratios of river sands have been tentatively related to the occurrence of arsenic in alluvial groundwater. The continent-wide study of Potter (1994) identified five mineral associations (Figure 10.9) and offers insight into the alluvial aquifers formed from them. The Pacific Association comprises very immature sands ($Q_{21}F_{15}R_{64}$), low in quartz, where half the rock fragments are either andesite or devitrified volcanic glass, and often display signs of hydrothermal alteration. The Argentine Association is similar, but contains even more (63%) volcanic rock. The Transitional Association occurs on the lowlands to the east of the Andes, and contains more quartz (60%), while the rock fragments are dominantly metamorphic. The Caribbean Association, which includes only one large river, the Magdalena, is similar to the Transitional Association. The most extensive association, the Brazilian ($Q_{86}F_7R_7$), includes the whole of the Amazon, Orinoco and Parana catchments, and comprises the most mature sands, strongly enriched in quartz (median 92%), and includes some of the world's purest modern sands (Potter, 1994).

The Pacific and Brazilian associations represent opposites. Pacific sands are the most immature and rich in volcanic material. They originate at high altitude, where there is little chemical weathering, and travel by short, steep routes to be deposited on a narrow coastal plain, where little organic matter accumulates. Groundwater in such sediments is likely to be oxic and alkaline, and favour AD, similar to the As-affected Basin-and-Range province of the USA. Sands of the Brazilian Association originate on the Brazilian and Guyanan shields, where weathering is so intense that potential fluvial sediment is reduced to almost pure quartz. Thus, in spite of a favourable climate and depositional environment, there is probably either insufficient arsenic to contaminate groundwater or it is so tightly bound to detrital haematite or limonite as to be unavailable. Sands of the Transitional Association are derived from sediments recycled from erosion of the Andes (DeCelles and Hertel, 1989), where weathering has been sufficient to alter the original composition of these sands, but not sufficient to destroy the igneous and metamorphic rock fragments.

The Amazonian foreland basins

Reports of arsenic are notably absent from the foreland basins that run along the eastern side of the Andes. These basins have certain features

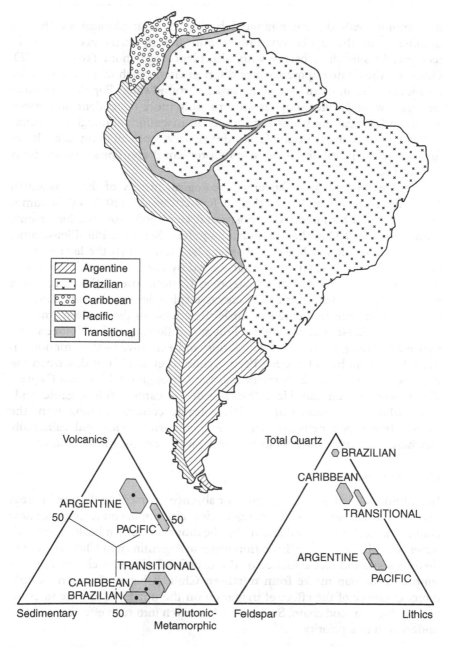

Figure 10.9 Sand mineral associations in South America. Both the quartz:feldspar:rock (QFR) ratios of the sands, and the proportions of volcanic, sedimentary and metamorphic rocks, reflect the potential content and/or availability of arsenic.
Source: Potter (1994)

in common with the contaminated basins in Asia: physical weathering dominates in the upper catchment; and the products accumulate in tectonically subsiding basins with abundant vegetation, favouring RD. However, the demographic settings differ greatly, which might account for non-identification of an arsenic hazard in groundwater. Population densities are low, and water supplies are probably more dependent on surface water, and agriculture is less dependent on irrigation, although this situation may change in the future. Groundwater development in this area therefore opens the possibility of an arsenic problem if appropriate precautions are not taken.

The late Tertiary (post-Barreiras) geological history of the Amazonian foreland was described by De Fatima Rossetti et al. (2005) and Schumm et al. (2000), who indicated depositional conditions suitable for arsenic mobilisation by RD in shallow alluvial aquifers. Since the Plio-Pleistocene, western Amazonia has been a subsiding basin, in which the lacustrine to marine Solimoes Formation was succeeded by the Ica Formation, derived from both the Andes and the Amazonian Craton. After 40 ka there was a major increase in deltaic or fluvial crevasse-splay deposition, indicating the drainage had been reoriented towards the course of the modern Amazon (De Fatima Rossetti et al., 2005). This was followed, in the Holocene, by massive flooding, lobate sand deposition and extensive peat formation. In the sub-Andean belt of eastern Peru, Schumm et al. (2000) described the Marañon, Ucayali and Beni rivers that flow through the Ucamara Depression to join the Amazon. Here, 'black-water' streams rich in organic acids meet 'white' silty rivers with a high volcanic content, coming from the Andes. Interaction between layers of organic-rich muds and minimally weathered volcanic sands could be conducive to arsenic mobilisation.

Irrigation and agriculture

In addition to verifying the presence or absence of arsenic pollution in areas where groundwater has not been tested, it is also important to consider how contaminated water is used and its implications for human health. Groundwater is used as a source of irrigation water in Argentina and Chile. Although there is some indirect evidence of the beneficial effects of changing water supply on human intake from northern Chile (Chapter 5), there is little direct evidence of the effect of irrigation on the uptake of arsenic in crops and the human food chain. Surveys and research into such effects should be undertaken as a priority.

Central America and the Caribbean

Similar hydrogeochemical conditions to those in the Amazonian foreland basin probably apply widely along the Isthmus of Panama and the larger

Caribbean islands such as Cuba and Hispaniola. The region is also likely to be rich in geothermal arsenic.

10.6.2 Africa and Australasia

Niger Delta

The evidence presented regarding contamination in the Niger Delta is contradictory. Similarities with South Asian river systems have been cited to suggest that groundwater of the Niger Delta might also be contaminated. Allen (1970) and Oomkens (1974) identified a sedimentary sequence comprising (a) alluvial valley-fill sand and gravel at depths of 30–60 m; (b) coastal plain deposits, up to 25 m thick, comprising a lower unit of lagoonal and mangrove muds and an upper sandy unit; and (c) fluvio-marine and coastal deposits, up to 35 m thick. Oomkens (1974) noted that 'silt and clay, rich in plant debris' formed 16% of the cores extracted, and also identified a well-developed soil horizon at the base (−44 m) of the Late Quaternary delta. The delta is surrounded by Precambrian basement (migmatites, gneisses, schists, granites and dolerites), Cretaceous sandstones, limestones and shales, and younger volcanics in the east.

Groundwater is abstracted from wells 30–300 m deep in light grey to yellow fluvial, tidal channel and coastal beach sands that form semi-confined aquifers of high transmissivity (1000–10,000 m²/day) (Amajor, 1991). The interbedded clays are mainly kaolinitic and pass from yellowish or reddish brown near the surface to light and dark grey at the base, with peat and lignite layers up to 6 m thick. The water table is normally within 6 m of the surface. Groundwater quality is generally good, but with known problems of high chloride and iron (Amajor, 1991). Groundwaters are moderately mineralised (EC 350–600 μS/cm) and subneutral (pH 6.0–7.0), and most low-Cl waters contain high Fe and low SO_4, suggesting iron reduction (Amadi et al., 1989). Thus conditions in the Niger Delta appear in many ways to be favourable for RD. However, the main outstanding question, as discussed below in a regional context, appears to be whether there is a significant source of arsenic within the river sediments. The Niger has a low gradient, and drains large areas of ancient rocks with little tectonic activity. As discussed in Chapter 3, long and intense weathering may have removed, or rendered unavailable, arsenic in the source rocks, but this remains a hypothesis that needs to be tested through field investigation.

Other alluvial basins

Other deltas and river systems of tropical Africa such as the Congo, Zambezi and Senegal rivers are also considered to present similar risks to the Niger.

The available evidence is that Africa and Australasia are the least arsenic-affected continents. Africa and Australia (but not New Zealand) comprise mostly ancient landscapes with extensive duricrusted surfaces and deep weathering profiles, and subdued topography. The major alluvial systems (e.g. Thomas, 2003; Goudie, 2005) have low gradients and derive much of the suspended load from the weathered mantle that underlies these surfaces. The suspended sediment in these rivers is rich in quartz sand and/or saprolite, and is likely to be depleted in available As, and hence the apparent absence of pollution may be substantially correct.

Despite these generalities, not all of Africa and Australia is formed of ancient rocks and landforms, and even ancient rocks can become important sources of arsenic if they have been recently and rapidly uplifted. The mountainous belts of southeastern Australia, the Atlas Mountains of northeast Africa, and a number of volcanic massifs within Africa (e.g. the Ruwenzori, southwest Cameroon[16], Ahaggar and Tibesti massifs) are potential sources of As-rich sediment. There is a possibility of arsenic pollution in alluvial basins around these highlands, with mobilisation by RD in humid climates and AD in more arid areas. The discovery of arsenic in the Okavango Delta is a case in point. The East African Rift Valley has no real parallel. It is volcanically active, and is also noted for the presence of alkaline lakes. Traces of arsenic were noted in Ethiopia, but generally there are few detailed data on groundwater quality, and the region should be considered suspect until properly surveyed.

NOTES

1 Along with India, all were once part of the supercontinent of Gondwanaland.
2 Hidroarsenicismo Cronico Regional Endemico (chronic endemic regional hydroarsenicism)
3 Analysed after dispersal using sodium hexametaphosphate and ultrasonic vibration.
4 The Pampean loess has a higher volcanic content than loess in North America, France and China.
5 The permeabilities (10 m/day) and recharge rates (30–100 mm/year) cited by Smedley et al. (2002) are not compatible. Assuming horizontal flow, outflow can be estimated in two ways. First, using the reported saturated thickness of 75 m, and hydraulic gradient (0.0005), the outflow would be 137 m^3/year per metre width. Alternatively, recharge of 30 mm/year spread over a 100 km flow length would generate an outflow of 3000 m^3/year, and require a hydraulic gradient of 0.25.
6 Presumably from the unsaturated zone.
7 Social factors may have contributed to the slow pace of mitigation in northern areas such as Santiago del Estero, where communities are smaller, poorer and more isolated, making communal supplies less feasible (O. Sracek, personal communication, 2007).
8 Due to percolating waters near the Earth's surface.

9   Borgono et al. (1977) reported the population of the city of Antofagasta as 130,000, Ferreccio and Sancha (2006) report 258,000, indicating rapid growth of the city.

10 Plants with deep roots that reach to the water table.

11 Dental and skeletal fluorosis have been documented in the area.

12 With a rural population of around 15 million mainly dependent on ground-water, this would suggest that 1.5 M people drink water with >10 ppb As.

13 These soils contain abundant pyrite, which is stable when anaerobic, but can be oxidised through drainage, releasing sulphate and acidity.

14 Because the highest pH was only 7.6, significant desorption is questionable.

15 Groundwater Research Leader, GNS Science.

16 Subsequently confirmed by Mbotake (2006).

Chapter Eleven

Synthesis, Conclusions and Recommendations

11.1 Scale and Impact of Arsenic Pollution

11.1.1 Global extent of arsenic pollution and exposure

At the beginning of this book (Figure 1.1) we showed the geographical range of As-contaminated waters, in more than 70 countries on six continents, but with little comment about their nature. In subsequent chapters we have explored the causes and human impacts of contamination. The affected areas differ enormously in their geographical extent, health effects and geochemistry. Tables 11.1 and 11.2 summarise the human impact in terms of the numbers of people drinking water with more than 10 and 50 ppb As, whether contaminated water is used to irrigate food crops, and to what extent As exposure is translated into physical illness. There are, of course, major difficulties in compiling such a table because of the different definitions and the variable quality of data. Many of the smaller occurrences of contamination lack medical diagnoses and quantitative exposure assessments. However, from a global perspective (Figure 11.1), these make little difference because the smaller occurrences impact on only a few thousands, or at most a few tens of thousands of people, whereas in the most severely affected countries the exposed populations are counted in millions, or even tens of millions. Nevertheless, there are several reasons why the numbers in Table 11.1 should be treated with caution. First, many areas are incompletely surveyed, and second, in the areas that have been surveyed, exposure has been modified by switching water sources or installing water treatment. Hence the exposed population estimates are best understood as the maximum number of people who have been exposed to high levels of arsenic during recent decades[1].

Table 11.1 Summary of estimated peak arsenic exposure in drinking water by country; see Chapters 5 and 8 to 10 for details of individual occurrences

Country	Geographical class‡	Concentration class§	Exposed population (millions) >50ppb	>10ppb	Irrigation used	Worst clinical symptom	Notes
Asia							
Afghanistan	B	A	?	0.5		None reported	All at Ghazni
Bangladesh	C	BC	27.0	50.0	Y	Death	
Cambodia	C	BC	0.5	0.6		Skin lesions	Large exposed population
China	C	B	5.6	14.7	Y	Death	Sun (2004)
India	C	B	11.0	30.0		Death	After Nickson et al. (2007)
Indonesia	A	?				N.I.	
Iran	A	C				Skin lesions	
Japan	B	A				None reported	
Kazakhstan	B	B	0.0	0.0		N.I.	
Lao PDR	C	B	*	*		N.I.	Could be large
Malaysia	A	?				N.I.	
Mongolia	C	BC		0.1		Skin lesions	
Myanmar	C	B	2.5	>2.5		Skin lesions	
Nepal	C	B	0.55	2.5	Y	Skin lesions	
Pakistan	C	B	2.0	5.0	Y	Skin lesions	Punjab only

(cont'd)

Table 11.1 (cont'd)

Country	Geographical class[‡]	Concentration class[§]	Exposed population[†] (millions) >50ppb	>10ppb	Irrigation used	Worst clinical symptom	Notes
Russia	B	C				N.I.	Thermal and mineral waters
Sri Lanka	A	?				Death	
Saudi Arabia	A	A				N.I.	
Taiwan	C	BC		0.06		Death	Southwest Taiwan only
Thailand	B	A	0.015	>0.015		Skin lesions	
Turkey	A	C				Skin lesions	
Vietnam	C	B	1.5	>1.5		Biomarker	
Subtotal			50.6	107.5			
Europe							
Belgium	A	A	0.0			N.I.	
Croatia	B	B	0.2	0.20		Skin lesions	
Czech Republic	A	C				N.I.	
Denmark	A	A	0.0			N.I.	
Finland	C	A				Susp. Cancer	
France	B	AB	0.02	0.2		None reported	
Germany	B	A				None reported	
Greece	B	A		0.005		None reported	
Hungary	C	B	0.5	>0.5		Cancer	

Italy	B	A			Y	N.I.	
Lithuania	A	A	0.0			N.I.	
Netherlands	A	A				None reported	
Norway	A	A	0.0			None reported	
Poland	A	B				Susp. Cancer	Historic case
Romania	B	AB				Skin lesions	
Serbia	C	?				N.I.	
Slovakia	C	B				N.I.	
Slovenia	B	AB				N.I.	
Spain	B	AB				None reported	
Sweden	B	A				None reported	
UK	A	A	0.0	0.0		None reported	
Subtotal			*0.7*	*0.9*			
North America							
Canada	B	A				Death	
Cuba	A	?				N.I.	
Mexico	C	B	0.4	2.0	Y	Death	Region Lagunera only
USA	C	A	3.0	29.6		Suspected cancer	
Subtotal			*3.4*	*31.6*			
South America							
Argentina	C	C	2.0	2.0	Y	Death	
Bolivia	C		0.025	>0.025		Skin lesions	
Brazil	A					Biomarkers	
Chile	B	C	0.5	>0.5	Y	Death	

(cont'd)

Table 11.1 (cont'd)

Country	Geographical class‡	Concentration class§	Exposed population† (millions)		Irrigation used	Worst clinical symptom	Notes
			>50 ppb	>10 ppb			
Costa Rica	A	?				N.I.	
Ecuador	A	C				N.I.	
El Salvador	B	BC	0.3	>0.3		N.I.	
Guatemala	A	?				N.I.	
Honduras	A	?				N.I.	
Nicaragua	A	AB		0.001		Skin lesions	
Peru	A	B				N.I.	
Uruguay	B	A				N.I.	
Subtotal			2.8	2.8			
Africa							
Botswana	A	A				None reported	
Burkina Faso	B	?				Skin lesions	
Cameroon	A	?				N.I.	
Ethiopia	A	A				N.I.	
Ghana	C	B		1.5		Skin lesions	
Nigeria	A	?				N.I.	
Subtotal			0.0	1.5			

Australasia					
Australia	A	A			Not known
New Zealand	B	AB		0.1	Animals only
Subtotal			0.0	0.1	
Oceanic Areas					
Iceland	A	B			N.I.
USA (Hawaii)	A	B			N.I.
Subtotal			0.0	0.0	
TOTAL			**57.5**	**144.4**	

N.I., no information on clinical effects, whereas 'not reported' suggests effects were looked for but not found.

†Population estimates are minima in that not all sources may have been exposed; but the estimates are also the largest reported credible estimates, although they may have changed due to mitigation or population growth. Where actual exposure estimates are not given, '*' indicates that it is suspected that exposure could be on the scale of hundreds of thousands to millions; and blank cells indicate no estimate is possible based on available information.

‡A, local impact, e.g. single village, town or equivalent; B, subregional, e.g. single city, group of towns or small catchment; C, major regional occurrence, covering large swathes of province or country.

§A, water generally 10–50 ppb As; B, As frequently >50 ppb, but rarely >200 ppb; C, As routinely >50 ppb, and frequently >200 ppb.

Table 11.2   Most severely arsenic affected countries; see text for discussion

Exposed population (millions)			*Exposed population (millions)*		
Country	*>50 ppb*	*>10 ppb*	*Country*	*>50 ppb*	*>10 ppb*
Bangladesh	27	50	Vietnam	1.5	?
India	11	30	Nepal	0.55	2.5
China	5.6	15	Cambodia	0.5	0.6
USA	3.0	30	Hungary	0.5	?
Myanmar	2.5	?	Chile*	0.5	?
Pakistan	2.0	5.0	Mexico	0.4	2.0
Argentina	2.0				

*In Chile, although arsenic originates from springs, the contaminated water is abstracted from rivers.

Around two-thirds of the people drinking water with >50 ppb As live in just two countries: Bangladesh and India. Further, because of general health and nutrition issues, these countries probably contain a disproportionately high number of the persons suffering from arsenicosis. China, in third place, is also severely impacted in terms of both exposure and disease. The USA, in fourth place, has a very low level of arsenical disease, which may be attributable to a combination of nutrition, low per capita intake of well-water, more widespread use of water treatment, and a lower proportion of high As concentrations. In addition to the numbers of people drinking water exceeding specific thresholds, it is important to recall that most health effects follow a dose–response curve. The available data do not allow comparisons of the numbers of people within specific concentration bands. However, for mapping and general characterisation purposes, we have divided the affected regions into three semi-quantitative classes:

A   contaminated groundwaters generally contain concentrations of 10–50 ppb;
B   arsenic concentrations frequently exceed 50 ppb, but rarely exceed about 200 ppb;
C   arsenic concentrations routinely exceed 50 ppb, and frequently exceed 200 ppb.

Due to inconsistencies in the format of data sets, it is not appropriate to define precise boundaries, but transitional classes, AB and BC, were assigned based on judgement. The occurrences have also been divided into a set of

a) >50 ppb As

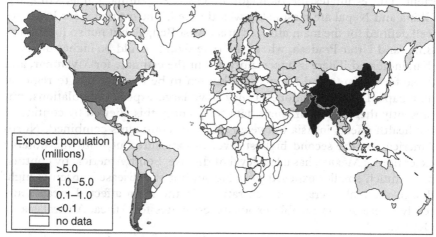

b) >10 ppb As

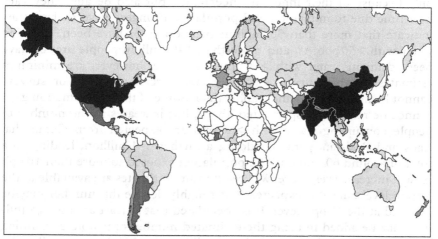

Figure 11.1 Global distribution of population affected by arsenic contamination. Countries are shaded based on the estimated exposed populations in Table 11.1, with no lower threshold.

geographical classes reflecting the areal extent of contamination, although even these do not convey the continuity of pollution. The classes are:

A local impact, e.g. single village, town or equivalent;
B subregional occurrence, e.g. a single city, group of towns or small catchment;
C major regional occurrence, covering large swathes of a province or country.

The population estimates in Tables 11.1 and 11.2 require further comment. The estimates for Bangladesh, USA, Argentina, Chile, Hungary, China and Nepal are reasonably well defined. The estimates for India are well defined for the main affected area, West Bengal, but not so for Assam, Bihar and Uttar Pradesh, where the true figures could be higher or lower than indicated. There is uncertainty about the estimate for Myanmar, and those for Pakistan and Mexico are known to be too low, due to regional data gaps. Laos and Indonesia may have large exposed populations, but presently there are insufficient data to quantify this. Viewed by continent, the health effects in Asia outweigh all other continents combined. North America has the second highest level of exposure but, with the notable exception of Mexico, has a low level of disease. South America, by contrast has a much smaller exposed population, but the disease burden is high, due to the high average concentrations in the main affected areas. Currently, there are no reliable exposure estimates for Africa, Australasia or Oceania.

The exposed population estimates should be treated with caution not only because of their inherent uncertainty, but also because they vary over time due to mitigation and population changes. Nevertheless, they indicate that more than 50 million people are, or have been, drinking water with >50 ppb As, and more than 140 million people are, or have been, drinking water with >10 ppb As. These, however, are minimum estimates because surveys of many areas are incomplete, or surveys cannot be matched to demographic data. Some of these information gaps cannot be reasonably speculated about, but increases in the number of people consuming water with >50 ppb are expected from Cambodia, Laos and Pakistan, perhaps adding a further 3–4 million, leading to a total of around 60 million. The population exposed to more than 10 ppb As will increase even more. Where exposure estimates are available at the 50 ppb level only, it is expected that roughly double this number may be exposed at the 10 ppb level. It is speculated that at least another 15 million may be added to bring the estimated number of people consuming more than 10 ppb As to around 150 million people. This may still be an underestimate.

11.1.2   Health, social and economic impacts

Exposure pathways

Although arsenic exposure may occur by inhalation (but not dermal absorption), in relation to contaminated waters, ingestion of water and food are the only important means of exposure. In drinking water, the only important forms of arsenic are trivalent arsenite and pentavalent arsenate. Arsenate dominates in oxidising waters and arsenite in reducing waters. At acute doses, arsenate is less toxic, but at low doses the difference is probably not important because it is converted to arsenite in the human gut. Organic forms are important in some foods, but because they are generally less toxic, exposure is normally assessed in terms of total inorganic arsenic. The FAO and WHO recommend a maximum daily intake (MDI) of inorganic As of 130 μg/day for adults, which is equivalent to 2.6 L of water containing 50 ppb As.

Recent studies indicate that food makes a major contribution to the intake of inorganic As. Where this results from irrigated crops, it is probable that the As contents have increased over time due to accumulation of arsenic in the soil. Injudicious use of such snapshot evidence may both exaggerate historic exposure and underestimate future exposure. Nevertheless, in West Bengal, Uchino et al. (2006) found that in people with arsenic skin manifestations, over half their current daily intake of arsenic came from food. The UK and Australia have a maximum hygiene standard of 1000 μg/kg As for food, although most countries have no such standard. This may be appropriate for typical western diets, but is not protective of health in subsistence rice economies, where the daily consumption of rice, containing up to 400 μg/kg As, may be as high as 400 g/d, of which up to 90% of the arsenic may be inorganic. This is sufficient to exceed the MDI with no contribution from water. Notwithstanding the importance of exposure from food, interventions to reduce exposure through drinking water are simpler and quicker than intervening in agriculture, which, although essential in many areas, takes longer to implement and is gradual in its impact. Water-supply interventions should also reduce intake from food because of its role in cooking.

Clinical effects and disease burden

The clinical effects of chronic arsenic poisoning include skin lesions, diseases of the heart, lungs, kidney and liver, multiple cancers, gangrene and death. The severity and causation[2] of these effects is established beyond reasonable doubt. Most effects follow distinct dose–response relationships, all symptoms have long latency periods, and the development of symptoms is progressive with continued exposure. In Bangladesh, Chen and Ahsan (2004) predicted that arsenic in drinking water will cause 'at least a doubling of lifetime mortality risk from liver, bladder, and lung cancers'. Symptomatic treatment is possible, but there is no cure other than to remove exposure. Early symptoms may be reversible, and improvements in the condition of skin lesions and ischaemia have been documented. However, there is evidence of skin lesions appearing after a safe drinking water source has been established, and cancers developing even decades after removal from exposure, and in Chile it has been shown that there have been four times as many deaths (from heart attacks and lung and bladder cancer) after a new water supply was commissioned than during the 13 years of extreme (800 ppb) exposure (Yuan et al., 2007). Even pre-natal exposure may cause disease in adulthood (Smith et al., 2006). Removing exposure from arsenic in drinking water is essential and urgent, but will not in itself prevent a future burden of fatal disease. Delay in implementing safe water supplies will lead to an increased prevalence of arsenicosis, worsened symptoms for those already affected and additional deaths. To reduce suffering and future impacts, interventions should be prioritised on the basis of arsenic concentration and, ideally, cumulative exposure.

There are major geographical differences in the health impacts of arsenic in drinking water. Clinical symptoms are particularly common in Bangladesh, India and parts of China, but apparently rare in the USA and many European countries. The rarity of symptoms in Vietnam and Cambodia is thought to be due to the shorter duration of exposure, and if correct, the incidence of arsenicosis will increase rapidly in the near future. However, the low incidence of arsenicosis in the USA and Europe is attributed to lower water consumption, diet and better nutrition. Other chemicals may affect the toxicity of arsenic: zinc deficiency or high concentrations of organic acids can exacerbate the effects of arsenic; however, selenium, toxic in its own right, reduces the toxicity of arsenic, and vice versa. Although there is no known interaction, fluoride and arsenic often co-occur, and so must add to the health burden.

There has been some doubt with regard to the health effects of low-level exposure, particularly in the range of 10–50 ppb As. However, there is increasing evidence of actual harm at concentrations of <50 ppb, both from the USA (Knobeloch et al., 2006; Meliker et al., 2007) and from Bangladesh (Ahsan et al., 2006). In Asia, although it may be argued that As intake from food is partly responsible, this merely strengthens the argument for adopting a lower drinking water standard in countries where food is an important source of exposure.

Social and economic effects

Although some economic effects of chronic arsenic poisoning are universal, the social effects are culturally specific. The universal effects include medical costs incurred, reduced economic output of workers, and impaired intellectual development of children[3]. Social assessments in West Bengal and Bangladesh show that, unlike the clinical burden, social effects are experienced disproportionately by women, who face involuntary divorce, rejection of marriage offers, and exclusion from education and other social activities. Exclusion may even follow from owning a polluted well or having a family member who suffers from arsenicosis. Mistaken beliefs, such as that arsenicosis is contagious, exacerbate these effects. The poorest members of communities are more likely to be clinically affected, not only because of poor nutrition, but also because they face more difficulty in gaining access to existing safe wells.

11.1.3 Drinking water standards

The US Public Health Service set a standard of 50 ppb As in 1942, and as early as 1962 specified 10 ppb as a goal. In 1993, the WHO reduced its guideline value for arsenic in drinking water from 50 ppb to 10 ppb, based mainly on epidemiological data from Taiwan, which suggested that if a linear extrapolation was applied, which is often done for known carcinogens, the guideline value could have been as low as 1.7 ppb. However, at the time laboratories could not reliably determine this concentration, and a provisional guideline of 10 ppb was set. Germany adopted this as a standard in 1996, and the EU in 2003. In the USA, after protracted and sometimes bizarre deliberations, the EPA adopted 10 ppb in 2006.

Most affected countries still apply a standard of 50 ppb As, although this has been a matter of contention as well as differing objectives. In Bangladesh, implementing a 10 ppb standard would mean that around 45% of all the wells in the country (about 5 million of them) ought to be condemned. For these and other reasons, Smith and Hira-Smith (2004) recommended that 'Developing countries with large populations exposed to arsenic in water might reasonably be advised to keep their arsenic drinking water standards at 50 µg/l.' However, Mukherjee et al. (2005) attacked this as an example of double standards by developed countries. This type of debate confuses means with ends. Both parties wish to see drinking water with <10 ppb supplied, and the argument is best resolved by a more flexible approach of defining two levels of compliance where a higher concentration is permitted under certain circumstances and on a strictly time-limited basis. Nevertheless, an additional reason for early adoption of a lower standard is necessary because of the additional exposure from food.

11.2 Chemistry, Cause and Prediction

11.2.1 Hydrogeochemical mechanisms

Where sufficient data were available, the cases of As contamination shown in Figure 1.1 were assigned to the four mobilisation mechanisms described earlier in the book: (a) reductive dissolution (RD), (b) alkali desorption (AD), (c) sulphide oxidation (SO) and (d) geothermal arsenic. Reductive dissolution (69 cases) was both the most numerous and, in terms of human impact, by far the most important. Reductive dissolution probably accounts for almost all major cases of As pollution in Asia, and is also the main source of As exposure from food, due to groundwater irrigation. Numerically, geothermal arsenic (36) is the second most common, however, it has caused significant human impacts only in Chile and Bolivia. Alkali desorption is the second most important reported cause in exploited aquifers, and occurs in the most diverse geological settings. Desorption at high pH is a well-known process, but often the field data from which conclusions were reached are rather ambiguous, and some may be reinterpreted when more rigorous studies are undertaken. Sulphide oxidation (25) tends to produce spatially restricted but often intense, pollution, and mainly in bedrock aquifers. In 62 cases worldwide, no mechanism could be assigned, mostly due to lack of geochemical data.

Arsenic occurrences in some bedrock aquifers warrant further research, such as Chhattisgarh (India), Burkina Faso and Ghana, the Triassic sandstones of Germany, and the Madrid and Duero Basins in Spain. The role of extreme concentrations of organic acids, such as in China and Hungary, also warrant further research, as do the occurrences of arsenic in Iran and Turkey, which may be indicative of more extensive contamination in the Alpine–Himalayan belt.

11.2.2 Geochemical mechanisms and their geological context

The four mobilisation mechanisms occur in fairly well-defined geological–climatic associations, as summarised in Table 11.3. Reductive dissolution occurs predominantly in young alluvial or glacial sediments, and preferentially under more humid climates, where abundant organic matter drives reduction of iron oxides. Geothermal arsenic occurs most commonly in regions of Tertiary to recent volcanic activity or mountain building. Alkali desorption occurs in diverse settings, but is more common in drier climates. In so far as it affects aquifers, sulphide oxidation occurs mainly in older bedrock aquifers, and is more related to local geological factors, such as sulphide mineralisation, than to large-scale geological or climatic parameters.

There is a strong association between arsenic in groundwater and certain tectonic and/or geomorphological settings. Not only does geothermal arsenic occur within Tertiary orogenic belts, but most contaminated alluvial aquifers occur in foreland basins. These areas are characterised by

Table 11.3 Geology–climate–process matrix

Aquifer Geology	Process	Climate		
		Cool–temperate	Humid: tropical and subtropical	Arid and semi-arid: warm–hot
Alluvium (deltaic,	AD	★	–	★★
lacustrine and aeolian)	GT	★	★	–
	RD	★★★	★★★	★★
	SO	–	–	★
Alluvial–volcaniclastic	AD	★★	–	★★
	GT	–	–	–
	RD	–	–	–
	SO	–	–	–
Glacial, and fluvio-	AD	–	–	–
glacial sediments	GT	★	–	–
	RD	★★★	–	–
	SO	–	–	–
Tertiary,	AD	–	–	★★
intracontinental	GT	★	–	★
sedimentary basins	RD	–	–	–
	SO	–	–	★
Tertiary–recent,	AD	–	–	★
volcanic rocks	GT	★★	★★	★★
	RD	–	–	–
	SO	★	–	–
Palaeozoic–	AD	★★	–	–
Mesozoic sedimentary	GT	★	–	–
rocks	RD	★★	–	–
	SO	–	–	–
Palaeozoic–Mesozoic	AD	★★	–	–
igneous and	GT	–	–	–
metamorphic rocks	RD	–	–	–
	SO	–	–	★
Precambrian–	AD	★★	–	–
Palaeozoic crystalline	GT	–	–	–
bedrock	RD	–	–	–
	SO	★★	★	★★

★★★ frequent; ★★ occurs; ★ rare; –, not reported; AD, alkali desorption; GT, geothermal arsenic; RD, reductive dissolution; SO, sulphide oxidation.

dominant physical weathering in the upper catchment, rapid sediment transport, and accommodation space in the lower catchment created by either tectonic subsidence inland or Quaternary sea-level fluctuations in the deltas. Where the lower catchment is humid, and organic matter is abundant, arsenic may be mobilised by RD, but under more arid conditions, the pH may be sufficiently elevated to mobilise arsenic by desorption.

Ancient crystalline bedrock is not naturally favourable to arsenic mobilisation, but exceptions occur in glaciated terrains where post-glacial marine flooding preceded isostatic uplift, such as in New England, British Columbia and southwest Finland. Most contaminated river basins drain young mountain belts, especially the Himalayas and Indo-Burman ranges. Severely contaminated deltas such as the Ganges–Brahmaputra, Irrawaddy, Mekong and Red rivers have superficial similarities with those of the Niger, Congo, Amazon or Orinoco. However, it appears that none of these latter basins is severely contaminated, and this is attributed to their tectonic stability, subdued topography and weathering history, which removed or immobilised arsenic.

11.2.3   A predictive model for arsenic pollution of groundwater

The rate of discovery of arsenic pollution in the past 10 years and, and the large parts of the world where water has apparently not been tested, suggests that more discoveries will be made, and begs the question as to where else arsenic will be discovered. The understanding of the distribution of arsenic developed in earlier chapters allows predictions of where arsenic pollution is likely to be found, based first on the geological–climatic–process matrix described above (Table 11.3), and second on the indicators of sediment and water quality in major rivers, as explained in Chapter 3. We emphasise, however, that these are guidelines, not rules, for identifying arsenic contamination.

Arsenic mobilisation by reductive dissolution

Arsenic contamination occurs in humid alluvial basins draining young mountains with high and cool upper catchments such as occur in the South and Southeast Asian Arsenic Belt (SSAAB). Apparent gaps include parts of the upper reaches of the Yangtze–Kiang and Xijiang basins in China, and the alluvial basins of Indonesia and Malaysia, where volcanic rocks form the upper catchments. In China, Vietnam, Thailand and Myanmar, smaller rivers adjacent to, and tributaries of, major contaminated river basins should be surveyed. In southern Europe, arsenic can be expected in alluvial basins draining the Alps and Carpathians. To date, severe contamination has been mapped on the Great Hungarian Plain and the Po Delta, and may occur in the deltas of the Danube, Rhine and Rhone rivers. By comparison with North America, arsenic contamination is expected in fluvio-glacial aquifers in northern Europe, particularly on the Baltic plains of Lithuania, Poland and Belarus. Similar conditions may also apply in northeast Asia. In South America, it is suspected that there may be extensive arsenic pollution in the Amazonian foreland basins, in Colombia, and further north along the Isthmus of Panama.

Arsenic mobilisation by alkali desorption

The global distribution of arsenic mobilised by AD appears erratic, and the evidence may be significantly incomplete[4]. The volcanic-loessal aquifers in Argentina have no equivalents elsewhere, but the mapped extent of contamination is much smaller than the extent of the Pampean loess. By contrast, occurrences such as the Basin-and-Range Province (USA) may have many unrecognised equivalents around the world in semi-arid, subsiding alluvial basins adjacent to young mountain chains. This may account for the occurrences in northwest Mexico, and similar conditions can be anticipated along the Pacific Plains of South America, from Ecuador to Chile. Similar conditions probably occur in large areas of West Asia and the Middle East, from Turkey to Iran, and along the Red Sea coast of the Arabian Peninsula. In each of these areas, there is little evidence of testing for arsenic in water. Alkali desorption is also associated with glaciated bedrock inundated by the sea at the end of the Pleistocene. Such conditions may also be encountered in the eastern Baltic states, Scotland, Siberia and Kamchatka, New Zealand and the southern tip of South America. Alkali desorption may also occur in rift valleys, such as the East African Rift Valley, where sodic and alkaline water bodies are common.

Arsenic mobilisation by sulphide oxidation

Sulphide oxidation does not follow the same global patterns as the other mechanisms, but normally requires that there has been hydrothermal sulphide mineralisation, although marine sulphides may also form suitable sources. In addition, the sulphide minerals must occupy a position in groundwater flow systems where they lie within the zone of water-table fluctuation. For these reasons, it is not practical to make global predictions of areas where sulphide oxidation is expected. Sulphide oxidation also occurs with acid-sulphate soils, oxidised when swamps are drained. However, this rarely results in the pollution of exploited aquifers.

Areas where extensive arsenic pollution is not expected

Because of the history of weathering and landscape development, it is considered unlikely that extensive arsenic pollution by either reductive dissolution or alkali desorption occurs in the alluvial basins draining the Gondwanan terrain of Africa, Australia, eastern South America and peninsular India. Local exceptions will occur in areas of intense sulphide mineralisation (e.g. southwest Ghana; Chhattisgarh) and areas of recent mountain building or volcanicity in Africa such as the Atlas Mountains, the Tibesti and Ahaggar Massifs, southwest Cameroon and the East African Rift Valley. Exceptions will also occur where there is geothermal activity.

From apparent to real risk

The preceding paragraphs indicate where geochemical conditions may favour mobilisation of arsenic. This, however, ignores the chain of causation that runs from the existence of a hazard in groundwater to actual exposure to arsenic through water or food. For various reasons, the presence of arsenic in groundwater may not be translated into actual harm. In most aquifers, arsenic is variably distributed with depth, and well construction will affect the concentrations at which arsenic is pumped from the ground. If water is aerated or stored prior to use, coprecipitation with iron hydroxides may reduce the concentrations. On the other hand, exposure from irrigated agriculture may double arsenic intake. Lifestyle and diet further modify exposure, and the consequences of exposure. Low income favours increased consumption of untreated well-water. Active, outdoor working lives and hot climate will increase the total intake of water. How food is cooked, particularly the quantity and quality of cooking water, may increase or decrease the quantity of arsenic ingested. Finally, the clinical manifestations will be affected by the general state of health and nutrition of the population. Each step described above should be understood for each specific case of contamination, because each represents an opportunity to reduce the impact on human health.

11.3   Agricultural Impacts, Prospects and Needs

Preamble

Natural arsenic affects agriculture in two situations. The first is where the source of arsenic is the soil itself, and the second is where arsenic is applied in irrigation water. In the first case, the store of arsenic continuously declines. Arsenic in irrigation water is a progressive, and potentially more serious, problem. Only in unusual situations (e.g. Chhattisgarh, India) are natural soil-As concentrations high enough to contaminate crops for long periods. Irrigation water drawn from underground is derived from two stores: arsenic already dissolved in groundwater, and arsenic bound to the aquifer minerals that may be released when the aquifer is recharged. The principal sink for arsenic in irrigation water is the soil, adsorbed to iron oxides. The other sinks are the plant parts that are harvested, and methylation losses to the atmosphere. Any arsenic that escapes these sinks is recycled through the aquifer but the amounts are thought to be small, and hence irrigation involves a net transfer of arsenic from groundwater to the land surface. A critical distinction, resulting from the Fe–As chemistry, is made between dryland crops grown in aerobic soils, and those grown in anaerobic, paddy-type soils, where As is more mobile. Quantitatively, As uptake and toxicity in paddy rice is the greatest single problem relating to arsenic and agriculture.

Arsenic accumulation and phytotoxicity

Information on As accumulation and toxicity in crops is derived from industrially polluted soils, soils contaminated by agrochemicals in the USA and Australia, and recent studies from Bangladesh and India. The American studies are most relevant to dryland crop production, whereas the Bengal studies mainly relate to paddy rice systems. Market- and field-based sampling of rice in Bangladesh and India have established that significant accumulation of As occurs in groundwater-irrigated soils, and that rice produced in these areas contains high levels of As. Although As–soil–water–plant relationships are highly complex and imperfectly understood, there is sufficient evidence that As levels in rice grain are causing transfers to the food chain and are of major health significance, and also that As concentrations in soil are reaching levels toxic to rice. Urgent action is required.

Toxicity and As uptake in grain are interlinked. The upper limit to As accumulation in rice is probably irrelevant, because farmers will cease cultivation, due to loss of yield, before that point is reached. Developing mitigation methods depends on understanding the processes that control arsenic transfer, and requires research including (a) better definition of arsenic accumulation rates in soils; (b) quantifying methylation losses; (c) examining regional differences between arsenic uptake in crops and soils; (d) identifying the correlation between arsenic in plant parts and soil; and (e) elucidating the role of iron plaque and its interactions with phosphate, sulphur fertilisation and the Fe:As ratio of soil and water.

Water resources and the magnitude of future problems

Irrigation with water containing 200–300 ppb adds about 1 mg/kg As per year to paddy soils. It appears that phytotoxic effects (yield reduction) become significant when soil-As rises to the order of 50 mg/kg (Duxbury and Panaullah, 2007). Hydrogeochemical studies in the Bengal Basin suggest that the store of dissolved As in the aquifers could be depleted in about 10–50 years, but that the larger store of adsorbed As will continue to release arsenic, albeit at declining concentrations, for centuries to come. Under the 'business as usual' scenario, potentially dangerous soil-As concentrations would become widespread on a timescale of 20–100 years after the onset of irrigation, and there is evidence from Bangladesh that this is already happening.

Mitigation: soil rehabilitation and reducing human exposure

In many As-affected areas, reducing human exposure to tolerable levels requires parallel action on drinking water and irrigated agriculture. The processes that lead to toxicity and As uptake in grain are complex and have no simple solutions. Much academic and practical research and extension will be needed, and optimum solutions will vary between regions. While it cannot be stopped, there are many approaches by which exposure can be reduced. Classified by their mode of action, proven or potential mitigation measures include:

1 identifying and avoiding contaminated irrigation sources;
2 actions to reduce or immobilise As already in soil;
3 actions to stop adding additional As to the soil;
4 actions to cope with As already in the soil and/or still being added to the soil, which can be divide into two categories:
    • reducing As uptake in crops,
    • reducing phytotoxicity and yield loss.

A precondition for reducing As uptake in irrigated crops is to survey all irrigation wells in affected areas, mainly using field test kits, and simultaneously disseminating information to farmers. Results should be compiled in a GIS and used for planning mitigation and as a baseline for monitoring. For logistical reasons, soil analyses would be collected only at a sample of sites.

Different solutions will be required for dryland crops and paddy rice. Methods used to reclaim industrially contaminated soils, where there is a regulatory driver, are currently at the point of transition from research studies to practical application for land with commercial or residential end-use. However, there is little prospect of these methods becoming economic for farmers to reclaim agricultural land, and even if they were, the issue of continued build-up of As from future irrigation would remain.

In Bangladesh, India and other parts of Asia, the existing practice whereby farmers in low-lying areas sell their soil for use in brick-making or embankment construction could be adapted for As mitigation. The root zone of paddy rice, where As accumulates, is only 10–15 cm deep, and so little soil needs to be excavated. There is potential for governments or NGOs to intervene through soil-testing and subsidy to promote removal of the most hazardous agricultural soils.

Treating water, in the manner required for potable purposes, is not economic for irrigation of rice or wheat. On the other hand, oxidation and co-precipitation with natural iron in irrigation channels might be enhanced to reduce As concentrations at field level, and perhaps further enhanced by pumping initially to a canal or pond. Other possible solutions involve developing an alternative surface water or deep aquifer source, although most reliable local surface waters have already been developed. Developing deep groundwater may be the optimum solution for individual farms, but not necessarily for the community and society due to the danger of overpumping a limited resource. Establishing where, and how much, deep groundwater can be allocated to irrigation should be an important objective of water resource studies.

Interventions at the plant level involve selecting or breeding crop varieties that are more tolerant of As and/or take up less As into the grain, and investigating the use of soil amendments and fertilisation to reduce As uptake. Research should be conducted into methods of growing rice under aerated soil conditions, and requiring less irrigation water. A further alternative is switching to dryland crops, such as wheat or maize, under which conditions As is less mobile. This, however, is not possible on all rice-growing land, and it will only delay, not prevent, the onset of significant As uptake or phytotoxicity.

Management needs

Arsenic contamination of soils and crops is complex, and all three mitigation approaches (soil, water and plant based) should be pursued in parallel. This will require a variety of implementation, research and education projects, and will need a body to coordinate the programme. A major programme of agricultural extension will be required to explain the issues and achieve the participation of farmers. Studies of As uptake by livestock and its implications should also be undertaken.

11.4 Water-supply Mitigation

There are three basic approaches to water-supply mitigation: continued use of the uncontaminated parts of polluted aquifers; treatment of contaminated water; and development of surface water sources. Whichever approach is followed, the starting point is always to survey and categorise polluted water sources, and to identify and commence symptomatic treatment of patients.

A common error has been to focus excessively on particular technologies or water sources (i.e. confusing ends with means) rather than the outcome of mitigation – the quality, quantity, cost, reliability and environmental impact. The impact of improvements should be measured ultimately in terms of their effect on human health and not only on water quality parameters.

11.4.1   Surveys, information and monitoring

Arsenic surveys

A range of surveys is required. Initially there should be a rapid and systematic regional reconnaissance of water sources, considering the hydrogeological conditions, and depth of wells, and analysing a subset of samples for all credible and mandatory water quality problems, and also possible changes in drinking water standards. Without compromising quality, the reconnaissance survey must be completed quickly in order to design follow-up medical and water-well surveys. Normally, this will involve 'blanket' testing of all wells in affected areas, although in some cases a second round of systematic sampling may be appropriate.

The use of As field test kits has been controversial. Field test kits are semi-quantitative, but quick and cheap, require less skill and the results can be instantaneously reported to water users, but they are inherently less accurate than laboratory methods. When first used for large-scale testing in Bangladesh, the kits could not reliably identify water containing 50–200 ppb As. Field test kits have been much improved, and can reliably detect the presence of As below 50 ppb, although their precision is less than ideal, and they are not yet proven reliable at the 10 ppb level. Therefore, where the standard is 10 ppb, or if this may be adopted in the foreseeable future (which it probably should be), then the uncontrolled use of field test kits is not acceptable. The optimum design will involve a combination of field test kits and collecting and storing a water sample from every well. Initially, all samples containing any trace of arsenic should be analysed together with random samples for quality control purposes. Later, samples showing no trace of arsenic may be tested for compliance with the 10 ppb level. Systematic, but not comprehensive, sampling of hair, nails and urine as biomarkers of exposure should be undertaken to provide a baseline for assessing mitigation.

Awareness raising and information campaigns

Governments should develop an arsenic information strategy that operates across sectors and at multiple levels from national to household level. The survey is the first opportunity to inform individuals about the dangers of arsenic pollution and means of mitigating it. Unfortunately, some governments have chosen not to do this, which has a series of negative consequences, including lack of demand for action by government, reduced activity within the community and ineffective participation in government-led projects. Ideally, arsenic information campaigns should be presented in the context of an integrated health education, sanitation and hygiene programme. Where there is a low level of literacy and/or formal education, much care is needed in preparing, and field testing, educational materials. In such situations, school children can be effective in disseminating information. The social organisation of water supply, and especially the role of women, should be understood and reflected in the design of the campaign.

Socio-economic considerations

The presence of arsenic in water adds significantly to the cost of safe water, and there are doubts about both the ability and the willingness to pay for water supply in rural economies of South Asia. Despite past failures to collect revenues, there are examples that demonstrate willingness to pay where the benefits are understood and the water supply is reliable and of good quality. Ability to pay does not necessarily prove willingness to pay. In New Mexico (USA), for instance, there was strong resistance to paying additional taxes to conform to the 10 ppb standard, partly explained by a historical resistance to federal intervention, but also by the inability to see tangible health benefits.

Monitoring

If surveys are the basis for designing a mitigation programme, monitoring is the basis for its management. As people become aware of arsenic, they begin to switch sources, and as mitigation progresses, tracking the exposed population becomes increasingly difficult. The design of a monitoring programme is complicated, and *inter alia* must consider:

- water quality testing at existing and new wells used for potable sources;
- monitoring of the water resource;
- tracking the number and location of mitigation devices installed by all agencies;
- monitoring arsenic and/or microbiological quality at mitigation devices, plus the operational status and number of persons served;
- monitoring of selected contaminated wells used for non-potable sources, which may be conveniently combined with monitoring of raw water quality at treatment plants;
- surveys to determine actual safe-water coverage in randomly selected villages;

- systematic sampling of hair, nails and urine as biomarkers of exposure, particularly where food is suspected to make a substantial contribution to exposure, in order to assess the effectiveness of mitigation.

11.4.2   Mitigation options

Safe groundwater solutions

Few aquifers are completely contaminated by arsenic, and so switching to a nearby safe well is often the simplest and quickest solution. However, there is often resistance to sharing private wells because of social reasons or fears for the security of the supply, whereas public or community-owned wells are more easily shared (e.g. van Geen et al., 2003). Dug wells usually have low As concentrations, but are prone to faecal contamination unless chlorinated. A key technical issue influencing the continued use of shallow aquifers is to know how long safe wells located close to contaminated wells will remain safe. Many shallow wells become polluted over time and, although theoretically this might be predicted, it is generally not practical to do so, and the only realistic solution is regular monitoring of safe sources.

In many locations, continued use of shallow aquifers is not an option. For example, Bangladesh had more than 2000 villages where every shallow well was polluted. Deep wells are popular, probably because from the users' perspective they are familiar, but they draw water from aquifers for which the safe yield is not known. In Bangladesh, deep wells have provided 90% of mitigation to date, and are at the centre of mitigation plans in West Bengal. Hence, discussions about whether, in principle, deep wells *ought* to be used are pointless. Research is urgently needed to determine the yield of these aquifers, and to improve the quality of construction to prevent faecal contamination, salinity or As seeping along the annulus or through leaking or corroded joints in the casing.

Surface water solutions

Surface water may be developed from local ponds and streams, by rainwater harvesting, or by long distribution systems from reservoirs or major rivers. It should be remembered that most hand-tubewell projects were installed to relieve the burden of diarrhoeal disease from polluted surface water sources. For treatment, ponds are preferred to streams because of their lower sediment and turbidity contents, but both are more susceptible to drought than groundwater and both require treatment. The pond sand filter (PSF), preferably preceded by a roughing filter, is the most popular treatment system, but this does not eliminate microbial pollution (Ahmed et al., 2005). Ponds are also prone to contamination by pesticides and PSF technology requires serious community support for operation and maintenance. Rainwater systems have the best microbiological quality amongst surface water options, but may be affected by heavy metals and hydrocarbons, are expensive and work best for better-off households with large metal roofs. Large-scale surface water treatment and distribution is likely to be a last resort or very long-term solution, to be developed if more easily implemented systems fail. Such schemes require massive investment, and take many years to plan and construct; nevertheless, it would be prudent to undertake preliminary planning studies as part of a flexible and integrated water-supply strategy.

Arsenic removal

There are so many methods that could remove arsenic from water that claims of competing manufacturers and promoters must be treated with caution. The key factors to consider in selecting a treatment method are (in order of importance): raw water quality; demographic setting (i.e. household, community or municipal); and cost. Raw water quality issues include:

1 Source water containing hundreds of ppb of arsenic can often be reduced by drilling the well to a different depth. If this is not possible, treatment methods that achieve 90–95% As removal may comply with 50 ppb, but not 10 ppb.
2 Contaminated waters with high Fe concentrations represent both a problem and an opportunity for cost-effective treatment using modified Fe-removal (oxidation) plants or coagulation-filtration, but the plants require regular backwashing.
4 Low-Fe groundwaters may also be treated by coagulation, but also offer possibilities of using ion-exchange, reverse osmosis (RO) and synthetic adsorbents. The latter are becoming increasingly popular due to ease of use and falling costs, but their cost is proportional to As concentration. Ion-exchange is unfavourable for high sulphate concentrations, whereas RO is attractive for high sulphate waters or where the total mineralisation is high.
5 If waters also require removal of other contaminants such as fluoride, boron, selenium and salinity, methods that remove all contaminants in a single process will be preferred.

The various technologies have different requirements in terms of personnel, capital investment, support services and waste disposal. For municipal systems, skilled operators and technical support should be available, and so all technologies may be considered, and optimising techniques such as pre-oxidation and/or pH adjustment can be employed. Some technologies, such as coagulation with microfiltration, are only competitive for very large systems. Community systems in poor countries pose most difficulties. The users cannot afford skilled, full-time operators, and they lack access to support services. In low-Fe waters, synthetic iron adsorbents require less maintenance and are less dependent on pre-oxidation and pH adjustment than other adsorbents. High-Fe waters may require daily backwashing to prevent clogging. In West Bengal, community-operated ARPs generally have poor performance records, although some work well where there is attention to social organisation before construction and to support operation and maintenance (e.g. Sarkar et al., 2005).

Selecting household devices introduces further restrictions. In the USA, fixed-bed adsorbers and RO have provided practical, low-maintenance solutions. In Asia, clogging by Fe-rich waters and unreliable electricity supplies make such technologies impractical, but gravity-flow columns that combine zero-valent Fe with a conventional sand filter, such as the award-winning Sono Filter in Bangladesh and the Kanchan Filter in Nepal, have been successful. However, there is normally no monitoring, so it is difficult to judge their long-term effectiveness.

In situ arsenic removal, which involves the cyclic injection and withdrawal of aerated water, deserves special mention. The technique is well established for Fe and Mn removal in Germany and The Netherlands, and is also known to remove low-level As, but has not been tested in highly contaminated aquifers. Potentially the method is cheap, requires no chemicals, and generates no waste. Feasibility studies of *in situ* methods in Fe-rich aquifers in South Asia are strongly recommended.

Water-supply options in Bangladesh

Optimum water-supply solutions will vary between regions depending on local hydrological and socio-economic conditions, and general recommendations may be misleading. With these reservations, Table 11.4 compares the main mitigation options for community supply in Bangladesh in terms of both (average) health impact and cost. The alternative water sources are all effective in reducing the arsenic risk, but without chlorination only deep wells and rainwater systems have an acceptable pathogen risk. However, the average cost of water from rainwater systems is 14 times higher. Quantitative health risk estimates are not available for As removal devices, and while neither risk will be insignificant, they should be much preferred to the continued use of polluted shallow wells. The costs of coagulation and adsorbent systems are intermediate between deep wells and rainwater systems, while the costs for air-oxidation IRPs, though only applicable to waters with a high Fe:As ratio, are very competitive. However, the performance of most community treatment systems has been very poor, and will require much effort in supporting operation and maintenance to gain popularity.

Table 11.4 Comparison of community water-supply options in Bangladesh

| Technology | Disease burden (DALY)* | | Cost ($/m³) |
	Pathogens	Arsenic	
Shallow wells (base case)	<10	400	<0.05
Alternative water sources			
Dug well	9400	<1	0.26
Deep well	<10	<1	0.15
Pond sand filter	2800	<0.1	0.16
Rainwater harvesting	<10	<1	2.13
Arsenic removal devices			
Coagulation – filtration	–	–	1.20[†]
GFO/GFH	–	–	1.13[†]
Iron removal plant[‡]	–	–	0.05[†]

DALY, disability adjusted life years per million persons per year.
*DALY values not calculated for treatment systems.
[†]Costs for treatment are in addition to the tubewell.
[‡]Using air oxidation.
Sources: Ahmed et al. (2005); World Bank (2005)

11.4.3 Aquifer clean-up

Regulation in North America and the European Union requires that polluted aquifers are restored to either their pristine condition or to drinking
water standards. This is difficult and expensive, and has led to a shift away
from active treatment towards monitored natural attenuation. Such
approaches are applicable to industrial pollution, but as a deliberate means of
cleaning-up regional aquifer pollution, would not stand up to a cost-benefit
test. Nevertheless, to provide a basis for permanent safe water supplies, it is
appropriate to encourage all measures that contribute to long-term clean-
up of the aquifers. For instance, it is known that nature removes arsenic
from the aquifers on a timescale of tens of thousands of years, and thus it is
rational to try to accelerate natural attenuation processes of oxidation,
adsorption and flushing. On a much shorter timescale, groundwater irrigation is contributing to cleaning up shallow aquifers, albeit by transferring
exposure from drinking water to food via the soil. In the Bengal Basin, older
and deeper strata have the ability to adsorb arsenic, and the deep and shallow abstraction horizons are separated by 50–150 m of sediment that has
some capacity to permanently sequester arsenic. Therefore, shifting part of
groundwater abstraction to deep aquifers could be a strategy for cleaning

up shallow groundwater. Even if arsenic were to break through into deep aquifers, it would take many years and the concentrations will be much lower than in shallow aquifers, such that the cost of treating deep groundwater, if it became necessary, would be delayed by many years and would be cheaper than treating shallow groundwater. Unfortunately, at present there is insufficient knowledge to justify such a policy.

11.5 Sustainability Issues

11.5.1 Migration of arsenic in groundwater

The lateral and vertical migration of arsenic in the subsurface is central to many sustainability issues. Direct evidence for the quantifiable migration of arsenic in aquifers is almost completely lacking, but the movement of arsenic in aquifers is indicated by temporal trends in the As concentration of wells. It is beyond reasonable doubt that many wells will increase in concentration. However, it is not practical to predict which wells will change, by how much and when, and so safe wells must be regularly monitored, with a frequency that reflects proximity to polluted wells.

Assessments of the safe yield of aquifers are founded on predictions (or assumptions) of As migration, or rather its retardation by natural attenuation, over scales of tens of metres to kilometres, and therefore involve great uncertainty. Mathematical models exist to predict the attenuation of arsenic, and common minerals such as iron oxides have the capacity to adsorb arsenic. However, without calibration, these models cannot be applied with confidence to predict the security of vulnerable aquifers, and will require detailed studies of the sorption characteristics of actual aquifer and aquitard materials, supported by modelling and intensive monitoring.

11.5.2 Sustainability of groundwater irrigation

The sustainability of groundwater irrigation in As-affected areas depends on the relative rates of arsenic addition to soils and the declining store of arsenic in the aquifer (Figure 11.2). Arsenic in irrigation water is mainly adsorbed to iron oxides, although some is lost by volatilisation and by plant uptake. Arsenic uptake by grain appears to be more progressive than the development of phytotoxic effects, which may have a threshold effect beyond which the loss of yield increases rapidly until the crop is abandoned. New crop varieties may have a reduced tendency to take up arsenic or be more resistant to arsenic toxicity, but this will not eliminate the problem. The critical question is whether As concentrations in groundwater will decline

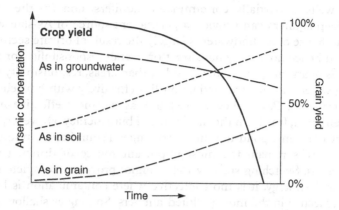

Figure 11.2   Sustainability of groundwater irrigation. No units are used for As concentration as the graphs only indicate the trends over time relative to the starting condition where an insignificant amount of arsenic has accumulated. Likewise, grain yield is expressed relative to the initial yield.

to negligible levels before soil concentrations result in excessive uptake or loss of yield. Outcomes will vary, but at concentrations of hundreds of ppb it is unlikely that irrigation can be sustainable. At lower concentrations, there is an increasing possibility that the rate of accumulation in the soil will be sufficiently slow that volatilisation and harvesting losses are quantitatively significant, and that As-tolerant crop varieties can be developed before unacceptable loss of yield or exposure from food develop.

Where continued irrigation is perceived to be unsustainable, the only practical options are to return to rainfed cropping, change the source of irrigation water, or periodically remove the topsoil. For economic reasons, it is unlikely the ARPs will ever be used to supply irrigation water. New wells may be drilled into deeper aquifers (in the Bengal Basin about 100–250 m deeper) but, for the foreseeable future, this is unlikely to be economic without subsidy, and also raises other sustainability questions as discussed below. On the other hand, drilling new wells slightly deeper (say 10–50 m) in the same aquifer could reduce As concentrations without threatening the deep aquifers, and could significantly extend the production of irrigated crops.

11.5.3   Sustainability of abstraction in the Bengal Basin

The alluvium of the Bengal Basin is the most important As-affected aquifer in the world, and serves as a model for other affected alluvial aquifers. The critical water management issues relating to arsenic are: (a) the continued use of aquifers for water supply and irrigation; (b) the long-term safety of shallow wells in partially contaminated aquifers; and (c) the extent to which deep aquifers can provide a permanent source of As-safe water. In Bangladesh, use of groundwater is largely the result of private sector investment, and hence no agency has direct or overall responsibility for the consequences of arsenic pollution. Outside urban areas, responsibility for rural drinking water and tubewell irrigation lies effectively with households and informal groups. Past policy viewed this as the most effective means of implementation, free from the hindrance of bureaucracy. However, with the discovery of arsenic pollution this is no longer a sound assumption.

Shallow wells remain the most important source of drinking water in affected areas. Switching shallow wells cannot provide a complete solution. Indeed, as a strategy, it is most effective where contamination is least, and totally ineffective in the most polluted aquifers. So long as shallow wells are used, there is a need to monitor them, but presently no organisation is equipped to perform this work. At the planning level, there is a need to predict the trends of As concentration, and hence the abandonment of shallow wells.

So far, community As-removal devices have met with limited success. The availability of small surface water sources varies enormously between regions and they are often already heavily exploited, thus deep groundwater has generally been the preferred source for mitigation. To date, 90% of mitigation in Bangladesh has involved installing wells in deep aquifers, for which the recharge mechanism, and hence safe yield, is not known. Given that national policy explicitly prefers surface water over groundwater, it follows that policy and practice should be reassessed and reconciled. Overpumping of deep aquifers is most likely if they are used for irrigation. Deep aquifers are threatened by arsenic drawn down from above and by saline water drawn either from above or nearer the coast. Research is needed to quantify the rates of recharge and As migration in deep aquifers. The yields of deep aquifers need to be understood on a regional basis. Routine monitoring of selected water sources and multilevel piezometers to identify overpumping, and the legal basis to control it, should be put in place before damage occurs.

Tubewell irrigation has been the single most important factor in attaining food grain self-sufficiency in Bangladesh. However, due to the build-up of As in irrigated soils, 'business-as-usual' will not be possible in many areas. The aggregate impact will be greatest in central Bangladesh, where intensive tubewell irrigation and As contamination coincide, and where excessive As uptake and phytotoxicity have already been noted. The most appropriate solution will be to switch the source of irrigation water but, as with drinking water supply, most local surface-water sources have already been exploited, large surface-water schemes have poor performance records, and switching to deep groundwater is expensive as well as putting potable supplies at risk.

11.5.4 Institutional and management needs

Arsenic investigations and mitigation require coordination. Where sophisticated water management bureaucracies exist and the extent of contamination is small, or knowledge of the problem has emerged gradually over a long period, a dedicated organisation may be unnecessary. However, where less-sophisticated bureaucracies have recently discovered massive cases of pollution, the case for creating a coordinating body is stronger. The organisation should be staffed by a combination of staff seconded from line agencies, NGOs and recognised experts, who would disseminate best practice from around the world. The agency should coordinate activities within government, and between government and NGOs, and also take a lead in public information programmes and overall monitoring of mitigation to ensure conformance with higher objectives. The agency should not play an important role in implementing mitigation, other than in demonstrating new technologies. Each ministry or department should be helped to adopt policies that are both consistent and sufficient as a whole. Any organisation created to coordinate arsenic investigations and mitigation should have a time-bound existence, wherein redundancy is an objective. Careful consideration also should be given to the legal and public accountability of the agency.

Many poor As-affected countries have no comprehensive plan to identify and mitigate contaminated water supplies and to reduce exposure from food. Although implementation can be delegated to the market, an unregulated market is unlikely to reach the poorest members of society and, in any case, will tend to reach the most vulnerable members of society last. All affected countries should adopt a national plan to eliminate exposure to dangerous levels of arsenic within a specified time, and implement a monitoring system that will inform all members of society whether this is being achieved.

11.6 Geographical Perspectives

11.6.1 Africa and Australasia

Africa and Australasia are the least affected continents. In Australia, there are many cases of anthropogenic soil contamination, but no natural occurrences with significant health impacts, and it is unlikely that major new discoveries will be found. In New Zealand, problems associated with geothermal arsenic and alluvial aquifers are well known and understood.

The only well-documented occurrence of arsenic pollution in Africa is in Ghana, although a significant problem is emerging in Burkina Faso, but the extent of health impacts are yet to be confirmed. There is little evidence that mitigation programmes have gone beyond the survey and awareness-raising stages. Throughout most of Africa, relatively little use is made of groundwater for irrigation, and so it is unlikely the food will add greatly to human exposure. Despite minor reports from Botswana, Cameroon and Nigeria, no problems equivalent to those in Asia have been reported from the major river basins. However, over vast areas of the continent, there are apparently no data on arsenic in groundwater, and reconnaissance surveys are urgently required.

11.6.2 Asia

Asia is the most severely arsenic-affected continent. About 88% of the 57 million people known to have been exposed to >50 ppb As in drinking water live in Asia, and moreover, the number of arsenicosis victims is likely to be disproportionately high due to the combination of poverty and exposure from food. The greatest concentration of human suffering due to arsenic in groundwater occurs in a semi-continuous band of alluvial basins including the Indus, Ganges, Brahmaputra, Irrawaddy, Mekong and Red rivers, that drain the Himalayas. The alluvial plains are densely populated by poor and malnourished agricultural communities heavily dependent on shallow groundwater for drinking and irrigation water. The affected aquifers contain anoxic, Fe-rich groundwater in which As is mobilised by RD. The similarities of As occurrence in these basins are greater than their differences, and hence there are opportunities for sharing knowledge, experience and research costs. Within this belt, many river basins have been incompletely surveyed, or simply not surveyed at all, and until proven otherwise must be expected to be contaminated. Pollution mapping appears to be most incomplete in Pakistan, Myanmar, Laos and some of the hill states of northeast India.

The most severely polluted areas of China are semi-arid Shanxi and Inner Mongolia provinces, and hyperarid Xinjiang province. Severe health impacts have been recorded in all three areas, and groundwater is also used for irrigation in these areas. In Shanxi and Inner Mongolia there is evidence for both RD and AD occurring in different parts of the aquifers. Hot springs on the Qinghai–Tibet plateau contain the highest natural arsenic concentrations in the world (up to 126 ppm) but, due to the nature of the terrain, the human impacts are small. Arsenic contamination has been recorded in 16 other provinces of China, but few details are available of the extent, causes or impacts.

Arsenic pollution has been known longer in Taiwan than elsewhere, and as a consequence exposure has been much reduced following construction of reservoirs and distribution to affected villages. There are many occurrences of natural arsenic in Japan, but all are relatively small, well studied, and managed sufficiently well to prevent major health impacts. On a global scale, Japan lies on the circum-Pacific Ring of Fire, extending along the western coast of the Americas, through Kamchatka, Japan and Taiwan, before apparently petering out in the island arcs that form the Philippines, Indonesia, Malaysia and Papua New Guinea (see Figure 8.1). Conditions therefore appear to be favourable for both geothermal arsenic and arsenic mobilised by RD, and it is likely that more occurrences will be identified. Apparently isolated cases in southwest Asia may be indicative of more extensive pollution along the Alpine–Himalayan chain from Tibet to Turkey. Arsenic may also be mobilised by RD in glacial deposits adjacent to the young mountain belts in the far northeast of Asia.

11.6.3   Europe

Although nearly 50 bodies of naturally contaminated groundwater have been identified in Europe, only alluvial groundwater in Hungary is associated with major health effects. A probable link to excess bladder cancer has been identified in Finland, but elsewhere the reported occurrences are of relatively small size and/or low concentration. Mitigation has mostly consisted in installing ARPs at existing water sources. In Hungary, exposure to water with >50 ppb has been largely eliminated, and efforts to comply with the 10 ppb standard are in progress. Arsenic contamination in Europe has a wide variety of causes. Reductive dissolution is responsible for arsenic beneath the Great Hungarian Plain and the Po Basin in northern Italy. In southern Italy, however, geothermal and volcanic sources are more important. North and west of the Alps, most contamination is attributed to SO or AD in bedrock aquifers. The apparent absence of As contamination in fluvio-glacial aquifers is surprising, and may be due to a lack of testing and a greater reliance on surface water sources.

11.6.4   North America

In North America, the USA contains the greatest diversity of arsenic occurrence, but Mexico is the worst affected in terms of arsenicosis. In Canada, bedrock aquifers are affected on both the eastern and western coasts, and significant numbers of arsenicosis patients were identified in Nova Scotia in the 1970s. In the USA, the existence of clinical effects in the exposed population has been disputed. Although they are probably present, this in itself is proof of their low incidence relative to such widespread exposure. Arsenic occurrences in the USA can be divided into four main groups. In New England, arsenic is mobilised by AD in crystalline bedrock aquifers that mainly provide private supplies. Around the Great Lakes and in the Mid-West, As is mobilised mainly by RD in fluvio-glacial sands and gravels. In the northwest, conditions are complex, but include a contribution from geothermal sources. In the dry southwest, As is extensively mobilised by AD in the Basin-and-Range province. It is unlikely that any major occurrences of As have been overlooked in the USA. In Mexico, most known clinical symptoms including cancer and death have been reported; however, the extent, geochemistry and health impacts of arsenic are poorly documented outside a few areas such as the Region Lagunera and the Zimapán Valley.

11.6.5 South and Central America

Arsenic pollution has resulted in severe health impacts on the Pampean plains of Argentina and on the Pacific plains of Chile. The former results from reactions with volcanic loess interbedded with alluvial sands, and produced very high concentrations arsenic, fluoride and sometimes selenium. The problem has been known since the 1920s, and mitigation has been slow, but treatment systems are being implemented. These waters are also used for irrigation, but there is no information about its consequences. In Chile, pollution results from hot springs leaking into Andean rivers that are exploited for water supply at coastal cities. The worst case was at Antofagasta where there was a single source of supply, so both the onset of exposure and its reduction after commissioning of a treatment plant in 1971 occurred suddenly and simultaneously across the exposed population. Rivers are affected by arsenic elsewhere on Pacific plains, and it is likely that alluvial groundwater is also affected in these areas. The remainder of South America is remarkable for the almost complete absence of reports of arsenic. Most of this area comprises plateaus of, and the alluvial plains that drain, the Brazilian and Guyanan shields, where weathering has removed or rendered arsenic unavailable. However, it is suspected that major occurrences of arsenic, mobilised by RD, may occur in the Amazonian foreland basin, and perhaps also in parts of Colombia, Venezuela and along the Isthmus of Panama.

11.7　The Politics of Arsenic Pollution and Mitigation

Sadly the discovery of arsenic pollution has often been accompanied by predictable political responses. Too often, the initial response of government has been to deny the existence of the problem, and then to blame the people who reported it. A further response has been a reluctance to share knowledge of arsenic with the affected population, either for fear of 'frightening' them or perhaps for fear of being held accountable. This is regrettable because it is very difficult to implement mitigation without strong political support.

Political problems apply at national and international levels. International agencies have been accused of double standards for not advocating the same drinking water standards in developing and developed countries. Pollution incidents affecting water supplies in developed countries are often responded to by free distribution of tankered water until a permanent solution can be effected. No such concerns are shown for the rural poor in the developing world. The lack of political will in developing countries is mirrored in the behaviour of the rich countries. To date, the response has been disproportionate to the suffering in many poor countries, and commitments of international aid have been inadequate to mitigate the problems in South and Southeast Asia.

The concerns of rich countries are exemplified in the court case brought against the British Geological Survey (BGS; see Annex 8.1) for their failure to identify arsenic in Bangladesh[6]. This case was eventually dismissed, albeit by the highest court in the land, without the BGS[7] standing trial. Although trial may not be the most appropriate means to address such questions, the net result is that the BGS has never been properly held to account, and hence there is no obligation to learn lessons. Had this oversight occurred in Britain, there would almost certainly have been a Public Enquiry that would have gone far beyond any possible failings of the BGS and examined the failings of an entire generation of professionals and the institutions within which they worked. Had such an enquiry taken place, it is equally hard to imagine that it would not have mandated governments and agencies to test more widely for arsenic and other toxic elements. However, the case also provides an excellent demonstration of the socially constructed and poorly regulated risks typified by Beck's (1992) 'risk society', including the characteristic travesty that attribution of responsibility is frequently difficult to achieve (Atkins et al., 2006).

Most of the undiscovered cases of arsenic contamination are undoubtedly in poor countries that lack the capability to initiate the required investigations. International agencies, which are aware of the experience of Bangladesh, India, China, Taiwan, Vietnam, Nepal, Argentina, Mexico and others, should ensure that these surveys take place. Some, notably UNICEF, are attempting to do this, but none with the appropriate urgency or allocation of resources. There is no question that the BGS and other agencies had good intentions, but in the words of the proverb 'the road to hell is paved with good intentions'.

11.8 Ten Priority Actions

1 Severe current and future human impacts of arsenic poisoning are beyond doubt, and therefore urgent action must be taken to reduce exposure and provide access to safe water, which should be considered a basic human right. Delaying mitigation will increase death and disease.

2 In suspect areas that have not yet been tested, there is an urgent need to carry out reconnaissance surveys to determine the location, scale and causes of contamination.

3 Water-supply interventions must be prioritised in the worst affected areas (e.g. the >2000 villages in Bangladesh where every well is contaminated), and the affected people must be educated about the nature of arsenic poisoning, water-related health matters, and the most practical means of reducing exposure to arsenic.

4 The contribution of food to arsenic exposure must be quantified to assess the combined impact of food and water on human health.

5 The impact of arsenic on irrigated agriculture must be investigated, and measures introduced to reduce the accumulation of arsenic in irrigated crops. For the poorest and most malnourished societies, action research should be conducted to reduce suffering by intervening in dietary and culinary practices. Reducing poverty will reduce the impact of arsenic poisoning.

6 The sustainability of pumping from deeper alluvial aquifers needs to be assessed, especially in coastal areas where safe aquifers are overlain by contaminated aquifers.

7 Where arsenic surveys have been completed, a permanent, local and affordable capability to test water supplies for arsenic must be established. Organisations must be created to coordinate and monitor arsenic mitigation, and be charged with producing, and publicising the progress of, quantitative and time-bound plans to eliminate arsenic exposure.

8 The institutional capacity to understand, plan, implement, support and monitor arsenic mitigation must be developed, and should include the training of future practitioners in schools and universities.

9 More funds should be allocated to arsenic mitigation, following a plan that is proportional to the degree of human suffering and maintenance of the natural resource base in each affected country.

10 The WHO guideline value of 10 ppb As should be implemented as a national drinking water standard through a realistic and phased time-bound plan.

NOTES

1 This ambiguity may overestimate the number of water supplies requiring mitigation, but as shown by the experience of northern Chile (section 5.14), quite reasonably reflects the numbers of people at risk of developing fatal cancers, heart attacks and bronchiectasis.
2 With the exception of Blackfoot Disease in southwest Taiwan.
3 Which must feed back into poorer future economic development.
4 And possibly also prone to errors of interpretation as noted earlier.
5 Also in Vietnam, though no court case followed.
6 Technically, their parent organisation, the Natural Environmental Research Council, would have stood trial.

References

AAN. (2000) *Arsenic Contamination in Groundwater and Hydrogeological Background in Samta Village, Western Bangladesh.* Report of the Asian Arsenic Network, July, 31 pp.

Abbgy, A., Kelly, T. Lawrie, C. & Riggs, K. (2002a) *AS 75 Arsenic Test Kit: Environmental Technology Verification Report.* Columbus, OH: ETV Advanced Monitoring Systems Center.

Abbgy, A., Kelly, T. Lawrie, C. & Riggs, K. (2002b) *Quick TM Arsenic Test Kit: Environmental Technology Verification Report.* Columbus, OH: ETV Advanced Monitoring Systems Center.

Abedin, M.J., Cresser, M.S., Meharg, A.A., Feldmann, J. & Cotter-Howells, J.C. (2002) Arsenic accumulation and metabolism in rice. *Environmental Science and Technology* 36, 962–968.

Abrahams, P.W. & Thornton, I. (Eds) (1987) Distribution and extent of land contaminated by arsenic and associated metals in mining regions of Southwest England. *Transactions of the Institute of Mining and Metallurgy, Section B: Applied Earth Science* 96, B1–B8.

Acharyya, S.K. & Shah, B.A. (2007) Arsenic-contaminated groundwater from parts of Damodar fan-delta and west of Bhagirathi River, West Bengal, India: influence of fluvial geomorphology and Quaternary morphostratigraphy. *Environmental Geology* 52(3), 489–501.

Acharyya, S.K., Chakraborty, P., Lahiri, S., Raymahashay, B.C., Guha, S. & Bhowmik, A. (1999) Arsenic poisoning in the Ganges delta. *Nature* 401, 545–545.

Acharyya, S.K., Lahiri, S., Raymahashay, B.C. & Bhowmik, A. (2000) Arsenic toxicity of groundwater in parts of the Bengal Basin in India and Bangladesh: the role of Quaternary stratigraphy and Holocene sea-level fluctuations. *Environmental Geology* 39, 1127–1137.

Acharyya, S.K., Shah, B.A., Ashyiya, I.D. & Pandey. Y. (2005) Arsenic contamination in groundwater from parts of Ambagarh-Chowki block, Chhattisgarh, India: source and release mechanism. *Environmental Geology* 49(1), 148–158.

Adams, J. (1995) *Risk*. London: UCL Press.

Aggarwal, P.K., Basu, A.R. & Poreda, R.J. (2000) *Isotope Hydrology of Groundwater in Bangladesh: Implications for Characterisation and Mitigation of Arsenic in Groundwater*. Vienna: International Atomic Energy Agency, TC Project BGD/8/016, 23 pp.

Aggarwal, P.K., Basu, A.R. & Kulkarni, K.M. (2003) Comment on 'Arsenic Mobility and Groundwater Extraction in Bangladesh' (I). *Science* **300**(5619), 584.

Aggett, J. & O'Brien. G.A. (1985) Detailed model for the mobility of arsenic in lacustrine sediments based on measurements in Lake Ohakuri. *Environmental Science and Technology* **19**, 231–238.

AGMI. (2004) *Quarterly Report on Environmental monitoring at the Puriton Closed Landfill, near Bridgwater, Somerset*. Cambridge, UK: Arcadis Geraghty & Miller International Ltd.

Aguirre, R.J., K. Banerjee, A. Balczewski & W. Driehaus. (2006) Arsenic adsorption technology – a review of long-term performance in full-scale applications from Stadtholdendorf to Phoenix. In: Bundschuh, J., Armienta, M.A., Bhattacharya, P., Matschullat, J., Birkle, P. & Rodriguez, R. (Eds) *Natural Arsenic in Groundwaters of Latin America*. Freiberg: Bergakademie, Abstract Volume.

Agusa, T., T. Kunito, J. Fujihara, et al. (2006) Contamination by arsenic and other trace elements in tube-well water and its risk assessment to humans in Hanoi, Vietnam. *Environmental Pollution* **139**(1), 95–106.

Ahmad, T.A., M.A. Kahlowm, M.A. Tahir & H. Rashid. (2004) Arsenic contamination: an emerging issue in Pakistan. UNICEF and Pakistan Council of Research in Water Resources. Presented at *30th WEDC International Conference*, Ventiane, Lao PDR.

Ahmed, K.M. (2003) Arsenic contamination of groundwater and a review of the situation in Bangladesh. In: Rahman, A.A. & Ravenscroft, P. (Eds) *Groundwater Resources and Development in Bangladesh*. Bangladesh Centre for Advanced Studies. Dhaka: University Press Ltd, pp. 275–295.

Ahmed, K.M., M.N. Imam, S.H. Akhter, et al. (1998) Mechanism of arsenic release to groundwater: geochemical and mineralogical evidence. International Conference on *Arsenic Pollution on Groundwater in Bangladesh: Causes, Effects and Remedies*. Dhaka Community Hospital, 8–12 February.

Ahmed, M.F. (2002) Alternative water supply options in Bangladesh. Theme Paper. *International Workshop on Arsenic Mitigation in Bangladesh*, Dhaka. Ministry of Local Government, Rural Development and Cooperatives, 86 pp.

Ahmed, M.F. (2003) Treatment of arsenic contaminated water. In: M.F. Ahmed (Ed.) *Arsenic Contamination: Bangladesh Perspective*. ITN – Bangladesh Centre for Water Supply and Waste Management, BUET, Bangladesh, pp. 354–403.

Ahmed, M.F., S.A.J. Shamsuddin, S.G. Mahmud, H. Rashid, D. Deere & G. Howard. (2005) *Risk Assessment of Arsenic Mitigation Options (RAAMO)*. Dhaka, Bangladesh: Arsenic Policy Support Unit (APSU).

Ahsan, H., Chen, Y. Parvez, F., et al. (2006) Arsenic exposure from drinking water and risk of premalignant skin lesions in Bangladesh: baseline results from the Health Effects of Arsenic Longitudinal Study. *American Journal of Epidemiology* **163**, 1138–1148.

AIT. (1981) *Investigation of Land Subsidence Caused Deep Well Pumping in the Bangkok Area: Comprehensive Report 1978–1981.* Division of Geotechnical and Transportation Engineering, Asian Institute of Technology for the Office of the Environment Board, Thailand.

Aiuppa, A., W. D'Alessandro, C. Federico, B. Palumbo & M. Valenza. (2003) The aquatic geochemistry of arsenic in volcanic groundwaters from southern Italy. *Applied Geochemistry* 18(9), 1283–1296.

Akter, K.F., G. Owens, D.E. Davey & R. Naidu. (2005a) Arsenic speciation and toxicity in biological systems. *Reviews in Environmental Contamination Toxicology* 184, 97–149.

Akter, K.F., Z. Chen, L. Smith, D. Davey & R. Naidu. (2005b) Speciation of arsenic in ground water samples: A comparative study of CE-UV, HG-AAS and LC-ICP-MS. *Talanta* 68(2), 406–415.

Allen, J.R.L. (1970) Sediments of the modern Niger Delta: a summary and review. In: Morgan, J.P. (Ed.). *Deltaic Sedimentation.* Tulsa, OK: Society of Economic Paleontologists and Mineralogists, Special Publication 15, pp. 138–151.

Al-Rmalli, S.W., C.F. Harrington, M. Ayub & P.I. Haris. (2005) A biomaterial based approach for arsenic removal from water. *Journal of Environmental Monitoring* 7, 279–282.

Amadi, P.A., C.O. Ofoegbu & T. Morrison. (1989) Hydrogeochemical assessment of groundwater quality on parts of the Niger Delta, Nigeria. *Environmental Geology and Water Science* 14(3), 195–202.

Amajor, L.C. (1991) Aquifers in Benin Formation (Miocene–recent), eastern Niger Delta, Nigeria: lithostratigraphy, hydraulics and water quality. *Environmental Geology and Water Science* 17(2), 85–101.

Amorosi, A., M.C. Centineo, E. Dinelli, F. Lucchini & F. Tateo. (2002) Geochemical and mineralogical variations as indicators of provenance changes in Late Quaternary deposits of SE Po Plain. *Sedimentary Geology,* 151(3–4), 273–292.

Anawar, H.M., K Komaki, J. Akai, et al. (2002) Diagenetic control on arsenic in sediments of the Meghna River delta, Bangladesh. *Environmental Geology* 41, 816–825.

Anawar, H.M., J. Akai & H. Sakugawa. (2004) Mobilization of arsenic from subsurface sediments by effect of bicarbonate ions in groundwater. *Chemosphere* 54(6), 753–762.

Ant, J., K. Rudnitski, B. Schmidt, E. Speelman & S. Nobouphasavanh. (1997) *Environmental Risk Assessment of Spraying Landfill Leachate on the Guelph Turfgrass Institute (GTI) Site: Focus on Lead and Arsenic.* Report to City of Guelph, Ontario, Canada.

Appelo, C.A.J. & W.W.J.M. de Vet. (2003) Modelling insitu iron removal from groundwater with trace elements such as As. In: Welch, A.H. & Stollenwerk, K.G. (Eds) *Arsenic in Groundwater: Geochemistry and Occurrence.* New York: Springer-Verlag, pp. 379–401.

Appelo, C.A.J. & D., Postma. (1996) *Geochemistry, Groundwater and Pollution.* Rotterdam: Balkema.

Appelo, C.A.J., B. Drijver, R. Hekkenberg & M. De Jonge. (1999) Modeling of *in situ* iron removal from groundwater. *Ground Water* 37, 811–817.

Appelo, C.A.J., M.J.J. Van Der Weiden, C. Tournassat & L. Charlet. (2002) Carbonate ions and arsenic dissolution by groundwater. *Environmental Science and Technology* **36**, 3096–3103.

Appleyard, S.J., J. Angeloni & R. Watkins. (2006) Arsenic-rich groundwater in an urban area experiencing drought and increasing population density, Perth, Australia. *Applied Geochemistry* **21**(1), 83–97.

APSU. (2005) *Progress with Provision of Arsenic Mitigation Options to the end of November 2005.* Dhaka, Bangladesh: Arsenic Policy Support Unit.

Armienta, M.A. (2003) Arsenic groundwater pollution in Mexico. *Medical Geology Newsletter* **6**, 4–6.

Armienta, M.A., R. Rodriguez, A. Aguayo, N. Ceniceros, G. Villaseñor & O. Cruz. (1997b) Arsenic contamination of groundwater at Zimapan, Mexico. *Hydrogeology Journal* **5**, 39–46.

Armienta, M.A., L.K. Ongley, R. Rodriguez, G. Villaseñor & H. Mango. (2001) The role of arsenic-bearing rocks in groundwater pollution at Zimapan Valley, Mexico. *Environmental Geology* **40**, 571–581.

Arnórsson, S. (2004) Environmental impact of geothermal energy utilization. *Geological Society of London Special Publication* **236**, 297–336.

Asnachinda, P. (1997) Hydrogeochemistry of the Chiang Mai Basin, northern Thailand. *Journal of Asian Earth Sciences* **15**(2–3), 317–326.

ATSDR. (2005) *Toxicological Profile for Arsenic* (Draft for Public Comment). Agency for Toxic Substances and Disease Registry, Atlanta, GA: U.S. Department of Health and Human Services, Public Health Service.

Atkins, P.J., M.M. Hassan & C.E. Dunn. (2006) Toxic torts: arsenic poisoning in Bangladesh and the legal geographies of responsibility. *Transactions of the Institute of British Geographers* **31**(3), 272–285.

Attaran, A. (2006) Will Negligence Law Poison the Well of Foreign Aid? A Case Comment on: Binod Sutradhar v. Natural Environment Research Council. *Global Jurist Advances* **6**(1), 3.

AWWA. (1999) *Water Quality and Treatment: a Handbook of Community Water Supplies,* 5th edn. American Water Works Association. McGraw-Hill, USA.

Ayotte, J.D., D.L. Montgomery, S.M. Flanagan & K.W. Robinson. (2003) Arsenic in groundwater in Eastern New England: occurrence, controls, and human health implications. *Environmental Science and Technology* **37**(10), 2075–2083.

Ayotte, J.D., Baris, D., Cantor, K.P., et al. (2006a) Bladder cancer mortality and private well use in New England: an ecological study. *Journal of Epidemiology and Community Health* **60**, 168–172.

Ayotte, J.D., B.T. Nolan, J.R. Nuckols, et al. (2006b) Modeling the probability of arsenic in groundwater in New England as a tool for exposure assessment. *Environmental Science and Technology* **40**(11), 3578–3585.

Aziz, S.N., K.J. Boyle & M. Rahman. (2006) Knowledge of arsenic in drinking-water: risks and avoidance in Matlab, Bangladesh. *Journal of Health, Population and Nutrition* **24**(3), 327–335.

Backman, B. & P. Lahermo. (2004) Arsenic in groundwater. In: Loukola-Ruskeeniemi, K. & Lahermo, P. (Eds) *Arsenic in Finland: Distribution, Environmental Impacts and Risks.* Geological Survey of Finland, pp. 103–112.

Backman, B., L. Hiisvirta, M. Ilmasti & P. Lahermo. (1994) Occurrence of arsenic and other heavy metals and anions in drilled wells. *Vesitalous* 5, 11–18 [in Finnish].

BADC. (1992) *Deep Tubewell II Project, Final Report.* Report prepared by Mott MacDonald International and Hunting Technical Services for the Bangladesh Agricultural Development Corporation under assignment to the Overseas Development Administration (UK); 45 volumes.

Bado, A.A. (1939) Composition of water and interpretation of analytical results. *Journal of the American Water Works Association* 31, 1975–1977.

Bae, M., C. Watanabe, T. Inaoka, M. Sekiyama, N. Sudo, M.H. Bokul & R. Ohtsuka. (2002) Arsenic in cooked rice in Bangladesh. *The Lancet* 360(9348), 1839–1840.

Ballantyne, J.M. & J.N. Moore. (1988) Arsenic geochemistry in geothermal systems. *Geochimica Cosmochimica Acta* 52(2), 475–483.

Bang, S., M.D. Johnson, G.P. Korfiatis & X. Meng. (2005) Chemical reactions between arsenic and zero-valent iron in water. *Water Research* 39(5), 763–770.

Banks, D., H. Markland, P.V. Smith, et al. (2004) Distribution, salinity and pH dependence of elements in surface waters of the catchment areas of the Salars of Coipasa and Uyuni, Bolivian Altiplano. *Journal of Geochemical Exploration* 84, 141–166.

Barcelona, M.J., M.D. Varljen, R.W. Puls & D. Kaminski. (2005) Ground water purging and sampling methods: history vs. hysteria. *Ground Water Monitoring and Remediation* 25(1), 52–62.

Bates, M.N., O.A. Rey, M.L. Biggs, et al. (2004) Case-control study of bladder cancer and exposure to arsenic in Argentina. *American Journal of Epidemiology* 159(4), 381–9.

Bearak, B. (1998) Death by arsenic: a special report; new Bangladesh disaster: wells that pump poison. *New York Times*, Special Report. November 10.

Beck, U. (1992) *Risk Society: Towards a New Modernity.* London: Sage, 260 pp.

Beck, U. (1996) Risk society and the provident state. In: Lash, S., Szerszynski, B. & Wynne, B. (Eds) *Environment and Modernity.* London, Sage, pp. 27–43.

Beck, U. (1999) *World Risk Society.* Cambridge: Polity Press; 192 pp.

Belzile, N. & A. Tessier. (1990) Interactions between arsenic and iron oxyhydroxides in lacustrine sediments. *Geochimica Cosmochimica Acta* 54(1), 103–109.

Berg M., H.C. Tran, T.C. Nguyen, H.V. Pham, R. Schertenleib & W. Giger. (2001) Arsenic contamination of groundwater in Vietnam: A human health threat. *Environmental Science and Technology* 35, 132621–2626.

Berg, M., S. Luzi, P.T.K. Trang, P.H. Viet, W. Giger & D. Stüben. (2006a) Arsenic removal from groundwater by household sand filters: comparative field study, model calculations, and health benefits. *Environmental Science and Technology* 40(17), 5567–5573.

Berg, M., C. Stengel, P.T.K. Trang, et al. (2006b) Magnitude of arsenic pollution in the Mekong and Red River Deltas Cambodia and Vietnam. *Science of the Total Environment* 372(2–3), 413–425.

Bethke, C.M. & P.V. Brady. (2000) How the K_d aproach undermines groundwater clean-up. *Ground Water* 38(3), 435–443.

Bexfield, L.M. & L.N. Plummer. (2003) Occurrence of arsenic in ground water of the Middle Rio Grande Basin, central New Mexico. In: Welch, A.H. &

Stollenwerk, K.G. (Eds) *Arsenic in Groundwater: Geochemistry and Occurrence.* New York: Springer-Verlag, pp. 295–327.

Bhattacharjee, B. (2007) A sluggish response to humanity's biggest mass poisoning. *Science* 315, 1659–1661.

Bhattacharya, P., Chatterjee, D. & Jacks, G. (1997) Occurrence of arsenic-contaminated groundwater in alluvial aquifers from delta plains, Eastern India: options for safe water supply. *Water Resources Development* 3(1), 79–92.

Bhattacharya, P., Jacks, G. & Khan, A.A. (Eds). (2001a) *Groundwater Arsenic Contamination in the Bengal Delta Plain of Bangladesh.* Proceedings of the KTH-Dhaka University Seminar, KTH Special Publication, TRITA-AMI Report 3084.

Bhattacharya P., G. Jacks, G. Jana, A. Sracek, J.P. Gustaffson & D. Chatterjee. (2001b) Geochemistry of the Holocene alluvial sediment of the Bengal Delta Plain: implications on arsenic contamination in groundwater. In: Bhattacharya, P., Jacks, G. & Khan, A.A. (Eds) *Groundwater Arsenic Contamination in the Bengal Delta Plain of Bangladesh.* Proceedings of the KTH-Dhaka University Seminar, KTH Special Publication, TRITA-AMI Report 3084, pp. 21–40.

Bhattacharya, P., M. Claesson, J. Bundschuh, et al. (2006) Distribution and mobility of arsenic in the Río Dulce alluvial aquifers in Santiago del Estero Province, Argentina. *Science of the Total Environment* 358(1–3), 97–120.

Biacs, P. (2005) Clear water – food safety: drinking water in Hungary. *Powerpoint presentation at East-West Agrarian Forum,* 21 January 2005, Berlin.

Bin, D., Y. Xiaojing, D. Xiayun, et al. (2004) Epidemiological investigation on drinking water type of arsenicosis in Jinchuan County of Sichuan. *Journal of Preventative Medicine (China)* 20, 4 [in Chinese].

Blum, M.D. & T.E. Törnqvist. (2000) Fluvial responses to climate and sea-level change: a review and look forward. *Sedimentology* 47(1), 2–48.

Bolan, N.S., S. Mahimairaja, M. Megharaj, R. Naidu & D.C. Adriano (2006) Biotransformation of arsenic in soil and aquatic environments. In: Naidu, R., Smith, E., Owens, G., Bhattacharya, P. & Nadebaum, P. (Eds) *Managing Arsenic in the Environment: from Soil to Human Health.* Australia: CSIRO Publishing, pp. 433–454.

Bonnemaison, M. (2005) L'eau, facteur de liberation de l'arsenic naturel. *Geosciences* 2, 54–59.

Borba, R.P., B.R. Figueiredo & J. Matschullat. (2003) Geochemical distribution of arsenic in waters, sediments and weathered gold mineralized rocks from Iron Quadrangle, Brazil. *Environmental Geology* 44(1), 39–52.

Borges, J. & Y. Huh. (2006) Petrography and chemistry of the bed sediments of the Red River in China and Vietnam: provenance and chemical weathering. *Sedimentary Geology* 194(3–4), 155–168.

Borgono, J.M., P. Vincent & H. Venturio. (1977) Arsenic in the drinking water of Antofagasta: epidemiological and clinical study before and after installation of a treatment plant. *Environmental Health Perspectives* 19, 103–105.

Börzsönyi, M., A. Bereczky, P. Rudnai, M. Csanady & A. Horvath. (1992) Epidemiological studies on human subjects exposed to arsenic in drinking water in Southeast Hungary. *Archives of Toxicology* 66(1), 77–78.

Boscolo, C. A. Ferronato, F. Mion & P. Vazzoler. (2005) Prezensa e monitoraggio del arsenico nelle aquae sotterannee del Veneto. In: *Presenza e diffusione dell'arsenico nel sottouolo e nelle risorse idriche italiane: nuovi strumenti di valutazione dinamiche di mobilizzazione*. I quaderni di Arpa. Agenzia Regionale Prevenzione e Ambiente dell Emilia-Romagna, pp. 51–66 [in Italian].

Bostick, B.C. & S. Fendorf. (2003) Arsenite sorption on troilite (FeS) and pyrite (FeS₂). *Geochimica Cosmochimica Acta* 67(5), 909–921.

Bostick, B.C., S. Fendorf & B.A. Manning. (2003) Arsenite adsorption on galena (PbS) and sphalerite (ZnS). *Geochimica Cosmochimica Acta* 67(5), 895–907.

Bottomley, D.J. (1984) Origins of some arseniferous groundwaters in Nova Scotia and New Brunswick, Canada. *Journal of Hydrology* 69, 223–257.

Boulet, R.,Y. Lucas, E. Fritsch & H. Paquet. (1997) Geochemical processes in tropical landscapes: role of soil covers. In: Paquet, H. & Clauer, N. (Eds) *Soils and Sediments: Mineralogy and Geochemistry*. Springer, Berlin, pp. 67–96.

Bowell, R.J. (1994) Arsenic speciation in soil porewaters from the Ashanti Mine, Ghana. *Applied Geochemistry* 9(1), 15–22.

Bowell, R.J. (2002) The hydrogeochemical dynamics of mine pit lakes. In: Younger, P.L. & Robins, N.S. (Eds) *Mine Water Hydrogeology and Geochemistry*. Geological Society of London Special Publication 198, 159–185.

Boyle, D.R., R.J.W. Turner & G.E.M. Hall. (1998) Anomalous arsenic concentrations in groundwaters of an island community, Bowen Island, British Columbia. *Environmental Geochemistry and Health* 20(4), 199–212.

Brammer, H. (1971) Coatings in seasonally flooded soils. *Geoderma* 6, 5–16.

Brammer, H. (1996) *The Geography of the Soils of Bangladesh*. Dhaka: University Press Ltd.

Brammer, H. (2000) *Agroecological Aspects of Agricultural Research in Bangladesh*. Dhaka: University Press Ltd.

Brammer, H. (2004) *Can Bangladesh be Protected from Floods?* Dhaka: University Press Ltd.

Bredberg, R.E. (2004) The Madoc-Bancroft geological corridor of Eastern Ontario. *Canadian Rockhound Magazine*; http://ilap.com/~bredberg/geo/madocg1.html.

Breit, G.N. (1998) The diagenetic history of Permian rocks in the Central Oklahoma Aquifer. *U.S. Geological Survey Water-Supply Paper* 2357-A, 45–69.

Breit, G.N. (2000) Arsenic cycling in eastern Bangladesh: the role of phyllosilicates. *Proceedings of the Annual Meeting of the Geological Society of America*, A-192.

Breit, G.N., H.A. Lowers, A.L. Foster, R.B Perkins, J.C.Yount, J.W.Whitney, M.N.I. Uddin & A. Muneem 2005) Redistribution of arsenic and iron in shallow sediment of Bangladesh. In: *Symposium on the Behaviour of Arsenic in Aquifers, Soils and Plants: Implications for Management*, Dhaka, 16–18 January. Centro Internacional de Mejoramiento de Maíz y Trigo and the U.S. Geological Survey.

Bundschuh, J., B. Farias, R. Martin, et al. (2004) Groundwater arsenic in the Chaco-Pampean Plain, Argentina: case study from Robles county, Santiago del Estero Province. *Applied Geochemistry* 19(2), 231–243.

Bundschuh, J., M.E. Garcia & P. Birkle. (2006) Rural Latin America – a forgotten part of the global groundwater arsenic problem? In: Bundschuh, J., Armienta, M.A., Bhattacharya, P., Matschullat, J., Birkle, P. & Rodriguez, R. (Eds) *Natural*

Arsenic in Groundwaters of Latin America. Freiberg: Bergakademie, Abstract Volume.

Burgess, W.G. & L. Pinto. (2005) Preliminary observations on the release of arsenic to groundwater in the presence of hydrocarbon contaminants in UK aquifers. *Mineral Magazine* **69**, 887–896.

Buschmann, J., M. Berg, C. Stengel, & M.L. Sampson. (2007) Arsenic and manganese contamination of drinking water resources in Cambodia: coincidence of risk areas with low relief topography. *Environmental Science and Technology* **41**(7), 2146–2152.

CABQ. (2005) *Water Quality Report 2005.* City of Albuquerque Water Utility Department. http://www.cabq.gov/waterquality/

Caldwell, B.K., J.C. Caldwell, S.N. Mitra & W. Smith. (2003) Tubewells and arsenic in Bangladesh: challenging a public health success story. *International Journal of Population Geography* **9**(1), 23–38.

Caldwell, B., R.M. Douglas, R. Murshed & G. Ranmuthugala. (2004) Clinicians' roles in management of arsenicosis in Bangladesh: interview study. *British Medical Journal* **328**, 493–494.

Campos, V. (2002) Arsenic in groundwater affected by phosphate fertilizers at São Paulo, Brazil. *Environmental Geology* **42**(1), 83–87.

Cano-Aguillera, I., Aguillera-Alvarado, A.F. & Guitierrez. M. (2004) Arsenic in groundwater: natural occurrence Guanajuato, Mexico: its impacts and low cost remediation. In: *32nd International Geological Congress, Pre-Congress Workshop BWO 06: Natural Arsenic in Groundwater,* 18–19 August, Florence.

Carl Bro. (2004) Implementation of the EU Water Framework Directive, Meeting 2006 deadlines. *Technical Note H. Review of the Impact of Human Activities on Groundwater.* Vilnius: Carl Bro (Denmark), Environmental Policy Center, Company of B. Paukštys Vandens Harmonija (LT).

Carrillo-Chávez, A., J.I. Drever & M. Martínez. (2000) Arsenic content and groundwater geochemistry of the San Antonio-El Triunfo, Carrizal and Los Planes aquifers in southernmost Baja California, Mexico. *Environmental Geology* **39**(11), 1295–1303.

Carter, J.M., S.K. Sando, T.S. Hayes & R.H. Hammond. (1998), Source, occurrence, and extent of arsenic in the Grass Mountain area of the Rosebud Indian Reservation, South Dakota. *U.S. Geological Survey Water-Resources Investigations Report* **97–4286**, 90 pp.

Castelli, A., S. Chiesa, G. Deriu, P.E. Vescovi, M. Zanotti & B. Zonca. (2005) Note sulla prezensa di arsenico nel sottosuolo e nellae aquae sotterannee della Lombardia. In: *Presenza e diffusione dell'arsenico nel sottouolo e nelle risorse idriche italiane: nuovi strumenti di valutazione dinamiche di mobilizzazione.* I quaderni di Arpa. Agenzia Regionale Prevenzione e Ambiente dell Emilia-Romagna, pp. 39–50 [in Italian].

Catling, D.H. (1993) *Rice in Deep Water.* London: Macmillan.

Caussy, D. (Ed.) (2005) A field guide for detection, management and surveillance of arsenicosis cases. WHO, New Delhi.

Caussy, D. & U. Than Sein. (2006) Health-risk assessment of arsenic contamination in the South-East Asia region. In: Naidu, R., Smith, E., Owens, G., Bhattacharya,

P. & Nadebaum, P. (Eds) *Managing Arsenic in the Environment: from Soil to Human Health*. Australia: CSIRO Publishing, pp. 483–493.

Cavar, S., T. Klapec, R.J. Grubesic & M. Valek. (2005) High exposure to arsenic from drinking water at several localities in eastern Croatia. *Science of the Total Environment* **339**, 277–282.

Cebrián, M.E., A. Albores, M. Aguilar & E. Blakely. (1983) Chronic arsenic poisoning in the north of Mexico. *Human Toxicology* **2**(1), 121–133.

Chakraborti, D., B.K. Biswas, T. Roy Chowdhury, et al. (1999) Arsenic groundwater contamination and sufferings of people in Rajnandgaon district, Madhya Pradesh, India. *Current Science* **77**, 502–504.

Chakraborti, D., G.K. Basu, B.K. Biswas, et al. (2001) Characterization of arsenic-bearing sediments of the Gangetic Delta of West Bengal, India. In: Chappell, W.R., Abernathy, C.O. & Calderon, R.L. (Eds) *Arsenic Exposure and Health Effects IV*. Oxford. Elsevier, pp. 27–52.

Chakraborti, D., M.M. Rahman, K. Paul, et al. (2002) Arsenic calamity in the Indian subcontinent: What lessons have been learned? *Talanta* **58**(1), 3–22.

Chakraborti, D., S.C. Mukherjee, S. Pati, et al. (2003) Arsenic groundwater contamination in Middle Ganga Plain, Bihar, India: a future danger? *Environmental Health Perspectives* **111**(9).

Chakraborti, D., E.J. Singh, B. Das, et al. (2008) Groundwater arsenic contamination in Manipur, one of the seven North-Eastern Hill states in India: a future danger. *Environmental Geology*, DOI 10.1007/s00254-007-1176-x.

Chakravarty, S., V. Dureja, G. Bhattacharyya, S. Maity & S. Bhattacharjee. (2002) Removal of arsenic from groundwater using low cost ferruginous manganese ore. *Water Research* **36**(3), 625–632.

Chapelle, F.H. (2001) *Ground-water Microbiology and Geochemistry*, 2nd edn. New York: Wiley.

Chapman, P.M. (2007) Determining when contamination is pollution — weight of evidence determinations for sediments and effluents. *Environment International* **33**(4), 492–501.

Chatterjee, A., D. Das & D. Chakraborti. (1993) A study of ground water contamination by arsenic in the residential area of Behala, Calcutta due to industrial pollution. *Environmental Pollution* **80**(1), 57–65.

Chen, A.S.C., K.A. Fields, T.J. Sorg & L. Wang. (2002) Field evaluation of As removal by conventional plants. *Journal of the American Water Works Association* **94**, 9.

Chen, C. & Wang, C. (1990) Ecological correlation between arsenic level in well water and age-adjusted mortality from malignant neoplasms. *Cancer Research* **50**, 5470–5474

Chen, C-J., T-L. Kuo & M-M. Wu. (1988) Arsenic and Cancers. *The Lancet* **331**(8582), 414–415.

Chen, H.-W., M.M. Frey, D. Clifford, L.S. McNeill & M. Edwards. 1999. Arsenic treatment considerations. *Journal of the American Water Works Association* **91**, 74–85.

Chen, K.P. & H.Y. Wu. (1962) Epidemiological studies on blackfoot disease in Taiwan: 2) A study of drinking water in relation to the disease. *Journal of the Formosan Medical Association* **61**(2), 611–618.

Chen, S-L., S.R. Dzeng & M-H. Yang. (1994) Arsenic species in groundwaters of the blackfoot disease area, Taiwan. *Environmental Science and Technology* **28**(5), 877–881.

Chen, Y. & H. Ahsan. (2004) Cancer burden from arsenic in drinking water in Bangladesh. *American Journal of Public Health* **94**(5), 741–744.

Chen, Z., Y-G. Zhu, W-J. Liu & A.A. Meharg. (2005) Direct evidence showing the effect of root surface iron plaque on arsenite and arsenate uptake into rice (*Oryza sativa*) roots. *New Phytologist* **165**(1), 91–7

Cheng, Z., A Van Geen, C. Jing, X. Meng, A. Seddique & K.M. Ahmed. (2004) Performance of a household-level arsenic removal system during 4-month deployment in Bangladesh. *Environmental Science and Technology* **38**(12), 3442–8.

Cherry, J.A., A.U. Shaikh, D.E. Tallman & R.V. Nicholson. (1979) Arsenic species as an indicator of redox conditions in groundwater. *Journal of Hydrology* **43**, 373–392.

Chery, L., J. Barbier & C. Arnaud. (1998) High heavy metal (Sb, As, Ba, Ni, Pb and Zn) concentrationsin drinking-water supplies: Relationship with the natural geochemical background and an aid in sanitary control. *Hydrogeologie* **4**, 57–62 [in French].

Chiou, H-Y., W-I. Huang, C-L. Su, S-F. Chang, Y-H. Hsu & C-J. Chen. (1997) Dose–response relationship between prevalence of cerebrovascular disease and ingested inorganic arsenic. *Stroke* **28**, 1717–1723.

Chiou, J-M., S-L. Wang, C-J. Chen, C-R. Deng, W. Lin & T-Y. Tai. (2005) Arsenic ingestion and increased microvascular disease risk: observations from the southwestern arseniasis-endemic area in Taiwan. *International Journal of Epidemiology* **34**, 936–943.

Chow, W.S., (1986) Investigation on the presence of excessive arsenic and fluoride in well water in Kg. Sekolah, Ulu Kepong [abstract]. In: *Geological Society of Malaysia Annual Conference, Kuala Lumpur, 28–29 April 1986. Warta Geologi* **12**(2), 94.

Christenson, S., D.L. Parkhurst & G.N. Breit. (1998) Ground-water-quality assessment of the Central Oklahoma Aquifer, Oklahoma: results of investigations. *U.S. Geological Survey Water-Supply Paper* **2357-A**, 107–117.

Claesson M. & J. Fagerberg. (2003) *Arsenic in groundwater of Santiago del Estero-Sources, mobility patterns and remediation with natural materials.* MSc thesis, KTH Stockholm, Sweden, 59 pp.

Clapperton, C.M. (1993) *Quaternary Geology and Geomorphology of South America.* Amsterdam: Elsevier.

Coccoziello, B., A.D. Donna, T.D. Meo, M.L. Impertrice, P. Mainolfi, G. Onorati & V. Romano. (2005) L'arsenico nellae aquae sotterannee della Compania. In: *Presenza e diffusione dell'arsenico nel sottouolo e nelle risorse idriche italiane: nuovi strumenti di valutazione dinamiche di mobilizzazione.* I quaderni di Arpa. Agenzia Regionale Prevenzione e Ambiente dell Emilia-Romagna, pp. 107–126 [in Italian].

Coetsiers, M. & K. Walraevens. (2006) Chemical chracterization of the Neogene aquifer, Belgium. *Hydrogeological Journal* **14**(8), 1556–1568.

Çöl, M., C. Çöl, A. Soran, B. S.Sayli & S. Öztürk. (1999) Arsenic-related Bowen's Disease, Palmar keratosis, and skin cancer. *Environmental Health Perspectives* **107**, 687–689.

Colak, M., U. Gemici & G. Tarcan. (2003) The effects of colemanite deposits on the arsenic concentrations of soil and ground water in Igdekoey-Emet, Kuetahya, Turkey. *Water, Air and Soil Pollution* **149**(1–4), 127–143.

Concha, G., B. Nermell & M. Vahter. (2006) Spatial and Temporal Variations in Arsenic Exposure via Drinking-water in Northern Argentina. *Journal of Health, Population and Nutrition* **24**, 2.

Conlon, T.D., K.C. Wozniak, D. Woodcock, et al. (2005) *Ground Water Hydrology of the Willamette Basin, Oregon*. Scientific Investigations Report 2005–5168, USGS and Oregon Water Resources Department.

Craw, D., D. Falconer & J. H. Youngson. (2003) Environmental arsenopyrite stability and dissolution: theory, experiment, and field observations. *Chemical Geology* **199**(1–2), 71–82.

Cresswell, R.G., J. Bauld, G. Jacobson, et al. (2001) A first estimate of ground water ages for the deep aquifer of the Kathmandu Basin, Nepal, using the radioisotope chlorine-36. *Ground Water* **39**(3), 449–457.

Csalagovitis, I. (1996) *Distribution of Arsenic Waters in Hungary; their Geological and Geochemical Environment and Formation*. Hungarian Geological Survey Annual Report, pp. 22–24.

Csanady, M., Z. Karpati & I. Csalagovits. (2005) *Arsenic in Drinking Water in Hungary*. National Institute of Hygiene and National Geological Institute. http://www.asia-arsenic.net/hungary/hungary-e.htm

Cullen, W. & K.J. Reimer. (1989) Arsenic speciation in the environment. *Chemistry Reviews* **89**, 713–764.

Cumbal, L.H., V. Aguirre, R. Tipan & C. Chavez. (2006) Monitoring concentrations, speciation and mobility of arsenic in geothermal sources of Ecuador's North-Center Andean Region. In: Bundschuh, J., Armienta, M.A., Bhattacharya, P., Matschullat, J., Birkle, P. & Rodriguez, R. (Eds) *Natural Arsenic in Groundwaters of Latin America*. Freiberg: Bergakademie, Abstract Volume.

Curray, J.R. & D.G. Moore. (1971) Growth of the Bengal deep sea fan and denudation of the Himalayas. *Geological Society of America Bulletin* **82**, 563–572.

Dakeishi, M., K. Murata & P. Grandjean. (2006) Long-term consequences of arsenic poisoning during infancy due to contaminated milk powder. *Environmental Health* **5**, 31.

Das, D., A. Chatterjee, G. Samanta, et al. (1994) Arsenic in groundwater in six districts of West Bengal, India: the biggest arsenic calamity in the world. *Analyst* **119**, 168–170.

Das D., A. Chatterjee, G. Samanta, B.K. Mandal, T.R. Chowdhury, C.R. Chanda, P.P. Chowdhury, G.K. Basu & D.Chakraborti. (1996) Arsenic in groundwater in six districts of West Bengal, India. *Environmental Geochemistry and Health* **18**(1), 5–15.

Datta, D.V. (1976) Arsenic and non-cirrhotic portal hypertension. *The Lancet* **307**(7956) 433.

Datta, D.V. & M.K. Kaul. (1976) Arsenic content of drinking water in villages in Northern India: a concept for arsenicosis. *Journal of the Association of Physicians India* **24**, 599–604.

Davies, J. & C. Exley. (1992) *Hydrochemical Character of the Main Aquifer Units of Central and Northeastern Bangladesh and Possible Toxicity of Groundwater to Fish and Humans*. Keyworth: British Geological Survey Technical Report WD/92/43R.

Davies, J. (1994) The hydrogeochemistry of alluvial aquifers in central Bangladesh. In: Nash, H. & McCall, G.J.H. (Eds) *Groundwater Quality*. London: Chapman and Hall.

Davis, C. (2003) Arsenic mitigation in Bangladesh: progress of the UNICEF–DPHE Arsenic Mitigation Project 2002. In: Chappell, W.R., Abernathy, C.O., Calderon, R.L. & Thomas, D.J. (Eds) *Arsenic Exposure and Health Effects V*. Amsterdam: Elsevier, pp. 421–437.

Dawson, A.G. (1992) *Ice Age Earth: Late Quaternary Geology and Climate*. London: Routledge, 293 pp.

De, L., G. Liu, P. Sui, et al. (2006) Investigation and analysis on the distribution of high arsenic and high fluoride in Wusu City. *Chinese Journal Endemiology* 25(1), 61–64.

De Fatima Rossetti, D., P.M. de Toledo & A.M. Góes. (2005) New geological framework for Western Amazonia (Brazil) and implications for biogeography and evolution. *Quaternary Research* 63(1), 78–89.

DeCelles, P.G. & F. Hertel. (1989) Petrology of fluvial sands from the Amazonian foreland basin, Peru and Bolivia. *Geological Society of America Bulletin* 101(12), 1552–1562.

DEFRA and EA. (2002a) *Soil Guideline Value for Arsenic Contamination*. London: Department for the Environment, Food and Rural Affairs and the Environment Agency.

DEFRA and EA. (2002b) *Contaminants in Soil: Collation of Toxicological Data and Intake Values for Humans. Arsenic*. London: R&D Tox. 1, Department for the Environment, Food and Rural Affairs and the Environment Agency.

Del Razo, L.M., M.A. Arellano & M.E. Cebrián. (1990) The oxidation states of arsenic in well-water from a chronic arsenicism area of Northern Mexico. *Environmental Pollution* 64(2), 143–153.

Del Razo, L.M., J.C. Corona, G. García-Vargas, A. Albores & M.E. Cebrián. (1993) Fluoride levels in well-water from a chronic arsenicism area of Northern Mexico. *Environmental Pollution* 80(1), 91–94.

Del Razo, L.M., G.G. Garcia-Vargas, M.F. Sanmiguel, M. Rivera, M.C. Hernandez & M.E. Cebrián. (2002) Arsenic levels in cooked food and assessment of adult dietary intake in the region of Lagunera, Mexico. *Food and Chemical Toxicology* 40, 1423–1431.

DeMarco, M.J., A.K. SenGupta & J.E. Greenleaf. (2003) Arsenic removal using a polymeric/inorganic hybrid sorbent. *Water Research* 37(1), 164–176

Deschamps, E., V.S.T. Ciminelli & W.H. Höll. (2005) Removal of As(III) and As(V) from water using a natural Fe and Mn enriched sample. *Water Research* 39(20), 5212–5220.

Diaz, O.P., I. Leyton, O. Munoz, et al. (2004) Contribution of water, bread, and vegetables (raw and cooked) to dietary intake of inorganic arsenic in a rural village of Northern Chile. *Journal of Agricultural and Food Chemistry* 52(6), 1773–1779.

Ding, Z., B. Zheng, J. Long, et al. (2001) Geological and geochemical characteristics of high arsenic coals from endemic arsenosis areas in southwestern Guizhou Province, China. *Applied Geochemistry* 16(11–12), 1353–1360.

Dittmar, J., A. Voegelin, L.C. Roberts, et al. (2007) Spatial Distribution and Temporal Variability of Arsenic in Irrigated Rice Fields in Bangladesh. 2. Paddy Soil. *Environmental Science and Technology* **41**(17), 5967–5972.

Dittmar, T. (2004) Hydrochemical processes controlling arsenic and heavy metal contamiantion in the Elqui river system. *Science of the Total Environment* **325**, 193–207.

Dixit, S. & J.G. Hering. (2003) Comparison of Arsenic(V) and Arsenic(III) sorption onto iron oxide minerals: implications for arsenic mobility. *Environmental Science and Technology* **37**, 4182–4189.

Dobrzynski, D. (2007) Chemical diversity of groundwater in the Carboniferous-Permian aquifer in the Unislaw Slaski–Sokolowsko area (the Sudetes, Poland); a geochemical modelling approach. *Acta Geologica Polonica* **57**(1), 97–112.

Doe, S. & McConvey, P. (2006) *Regional Groundwater Monitoring Network, Northern Ireland: Review of 2004 Monitoring Data.* Belfast: Environment and Heritage Service.

Dogan, M., Dogan, A.U., Celebi, C., & Baris, Y.I. (2005) Geogenic arsenic and a survey of skin lesions in Emet Region of Kutahya, Turkey. *Indoor-Built Environment* **14**(6), 533–536.

Dou, X., Y. Zhang, M. Yang, Y. Pei, X. Huang, T. Takayama & S. Kato. (2006) Occurrence of arsenic in groundwater in the suburbs of Beijing and its removal using an iron-cerium bimetal oxide adsorbent. *Water Quality Research Journal Canada* **41**(2), 140–146.

Dowling C.D., R.J. Poreda, A.R. Basu, S.L. Peters & P.K. Aggarwal. (2003) Geochemical study of arsenic release mechanisms in the Bengal Basin groundwater. *Water Resources Research* **38**, 1173–1190.

DPHE. (2000) *Deeper aquifers of Bangladesh.* Proceeedings of a Review Meeting. Department of Public Health Engineering with support from UNICEF and the Water and Sanitation Program (South Asia), 43 pp.

DPHE/BGS. (2001) *Arsenic Contamination of Groundwater in Bangladesh.* Department of Public Health Engineering and British Geological Survey. BGS Technical Report WC/00/19 (4 Volumes).

DPHE/MMI/BGS. (1999) *Groundwater Studies for Arsenic Contamination in Bangladesh. Rapid Investigation Phase. Final Report.* Mott MacDonald International Ltd and British Geological Survey. Report for Department of Public Health Engineering (Bangladesh) and Department for International Development (UK).

Drahota, P., T. Paces, Z. Pertold, M. Mihaljevic & P. Skrivan. (2006) Weathering and erosion fluxes of arsenic in watershed mass budgets. *Science of the Total Environment* **372**(1), 306–316.

Driehaus, W. (2000) Arsenic removal from drinking water: the GEH process. *AWWA Inorganic Contaminants Workshop,* Albuquerque, New Mexico, 28–29 February.

Driehaus, W. (2002) Arsenic removal – experience with the GEH process in Germany. *Journal of Water Supply: Research and Technology. AQUA* **2**(2), 275–280.

Duong, H.A., M. Berg, M.H. Hoang, H.V. Pham, H. Gallard, W. Giger & U. von Gunten. (2003) Trihalomethane formation by chlorination of ammonium- and bromide-containing groundwater in water supplies of Hanoi, Vietnam. *Water Research* **37**(13), 3242–3252.

Duxbury, J. & G. Panaullah. (2007) *Remediation of Arsenic for Agriculture Sustainability, Food Security and Health in Bangladesh*. Rome: Food and Agriculture Organisation Working Paper.

Duxbury, J.M. & Y.J. Zavala. (2005) What are safe levels of arsenic in food and soils? In: *Symposium on the Behaviour of Arsenic in Aquifers, Soils and Plants: Implications for Management*, Dhaka, 16–18 January. Centro Internacional de Mejoramiento de Maíz y Trigo and the U.S. Geological Survey.

DWASA. (1991) *Dhaka Region Groundwater and Subsidence Study. Final Report*. Engineering and Planning Consultants (Dhaka) and Sir M. MacDonald and Partners (UK). Report for Dhaka Water Supply and Sewerage Authority under assignment to the World Bank.

DWQR. (2006) *Drinking Water Quality in Scotland in 2005*. Annual Report by the Drinking Water Quality Regulator.

Edet, A.E. & O.E. Offiong. (2002) Evaluation of water quality pollution indices from heavy metal contamination monitoring. A case study from Akpabuyo-Odukpani area, Lower Cross River Basin (southeastern Nigeria). *GeoJournal* 57, 295–304.

Edmunds, W.M. & P.L. Smedley. (1996) Groundwater geochemistry and health: an overview. *Geological Society of London Special Publication* 113, 91–105.

Edmunds, W.M, J.M. Cook, D.G. Kinniburgh, D.L. Miles & J.M Trafford. (1989) *Trace Element Occurrence in British Groundwaters*. Keyworth: British Geological Survey Research Report SD/89/3.

Edwards, M.A. (1994) Chemistry of arsenic removal during coagulation and Fe–Mn oxidation. *Journal of the American Water Works Association* **September**, 64–77.

EFMA. (1999) Production of phosphoric acid. BAT booklet 4 (1995 rev. (1999). European Fertilizer Manufacturers Association, Brussels. http://www.efma.org.

Elless, M.P., C.Y. Poynton, C.A. Willms, M.P. Doyle, A.C. Lopez, D.A. Sokkary, B.W. Ferguson & M.J. Blaylock. (2005) Pilot-scale demonstration of phytofiltration for treatment of arsenic in New Mexico drinking water. *Water Research* 39(16), 3863–3872.

Embleton, C. (Ed.) (1984) *Geomorphology of Europe*. London: McMillan.

Engel, R.R. & A.H. Smith. (1994) Arsenic in drinking water and mortality from vascular disease: An ecologic analysis in 30 counties in the United States. *Archives of Environmental Health* 49(5), 418–427.

ENPHO. (2005) *Dissemination Workshop on 'Groundwater Quality Surveillance in Kathmandu and Lalitpur Municipality areas'*. 10 June, JICA Expert Office and Environment and Public Health Organization.

EPA. (2000) *Technologies and Costs for Removal of Arsenic from Drinking Water*. Washington, DC: EPA/815/R-00–028) US Environmental Protection Agency.

EPA. (2003a) *Design Manual: Removal of Arsenic from Drinking Water by Adsorptive Media*. Washington, DC: EPA 600/R-03/019) US Environmental Protection Agency.

EPA. (2003b) *Design Manual: Removal of Arsenic from Drinking Water by Ion Exchange*. Washington, DC: EPA 600/R-03/080) US Environmental Protection Agency.

EPA. (2003c) *Arsenic Treatment Technology: Evaluation Handbook for Small Systems*. Washington, DC: US Environmental Protection Agency, Office of Water, EPA 816-R-03-014.

EPA. (2006) *Point-of-Use or Point-of-Entry Treatment Options for Small Drinking Water Sysems.* Washington, DC: US Environmental Protection Agency, Office of Water, EPA 815-R-06-010.

Erickson, B. (2003) Field kits fail to provide accurate measure of arsenic in groundwater. *Environmental Science and Technology* 37(1), 35A–38A.

Erickson, M.L. & R.J. Barnes. (2005a) Well characteristics influencing arsenic concentrations in ground water. *Water Research* 39, 4029–4039.

Erickson, M.L. & R.J. Barnes. (2005b) Glacial sediment causing regional-scale elevated arsenic in drinking water. *Ground Water*, 43(6), 796–805.

Erickson, M.L. & R.J. Barnes. (2006) Arsenic concentration variability in public water system wells in Minnesota, USA. *Applied Geochemistry* 21(2), 305–317.

Espinoza, M.A. (2005) *Distribution of Arsenic Pollution in Groundwater of the South West Basin of Sebaco Valley, Matagalpa, Nicaragua.* http://www.portofentry.com/site/root/resources/case_study/2824.html

Espinoza, M.A. (2006) Distribution of natural arsenic contamination in groundwater of the southwest of the Sebaco-Matagalpa Valley. In: Bundschuh, J., Armienta, M.A., Bhattacharya, P., Matschullat, J., Birkle, P. & Rodriguez, R. (Eds) *Natural Arsenic in Groundwaters of Latin America.* Freiberg: Bergakademie, Abstract Volume.

ESRI. (1996) *ArcAtlas: Our Earth (GIS Data).* Redlands, CA: Environmental Systems Research Institute.

FAO. (1988) *Land Resources Appraisal of Bangladesh for Agricultural Development. Report 2: Agroecological Regions of Bangladesh.* Rome: Food and Agriculture Organization,

FAO. (2005) *World River Sediment Yields Database.* Rome: Food and Agriculture Organization. http://www.fao.org/ag/agL/AGLW/sediment

Farías, S.S., V.A. Casaa, C. Vázqueza, L. Ferpozzic, G.N. Puccia & I.M. Cohen. (2003) Natural contamination with arsenic and other trace elements in ground waters of Argentine Pampean Plain. *Science of the Total Environment* 309(1–3), 187–199.

Farina, M., M. Marcaccio & G. Martinelli. (2005) La prezensa di arsenico nellae aquae sotterannee del'Emilia-Romagna. In: *Presenza e diffusione dell'arsenico nel sottouolo e nelle risorse idriche italiane: nuovi strumenti di valutazione dinamiche di mobilizzazione.* I quaderni di Arpa. Agenzia Regionale Prevenzione e Ambiente dell Emilia-Romagna, pp. 67–78 [in Italian].

Farooqi, A., H. Masuda & N. Firdous. (2007) Toxic fluoride and arsenic contaminated groundwater in the Lahore and Kasur districts, Punjab, Pakistan and possible contaminant sources. *Environmental Pollution* 145(3), 839–849.

Feeney, R. & S.P. Kounaves. (2002) Voltammetric measurement of arsenic in natural waters. *Talanta* 58(1), 23–31.

Ferguson, J.F. & J. Gavis. (1972) A review of the arsenic cycle in natural waters. *Water Research* 6(11), 1259–1274.

Ferreccio, C. & A.M. Sancha. (2006) Arsenic exposure and its impact on health in Chile. *Journal of Health, Population and Nutrition* 24(2), 164–175.

Fetter, C.W. (1999) *Contaminant Hydrogeology*, 2nd edn. New Jersey: Macmillan.

Fetter, C.W. (2001) *Applied Hydrogeology*, 4th edn. New Jersey: Prentice-Hall.

Focazio, M.J., A.H. Welch, S.A. Watkins, D.R. Helsel, & M.A. Horn. (2000) *A Retrospective Analysis on the Occurrence of Arsenic in Ground-Water Resources of the*

United States and Limitations in Drinking-Water-Supply Characterizations. Washington, DC: US Geological Survey, Water-Resources Investigation Report 99–4279.

Foust, R.D., P. Mohapatra, A.M. Compton-O'Brien & J. Reifel. (2004) Groundwater arsenic in the Verde Valley in Central Arizona, USA. *Applied Geochemistry* 19(2), 251–255.

Fowler, B.A. (1977) International conference on environmental arsenic: an overview. *Environmental Health Perspectives* 19, 239–242.

Frans, R. (1988) *Influence of MSMA on Straighthead, Arsenic Uptake and Growth Response in Rice (Oryza sativa).* University of Arkansas, Division of Agriculture, Agriculture Research Station

Frengstad, B., A.K.M. Skrede, D. Banks, J.R. Krog & U. Siewers. (2000) The chemistry of Norwegian groundwaters: III. The distribution of trace elements in 476 crystalline bedrock groundwaters, as analysed by ICP-MS techniques. *Science of the Total Environment* 246(1), 21–40.

Frost, F.J., D.F.K. Pierson, L. Woodruff, B. Raasina, R. Davis & J. Davies. (1993) A seasonal study of arsenic in groundwater, Snohomish County, Washington, USA. *Environmental Geochemistry and Health* 15(4), 209.

Fujino, Y., X. Guo, J. Liu, L. You, M. Miyatake, T. Yoshimura and Japan Inner Mongolia Arsenic Pollution (JIAMP) Study Group. (2004) Mental health burden amongst inhabitants of an arsenic-affected area in Inner Mongolia, China. *Social Science and Medicine* 59(9), 1969–1973.

Fytianos, K. & C. Christophoridis. (2004) Nitrate, arsenic and chloride pollution of drinking water northern Greece. Elaboration by applying GIS. *Environmental Monitoring and Assessment* 93(1–3), 55–67.

Gaillardet, J., B. Dupré, P. Louvat & C. J. Allègre. (1999) Global silicate weathering and CO_2 consumption rates deduced from the chemistry of large rivers. *Chemical Geology* 159, 1–4, 3–30.

Gao, S., J. Ryu, K.K. Tanji & M.J. Herbel. (2007) Arsenic speciation and accumulation in evapoconcentrating waters of agricultural evaporation basins. *Chemosphere* 67(5), 862–871.

Garai, R., A.K. Chakraborti, S.B. Dey & K.C. Saha. (1984) Chronic arsenic poisoning from tubewell water. *Journal of the Indian Medical Association* 82, 34–35.

García, M.G., O. Sracek, D.S. Fernández & M. del Valle Hidalgo. (2006b) Factors affecting arsenic concentration in groundwaters from Northwestern Chaco-Pampean Plain, Argentina. *Environmental Geology* 52(7), 1261–1275.

Garcia-Sanchez, A. & E. Alvarez-Ayuso. (2003) Arsenic in soils and waters and its relation to geology and mining activities (Salamanca Province, Spain). *Journal of Geochemical Exploration* 80(1), 69–79.

Garcia-Sanchez, A., A. Moyano & P. Mayorga. (2005) High arsenic contents in groundwater of Central Spain. *Environmental Geology* 47, 847–854.

Gbadebo, A.M. & A.S Mohammed. (2004) Arsenic pollution in aquifers located within the limestone areas of Ogunstate, South-Western Nigeria. In: *32nd International Geological Congress, Pre-Congress Workshop BWO 06: Natural Arsenic in Groundwater,* 18–19 August, Florence.

Gemicic, U. & G. Tarcan. (2004) Hydrogeological and hydrogeochemical features of the Heybeli Spa, Afyon, Turkey: Arsenic and the Other Contaminants in the

Thermal Waters. *Bulletin of Environmental Contamination and Toxicology* 72(6), 1107–1114.

Ghosh, A., A.E. Sáez & W. Ela. (2006a) Effect of pH, competitive anions and NOM on the leaching of arsenic from solid residuals. *Science of the Total Environment* 363(1–3), 46–59.

Ghosh, A., M. Mukiibi, A.E. Saez & W.P. Ela. (2006b) leaching of arsenic from granular ferric hydroxide residuals under mature landfill conditions. *Environmental Science and Technology* 40(19), 6070–6075.

Ghurye, G.L, D.A. Clifford & A.R. Tripp. (1999) Combined arsenic and nitrate removal by ion exchange. *Journal of the American Water Works Association* 91(10), 85–96.

Giménez, J., M. Martínez, J. de Pablo, M. Rovira & L. Duro. (2007) Arsenic sorption onto natural hematite, magnetite, and goethite. *Journal of Hazardous Materials* 141(3), 575–580.

Giuliano, G. (1995) Ground water in the Po Basin: some problems relating to its use and protection. *Science of the Total Environment* 171(1–3), 17–27.

Giuliano, G., E. Preziosi & R. Vivona. (2005) Valutazione della qualita dellae aquae sotterannee a scopi idroptabiliti: il caso del Lazio settentrionale. In: *Presenza e diffusione dell'arsenico nel sottouolo e nelle risorse idriche italiane: nuovi strumenti di valutazione dinamiche di mobilizzazione*. I quaderni di Arpa. Agenzia Regionale Prevenzione e Ambiente dell Emilia-Romagna, pp. 97–106 [in Italian].

Glass, R.L. (1996) Ground-water conditions and quality in the western part of Kenai Peninsula, south-central Alaska. *U.S. Geological Survey Open-File Report* 96–466, 66 pp.

Glass, R.L. (2001) *Ground-Water Quality, Cook Inlet Basin, Alaska, 1999*. Reston, VA: U.S. Geological Survey, WRIR 01–4208.

GOB. (2004) *National Policy for Arsenic Mitigation*. Government of Bangladesh. http://www.sdnpbd.org/sdi/policy/doc/arsenic_policy.pdf.

Goldberg, S. (2002) Competitive adsorption of arsenate and arsenite on oxides and clay minerals. *Soil Science Society of America Journal* 66, 413–421.

Goldberg, G., J. Lepper & H.G. Roehling. (1995) Geogenic arsenic in rocks and groundwater of the Bunter Sandstone in Lower Saxony. *Zeitschrift für Angewandte Geologie* 41(2), 118–124 [in German].

Goldsmith, J.R., M. Deane, J. Thom & G. Gentry. (1972) Evaluation of health implications of elevated arsenic in well waters. *Water Research* 6(10), 1133–1136.

Gómez, J.J., J. Lillo & B. Sahún. (2006) Naturally occurring arsenic in groundwater and identification of the geochemical sources in the Duero Cenozoic Basin, Spain. *Environmental Geology* 50(8), 1432–0495

Gong, Z., X. Lu, M. Ma, C. Watt & X.C. Le. (2002) Arsenic speciation analysis. *Talanta* 58(1), 77–96.

Goodbred S.L. Jr., & S.A. Kuehl. (2000a) The significance of large sediment supply, active tectonism, and eustasy on margin sequence development: Late Quaternary stratigraphy and evolution of the Ganges-Brahmaputra delta. *Sedimentary Geology* 133, 227–248.

Goodbred, S.L. Jr., & S.A. Kuehl. (2000b) Enormous Ganges–Brahmaputra sediment discharge during strengthening early Holocene monsoon. *Geology* 28, 1083–1086.

Goodbred, S.L. Jr., S.A. Kuehl, M.S. Steckler & M.H. Sarker. (2003) Controls on facies distribution and stratigraphic preservation in the Ganges–Brahmaputra delta sequence. *Sedimentary Geology* **155**(3–4), 301–316.

Goudie, A.S. (2005) The drainage of Africa since the Cretaceous. *Sedimentology* **67**, 437–456.

Grafe, M., M.J. Eick & P.R. Grossl. (2001) Adsorption of arsenate (V) and arsenite (III) on goethite in the presence and absence of dissolved organic carbon. *Soil Science Society of America Journal* **65**, 1680–1687.

Grafe, M., M.J. Eick, P.R. Grossl & A.M. Saunders. (2002) adsorption of arsenate and arsenite on ferrihydrite in the presence and absence of dissolved organic carbon. *Journal of Environmental Quality* **31**, 1115–1123.

Grantham, D.A. & J.F. Jones. (1977) Arsenic contamination of water wells in Nova Scotia. *Journal of the American Water Works Association* **69**, 653–657.

Griffiths, J.K., P. Shand & J. Ingram. (2003) Baseline Report Series: 8) The Permo-Triassic Sanstones of Manchester and East Cheshire. BGS Report CR/03/265N for the Environment Agency.

Griffiths, J.K., P. Shand & J. Ingram. (2005) *Baseline Report Series: 19. The Permo-Triassic Sanstones of Liverpool and Rufford.* Keyworth: British Geological Survey Report CR/05/131N for the Environment Agency.

Griffiths, J.K., P. Shand & P. Marchant. (2006) *Baseline Report Series: 23. The Lincolnshire Limestone.* Keyworth: British Geological Survey Report CR/06/060N for the Environment Agency.

Grimmett, R.E.R. & I.G. McIntosh. (1939) Occurrence of arsenic in soils and waters in the Waiotapu Valley, and its relation to stock health. *New Zealand Journal of Science and Technology* **21**, 138–150.

Grossier, P. & M. Ledrans. (1999) Arsenic in drinking water: a primary approach to assess exposure of the French population. *Techniques Sciences Methodes. Genie Urbain-Genie Rural* **2**, 27–32 [in French].

Guha Mazumder, D.N. (2003) Criteria for case definitions of arsenicosis. In: Chappell, W.R., Abernathy, C.O., Calderon, R.L. & Thomas, D.J. (Eds) *Arsenic Exposure and Health Effects V.* Amsterdam: Elsevier, pp. 117–134.

Guha Mazumder, D.N., A.K. Chakraborty, A. Ghose, J.D. Gupta, D.P. Chakraborty, S.B. Dey & N. Chattopadhay. (1988) Chronic arsenic toxicity from tubewell water in rural West Bengal. *Bulletin of the World Health Organization* **66**(4), 499–506.

Guha Mazumder, D.N., J. Das Gupta, A.K. Chakraborty, A. Chatterjee, D. Das & D. Chakraborti. (1992) Environmental pollution and chronic arsenicosis in South Calcutta. *Bulletin of the World Health Organization* **70**(4), 481–485.

Guha Mazumder, D.N., R. Haque, N. Ghosh, et al. (1998) Arsenic levels in drinking water and the prevalence of skin lesions in West Bengal, India. *International Journal of Epidemiology* **27**, 871–877.

Guha Mazumder, D.N., R. Haque, N. Ghosh, et al. (2000) Arsenic in drinking water and the prevalence of respiratory effects in West Bengal, India. *International Journal of Epidemiology* **29**, 1047–1052.

Guha Mazumder, D.N., N. Ghose, K. Mazumder, et al. (2003) Natural history following arsenic exposure: a study in an arsenic endemic area of West Bengal, India.

In: Chappell, W.R., Abernathy, C.O., Calderon, R.L. & Thomas, D.J. (Eds) *Arsenic Exposure and Health Effects V*. Amsterdam: Elsevier, pp. 381–389.

Guo, H. & Y. Wang. (2005) Geochemical characteristics of shallow groundwater in Datong basin, northwestern China. *Journal of Geochemical Exploration* **87**(3), 109–120.

Guo, H., Y. Wang, G.M. Shpeizer & S. Yan. (2003) Natural occurrence of arsenic in shallow groundwater, Shanyin, Datong Basin, China. *Journal of Health, Part A: Toxic/Hazardous Substances in Environmental Engineering* **A38**(11), 2565–2580.

Guo, X., Y. Fujino, X. Ye, J. Liu, T. Yoshimura & JI Study Group. (2006) Association between multi-level inorganic arsenic exposure from drinking water and skin lesions in China. *International Journal of Environmental Research and Public Health* **3**(3), 262–7.

Gurung, J.K., H. Ishiga & M.S. Khadka. (2005) Geological and geochemical examination of arsenic contamination in groundwater in the Holocene Terai Basin, Nepal. *Environmental Geology* **49**(1), 98–113.

Gurzau, E.S. & A.E Gurzau. (2001) Arsenic in drinking water from groundwater in Transylvania: an overview. In: Chappell, W.R., Abernathy, C.O. & Calderon, R.L. (Eds) *Arsenic Exposure and Health Effects IV*. Oxford. Elsevier, pp. 181–184.

Habuda-Stanić, M., M. Kuleš, B. Kalajdžić & Ž. Romić. (2007) Quality of groundwater in eastern Croatia – the problem of arsenic pollution. *Desalination* **210**(1–3), 157–162.

Hadi, A. (2003) Fighting arsenic at the grassroots: experience of BRAC's community awareness initiative in Bangladesh. *Health Policy and Planning* **18**(1), 93–100.

Hakala, E. & A. Hallikainen. (2004) Exposure of the Finnish population to arsenic, effects and health risks. In: Loukola-Ruskeeniemi, K. & Lahermo, P. (Eds) *Arsenic in Finland: Distribution, Environmental Impacts and Risks*. Geological Survey of Finland, pp. 153–166 [in Finnish].

Hall, K.J. (2005) Arsenic in Groundwater in Coastal British Columbia. *Conference on Arsenic in Groundwater: Bangladesh Experience*, University of British Columbia, 24 October.

Hammer, M.J. & M.J. Hammer Jr. (2001) *Water and Wastewater Technology*, 4th edn. New Jersey:Prentice-Hall.

Han, F.X., Y. Su, D.L. Monts, M.J. Plodinec, A. Banin & G.E. Triplett. (2003) Assessment of global industrial-age anthropogenic arsenic contamination. *Naturwissenschaften* **90**(9), 395–401.

Hanchett, S. (2004) Social Aspects of the Arsenic Contamination of Drinking Water: A review of knowledge and practice in Bangladesh and West Bengal. Report for the Arsenic Policy Support Unit, Local Government Division, Government of Bangladesh.

Hanchett, S., Q. Nahar, A. van Agthoven, C. Geers & M.F. Jamil Rezvi. (2002) Increasing awareness of arsenic in Bangladesh: lessons from a public education programme. *Health Policy and Planning* **17**, 393–401.

Harvey C.F., C.H. Swartz, A.B.M. Badruzzaman, et al. (2002) Arsenic mobility and groundwater extraction in Bangladesh. *Science* **298**, 1602–1606.

Harvey, C.F., K.N. Ashfaque, W. Yu, et al. (2006) Groundwater dynamics and arsenic contamination in Bangladesh. *Chemical Geology* **228**(1–3), 112–136.

Hasnat, M.A. (2005) *Assessment of arsenic mitigation options: pregnancy outcomes and nutritional status due to chronic arsenic exposure in Bangladesh.* Unpublished PhD thesis, Australian National University, Canberra.

Hassan, M.M., P.J. Atkins & C.E. Dunn. (2005) Social implications of arsenic poisoning in Bangladesh. *Social Science and Medicine* **61**(10), 2201–2211.

Havelaar, A.H. & J.M. Melse. (2003) *Quantifying Pulic Health Risk in the WHO Guidelines for DrinkingWater Quality.* Bilthoven: Rijksinstituut voorVolksgezondheid en Milieu, RIVM Report 734301022/2003.

Heikens, A. (2006) *Arsenic Contamination of Irrigation Water, Soil and Crops in Bangladesh: Risk Implications for Sustainable Agriculture and Food Safety in Asia.* Rome: Food and Agriculture Organisation, FAO-RAP Publication 2006/20.

Heikens, A., G.M. Panaullah & A.A. Meharg. (2007) Review of arsenic behaviour from groundwater and soil to crops and potential impacts on agriculture and food safety. *Reviews of Environmental Contamination and Toxicology* **189**, 43–87.

Heinrichs, G. & P. Udluft. (1999) Natural arsenic in Triassic rocks: a source of drinking water contamination in Bavaria, Germany. *Hydrogeology Journal* 7, 468–476.

Hem, J.D. (1977) Reactions of metal ions at surface of hydrous iron oxides. *Geochimica Cosmochimica Acta* **41**, 527–538.

Hem J.D. (1985) *Study and Interpretation of the Chemical Characteristics of Natural Water,* 3rd edn. Reston, VA: U.S. Geological Survey Water Supply Paper 2254,

Hering, J.G., P-Y. Chen & J.A. Wilkie. (1997) Arsenic removal from drinking water by coagulation: the rate of adsorption and effects of source water composition. In: Abernathy, C.O., Calderon, R.L. & Chappell, W.R. (Eds). *Arsenic Exposure and Health Effects II.* Oxford: Elsevier, pp. 369–381.

Hernández-García, M.E. & E. Custodio. (2004) Natural baseline quality of Madrid Tertiary Detrital Aquifer groundwater (Spain): a basis for aquifer management. *Environmental Geology* **46**(2), 173–188.

Hingston, J.A., C.D. Collins, R.J. Murphy & J.N. Lester. (2001) Leaching of chromated copper arsenate wood preservatives: a review. *Environmental Pollution* **111**(1), 53–66.

Hinkle, J. (1997) *Quality of Shallow Ground Water in Alluvial Aquifers of the Willamette Basin, Oregon, 1993–95.* Reston, VA: U.S. Geological Survey, Water-Resources Investigations Report 97-4082-B.

Hinkle, S.R. & D.J. Polette. (1999) *Arsenic in Ground Water in the Williamette Basin, Oregon.* Reston, VA: U.S. Geological Survey, Water-Resources Investigations Report 98–4205.

Hira-Smith, M.M., Y. Yuan, X. Savarimuthu, et al. (2007) Arsenic concentrations and bacterial contamination in a pilot shallow dugwell program in West Bengal, India. *Journal of Environmental Science and Health, Part A: Toxic/Hazard Substances and Environmental Engineering* **42**(1), 89–95.

Hiscock, K. (2005) *Hydrogeology: Principles and Practice.* Oxford: Blackwell.

Hlavay, J. & K. Polyak. (1997) Removal of arsenic ions from drinking water by novel type absorbents. In: Abernathy, C.O., Calderon, R.L. & Chappell, W.R. (Eds) *Arsenic Exposure and Health Effects II.* Oxford: Elsevier, pp. 382–392.

Höhn, R., M. Isenbeck-Schröter, D.B. Kent, et al. (2006) Tracer test with As(V) under variable redox conditions controlling arsenic transport in the presence of elevated ferrous iron concentrations. *Journal of Contamination Hydrology* **88**(1–2), 36–54.

Hopenhayn, C., H.M. Bush, A. Bingcang & I. Hertz-Picciotto. (2006) Association between arsenic exposure from drinking water and anemia during pregnancy. *Journal of Occupation and Environmental Medicine* **48**(6), 635–643.

Hopenhayn-Rich, C., M.L. Biggs, A. Fuchs & A.H. Smith. (1996) Bladder cancer mortality associated with arsenic in drinking water in Cordoba, Argentina. *Epidemiology* **7**, 117–124,

Hopenhayn-Rich, C., M.L. Biggs & A.H. Smith. (1998) Lung and kidney cancer mortality associated with arsenic in drinking water in Cordoba, Argentina. *International Journal of Epidemiology* **27**(4), 561–9.

Hoque B.A. (1998) *Biological Contamination of Tubewell Water*. Bangladesh: Environmental Health Programme Report, International Centre for Diarrhoeal Disease Research.

Hoque, B.A, M.M. Hoque, T. Ahmed, et al. (2004) Demand-based water options for arsenic mitigation: an experience form rural Bangladesh. *Public Health* **118**, 70–77.

Hoque, B.A., S. Yamaura, A. Sakai, et al. (2006) Arsenic mitigation for water supply in Bangladesh: appropriate technological and policy perspectives. *Water Quality Research Journal, Canada* **41**(2), 226–234.

Horneman, A., A. van Geen, D.V. Kent, et al. (2004) Decoupling of As and Fe release to Bangladesh groundwater under reducing conditions. Part I: Evidence from sediment profiles. *Geochimica Cosmochimica Acta* **68**, 3459–3473.

Hossain, M.A., M.K. Sengupta, S. Ahamed, et al. (2005) Ineffectiveness and poor reliability of arsenic removal plants in West Bengal, India. *Environmental Science and Technology* **39**(11), 4300–4306.

Hossain, M.A., A. Mukherjee, M.K. Sengupta, et al. (2006) Million dollar arsenic removal plants in West Bengal, India: Useful or Not? *Water Quality Research Journal, Canada* **41**(2), 216–225.

Hossain, M.B. (2005) Arsenic distribution in soil and water of a STW command area. In: *Symposium on the Behaviour of Arsenic in Aquifers, Soils and Plants: Implications for Management*, Dhaka, 16–18 January. Centro Internacional de Mejoramiento de Maíz y Trigo and the U.S. Geological Survey.

Hossain, M.K., M.M. Khan, M.A. Alam, et al. (2005) Manifestation of arsenicosis patients and factors determining the duration of arsenic symptoms in Bangladesh. *Toxicology and Applied Pharmacology* **208**(1), 78–86.

Hounslow, A.W., (1980) Ground-water geochemistry: arsenic in landfills. *Ground Water* **18**(4), 331–333.

Hsu, K-H., J.R. Froines & C-J. Chen. (1997) Studies of arsenic ingestion from drinking water in northeastern Taiwan: chemical speciation and urinary metabolites. In: Abernathy, C.O., Calderon, R.L. & Chappell, W.R. (Eds). *Arsenic Exposure and Health Effects II*. Oxford: Elsevier, pp. 190–209.

Hu, Y., J.H. Li, Y.G. Zhu, Y.Z. Huang, H.Q. Hu & P. Christie. (2005) Sequestration of As by iron plaque on the roots of three rice (Oryza sativa L.) cultivars in a low-P soil with or without P fertilizer. *Environmental Geochemistry and Health* **27**(2), 169–76

Hu, Z-Y., Y-G. Zhu, M. Li., L-G. Zhang, Z-H. Cao & F.A. Smith. (2007) Sulfur (S)-induced enhancement of iron plaque formation in the rhizosphere reduces arsenic accumulation in rice (Oryza sativa L.) seedlings. *Environmental Pollution* 147(2), 387–393.

Huang, R-Q., S-F. Gao, W-L. Wang, S. Stuanton & G. Wang. (2006) Soil arsenic availability and the transfer of soil arsenic to crops in suburban areas in Fujian Province, southeast China. *Science of the Total Environment* 368(2–3), 531–541.

Huang, W.W., J.M. Martin, P. Seyler, J. Zhang & X. M. Zhong. (1988) Distribution and behaviour of arsenic in the Huang He (Yellow River) estuary and Bohai sea. *Marine Chemistry* 25(1), 75–91.

Hug, S.J., L. Canonica, M. Wegelin, D. Gechter & U. von Gunten. (2001) Solar oxidation and removal of arsenic at circumneutral pH in iron containing waters. *Environmental Science and Technology* 35(10), 2114–2121.

Hughes, M.F. (2002) Arsenic toxicity and potential mechanisms of action. *Toxicology Letters* 133(1), 1–16.

Huisman, L. & W.E. Wood. (1974) *Slow Sand Filtration*. Geneva: World Health Organization.

Hung, D.Q., O. Nekrassova & R.G. Compton. (2004) Analytical methods for inorganic arsenic in water: a review. *Talanta* 64(2), 269–277.

Huntsman-Mapila, P., T. Mapila, M. Letshwenyo, P. Wolski & C. Hemond. (2006) Characterization of arsenic occurrence in the water and sediments of the Okavango Delta, NW Botswana. *Applied Geochemistry* 21(8), 1376–1391.

Huq, S.M.I., A. Rahman, N. Sultana & R. Naidu. (2003) Extent and severity of arsenic contamination in soils of Bangladesh. In: Ahmed, M.F., Ali, A.& Adeel, Z. (Eds) *BUET-UNU International Symposium on Fate of Arsenic in the Environment*. Dhaka, Bangladesh, 5–6 February. http://www.unu.edu/env/arsenic/BUETSympo siumProc.htm

Huq, S.M.I., U.K. Shila & J.C. Joardar. (2006) Arsenic mitigation strategy for rice, using water regime management. *Land Contamination and Reclamation* 14(4), 805–813.

Hussam, A., M. Alauddin, A.H. Khan, S.B. Rasul & A.K.M. Munir. (1999) Evaluation of arsine generation in arsenic field kit. *Environmental Science and Technology* 33(20), 3686–3688.

Ingebritsen, S.E. & W.E. Sanford. (1998) *Groundwater in Geologic Processes*. Cambridge University Press.

Inskeep, W.P., T.R. McDermott & S. Fendorf. (2002) Arsenic (V)/(III) cycling in soils and natural waters: chemical and microbiological processes. In: Frankenberger W.T. (Ed.) *Environmental Chemistry of Arsenic*. New York: Marcel Dekker, pp. 185–215.

Iriondo, M. (1993) Geomorphology and Late Quaternary of the Chaco (South America). *Geomorphology* 7, 289–303.

Islam, F.S., A.G. Gault, C. Boothman, et al. (2004) Role of metal-reducing bacteria in arsenic release from Bengal delta sediments. *Nature* 430, 68–71.

Islam, F.S., C. Boothman, A.G. Gault, D.A. Polya & J.R. Lloyd. (2005) Potential role of the Fe(III)-reducing bacteria *Geobacter* and *Geothrix* in controlling arsenic solubility in Bengal delta sediments. *Mineral Magazine* 69, 865–875.

Islam, M.R., W.P. Lahermo, R. Salminen, S. Rojstaczer & V. Peuraniemi. (2000) Lake and reservoir water quality affected by metals leaching from tropical soils, Bangladesh. *Environmental Geology* **39**(10), 1083–1089.

Islam, M.R., M. Jahiruddin, G.K.M.M. Rahman, et al. (2005) Arsenic in paddy soils of Bangladesh: levels, distribution and contribution of irrigation and sediments. In: *Symposium on the Behaviour of Arsenic in Aquifers, Soils and Plants: Implications for Management*, Dhaka, 16–18 January. Centro Internacional de Mejoramiento de Maíz y Trigo and the U.S. Geological Survey.

IUSS Working Group. (2006) *World Reference Base for Soil Resources 2006*. Rome: Food and Agriculture Organisation, World Soil Resources Report 103.

IWACO. (1994) *Jabatobek Water Resources Management Study*; Vol. 7. Report prepared for the Directorate of Water Resources Development (Indonesia) by IWACO Consultants (The Netherlands).

Jahiruddin, M., M.R. Islam, M.A.L. Shah, M.A. Rashid, M.H. Rashid & M.A. Ghani. (2005) Arsenic in the water–soil–crop systems: PETRRA-BRRI-BAU-AAS study. In: *Symposium on the Behaviour of Arsenic in Aquifers, Soils and Plants: Implications for Management*, Dhaka, 16–18 January. Centro Internacional de Mejoramiento de Maíz y Trigo and the U.S. Geological Survey.

Jain, A. & R.H. Loeppert. (2000) Effect of competing anions on the adsorption of arsenate and arsenite by ferrihydrite. *Journal of Environmental Quality* **29**, 1422–1430.

Jain, C.K. & I. Ali. (2000) Arsenic: occurrence, toxicity and speciation techniques. *Water Research* **34**(17), 4304–4312.

Jekel, M.R. (1996) New WHO recommendations for water quality standards. Impact on water treatment practices. National Report: Germany. *Journal of Water Supply: Research and Technology. AQUA* **14**(3–4), 50–51.

Jekel, M. (2002) Actual problems related to inorganic water compounds. *Journal of Water Supply: Research and Technology. AQUA* **2**(1), 1–9.

Jekel, M. & R. Seith. (2002) Comparison of conventional and new techniques for the removal of arsenic in a full scale water treatment plant. *Journal of Water Supply: Research and Technology. AQUA* **18**(1), 628–631.

Jelinek, C.F. & P.E. Corneliussen. (1977) Levels of arsenic in the United States food supply. *Environmental Health Perspectives* **19**, 83.

Jessen, S., F. Larsen, C.B. Koch & E. Arvin. (2005) Sorption and desorption of arsenic to ferrihydrite in a sand filter. *Environmental Science and Technology* **39**(20), 8045–8051.

JICA. (2004) *Arsenic Contamination of Deep Tubewells in Sharsha Upazila*. JICA/AAN Arsenic Mitigation Project. Report 1. Japanese International Cooperation Agency and Asian Arsenic Network.

Jing, C., S. Liu, M. Patel & X. Meng. (2005) Arsenic leachability in water treatment adsorbents. *Environmental Science and Technology* **39**(14), 5481–5487.

Johnston, R.B. & M.H. Sarker. (2007) Arsenic mitigation in Bangladesh: national screening data and case studies in three upazilas. *Journal of Environmental Science and Health, Part A* **42**(12), 1889–1896.

Joshi, A. & M. Chaudhuri. (1996) Removal of arsenic from ground water by iron oxide-coated sand. *Journal of Environmental Engineering* **122**(8), 769–771.

Juntunen, R., S. Vartiainen & A. Pullinen. (2004) Arsenic in water from drilled bedrock wells in Pirkanamaa, southern Finland. In: Loukola-Ruskeeniemi, K. & Lahermo, P. (Eds) *Arsenic in Finland: Distribution, Environmental Impacts and Risks.* Geological Survey of Finland, pp. 111–122 [in Finnish].

Kabata-Pendias, A. (2001) *Trace Elements in Soils and Plants.* Boca Raton, FL: CRC Press.

Kabir, A., R. Johnston, R. Ogata & S. Tsushima. (2005) *Practical Approach for Efficient Safe Water Option.* JICA and UNICEF, Bangladesh.

Karcher, S., L. Caceres, M. Jekel & R. Contreras. (1999) Arsenic removal from water supplies in northern Chile using ferric chloride coagulation. *Water and Environmental Management* **13**(3), 164–169.

Karro, E. & P. Lahermo. (1999) Occurrence and chemical characteristics of groundwater in Precambrian bedrock in Finland. *Geological Survey of Finland – Special Paper* **27**, 85–96.

Kasse, C. (1998) Depositional model for cold-climate tundra rivers. In: Benito, G., Baker, V.R. and Gregory, K.J. (Eds) *Palaeohydrology and Environmental Change.* Chichester: Wiley, pp. 83–97.

Katsoyiannis, I.A. & A.I. Zouboulis. (2004) Application of biological processes for the removal of arsenic from groundwaters. *Water Research* **38**(1), 17–26.

Katsoyiannis, I., A. Zouboulis, H. Althoff & H. Bartel. (2002) As(III) removal from groundwaters using fixed-bed upflow bioreactors. *Chemosphere* **47**(3), 325–332.

Kavaf, N. & M.T. Nalbantcilar. (2007) Assessment of contamination characteristics in waters of the Kütahya Plain, Turkey. *CLEAN – Soil, Air, Water* **35**(6), 585–593.

Kelepertsis, A., D. Alexakis & K. Skordas. (2006) Arsenic, antimony and other toxic elements in the drinking water of eastern Thessaly in Greece and its possible effects on human health. *Environmental Geology* **50**(1), 76–84.

Kelly, W.R., T.R. Holm, S.D. Wilson & G.S. Roadcap. (2005) Arsenic in glacial aquifers: sources and geochemical controls. *Ground Water* **43**(4), 500–510.

Kevekordes, S., R. Suchenwirth, T. Gebel, J. Demuth, H. Dunkelberg & H. Küntzel. (1998) Drinking water supply with reference to geogenic arsenic contamination. *Gesundheitswesen* **60**(10), 576–9 [in German].

Kim, M-J., J. Nriagu & S. Haack. (2000) Carbonate ions and arsenic dissolution by groundwater. *Environmental Science and Technology* **34**, 3094–3100.

Kim, M-J, J. Nriagu & S. Haack. (2002) Arsenic species and chemistry in groundwater of southeast Michigan. *Environmental Pollution* **120**(2), 379–390.

Kinniburgh, D.G. & W. Kosmus. (2002) Arsenic contamination in groundwater: some analytical considerations. *Talanta* **58**(1), 165–180.

Kirk, M.F., T.R. Holm, J. Park, et al. (2004) Bacterial sulfate reduction limits natural arsenic contamination in groundwater. *Geology* **32**(11), 953–956.

Klump, S., R. Kipfer, O.A. Cirpka, et al. (2006) Groundwater dynamics and arsenic mobilization in Bangladesh assessed using noble gases and tritium. *Environmental Science and Technology* **40**(1), 243–250.

Knobeloch, L.M., K.M. Zierold & H.A. Anderson. (2006) Association of arsenic-contaminated drinking-water with prevalence of skin cancer in Wisconsin's Fox River Valley. *Journal of Health, Population and Nutrition* **24**(2), 206–213.

Kohnhorst, A., L. Allan, P. Pokethitiyoke & S. Anyapo. (2002) Groundwater arsenic in central Thailand. *28th World Economic Development Congress International Conference*, Kolkata, India.

Kolker, A., S.K. Haack, W.F. Cannon, et al. (2003) Arsenic in southeastern Michigan. In: Welch, A.H. & Stollenwerk, K.G. (Eds) *Arsenic in Groundwater: Geochemistry and Occurrence*. New York: Springer-Verlag, pp. 281–294.

Kondo, H., Y. Ishiguro, K. Ohno, M. Nagase, M. Toba & Takagi. (1999) Naturally occurring arsenic in the groundwaters in the southern region of Fukoka Prefecture, Japan. *Water Research* 33(8), 1967–1972.

Korngold, E., N. Belayev & L. Aronov. (2001) Removal of arsenic from drinking water by anion exchangers. *Desalination* 141(1), 81–84.

Kortatsi, B. (2007) Hydrochemical framework of groundwater in the Ankobra Basin, Ghana. *Aquatic Geochemistry* 13(1), 41–74.

Kortatsi, B.K., C.K. Tay, G. Anornu, E. Hayford & G.A. Dartey. (2007) Hydrogeochemical evaluation of groundwater in the lower Offin basin, Ghana. *Environmental Geology* 53(8), 1651–1662.

Korte N.E. (1991) Naturally occurring arsenic in groundwaters of the midwestern United-States. *Environmental Geology and Water Science* 18(2), 137–141.

Kortsenshteyn V.N., A.P. Karaseva & A.K. Aleshina. (1973) Distribution of arsenic in deep ground water of the Middle Caspian Artesian Basin. *Geokhimiya* 4, 612–617 [in Russian].

Kralj, P. (2004) Chemical composition of low temperature (<20–40°C) thermal waters in Slovenia. *Environmental Geology* 46(5), 635–642.

Kubota, Y., D. Yokota & Y. Ishiyama. (2003) Arsenic concentration in hot spring waters from the Nigata Plain and Shinji Lowland, Japan. Part 2: source supply of arsenic in arsenic contaminated ground water problem. *Earth Science (Chikyu Kagaku)* 55, 11–22.

Kumar, P.R., S. Chaudhari, K.C. Khilar & S.P. Mahajan. (2004) Removal of arsenic from water by electrocoagulation. *Chemosphere* 55(9), 1245–1252.

Kuntzel, H. (1987) Problems of natural arsenic contents in groundwater and drinking-water of southern Lower Saxony. *Zentralblatt fuer Bakteriologie und Hygiene* 183(5–6), 487. (abstract)

Kurttio, P., H. Komulainen, E. Hakala, H. Kahelin & J. Pekkanen. (1998) Urinary excretion of arsenic species after exposure to arsenic present in drinking water. *Archives of Environmental Contamination and Toxicology* 34(3), 297–305.

Kurttio, P., E. Pukkala, H. Kahelin, A. Auvinen & J. Pekkanen. (1999) Arsenic concentrations in well water and risk of bladder and kidney cancer in Finland. *Environmental Health Perspectives* 107(9), 1–8.

Lai, M-S., Y-M. Hsueh, C-J. Chen, et al. (1994) Ingestion of inorganic arsenic and prevalence of diabetes mellitus. *American Journal of Epidemiology* 139, 484–492.

Lambeck, K., T.M. Esat & E-K. Potter. (2002) Links between climate and sea levels for the past three million years. *Nature* 419, 199–206.

Lamm, S.H., A. Engel, M.B. Kruse, et al. (2004) Arsenic in drinking water and bladder cancer mortality in the United States: an analysis based on 133 US counties and 30 years of observation. *Journal of Occupation and Environmental Medicine* 46(3), 298–306.

Lamm, S.H., A. Engel, C.A. Penn, R. Chen & M. Feinleib. (2006a) Arsenic cancer risk confounder in southwest Taiwan data set. *Environmental Health Perspectives* 114(7), 1077–82.

Lamm, S.H., R. Wilson, S. Lai, et al. (2006b) Skin cancer, skin lesions, and the inorganic arsenic content of well water in Huhhot, Inner Mongolia. *American Association of Cancer Research Meeting Abstracts* **April**, 1070–1071.

Langmuir, D. (1997) *Aqueous Environmental Geochemistry*. New York: Prentice-Hall.

Laparra, J.M., D. Velez, R. Barbera, R. Farre & R. Montoro. (2005) Bioavailability of inorganic arsenic in cooked rice: practical aspects for human health risk assessments. *Journal of Agricultural and Food Chemistry* 53(22), 8829–33.

Lauren, J.G. & J.M. Duxbury. (2005) Management strategies to reduce arsenic uptake by rice. In: *Symposium on the Behaviour of Arsenic in Aquifers, Soils and Plants: Implications for Management*, Dhaka, 16–18 January. Centro Internacional de Mejoramiento de Maíz y Trigo and the U.S. Geological Survey.

Lawrence, A.R., D.C. Gooddy, M. Kanatharan & V. Ramnarong. (2000) Groundwater evolution beneath Hat Yai, a rapidly developing city in Thailand. *Hydrogeology Journal* 8, 564–575.

Lee, J.U., S.W. Lee, K.W. Kim & C.H. Yoon. (2005) The effects of different carbon sources on microbial mediation of arsenic in arsenic-contaminated sediment. *Environmental Geochemistry and Health* 27(2), 159–6.

Lee, S.W., J.Y. Kim, J.U. Lee, I. Ko, & K.W. Kim. (2004) Removal of arsenic in tailings by soil flushing and the remediation process monitoring. *Environmental Geochemistry and Health* 26(4), 403–409.

Leon, L.F.M. (2004) Arsenic occurrence in a hard rock aquifer: a factorial approach to the optimisation of the groundwater monitoring network. In: *32nd International Geological Congress, Pre-Congress Workshop BWO 06: Natural Arsenic in Groundwater*, 18–19 August, Florence.

Leupin, O.X. & S.J. Hug. (2005) Oxidation and removal of arsenic (III) from aerated groundwater by filtration through sand and zero-valent iron. *Water Research* 39(9), 1729–1740.

Leupin, O.X., S.J. Hug & A.B. Badruzzaman. (2005) Arsenic removal from Bangladesh tube well water with filter columns containing zerovalent iron filings and sand. *Environmental Science and Technology* 39(20), 8032–7.

Levy, D.B., J.A. Schramke, K.J. Esposito, T.A. Erickson & J.C. Moore. (1999) The shallow ground water chemistry of arsenic, fluorine, and major elements: eastern Owens Lake, California. *Applied Geochemistry* 14(1), 53–65.

Li, C., P. Wang, H. Sun, J. Zhang, D. Fan & B. Deng. (2002) Late Quaternary incised-valley fill of the Yangtze delta (China): its stratigraphic framework and evolution. *Sedimentary Geology* 152(1–2), 1 133–158.

Li, W., Z. Zhou, L. Zhao, J. Zhang, X. Wang & Y. Wang. (2006) Investigation of endemic arsenism in areas Anhui Province of China. *Anhui Journal of Preventative Medicine* 12(4), 193–196 [in Chinese].

Li, Y., Y. Xia, K. Wu, et al. (2006) Neurosensory effects of chronic exposure to arsenic via drinking water in Inner Mongolia: I. signs, symptoms and pinprick testing. *Journal of Water and Health* 4, 29–37.

Lianfang, W. & H. Jhianzong. (1994) Chronic arsenism from drinking water in some areas of Xinjiang, China. In: Nriagu, J.O. (Ed.). (1994) *Arsenic in the Environment. Vol. 2: Human Health and Ecosystem Effects.* New York: Wiley, pp. 159–172.

Liao, C-M., B-C. Chen, S. Singh, M-C. Lin, C-W. Liu & B-C. Han. (2003) Acute toxicity and bioaccumulation of arsenic in tilapia (*Oreochromis mossambicus*) from a blackfoot disease area in Taiwan. *Environmental Toxicology* 18(4), 252–259.

Liebe, P. (2002) *Guide to Groundwater in Hungary.* Hungarian Ministry of Environment and Water. *http://www.kvvm.hu/szakmai/karmentes/kiadvanyok/fav/fava/fava_index.htm.*

Lien, H.L. & R.T. Wilkin. (2005) High-level arsenite removal from groundwater by zero-valent iron. *Chemosphere* 59(3), 377–86.

Lin, Z. & R.W. Puls. (2003) Potential indicators for the assessment of arsenic natural attenuation in the subsurface. *Advances in Environmental Research* 7(4), 825–834.

Lin, N-F., J. Tang & J-M. Bian. (2002) Characteristics of environmental geochemistry in the Arseniasis area of the Inner Mongolia of China. *Environmental Geochemistry and Health* 24(3), 249–259 [in Chinese].

Lindberg, A-L., W. Goessler, E. Gurzau, et al. (2006) Arsenic exposure in Hungary, Romania and Slovakia. *Journal of Environmental Monitoring* 8(1), 203–208. Epub: 2005 Dec 01.

Liu, C-W., C-S. Jang & C-M. Liao. (2004) Evaluation of arsenic contamination potential using indicator kriging in the Yun-Lin aquifer (Taiwan). *Science of the Total Environment* 321(1–3), 173–188.

Liu, C-W., S-W. Wang, C-S. Jang & K-H. Lin. (2006) Occurrence of arsenic in ground water in the Choushui River alluvial fan, Taiwan. *Journal of Environmental Quality* 35, 68–75.

Liu, J., G. Li, W. Liu, et al. (2003) Analysis of endemic arsenism distribution in Liaoning Province. *Chinese Journal of Endemiology* 22(6), 528–529

Liu, W.J., Y.G. Zhu, Y. Hu, et al. (2006a) Arsenic sequestration in iron plaque, its accumulation and speciation in mature rice plants (*Oryza sativa* L.). *Environmental Science and Technology* 40(18), 5730–5736.

Liu, X., S. Zhang, X. Shan & Y-G. Zhu. (2006b) Toxicity of arsenate and arsenite on germination, seedling growth and amylolytic activity of wheat. *Chemosphere* 61, 293–301.

Loeppert, R.H., N. White, B. Biswas & R. Drees. (2005) Mineralogy and arsenic bonding in Bangladesh rice paddy soils. In: *Symposium on the Behaviour of Arsenic in Aquifers, Soils and Plants: Implications for Management,* Dhaka, 16–18 January. Centro Internacional de Mejoramiento de Maíz y Trigo and the U.S. Geological Survey.

Lokuge, K.M., W. Smith, B. Caldwell, K. Dear & A.H. Milton. (2004) The effect of arsenic mitigation interventions on disease burden in Bangladesh. *Environmental Health Perspectives* 112(11), 172.

Lopez, D.L., L. Ransom, J. Moterrosa, T. Soriano, F. Barahona & J. Bundschuh. (2006) Volcanic pollution of arsenic and boron at Ilopango lake, El Salvador. In: Bundschuh, J., Armienta, M.A., Bhattacharya, P., Matschullat, J., Birkle, P. & Rodriguez, R. (Eds) *Natural Arsenic in Groundwaters of Latin America.* Freiberg: Bergakademie, Abstract Volume.

Loukola-Ruskeeniemi, K. & Lahermo, P. (Eds). (2004) *Arsenic in Finland: Distribution, Environmental Impacts and Risks.* Geological Survey of Finland, 176 pp [in Finnish].

Lowers, H.A., G.N. Breit, A.L. Foster, et al. (2007) Arsenic incorporation into authigenic pyrite, Bengal Basin sediment, Bangladesh. *Geochimica Cosmochimica Acta* 71(11), 2699–2717.

Lowney, Y.W., M.V. Ruby, R.C. Webster, R.A. Schoof & S.E. Holm. (2005) Percutaneous absorption of arsenic from environmental media. *Toxicology and Industrial Health* 21, 1–14.

Lu, F.J. (1990) Blackfoot disease: arsenic or humic acid? *The Lancet* 336(8707), 115–116.

Lu, S., J. Ma, C. Zhou, H. Zhang & X. Cheng. (2004) Research on arsenic content in inhabitants drinking water and endemic arsenic poisoning in Hebei province. *Chinese Journal of Endemiology* 23(1), 46–47 [in Chinese].

Ludwig, W. & J.L. Probst. (1998) River sediment discharge to the oceans; present-day controls and global budgets. *American Journal of Science* 298, 265–295.

Luo, Z.D., Y.M. Zhang, L. Ma, et al. (1997) Chronic arsenicism and cancer in Inner Mongolia – consequences of well-water arsenic levels greater than 50 μg/l. In: Abernathy, C.O., Calderon, R.L. & Chappell, W.R. (Eds). *Arsenic Exposure and Health Effects II.* Oxford: Elsevier, pp. 54–72.

Lytle, D.A., T.J. Sorg & V.L. Snoeyink. (2005) Optimizing arsenic removal during iron removal: Theoretical and practical considerations. *Journal of Water Supply: Research and Technology. AQUA* 54, 545–560.

Ma, L.Q., K.M. Komar, C. Tu, W. Zhang, Y. Cai & E.D. Kennelley. (2001) A fern that hyperaccumulates arsenic. *Nature* 409, 579–579.

Maddison, D., R. Catala-Luque & D. Pearce. (2005) Valuing the Arsenic Contamination of Groundwater in Bangladesh. *Environmental and Resource Economics* 31(4), 459–476.

MAFF. (1993) *Code of Good Practice for the Protection of Soil.* London: Ministry of Agriculture, Fisheries and Food.

Maharjan, M., R.R. Shrestha, S.A. Ahmad, C. Watanabe & R. Ohtsuka. (2006) Prevalence of Arsenicosis in Terai, Nepal. *Journal of Health, Population and Nutrition* 24(2), 246–252.

Mahimairaja, S., N.S. Bolan, D.C. Adriano & B. Robinson. (2005) Arsenic contamination and its risk management in complex environmental settings. *Advances in Agronomy* 86, 1–82.

Mallick, S. & N.R. Rajagopal. (1996) Groundwater development in the arsenic-affected alluvial belt of West Bengal – some questions. *Current Science* 70(11), 956–958.

Mandal, B.K. & K.T. Suzuki. (2002) Arsenic round the world: a review. *Talanta* 58(1), 201–235.

Manganelli, A., C. Goso, R. Guerequiz, J.L. Fernández Turiel, M. García Vallès, D. Gimeno & C. Pérez. (2007) Groundwater arsenic distribution in Southwestern Uruguay. *Environmental Geology* 53(4), 827–834.

Manna, B. & U.C. Ghosh. (2005) Pilot-scale performance of iron and arsenic removal from contaminated groundwater. *Water Quality Research Journal, Canada* 40(1), 82–90.

Manning, B.A. & S. Goldberg. (1996) Modelling competitive adsorption of arsenate with phosphate and molybdate on oxide minerals. *Soil Science Society of America Journal* 60, 121–131.

Mantelli, F., S. Cavallieri & R. Palmieri. (2005) L'arsenico nellae aquae in Tuscana. In: *Presenza e diffusione dell'arsenico nel sottouolo e nelle risorse idriche italiane: nuovi strumenti di valutazione dinamiche di mobilizzazione*. I quaderni di Arpa. Agenzia Regionale Prevenzione e Ambiente dell Emilia-Romagna, pp. 79–96 [in Italian].

Marcaccio, M., G. Martinelli, R. Messori & L. Vicari. (2005) Processi di rilascio dell'arsenico nellae aquae sotterannee del'Emilia-Romagna. In: *Presenza e diffusione dell'arsenico nel sottouolo e nelle risorse idriche italiane: nuovi strumenti di valutazione dinamiche di mobilizzazione*. I quaderni di Arpa. Agenzia Regionale Prevenzione e Ambiente dell Emilia-Romagna, pp. 199–208 [in Italian].

Mason, B. (1966) *Principles of Geochemistry*, 2nd edn. New York: McGraw-Hill.

Mason, B. & Berry, L.G. (1978) *Elements of Mineralogy*. New York: Freeman.

Matisoff, G., C.J. Khourey, J.F. Hall, A.W. Varnes & W.H. Strain. (1982) The nature and source of arsenic in north-eastern Ohio groundwater. *Ground Water* 20, 446–456.

Matschullat, J., R.P. Borba, E. Deschamps, B.R. Figueiredo, T. Gabrio & M. Schwenk. (2000) Human and environmental contamination in the Iron Quadrangle, Brazil. *Applied Geochemistry* 15, 181–190.

Mazid Miah, M.A., M.S. Rahman, A. Islam, et al. (2005) Nationwide survey of arsenic in soils, water and crops in Bangladesh. In: *Symposium on the Behaviour of Arsenic in Aquifers, Soils and Plants: Implications for Management*, Dhaka, 16–18 January. Centro Internacional de Mejoramiento de Maíz y Trigo and the U.S. Geological Survey.

Mbotake, I.T. (2006) A preliminary study of sources of arsenic contamination in southwest Cameroon. *Journal of Environmental Hydrology* 14(December), Paper 25.

McArthur, J.M., P. Ravenscroft, S. Safiullah & M.F. Thirlwall. (2001) Arsenic in groundwater: testing pollution mechanisms for sedimentary aquifers in Bangladesh. *Water Resources Research* 37, 109–117.

McArthur, J.M., D.M. Banerjee, K.A. Hudson-Edwards, et al. (2004) Natural organic matter in sedimentary basins and its relation to arsenic in anoxic groundwater: the example of West Bengal and its worldwide implications. *Applied Geochemistry* 19, 1255–1293.

McArthur, J.M. P. Ravenscroft, D.M. Banerjee, et al. (2008) How palaeosols influence groundwater flow and arsenic pollution: a model from the Bengal Basin and its worldwide implication. *Water Resources Research*, DOI: 10.1029/2007WR006552.

McCleskey, R.B, D.K. Nordstrom & A.S. Maest. (2004) Preservation of water samples for arsenic(III/V) determinations: an evaluation of the literature and new analytical results. *Applied Geochemistry* 19(7), 995–1009.

McLaren, R.G., M. Megharaj & R. Naidu. (2006) Fate of arsenic in the soil environment. In: Naidu, R., Smith, E., Owens, G., Bhattacharya, P. & Nadebaum, P. (Eds) *Managing Arsenic in the Environment: from Soil to Human Health*. Australia: CSIRO Publishing, pp. 57–182.

McLaren, S.J. & N.D. Kim. (1995) Evidence for a seasonal fluctuation of arsenic in New Zealand's longest river and the effect of treatment on concentrations in drinking water. *Environmental Pollution* 90(1), 67–73.

McNeill, L.S. & M. Edwards. (1995) Soluble arsenic removal at water treatment plants. *Journal of the American Water Works Association* **87**(4), 105–113.

McNeill, L.S. & M. Edwards. (1997) Predicting arsenic removal during metal hydroxide precipitation. *Journal of the American Water Works Association* **89**(1), 75.

Meera, V. & M.M. Ahammed. (2006) Water quality of rooftop rainwater harvesting systems: a review. *Journal of Water Supply: Research and Technology. AQUA* **55**, 257–268.

Meharg, A.A. (2005) *Venomous Earth: How Arsenic Caused the World's Worst Mass Chemical Poisoning.* London: Macmillan.

Meharg, A.A. & M. Rahman. (2003) Arsenic contamination of Bangladesh paddy fields soils: implications for rice contribution to arsenic consumption. *Environmental Science and Technology* **37**, 229–234.

Melamed, D. (2004) *Monitoring Arsenic in the Environment: a Review of Science and Technologies for Field Measurement and Sensors.* Washington, DC: U.S. Environmental Protection Agency Report 542/R-04/002.

Meliker, J.R., R.L. Wahl, L.L. Cameron & J.O. Nriagu. (2007) Arsenic in drinking water and cerebrovascular disease, diabetes mellitus, and kidney disease in Michigan: a standardized mortality ratio analysis. *Environmental Health* **6**(1), 4.

Meltem, C. (2004) Arsenic concentrations in the surface, well, and drinking waters of the Hisarcik area, Turkey. *Human and Ecological Risk Assessment* **10**(2), 461–465.

Mench, M., J. Vangronsveld, C. Beckx & A. Ruttens. (2006) Progress in assisted natural remediation of an arsenic contaminated agricultural soil. *Environmental Pollution* **144**(1), 51–61.

Meng, X., S. Bang & G.P. Korfiatis. (2000) Effects of silicate, sulfate, and carbonate on arsenic removal by ferric chloride. *Water Research* **34**(4), 1255–1261.

Meng, X., G.P. Korfiatis, C. Christodoulatos & S. Bang. (2001) Treatment of arsenic in Bangladesh well water using a household co-precipitation and filtration system. *Water Research* **35**(12), 2805–2810.

Mettler S., M. Abdelmoula, E. Hoehn, R. Schoenenberger, P. Weidler & U. von Gunten. (2001) Characterization of iron and manganese precipitates from an in situ ground water treatment plant. *Ground Water* **39**(6), 921–30.

Mianpiang, Z. (1997) *An Introduction to Saline-alkaline Lakes on the Qinghai-Tibet Plateau.* Dordrecht: Kluwer.

Milliman, J.D. & J.D. Syvitski. (1992) Geomorphic/tectonic control of sediment discharge to the ocean: the importance of small mountainous rivers. *Journal of Geology* **100**, 525–544.

Misbahuddin, M. (2003) Consumption of arsenic through cooked rice. *The Lancet* **361**(9355), 435–436.

Miteva, E. (2002) Accumulation and effect of arsenic on tomatoes. *Communications in Soil Science and Plant Analysis* **33**(11–12), 1917–1926.

Mitra, S.R., D.N. Mazumder, A. Basu, et al. (2004) Nutritional factors and susceptibility to arsenic-caused skin lesions in West Bengal, India. *Environmental Health Perspectives* **112**(10), 1104–1109.

Mitrakas, M. (2001) A survey of arsenic levels in tap, underground and thermal mineral waters of Greece. *Fresenius Environmental Bulletin* **10**(9), 717–721.

MOH. (2004) *Survey Report on Arsenic Determination in Mongolia.* Ulaanbaatar: Ministry of Health, Public Health Institute.

Morell, I., M.V. Esteller & E. Gimenez. (2006) The presence of arsenic in arenaceous rocks: a case of study of an aquifer in the Spanish Mediterranean. In: Bundschuh, J., Armienta, M.A., Bhattacharya, P., Matschullat, J., Birkle, P. & Rodriguez, R. (Eds) *Natural Arsenic in Groundwaters of Latin America.* Freiberg: Bergakademie, Abstract Volume.

Morgan, J.P. (1970) Depositional processes in the deltaic environment. In: Morgan, JP (Ed.). *Deltaic Sedimentation.* Tulsa: Society of Economic Paleontologists and Mineralogists, Special Publication 15, pp. 31–46.

Morgan, J.P. & W.G. McIntire. (1959) Quaternary geology of the Bengal Basin, East Pakistan and India. *Geological Society of America Bulletin* 70, 319–342.

Morrison, S.J., D.R. Metzler & A.P. Dwyer. (2002) Removal of As, Mn, Mo, Se, U, V and Zn from groundwater by zero-valent iron in a passive treatment cell: reaction progress modelling. *Journal of Contaminant Hydrology* 56(1–2), 99–116.

Morse, B.S. (2001) Comment on 'The role of arsenic-bearing rocks in groundwater pollution at Zimapan Valley, Mexico' by Armienta and others. *Environmental Geology* 41(1–2), 241–243.

Mosaferi, M., M. Yunesian, A. Mesdaghinia, A. Nadim, S. Nasseri & A. H. Mahvi. (2003) Arsenic occurrence in drinking water of I.R of Iran: the case of Kurdistan Province. In: Ahmed, M.F., Ali, A.& Adeel, Z. (Eds) *BUET-UNU International Symposium on Fate of Arsenic in the Environment.* Dhaka, Bangladesh, 5–6 February. http://www.unu.edu/env/arsenic/BUETSymposiumProc.htm

MPO. (1987) *Groundwater Resources of Bangladesh.* Technical Report 5. Master Plan Organisation. Dhaka. Harza Engineering (USA), Sir M. MacDonald & Partners (UK), Meta Consultants (USA) and EPC Ltd (Bangladesh).

Mroczek, E.K. (2005) Contributions of arsenic and chloride from the Kawerau geothermal field to the Tarawera River, New Zealand. *Geothermics* 34(2), 218–233.

Mueller, S., R. Goldfarb & P. Verplanck. (2001) *Ground-water Studies in Fairbanks, Alaska; a Better Understanding of Some of the United States' Highest Natural Arsenic Concentrations.* Reston, VA: U.S. Geological Survey Report 111-01) http://pubs. usgs.gov/fs/fs-0111-01.

Mueller, S.H., R.J. Goldfarb, G.L. Farmer, et al. (2002) Trace, minor and major element data for ground water near Fairbanks, Alaska, 1999–2000. *U.S. Geological Survey Open-File Report* 02-0090. URL: <http://pubs.usgs.gov/of/2002/ofr-02-0090.

Mukherjee, A, M.K. Sengupta, M.A. Hossain, et al. (2005a) Are some animals more equal than others? *Toxicology* 208, 165–169.

Mukherjee, A., M.K. Sengupta, S. Ahamed, et al. (2005b) Comment on 'Reliability of a Commercial Kit To Test Groundwater for Arsenic in Bangladesh'. *Environmental Science and Technology* 39(14), 5501–5502.

Mukherjee, A.B., P. Bhattacharya, G. Jacks, et al. (2006) Groundwater arsenic contamination in India. In: Naidu, R., Smith, E., Owens, G., Bhattacharya, P. & Nadebaum, P. (Eds) *Managing Arsenic in the Environment: from Soil to Human Health.* Australia: CSIRO Publishing, pp. 553–594.

Mukherjee, S.C., K.C. Saha, S. Pati, et al. (2005) Murshidabad – one of the nine groundwater arsenic affected districts of West Bengal, India. Part II: dermatological, neurological and obstetric findings. *Clinical Toxicology* **43**, 835–848.

Murcott, S. (2001) A comprehensive review of low-cost tubewell water treatment technologies for arsenic removal. In: Chappell,W.R., Abernathy, C.O. & Calderon, R.L. (Eds) *Arsenic Exposure and Health Effects IV*. Oxford. Elsevier, pp. 419–429.

Naidu, R., Smith, E., Owens, G., Bhattacharya, P. & Nadebaum, P. (Eds). (2006) *Managing Arsenic in the Environment: from Soil to Human Health*. Australia: CSIRO Publishing.

Nandi, D., R. C. Patra & D. Swarup. (2005) Arsenic residues in hair samples from cattle in some arsenic affected areas of West Bengal, India. *Bulletin of Environmental Contamination and Toxicology* **75**(2), 251–256.

NASC/ENPHO. (2004) *The State of Arsenic in Nepal – 2003*. National Arsenic Steering Committee and the Environment and Public Health Organisation, 123 pp.

Nath, B., Z. Berner, S. B. Mallik, D. Chatterjee, L. Charlet, & D. Stueben. (2005) Characterization of aquifers conducting groundwaters with low and high arsenic concentrations: a comparative case study from West Bengal, India. *Mineralogy Magazine* **69**, 841–854.

Navas-Acien, A., A.R. Sharrett, E.K. Silbergeld, et al. (2005) Arsenic exposure and cardiovascular disease: a systematic review of the epidemiologic evidence. *American Journal of Epidemiology* **162**, 1037–1049.

Neuberger, C.S. & G.R. Helz. (2005) Arsenic(III) carbonate complexing. *Applied Geochemistry* **20**, 1218–1225.

Ngai, T., B. Dangol, S. Murcott & R.R. Shrestha. (2006) *Kanchan Arsenic Filter*. Massachusetts Institute of Technology, and Environment and Public Health Organization, Nepal.

NGO Forum. (2003) *Arsenic through Rhymes*. Dhaka: NGO Forum for Drinking Water and Sanitation. http://www.ngoforum-bd.org/publication.htm [in Bangla].

Nguyen,V.L., T.K.O. Ta & M. Tateishi. (2000) Late Holocene depositional environments and coastal evolution of the Mekong River Delta, Southern Vietnam. *Journal of Asian Earth Sciences* **18**(4), 427–439.

Nickson, R.T., J.M. McArthur, W. Burgess, K.M. Ahmed, P. Ravenscroft & M. Rahman. (1998) Arsenic poisoning of Bangladesh groundwater. *Nature* **395**, 338.

Nickson, R.T., J.M. McArthur, P. Ravenscroft,W.G. Burgess & K.M. Ahmed. (2000) Mechanism of arsenic poisoning of groundwater in Bangladesh and West Bengal. *Applied Geochemistry* **15**, 403–413.

Nickson, R.T., J.M. McArthur, B. Shrestha, T.O. Kyaw-Myint & D. Lowry. (2005) Arsenic and other drinking water quality issues, Muzaffargarh District, Pakistan. *Applied Geochemistry* **20**(1), 55–68.

Nickson, R.T., C. Sengupta, P. Mitra, et al. (2007) Current knowledge on arsenic in groundwater in five states of India. *Journal of Environmental Science and Health* **42**(12), 1707–1718.

Nicolli, D.M., J.M. Suriano, M.A. Gomez Peral, L.H. Ferpozzi & O.A. Baleani. (1989) Groundwater contamination with arsenic and other trace elements in an area of the Pampa, Province of Cordoba, Argentina. *Environmental Geology and Water Science* 14(1), 3–16.

Ning, R.Y. (2002) Arsenic removal by reverse osmosis. *Desalination* 143(3), 237–241.

Nordstrom, D.K. (2002) Worldwide occurrences of arsenic in groundwater. *Science* 296, 2143–2145.

Nordstrom, D.K., S. Mueller, R. Goldfarb, L. Farmer & R. Sanzalone (2006) Geochemistry and high arsenic concentrations in ground waters of Fairbanks, Alaska. *Internaional Geological Congress*, Delhi. February.

Norman, D.I., G.P. Miller, L. Branvold, et al. (2001) Arsenic in Ghana, West Africa, groundwaters. *U.S. Geological Survey Workshop on Arsenic in the Environment.* wwbrr.cr.usgs.gov/Arsenic/FinalAbsPDF/norman.pdf

Norra, S., Z.A. Berner, P. Agarwala, F. Wagner, D. Chandrasekharam & D. Stüben. (2005) Impact of irrigation with As rich groundwater on soil and crops: A geochemical case study in West Bengal Delta Plain, India. *Applied Geochemistry* 20(10), 1890–1906

NRC. (1999) *Arsenic in Drinking Water. Sub-Committee on Arsenic in Drinking Water Report, National Research Council.* Washington, DC: National Academy Press.

NRC. (2001) *Arsenic in Drinking Water: 2001 Update. Sub-Committee to Update the 1999 Arsenic in Drinking Water Report. National Research Council.* Goyer, R. (Chair). Washington, DC: National Academy Press.

NRDC. (2003) *Grading Drinking Water in US Cities: Albuquerque.* Natural Resources Defense Council. http://www.nrdc.org/water/drinking/uscities.asp.

NRECA. (1997) *Study of the Impact of the Bangladesh Rural Electrification Program on Groundwater Quality.* Bangladesh Rural Electrification Board. NRECA International with The Johnson Company (USA) and ICDDR,B (Bangladesh).

(Ed.)Nurun Nabi, A.H.M., M.M. Rahman & L.N. Islam. (2005) Evaluation of biochemical changes in chronic arsenic poisoning among Bangladeshi patients. *International Journal of Environmental Research and Public Health* 2(3–4), 385–393.

Obiri, S. (2007) Determination of heavy metals in water from boreholes in Dumasi in the Wassa West District of Western Region of Republic of Ghana. *Environmental Monitoring and Assessment* 130(1–3), 455–463.

O'Day, P.A., D. Vlassopoulos, R. Root & N. Rivera. (2004) The influence of sulfur and iron on dissolved arsenic concentrations in the shallow subsurface under changing redox conditions. *Proceedings of the National Academy of Science* 101, 13703–13708.

Oh, J.I., K. Yamamoto, H. Kitawaki, S. Nakao, T. Sugawara, M.M. Rahman & M.H. Rahman. (2000) Application of low-pressure nanofiltration coupled with a bicycle pump for the treatment of arsenic-contaminated groundwater. *Desalination* 132(1–3), 307–314.

Oke, S.A. (2003) Preliminary assessment of the impact of petroleum refinery, Kaduna, Northern Nigeria on the environment and human health. *Medical Geology Newsletter* 7, 11–13.

Oldfield, J.E. (2002) *Selenium World Atlas.* Grimbergen: Selenium–Tellurium Development Association, p. 83.

Olorunfemi, B.N., W.S. Fyfe, B. Kronberg & O. Imasuen. (1985) Clay diagenesis as a function of marine and nonmarine water flow, Niger Delta, Nigeria. *Journal of African Earth Science* 3(4), 399–408.

O'Neill, P. (1995) Arsenic. In: Alloway, B.J. (Ed.) *Heavy Metals in Soils*. New York: Wiley.

Onishi, H. & E.B. Sandell. (1955) Geochemistry of arsenic. *Geochimica Cosmochimica Acta* 7, 1–33.

Oomkens, E. (1974) Lithofacies relations in the Late Quaternary Niger Delta complex. *Sedimentology* 21, 195–222.

Oono, M., H. Masuda & M. Kusakabe. (2002) *Seasonal Change of Arsenic Concentrations in Groundwater at the South of Osaka Prefecture*. http://www-jm.eps.s.u-tokyo.ac.jp/2002cd-rom/pdf/b006/b006-p012_e.pdf.

Opar, A., A. Pfaff, A.A. Seddique, K.M. Ahmed, J.H. Graziano & A. van Geen. (2007) Responses of 6500 households to arsenic mitigation in Araihazar, Bangladesh. *Health and Place* 13(1), 164–172.

Oremland, R.S. & J.F. Stolz. (2003) The ecology of arsenic. *Science* 300, 939–944.

Oremland, R.S. & J.F. Stolz. (2005) Arsenic, microbes and contaminated aquifers. *Trends in Microbiology* 13(2), 45–49.

Ortega-Guerroro, M.A. (2004) Origin of high concentrations of of arsenic in groundwater at the La Laguna Region, Northern Mexico and implications for aquifer management. In: *32nd International Geological Congress, Pre-Congress Workshop BWO 06: Natural Arsenic in Groundwater*, 18–19 August, Florence.

Otto, D., L. He, Y. Xia, et al. (2006) Neurosensory effects of chronic exposure to arsenic via drinking water in Inner Mongolia: II. Vibrotactile and visual function. *Journal of Water and Health* 4(1), 39–48.

OU. (2006) *Water and well-being: Arsenic in Bangladesh*. Open University (UK) Course S250 Science in Context.

Ouvrard, S., M-O. Simonnot & M. Sardin. (2001) Removal of arsenate from drinking water with a natural manganese oxide in the presence of competing anions. *Journal of Water Supply: Research and Technology. AQUA* 1(2), 167–173.

Ouvrard, S; Simonnot, M-O. & M. Sardin. (2002) Key parameters controlling an adsorption process for the selective removal of arsenic from drinking water. *Journal of Water Supply: Research and Technology. AQUA* 2(5–6), 111–117.

Oyarzun, R., S. Guevara, J. Oyarzún, J. Lillo, H. Maturana & P. Higueras. (2006) The As-contaminated Elqui River Basin: a long lasting perspective (1975–1995) covering the initiation and development of Au–Cu–As mining in the High Andes of Northern Chile. *Environmental Geochemistry and Health* 28(5), 431–443.

Oyarzun, R., J. Oyarzún, J. Lillo, H. Maturana & P. Higueras. (2007) Mineral deposits and Cu–Zn–As dispersion–contamination in stream sediments from the semi-arid Coquimbo Region, Chile. *Environmental Geology* 53(2), 283–294.

Pandey, P.K., R.N. Khare, R. Sharma, S.K. Sar, M. Pandey & P. Binayake. (1999) Arsenicosis and deteriorating groundwater quality: Unfolding crisis in central-east Indian region. *Current Science* 77, 686–693.

Pandey, P.K., S. Yadav, S. Nair & A. Bhui. (2002) Arsenic contamination of the environment: a new persepctive from central-east India. *Environment International* 28, 235–245.

Pandey, P.K., R. Sharma, M. Roy, S. Roy & M. Pandey. (2006) Arsenic contamination in the Kanker district of central-east India: geology and health effects. *Environmental Geochemistry and Health* 28(5), 409–420.

Paoloni, J.D., M.E. Sequeira & C.E. Fiorentino. (2005) Mapping of arsenic content and distribution in groundwater in the southeast Pampa, Argentina. *Journal of Environmental Health* **67**(8), 50–3.

Parga, J.R; D.L. Cocke, J.L. Valenzuela, et al. (2005) Arsenic removal via electrocoagulation from heavy metal contaminated groundwater in La Comarca Lagunera Mexico. *Journal of Hazardous Materials* **124**(1–3), 247–254.

Pasquini, A. I., P.J. Depetris, D.M. Gaiero and J-L. Probst. (2005) Material sources, chemical weathering, and physical denudation in the Chubut River Basin (Patagonia, Argentina): Implications for Andean Rivers. *Journal of Geology* **113**, 451–469.

Patel, K.S., K. Shrivas, R. Brandt, N. Jakubowski, W. Corns & P. Hoffmann. (2005) Arsenic contamination in water, soil, sediment and rice of central India. *Environmental Geochemistry and Health* **27**(2), 131–45.

Paul, B.K. & V.L. Tinnon-Brock. (2006) Treatment delay period: The case of arsenicosis in rural Bangladesh. *Health and Place* **12**(4), 580–593.

Payne, K.B. & T.M. Abdel-Fattah. (2005) Adsorption of arsenate and arsenite by iron-treated activated carbon and zeolites: effects of pH, temperature, and ionic strength. *Journal of Environmental Science and Health, Part A* **40**(4), 723–749.

Pena, M.E., G.P. Korfiatis, M. Patel, L. Lippincott & X. Meng. (2005) Adsorption of As(V) and As(III) by nanocrystalline titanium dioxide. *Water Research* **39**(11), 2327–2337

Percival, J B., Y.T.J. Kwong, C.G. Dumaresq & F.A. Michel. (2004) Transport and attenuation of arsenic, cobalt and nickel in an alkaline environment (Cobalt, Ontario). *Geological Survey of Canada, Open File* **1680**.

Pershagen, G. (1983) The epidemiology of human arsenic exposure. In: Fowler, B.A. (Ed.) *Biological and Environmental Effects of Arsenic*. Amsterdam: Elsevier, pp. 199–232.

Peryea, P.J. (2002) Evaluation of five soil tests for predicting responses of apple trees planted in lead arsenate-contaminated soil. *Communications in Soil Science and Plant Analysis* **33**(1–2), 243–257.

Peters, S.C. & J.D. Blum. (2003) The source and transport of arsenic in a bedrock aquifer, New Hampshire, USA. *Applied Geochemistry* **18**(11), 1773–1787.

Petrusevski, B., S.K. Sharma, F. Kruis, P. Omeruglu & J.C. Schippers. (2002) Family filter with iron-coated sand: solution for arsenic removal in rural areas. *Journal of Water Supply: Research and Technology. AQUA* **2**(5–6), 127–133.

Peyton, G.R., T.R. Holm & J. Shim. (2006) *Development of Low Cost Treatment Options for Arsenic Removal in Water Treatment Facilities*. Illinois State Water Survey; MTAC Publication TR06-03.

Pfeifer, H-R., A. Gueye-Girardet, D. Reymond, et al. (2004) Dispersion of natural arsenic in the Malcantone watershed, Southern Switzerland: field evidence for repeated sorption-desorption and oxidation-reduction processes. *Geoderma* **122**(2–4), 205–234.

PHED. (1991) Arsenic pollution in groundwater in West Bengal. Public Health Engineering Department, Govt of West Bengal

Pierce, M.L. & C.M. Moore. (1982) Adsorption of arsenite and arsenate on amorphous Fe hydroxide. *Water Research* **16**, 1247–1253.

Planer-Friedrich, B., M. Armienta & A. Merkel. (2001) Origin of arsenic in the groundwater of the Rioverde basin, Mexico. *Environmental Geology* **40**(10), 1290–1298.

Pokhrel, D, T. Viraraghavan & L. Brau. (2005) Evaluation of treatment systems for the removal of arsenic from groundwater. *Practical Periodical of Hazardous, Toxic, and Radioactive Waste Management* **9**(3), 152–157.

Polizzotto, M.L., C.F. Harvey, S.R. Sutton & S. Fendorf. (2005) Processes conducive to the release and transport of arsenic into aquifers of Bangladesh. *Proceedings of the National Academy of Science* 10.1073/pnas.0509539103.

Polya, D.A., A.G. Gault, N. Diebe, P. et al. (2005) Arsenic hazard in shallow Cambodian groundwaters. *Mineral Magazine* **69**, 807–823.

Potter, P.E. (1978) Petrology and chemistry of modern big river sands. *Journal of Geology* **86**, 423–449.

Potter, P.E. (1994) Modern sands of South America: composition, provenance and global significance. *International Journal of Earth Science* **83**(1), 212–232.

Przygoda, G., J. Feldmann & W.R. Cullen. (2001) The arsenic eaters of Styria: a different picture of people who were chronically exposed to arsenic. *Applied Organometallurgy and Chemistry* **15**, 457–462.

Radu, T., J.L. Subacz, J.M. Phillippi & M.O. Barnett. (2005) Effects of dissolved carbonate on arsenic adsorption and mobility. *Environmental Science and Technology* **39**(20), 7875 –7882.

Rahman, A.A. & P. Ravenscroft (Eds). (2003) *Groundwater Resources and Development in Bangladesh – Background to the Arsenic Crisis, Agricultural Potential and the Environment.* Bangladesh Centre for Advanced Studies. Dhaka: University Press Ltd.

Rahman, M., M. Tondel, S.A. Ahmad & O. Axelson. (1998) Diabetes Mellitus Associated with Arsenic Exposure in Bangladesh. *American Journal of Epidemiology* **148**(2) 198–203.

Rahman, M., M. Tondel, I.A. Chowdhury & O. Axelson. (1999) Relations between exposure to arsenic, skin lesions and glucosuria. *Occupational Environmental Medicine* **56**, 277–281.

Rahman, M., M. Vahter, M.A. Wahed, et al. (2006) Prevalence of arsenic exposure and skin lesions. A population based survey in Matlab, Bangladesh. *Journal of Epidemiology and Community Health* **60**, 242–248.

Rahman, M.A., H. Hasegawa, M.A. Rahman, M.M. Rahman & M.A. Majid Miah. (2006) Influence of cooking method on arsenic retention in cooked rice related to dietary exposure. *Science of the Total Environment* **370**(1), 51–60.

Rahman, M.M., D. Mukherjee, M.K. Sengupta, et al. (2002) Effectiveness and reliability of arsenic field testing kits: are the million dollar screening projects effective or not? *Environmental Science and Technology* **36**(24), 5385–5394.

Rahman, M.M., M.K. Sengupta, S. Ahamed, et al. (2005a) Murshidabad: The magnitude of arsenic contamination in groundwater and its health effects to the inhabitants of the Jalangi – one of the 85 arsenic affected blocks in West Bengal, India. *Science of the Total Environment* **338**(3), 189–200.

Rahman, M.M., M.K. Sengupta, S. Ahamed, et al. (2005b) Status of groundwater arsenic contamination and human suffering in a Gram Panchayet (cluster of villages) in Murshidabad, one of the nine arsenic affected districts in West Bengal, India. *Journal of Water and Health* **3**(3), 283–96.

Rahman, M.M., M.K. Sengupta, S.C. Mukherjee, et al. (2005c) Murshidabad – one of the nine groundwater arsenic affected districts of West Bengal, India. Part I: magnitude of contamination and population at risk. Part II: dermatological, neurological and obstetric findings. *Clinical Toxicology* **43**(7), 823–834.

Raiswell, R., D.E. Canfield & R.A. Berner. (1994) A comparison of iron extraction methods for the determination of the degree of pyritisation and the recognition of iron-limited pyrite formation. *Chemical Geology* **111**, 101–110.

Rapant, S. & K. Krčmová. (2007) Health risk assessment maps for arsenic groundwater content: application of national geochemical databases. *Environmental Geochemistry and Health* **29**(2), 131–141.

Rasul, S.B., A.K.M. Munir, Z.A. Hossain, A.H. Khan, M. Alauddin & A. Hussam. (2002) Electrochemical measurement and speciation of inorganic arsenic in groundwater of Bangladesh. *Talanta* **58**(1), 33–43.

Ravenscroft, P. (2000) On the sustainability of groundwater pumping in arsenic affected areas of Bangladesh. *International Workshop on Control of Arsenic Contamination in Ground Water*, Calcutta, 5–6 January.

Ravenscroft, P. (2001) Distribution of groundwater arsenic in the Bangladesh related to geology. In: Bhattacharya, P., Jacks, G. & Khan, A.A. (Eds) *Groundwater Arsenic Contamination in the Bengal Delta Plain of Bangladesh*. Proceedings of the KTH-Dhaka University Seminar, KTH Special Publication, TRITA-AMI Report 3084, pp. 4–56.

Ravenscroft, P. (2003) An overview of the hydrogeology of Bangladesh. In: Rahman, A.A. & Ravenscroft, P. (Eds) *Groundwater Resources and Development in Bangladesh*. Bangladesh Centre for Advanced Studies. Dhaka: University Press Ltd, pp. 43–85.

Ravenscroft, P. & K.M. Ahmed. (1998) Regional hydrogeological controls on the occurrence of arsenic in groundwater in the Bengal Basin. International Conference on *Arsenic Pollution on Groundwater in Bangladesh: Causes, Effects and Remedies*. Dhaka Community Hospital, 8–12 February.

Ravenscroft, P., J.M. McArthur & A.A. Hoque. (2001) Geochemical and palaeohydrological controls on pollution of groundwater by arsenic. In: Chappell, W.R., Abernathy, C.O. & Calderon, R.L. (Eds) *Arsenic Exposure and Health Effects IV*. Oxford. Elsevier, pp. 53–77.

Ravenscroft P., W.G. Burgess, K.M. Ahmed, M. Burren & J. Perrin. (2005) Arsenic in groundwater of the Bengal Basin, Bangladesh: Distribution, field relations, and hydrogeological setting. *Hydrogeology Journal* **13**, 727–751.

Ravenscroft, P., R.J. Howarth & J.M. McArthur. (2006) Comment on 'Limited temporal variability of arsenic concentrations in 20 wells monitored for 3 years in Araihazar, Bangladesh'. *Environmental Science and Technology* **40**(5), 1716–1717.

Redman, A.D., D.L. Macalady & D. Ahmann. (2002) Natural organic matter affects arsenic speciation and sorption onto hematite. *Environmental Science and Technology* **36**(13), 2889–2896.

Redwine, J.C. (2001) Innovative technologies for remediation of arsenic in soil and groundwater. In: Chappell, W.R., Abernathy, C.O. & Calderon, R.L. (Eds) *Arsenic Exposure and Health Effects IV*. Oxford. Elsevier, pp. 453–462.

Reed, J.F. & M.B. Sturgis. (1936) Toxicity from arsenic compounds to rice on flooded soils. *Journal of the American Society of Agronomy* 28(6), 432–436.

Reimann, C., K. Bjorvatn, B. Frengstad, Z. Melaku, R. Tekle-Haimanot & U. Siewers. (2003) Drinking water quality in the Ethiopian section of the East African Rift Valley I—data and health aspects. *Science of the Total Environment* 311(1–3), 65–80.

Renshaw, C.E., B.C. Bostick, X. Feng, et al. (2006) Impact of land disturbance on the fate of arsenical pesticides. *Journal of Environmental Quality* 35, 61–67.

Rivero, S., J.A. Alvarez, V. Liberal & M.L. Esparza. (2000) Community participation in reducing risks by exposure to arsenic in drinking water. *Journal of Water Supply: Research and Technology. AQUA* 18(1–2), 618–620.

Roberts, L.C., S.J. Hug, J. Dittmar, et al. (2007) Spatial distribution and temporal variability of arsenic in irrigated rice fields in Bangladesh. 1. Irrigation water. *Environmental Science and Technology* 41(17), 5960–5966.

Robertson, F. (1989) Arsenic in ground-water under oxidizing conditions, southwest Unites States. *Environmental Geochemistry and Health* 11, 171–185.

Rodríguez, R.J., A. Ramos & A. Armienta. (2004) Groundwater arsenic variations: the role of local geology and rainfall. *Applied Geochemistry* 19(2), 245–250.

Roman, S. & V. Peuraniemi. (1999) The effect of bedrock, glacial deposits and a waste disposal site on groundwater quality in the Haukipudas area, Northern Finland. In: Chilton, J. (Ed.) *Groundwater in the Urban Environment.* Rotterdam: Balkema, pp. 329–334.

Román-Ross, G., G.J. Cuello, X. Turrillas, A. Fernández-Martínez & L. Charlet. (2006) Arsenite sorption and co-precipitation with calcite. *Chemical Geology* 233(3–4), 328–336.

Romero, L., H. Alonso, P. Campano, et al. (2003) Arsenic enrichment in waters and sediments of the Rio Loa (Second Region, Chile). *Applied Geochemistry* 18(9), 1399–1416.

Romero, F.M., M.A. Armienta & A. Carrillo-Chavez. (2004) Arsenic sorption by carbonate-rich aquifer material, a control on arsenic mobility at Zimapan, Mexico. *Archives of Environmental Contamination and Toxicology* 47(1), 1–13.

Romero, F.M., M.A. Armienta & G. González-Hernández. (2006) Solid-phase control on the mobility of potentially toxic elements in an abandoned lead/zinc mine tailings impoundment, Taxco, Mexico. *Applied Geochemistry* 22(1), 109–127.

Ronai, A. (1985) The Quaternary of the Great Hungarian Plain. In: Pesci, M. (Ed.) *Loess and the Quaternary.* Budapest: Akadamiai Kiadi, pp. 51–63,

Rosenboom, J.W. (2004) *Arsenic in 15 Upazilas of Bangladesh: Water Supplies, Health and Behaviour – an Analysis of Available Data.* DPHE, DFID, UNICEF.

Ross, Z., J.M. Duxbury, S.D. DeGloria, D. Narayan & R. Paul. (2006) Potential for arsenic contamination of rice in Bangladesh: spatial analysis and mapping of high risk areas. *International Journal of Risk Assessment Management* 6(4/5/6), 298–315

Rott, U. & M. Friedle. (1999) Subterranean removal of arsenic from groundwater. In: Chappell, W.R., Abernathy, C.O. & Calderon, R.L. (Eds) *Arsenic Exposure and Health Effects III.* Oxford: Elsevier, pp. 389–396.

Rott, U., C. Meyer & M. Friedle. (2002) Residue-free removal of arsenic, iron, manganese and ammonia from groundwater. Innovations in Conventional and

Advanced Water Treatment Processes. *Journal of Water Supply: Research and Technology. AQUA* 2(1), 17–24.

Roy Chowdhury, T., G.K. Basu, B.K. Mandal, et al. (1999) Arsenic poisoning of Bangladesh groundwater. *Nature* 401, 545–546.

Roychowdhury, T., T. Uchino, H. Tokunaga & M. Ando. (2002) Survey of arsenic in food composites from an arsenic-affected area of West Bengal, India. *Food and Chemical Toxicology* 40(11), 1611–1621

Roychowdhury, T., Tokunaga, T. Uchino & M. Ando. (2005) Effect of arsenic-contaminated irrigation water on agricultural land soil and plants in West Bengal, India. *Chemosphere* 58(6), 799–810.

Rushton, K.R. (2003) *Groundwater Hydrology: Conceptual and Computational Models.* Chichester: Wiley.

Ryker, S.J. (2003) Arsenic in ground water used for drinking in the United States. In: Welch, A.H. & Stollenwerk, K.G. (Eds) *Arsenic in Groundwater: Geochemistry and Occurrence.* New York: Springer-Verlag, pp. 165–178.

Sadiq, M. & I. Alam. (1996) Arsenic chemistry in a groundwater aquifer from the Eastern Province of Saudi Arabia. *Water, Air and Soil Pollution* 89, 67–76.

Saha, G.C. & M.A. Ali. (2007) Dynamics of arsenic in agricultural soils irrigated with arsenic contaminated groundwater in Bangladesh. *Science of the Total Environment* 379(2–3), 180–189.

Saha, K.C. (1984) Melanokeratosis from arsenical contamination of tubewell water. *Indian Journal of Dermatology* 29, 37–46.

Saha, K.C. (2003) Saha's grading of arsenicosis progression and treatment. In: Chappell, W.R., Abernathy, C.O., Calderon, R.L. & Thomas, D.J. (Eds) *Arsenic Exposure and Health Effects V.* Amsterdam: Elsevier, pp. 391–414.

Saito, Y., Z. Yang & K. Hori. (2001) The Huanghe (Yellow River) and Changjiang (Yangtze River) deltas: a review on their characteristics, evolution and sediment discharge during the Holocene. *Geomorphology* 41, 219–231.

Saltori, R. (2004) Arsenic contamination in Afghanistan preliminary findings. *Conference on Water Quality – Arsenic Mitigation,* Taiyuan, 23–26 November, UNICEF and Water and Sanitation Group (Afghanistan).

Sancha, A.M. (1999) Full scale application of coagulation processes for arsenic removal in Chile: a successful case study. In: Chappell, W.R., Abernathy, C.O. & Calderon, R.L. (Eds) *Arsenic Exposure and Health Effects III.* Oxford: Elsevier, pp. 373–378.

Sancha, A.M. (2006a) Estimate of the current exposure to total arsenic in Chile. In: Bundschuh, J., Armienta, M.A., Bhattacharya, P., Matschullat, J., Birkle, P. & Rodriguez, R. (Eds) *Natural Arsenic in Groundwaters of Latin America.* Freiberg: Bergakademie, Abstract Volume.

Sancha, A.M. (2006b) Review of coagulation technology for removal of arsenic: case of Chile. *Journal of Health, Population and Nutrition* 24, 3, 267–272.

Sancha, A.M. & M.L. Castro. (2001) Arsenic in Latin America: occurrence, exposure, health effects and remediation. In: Chappell, W.R., Abernathy, C.O. & Calderon, R.L. (Eds) *Arsenic Exposure and Health Effects IV.* Oxford. Elsevier, pp. 87–96.

Sancha, A.M. & P. Frenz. (1998) Exposure of the current exposure of the urban population in Northern Chile to arsenic. Proceedings of Symposium on

Interdisciplinary Persepective on Drinking Water Risk Assessment and Management, Santiago, IAHS Publ. No 260, pp. 3–8.

Sanyal, S.K. & Nasar, S.K.T. (2002) Arsenic contamination of groundwater in West Bengal (India): build-up in soil-crop systems. *International Conference on Water-related Disasters*, Kolkata, 5–6 December.

Sargent-Michaud, J., K.J. Boyle & A.E. Smith. (2006) Cost effective arsenic reductions in private well water in Maine. *Journal of the American Water Resources Association* 42, 1237–1245.

Sarkar, A. & R. Mehrotra. (2005) Social dimensions of chronic arsenicosis in West Bengal (India). *Epidemiology* 16(5), 68.

Sarkar, A.R. & O.T. Rahman. (2001) *In situ Removal of Arsenic: Experiences of the DPHE–Danida*. Dhaka: DPHE and Danida, 6 pp.

Sarkar, S., A. Gupta, R.K. Biswas, A.K. Deb, J.E. Greenleaf & A.K. SenGupta. (2005) Well-head arsenic removal units in remote villages of Indian subcontinent: field results and performance evaluation. *Water Research* 39, 2196–2206

Sattran, V. & U. Wnmenga. (2002) *Geology of Burkina Faso*. Czech Geological Survey, Prague.

Saxena, V.K. (2004) *Geothermal Resources of India*. New Delhi: Allied Publishers.

Schlottmann, J.L., E.L. Mosier & G.N. Breit. (1998) Arsenic, chromium, selenium, and uranium in the Central Oklahoma Aquifer. In: *Ground Water Quality Assessment of the Central Oklahoma Aquifer, Oklahoma*. Reston, VA: U.S. Geological Survey Water-Supply Paper 2357-A, pp. 119–179.

Schoen, A., B. Beck, R. Sharma & E. Dube. (2004) Arsenic toxicity at low doses: epidemiological and mode of action considerations. *Toxicology and Applied Pharmacology* 198(3), 253.

Schoof, R. A., L.J. Yost, E. Crecelius, K. Irgolic, W. Goessler, H-R. Guo & H. Greene. (1998) Dietary arsenic intake in Taiwanese districts with elevated arsenic in drinking water. *Human Ecology and Risk Assessment* 4(1), 117–135.

Schreiber, M.E, J.A. Sino & P.G. Freiberg. (2000) Stratigraphic and geochemical controls on naturally occurring arsenic in groundwater, eastern Wisconsin, USA. *Hydrogeology Journal* 8, 161–176.

Schreiber, M.E., M.B. Gotkowitz. J.A. Simo & P.G. Freiberg. (2003) Mechanisms of arsenic release to ground water from naturally occurring substances, Eastern Substances. In: Welch, A.H. & Stollenwerk, K.G. (Eds) *Arsenic in Groundwater: Geochemistry and Occurrence*. New York: Springer-Verlag, pp. 259–280.

Schroeder, D.M. (2006) *Field experience with the SONO Filters. Evaluation Report for SIM Bangladesh.* http://www.dwc-water.com/

Schumm, S.A., J.F. Dumont & J.M. Holbrook. (2000) *Active Tectonics and Alluvial Rivers*. Cambridge University Press.

Schwenzer, S.P., C.E. Tommaseo, M. Kersten & T. Kirnbauer. (2001) Speciation and oxidation kinetics of arsenic in the thermal springs of Wiesbaden spa, Germany. *Fresenius Journal of Analytical Chemistry* 371, 927–933.

Selvin, N., J. Upton, J. Simms & J. Barnes. (2002) Arsenic treatment technology for groundwaters. Innovations in Conventional and Advanced Water Treatment Processes. *Journal of Water Supply: Research and Technology. AQUA* 2(1), 11–16.

Senanayake, N., W.A.S. de Silva & M.S.L. Salgado. (1972) Arsenical polyneuropathy – a clinical study. *Ceylon Medical Journal* 17, 195.

Sengupta, M.K., S. Ahamed, M.A. Hossain, et al. (2004) Increasing time trends in hand tubewells and arsenic contamination in affected areas of West Bengal, India. In: *5th International Conference on Arsenic: Developing Country Perspectives on Health, Water and Environmental Issues,* 15–17 February, Dhaka, Bangladesh.

Sengupta, M.K., A. Mukherjee, S. Ahamed, M.A. Hossain, B. Das, B. Nayak & D. Chakraborti. (2006a) Comment on 'Limited temporal variability of arsenic concentrations in 20 wells monitored for 3 years in Araihazar, Bangladesh'. *Environmental Science and Technology* 40(5), 1714–1715.

Sengupta, M.K., M.A. Hossain, A. Mukherjee, S. Ahamed, B. Das, B. Nayak, A. Pal & D. Chakraborti. (2006b) Arsenic burden of cooked rice: traditional and modern methods. *Food and Chemical Toxicology* 44, 1823–1829.

Sengupta, S., P.K. Mukherjee, T. Pal & S. Shome. (2004) Nature and origin of arsenic carriers in shallow aquifer sediments of Bengal Delta, India. *Environmental Geology* 45(8), 1071–1081.

Senior, L.A. & Ronald A. Sloto. (2006) *Arsenic, Boron, and Fluoride Concentrations in Ground Water in and Near Diabase Intrusions, Newark Basin, Southeastern Pennsylvania.* Reston, VA: U.S. Geological Survey Scientific Investigations Report 2006–5261. http://pubs.usgs.gov/sir/2006/5261/

Seyler, P. & J.M. Martin. (1990) Distribution of arsenite and total dissolved arsenic in major French estuaries: Dependence on biogeochemical processes and anthropogenic inputs. *Marine Chemistry* 29, 277–294.

SGU. (2005) *Mineralmarknaden. Tema: Arsenik.* Sveriges Geologiska Undersokning, Per, publ. 2005:4 [in Swedish].

Shah, B.A. (2007) Role of Quaternary stratigraphy on arsenic-contaminated groundwater from parts of Middle Ganga Plain, UP–Bihar, India. *Environmental Geology* 53(7), 1553–1561.

Shamsudhoha, A.S.M., A. Bulbul & S.M.I. Huq. (2006) Accumulation of arsenic in green algae and its subsequent transfer to soil-plant system. *Bangladesh Journal of Microbiology* 22(2), 148–151.

Shand, P., R. Hargreaves & L.J. Brewerton. (1999) *The Natural (Baseline) Quality of Groundwaters in England and Wales – the Permo-Triassic Sandstones of Cumbria, North-West England.* Keyworth: British Geological Survey and Environment Agency.

Shand, P., J. Cobbing, R. Tyler-White, A. Tooth & A. Lancaster. (2003) *Baseline Report Series: 9. The Lower Greensand of southern England.* Keyworth: British Geological Survey Report CR/03/273N for the Environment Agency.

Sheppard, S.C. (1992) Summary of phytotoxic levels of soil arsenic. *Water, Air and Soil Pollution* 64(3–4), 539–550.

Shevade, S. & R.G. Ford. (2004) Use of synthetic zeolites for arsenate removal from pollutant water. *Water Research* 38(14–15), 3197–3204.

Shih, M-C. (2005) An overview of arsenic removal by pressure-driven membrane processes. *Desalination* 172(1), 85–97.

Shimada, N. (1996) Geochemical conditions enhancing the solubilization of arsenic into groundwater in Japan. *Applied Organometallic Chemistry* 10(9), 667–674.

Shivanna, K., U.K. Sinha, T.B. Joseph, S. Sharma & S.V. Navada. (2000) Isotope hydrological investigation in arsenic infested areas of West Bengal, India.

Proceedings of International Conference on Integrated Water Resources Management for Sustainable Development, 19–21 December, New Delhi.

Shrestha, R.R., M.P. Shrestha, N.P. Upadhyay, et al. (2003) Groundwater arsenic contamination in Nepal. In: Chappell, W.R., Abernathy, C.O., Calderon, R.L. & Thomas, D.J. (Eds) *Arsenic Exposure and Health Effects V*. Amsterdam: Elsevier, pp. 25–38.

Shroder, J.F. (1993) *Himalayas to the Sea: Geology, Geomorphology and the Quaternary*. London: Routledge.

Siabi, W.K. (2004) Application of Mwacafe plant for the removal of iron and manganese. *Proceedings of the 30th WEDC International Conference*, Vientiane, Lao PDR, pp. 632–636

Sidle, W.C. (2002) O-18(SO$_4$) and O-18(H$_2$O) as prospective indicators of elevated arsenic in the Goose River ground-watershed, Maine. *Environmental Geology* 42(4), 350–359.

Sidle, W.C. & R.A. Fischer. (2003) Detection of H-3 and Kr-85 in groundwater from arsenic-bearing crystalline bedrock of the Goose River basin, Maine. *Environmental Geology* 44(7), 781–789.

Sidle, W.C., B. Wotten & E. Murphy. (2001) Provenance of geogenic arsenic in the Goose River basin, Maine, USA. *Environmental Geology* 41(1–2), 62–73, 2001.

Siegel, M.D., F. Frost & K. Tollestrup. (2002) Ecological study of bladder cancer in counties with high levels of arsenic in drinking water. *Annals of Epidemiology* 12(7), 512–513.

Signes-Pastor, A., F. Burló, K. Mitra & A.A. Carbonell-Barrachina. (2006) Arsenic biogeochemistry as affected by phosphorus fertilizer addition, redox potential and pH in a west Bengal (India) soil. *Geoderma* 137(3–4), 504–510.

Simon, N., M. Cropper, A. Alberini & S. Arora. (1999) *Valuing Mortality Reductions in India: a Study of Compensating Wage Differential*. Washington, DC: World Bank, Working Paper WPS-2078.

Simsek, C., A. Elci, O. Gunduz & A. Erdogan. (2008) Hydrogeological and hydrogeochemical characterization of a karstic mountain region. *Environmental Geology* 54(2), 291–308.

Singh, A.K. (2004) Arsenic contamination in groundwater in northeastern India. In: *Proceedings of the 11th National Symposium on Hydrology with Focal Theme on Water Quality*, National Institute of Hydrology, Rorkee, India.

Singh, I.B. (1996) Geological evolution of the Ganga Plain – an overview. *Journal of the Paleontological Society India* 41, 99–137.

Slotnick, M.J., J.R. Meliker & J.O. Nriagu. (2006) Effects of time and point-of-use devices on arsenic levels in Southeastern Michigan drinking water, USA. *Science of the Total Environment* 369(1–3), 42–50.

Smedley, P.L. & W.M. Edmunds. (2002) Redox patterns and trace-element behavior in the East Midlands Triassic Sandstone Aquifer, U.K. *Ground Water* 40(1), 44–58.

Smedley, P.L. & D.G. Kinniburgh. (2002) A review of the source, behaviour and distribution of arsenic in natural waters. *Applied Geochemistry* 17(5), 517–568.

Smedley, P.L., W.M. Edmunds & K.B. Pelig-Ba. (1996) Mobility of arsenic in groundwater in the Obuasi gold-mining area of Ghana. In: Appleton, J.D., Fuge, R. &

McCall, G.J.H. (Eds) *Environmental Geochemistry and Health. Geological Society of London Special Publication* **113**, 163–181.

Smedley, P.L., H.B. Nicolli, D.M.J. Macdonald, A.J. Barros & J.O. Tullio. (2002) Hydrogeochemistry of arsenic and other inorganic constituents in groundwaters from La Pampa, Argentina. *Applied Geochemistry* **17**(3), 259–284.

Smedley, P.L., M. Zhang, G. Zhang & Z. Luo. (2003) Mobilisation of arsenic and other trace elements in fluvio-lacustrine aquifers of the Huhhot Basin, Inner Mongolia. *Applied Geochemistry* **18**(9), 1453–1477.

Smedley, P.L., I. Neumann & R. Farrell. (2004) *Baseline Report Series: 10. The Chalk of Yorkshire and North Humberside.* Keyworth: British Geological Survey Report CR/04/128 for the Environment Agency.

Smith, A.H. & M.M. Hira-Smith. (2004) Arsenic drinking water regulations in developing countries with extensive exposure. *Toxicology* **198**(1–3), 39–44.

Smith, A.H., M. Goycolea, R. Haque & M.L. Biggs. (1998) Marked increase in bladder and lung cancer mortality in a region of northern Chile due to arsenic in drinking water. *American Journal of Epidemiology* **147**(7), 660–669.

Smith, A.H., C. Hopenhayn-Rich, M.N. Bates, et al. (1992) Cancer risks from arsenic in drinking water. *Environmental Health Perspectives* **97**, 259–267.

Smith, A.H., E.O. Lingas & M. Rahman. (2000) Contamination of drinking-water by arsenic in Bangladesh: a public health emergency. *Bulletin of the World Health Organization* **78**(9), 1093–1103.

Smith, A.H., P.A. Lopipero, M.N. Bates & C.M. Steinmaus. (2002) Arsenic Epidemiology and Drinking Water Standards. *Science* **296**(5576), 2145–2146.

Smith, A.H., G. Marshall, Y. Yuan, et al. (2006) Increased mortality from lung cancer and bronchiectasis in young adults after exposure to arsenic in utero and in early childhood. *Environmental Health Perspectives* **114**(8), 1293–1296.

Smith, A.H., C. Steinmaus, Y. Yuan, J. Liaw & M.M. Hira-Smith. (2007) High concentrations of arsenic in drinking water result in the highest known increase in mortality attributable to any environmental exposure. *Royal Geographical Society Annual Conference, London, 29 September.* http://www.geog.cam.ac.uk/research/projects/arsenic/.

Smith, E., R. Naidu & A.M. Alston. (2002) Chemistry of Inorganic Arsenic in Soils: II. Effect of Phosphorus, Sodium, and Calcium on Arsenic Sorption. *Journal of Environmental Quality* **31**, 557–563.

Smith, J.V.S., J. Jankowski & J. Sammut. (2003) Vertical distribution of As(III) and As(V) in a coastal sandy aquifer: factors controlling the concentration and speciation of arsenic in the Stuarts Point groundwater system, northern New South Wales, Australia. *Applied Geochemistry* **18**(9), 1479–1496.

Smith, N.M., R. Lee, D.T. Heitkemper, K.D. Cafferky, A. Haque & A.K. Henderson. (2006) Inorganic arsenic in cooked rice and vegetables from Bangladeshi households. *Science of the Total Environment* **370**(2–3), 294–301.

Smith, S.D. & M. Edwards. (2005) The influence of silica and calcium on arsenate sorption to oxide surfaces. *Journal of Water Supply: Research and Technology. AQUA* **54**(4), 201–211.

Smith, S.J. (2005) *Naturally Occurring Arsenic in Ground Water, Norman, Oklahoma, 2004, and Remediation Options for Produced Water.* Reston, VA: U.S. Geological Survey Fact Sheet 2005–3111.

Soil Survey Staff. (1999) *Soil Taxonomy. A Basic System of Soil Classification for Making and Interpreting Soil Surveys*, 2nd edn. Agricultural Handbook 436. Washington, DC: Natural Resources Conservation Service, U.S. Department of Agriculture.

Somasundaram, M.V., G. Ravindran & J.H. Tellam. (1993) Ground-water pollution of the Madras urban aquifer, India. *Ground Water* 31(1), 4–11.

Song, S., A. Lopez-Valdivieso, D.J. Hernandez-Campos, C. Peng, M.G. Monroy-Fernandez & I. Razo-Soto. (2005) Arsenic removal from high-arsenic water by enhanced coagulation with ferric ions and coarse calcite. *Water Research* 40(2), 364–372.

Sorg, T.J. (2002) Iron treatment for arsenic removal neglected. *Opflow* 28(11), 15.

Spallholz, J.E., L.M. Boylan & M.M. Rahman. (2004) Environmental hypothesis: is poor dietary selenium intake an underlying factor for arsenicosis and cancer in Bangladesh and West Bengal, India? *Science of the Total Environment* 323(1–3), 21–32.

Sperlich, A., A. Werner, A. Genz, G. Amy, E. Worch & M. Jekel. (2005) Breakthrough behavior of granular ferric hydroxide (GFH) fixed-bed adsorption filters: modeling and experimental approaches. *Water Research* 39(6), 1190–1198.

Squibb, K.S. & B.A. Fowler. (1983) The toxicity of arsenic and its compounds. In: Fowler, B.A. (Ed.) *Biological and Environmental Effects of Arsenic*. Amsterdam: Elsevier, pp. 233–270.

Sracek, O., P. Bhattacharya, G. Jacks, J-P. Gustafsson & M. von Brömssen. (2004) Behavior of arsenic and geochemical modeling of arsenic enrichment in aqueous environments. *Applied Geochemistry* 19(2), 169–180.

Sracek, O., M. Novák, P. Sulovský, R. Martin, J. Bundschuh & P. Bhattacharya. (2007) Mineralogical Study of Arsenic-Enriched Aquifer Sediments at Santiago del Estero, Northwest Argentina. In: Bundschuh, J., Armienta, M.A., Bhattacharya, P., Matschullat, J., Birkle, P. & Rodriguez, R. (Eds) *Natural Arsenic in Groundwaters of Latin America*. Freiberg: Bergakademie, Abstract Volume.

Sriwana, T., M.J. van Bergen, S. Sumarti, et al. (1998) Volcanogenic pollution by acid water discharges along Ciwidey River, West Java (Indonesia). *Journal of Geochemical Exploration* 62(1–3), 161–182.

Stanger, G. (2005) A paleo-hydrogeological model for arsenic contamination in southern and south-east Asia. *Environmental Geochemistry and Health* 27(4), 359–68.

Stanger, G., T.V. Truong, K.S.L.T. M. Ngoc, T.V. Luyen & T. Tran. (2005) Arsenic in groundwaters of the Lower Mekong. *Environmental Geochemistry and Health* 27(4), 341–357.

Stauder, S., B. Raue & F. Sacher. (2005) Thioarsenates in sulfidic waters. *Environmental Science and Technology* 39(16), 5933–5939.

Steinberg, L.J. & J. Hering. (2001) Variations in arsenic concentrations within a ground-water distribution system. *World Water Congress 2001*, Hanford, CA, pp. 111, 411.

Steinmaus, C., Y. Yuan, M.N. Bates & A.H. Smith. (2003) Case-control study of bladder cancer and drinking water arsenic in the western United States. *American Journal of Epidemiology* 158(12), 1193–201.

Steinmaus, C.M., Y. Yuan & A.H. Smith. (2005) The temporal stability of arsenic concentrations in well water in western Nevada. *Environmental Research* 99(2), 164–168.

Steinmaus, C.M., C.M. George, D.A. Kalman & A.H. Smith. (2006) Evaluation of two new arsenic field test kits capable of detecting arsenic water concentrations close to 10 µg/L. *Environmental Science and Technology* **40**(10), 3362–3366.

Stocker, J., D. Balluch, M. Gsell, et al. (2003) Development of a set of simple bacterial biosensors for quantitative and rapid measurements of arsenite and arsenate in potable water. *Environmental Science and Technology* **37**(20), 4743–4750.

Stollenwerk, K.G. (2003) Geochemical processes controlling the transport of arsenic in groundwater: a review of adsorption. In: Welch, A.H. & Stollenwerk, K.G. (Eds) *Arsenic in Groundwater: Geochemistry and Occurrence*. New York: Springer-Verlag, pp. 67–100.

Stollenwerk, K.G., G.N. Breit, A.H. Welch, et al. (2007) Arsenic attenuation by oxidized aquifer sediments in Bangladesh. *Science of the Total Environment* **379**(2–3), 133–150.

Stoop, W.A., N. Uphoff & A. Kassam. (2002) A review of agricultural research issues raised by the system of rice intensification (SRI) from Madagascar: opportunities for improving farming systems for resource-poor farmers. *Agricultural Systems* **71**, 249–274.

STSL. (2006) Record arsenic treatment project in El Paso, Texas. *Water and Wastewater Newsletter* **April**. Severn Trent Services Ltd. http://www.severntrent-services.com/enews/vol13.html

Stüben, D., Z. Berner, D. Chandrasekharam & J. Karmakar. (2003) Arsenic enrichment in groundwater of West Bengal, India: geochemical evidence for mobilization of As under reducing conditions. *Applied Geochemistry* **18**(9), 1417–1434.

Stummeyer, J., V. Marchig & W. Knabe. (2002) The composition of suspended matter from Ganges–Brahmaputra sediment dispersal system during low sediment transport season. *Chemical Geology* **185**(1–2), 125–147.

Stuyfzand, P.J. (1991) Nonpoint sources of trace elements in potable groundwaters in the Netherlands. *Journal of Water Supply: Research and Technology. AQUA* **9**(3–4), SS10-11–SS10-15.

Subramanian, K.S., T. Viraghavan, T. Phommavong & S. Tanjore. (1997) Manganese greensand for removal of arsenic in drinking water. *Water Quality Research Journal, Canada* **32**(3), 551–561.

Sun., G. (2004) Arsenic contamination and arsenicosis in China. *Toxicology and Applied Pharmacology* **198**(3), 268–271.

Sun, G., J. Pi, B. Li, X. Guo, H. Yamauchi & T. Yoshida. (2001) Progress on researches of endemic arsenism in China: population at risk, intervention actions and related scientific issues. In: Chappell, W.R., Abernathy, C.O. & Calderon, R.L. (Eds) *Arsenic Exposure and Health Effects IV*. Oxford. Elsevier, pp. 79–85.

Sun, G., X. Li, J. Pi, Y. Sun, B. Li, Y. Jin & Y. Xu. (2006) Current Research Problems of Chronic Arsenicosis in China. *Journal of Health, Population and Nutrition* **24**(2), 176–181.

Swartz, C.H., N.K. Blute, B. Badruzzman, et al. (2004) Mobility of arsenic in a Bangladesh aquifer: Inferences from geochemical profiles, leaching data, and mineralogical characterization. *Geochimica Cosmochimica Acta* **15**(8), 22, 4539–4557.

Swash, P. (2003) *Field Evaluation of the Wagtech Arsenator.* Report by Imperial College London based on an evaluation in Myanmar in October 2003.

Swedlund, P.J. & J.G. Webster. (1999) Adsorption and polymerisation of silicic acid on ferrihydrite, and its effect on arsenic adsorption. *Water Research* 33; 3413–3422.

Sylvester, P., P. Westerhoff, T. Möller, M. Badruzzaman & O. Boyd. (2007) A hybrid sorbent utilizing nanoparticles of hydrous iron oxide for arsenic removal from drinking water. *Environmental Engineering and Science* 24(1), 104–112.

Szramek, K., L.M. Walter & P. McCall. (2004) Arsenic mobility in groundwater/surface water systems in carbonate-rich Pleistocene glacial drift aquifers (Michigan). *Applied Geochemistry* 19(7), 1137–1155.

Talukder, A.S.M.H.M. (2005) Effect of water management and phosphorus rates on the growth of rice in a high-arsenic soil-water system. In: *Symposium on the Behaviour of Arsenic in Aquifers, Soils and Plants: Implications for Management,* Dhaka, 16–18 January. Centro Internacional de Mejoramiento de Maíz y Trigo and the U.S. Geological Survey.

Tamasi, G. & R. Cini. (2004) Heavy metals in drinking waters from Mount Amiata (Tuscany, Italy). Possible risks from arsenic for public health in the Province of Siena. *Science of the Total Environment* 327(1–3), 41–51.

Tanabe, S., K. Hori, Y. Saito, S. Harutama, V.P. Vu & A. Kitamura. (2003) Song Hong (Red River) delta evolution related to millennium scale sea level changes. *Quaternaty Science Reviews* 22, 2345–2361.

Tanskanen, H., P. Lahermo & K. Loukola-Ruskeeniemi. (2004) Arsenic in groundwater in Kittiliä, Finnish Lapland. In: Loukola-Ruskeeniemi, K. & Lahermo, P. (Eds) *Arsenic in Finland: Distribution, Environmental Impacts and Risks.* Geological Survey of Finland, pp. 123–134 [in Finnish].

Tarvainen, T., P. Lahermo, T. Hatakka, et al. (2001) Chemical composition of well water in Finland – main results of the 'one thousand wells' project. *Special Paper – Geological Survey of Finland* 31, 57–76.

Taylor, R. & K. Howard. (1994) A tectono-geomorphic model of the hydrogeology of deeply weathered crystalline rock: Evidence from Uganda. *Hydrogeology Journal* 8(3), 279–294.

Thirunavukkarasu, O. S., T. Viraraghavan, K.S. Subramanian & S. Tanjore. (2002) Organic arsenic removal from drinking water. *Urban Water* 4(4), 415–421.

Thomas, D.J. (1994) Arsenic toxicity in humans: Research problems and prospects. *Environmental Geochemistry and Health* 16(3–4), 107–111.

Thomas, D.J., M. Styblo & S. Lin. (2001) The cellular metabloism and systemic toxcity of arsenic. *Toxicology and Applied Pharmacology* 176, 127–144.

Thomas, M.F. (1994) *Geomorphology in the Tropics: a Study of Weathering and Denudation in the Tropics.* New York: Wiley, 460 pp.

Thomas, M.F. (2003) Late Quaternary sedimentary fluxes from tropical watersheds. *Sedimentary Geology* 162, 63–81.

Thomson, B.M., T.J. Cotter & J.D. Chwirka. (2003) Design and Operation of Point-of-Use Treatment System for Arsenic Removal. *Journal of Environmental Engineering* 129, 561.

Thompson, T.S., M.D. Le, A.R. Kasick & T.J. Macaulay. (1999) Arsenic in Well Water Supplies in Saskatchewan. *Bulletin of Environmental Contamination and Toxicology* 63, 478–283.

Thornton, I. (1996) Sources and pathways of arsenic in the geochemical environment: health implications. In: Appleton, J.D., Fuge, R. & McCall, G.J.H. (Eds) *Environmental Geochemistry and Health*. Geological Society of London Special Publication 113, 153–161.

Tollestrup, K, F.J. Frost, M. Christiani, G.P. McMillan, R.L. Calderon & R.S. Padilla. (2005) Arsenic induced skin conditions identified in southwest dermatology practices: an epidemiologic tool? *Environmental Geochemistry and Health* 27, 47–53.

Tondel, M., M. Rahman, A. Magnuson, I.A. Chowdhury, M.H. Faruquee & S.A. Ahmad. (1999) The relationship of arsenic levels in drinking water and the prevalence rate of skin lesions in Bangladesh. *Environmental Health Perspectives* 107(9), 727–9.

Toner, P., J. Bowman, K Clabby, et al. (2004) *Water Quality in Ireland 2001–2003*. Wexford: Environmental Protection Agency.

Torres, I.S.I. & H. Ishiga. (2003) Assessment of geochemical conditions for the release of arsenic, iron and copper into groundwater in the coastal aquifer at Yumigahama, western Japan. In: Brebbia, C.A., Almorza, D. & Sales, D. (Eds) *Water Pollution VII: Modelling. Measuring and prediction*. Southampton: WIT Press.

Trafford, J.M., A.R. Lawrence, D.M.J. MacDonald, V.D. Nguyen, D.N. Tran & T.H. Nguyen. (1996) *Impact of Urbanisation on Groundwater Quality Beneath the City of Hanoi, Vietnam*. Keyworth: British Geological Survey Technical Report WC/96/22.

Tseng, C-H. (2005) Blackfoot Disease and arsenic: a never-ending story. *Journal of Environmental Science Health, Part C: Environmental, Carcinogenic and Ecotoxicological Reviews* 23(1), 55–74.

Tseng, C.H., C.K. Chong, C.J. Chen & T.Y. Tai. (1996) Dose–response relationship between peripheral vascular disease and ingested inorganic arsenic among residents in blackfoot disease endemic villages in Taiwan. *Atherosclerosis*, 120, 125–133.

Tseng, W.P. (1977) Effects and dose–response relationships of skin cancer and Blackfoot disease with arsenic. *Environmental Health Perspectives* 19, 109–119.

Tseng, W.P., H.M. Chu, J.L. Sung & J.S. Chen. (1961) A clinical study of blackfoot disease in Taiwan: an endemic peripheral vascular disease. *Memoirs of the College of Medicine, National Taiwan University* 7, 1–18.

Tun, K.M. (2002) assessment of arsenic content in ground water and the prevalence of arsenicosis in Thabaung and Kyonpyaw Townships in Ayeyarwaddy Division, Myanmar. Clinical Research Division, Department of Medical Research, Myanmar.

Tun, T.N. (2003) Arsenic contamination of water sources in rural Myanmar. *29th WEDC International Conference*, Abuja, Nigeria, pp. 219–221.

Uchino, T., T. Roychowdhury, M. Ando & H. Tokunaga. (2006) Intake of arsenic from water, food composites and excretion through urine, hair from a studied population in West Bengal, India. *Food and Chemical Toxicology* 44(4), 455–461.

UNESCO. (1974) *Explanatory Notes for the Hydrogeological Map of Europe (Warsaw)*. Paris: UNESCO.

UNICEF. (1998) *Progothir Pathey (on the Road to Progress): Achieving the Goals for Children in Bangladesh*. United Nations Children's Fund.

UNICEF. (2004) *Arsenic Contamination in Groundwater and Drinking Water Quality Surveillance Lao PDR.* United Nations Children's Fund.

UNICEF/DPHE. (1994) *Declining Water Level Study.* Report United Nations Children's Fund and Department of Public Health Engineering (Bangladesh) by Engineering and Planning Consultants (Dhaka) and Sir M. MacDonald and Partners (UK).

UN. (2001) *Synthesis Report on Arsenic in Drinking Water.* United Nations with UNICEF, UNIDO, IAEA and World Bank.

Vaaramaa, K. & J. Lehto. (2003) Removal of metals and anions from drinking water by ion exchange. *Desalination* **155**(2), 157–170.

Vaishya, R.C. & I.C. Agarwal. (1993) Removal of arsenic(III) from contaminated ground waters by Ganga sand. *Journal of Indian Water Works Association* **25**(3), 249–253.

Van Beek, C.G.E.M. (1980) A model for the induced removal of iron and manganese from groundwater in the aquifer. *Proceedings of the 3rd Water–Rock interaction Symposium,* Edmonton, Canada, pp. 29–31.

Van Geen, A., H. Ahsan, A.H. Horneman, et al. (2002) Promotion of well-switching to mitigate the current arsenic crisis in Bangladesh. *Bulletin of the World Health Organization* **80**(9), 732–737.

Van Geen A., K.M. Ahmed, A.A. Seddique & M. Shamsudduha. (2003) Community wells to mitigate the current arsenic crisis in Bangladesh. *Bulletin of the World Health Organization* **82**, 632–638.

Van Geen A., Y. Zheng, R. Versteeg, et al. (2003a) Spatial variability of arsenic in 6000 tubewells in a 25 km² area of Bangladesh. *Water Resources Research* **39**(5), 1140.

Van Geen, A., Y. Zheng, M. Stute & K.M. Ahmed. (2003b) Comment on 'Arsenic mobility and groundwater extraction in Bangladesh'. *Science* **300**(5619), 584.

Van Geen, A., J. Rose, S. Thoral, J.M. Garnier, Y. Zheng & J.Y. Bottlero. (2004) Decoupling of As and Fe release to Bangladesh groundwater under reducing conditions. Part II: Evidence from sediment incubations. *Geochimica Cosmochimica Acta* **68**, 3475–3486.

Van Geen, A., Z. Cheng, A.A. Seddique, et al. (2005) Reliability of a commercial kit to test groundwater for arsenic in Bangladesh. *Environmental Science and Technology* **39**(1), 299–303.

Vantroyen, B., J-F. Heilier, A. Meulemans, A. Michels, J-P. Buchet, S. Vanderschueren, V. Haufroid & M. Sabbe. (2004) Survival after a lethal dose of arsenic trioxide. *Journal of Toxicol. Clinical Toxicology* **42**(6), 889–895.

Varsányi, I. & L.Ó. Kovács. (2006) Arsenic, iron and organic matter in sediments and groundwater in the Pannonian Basin, Hungary. *Applied Geochemistry* **21**(6), 949–963.

Varsányi, I., Z. Fodre & A. Bartha. (1991) Arsenic in drinking water and mortality in the Southern Great Plain, Hungary. *Environmental Geochemistry and Health* **13**, 14–22.

Violante, A. & M. Pigna. (2002) Competitive sorption of arsenate and phosphate on different clay minerals and soils. *Soil Science Society of America Journal* **66**, 1788–1796.

Virtanen, K. (2004) Arsenic in peat in the Ostrobothnian area, Northern Finland. In: Loukola-Ruskeeniemi, K. & Lahermo, P. (Eds) *Arsenic in Finland: Distribution, Environmental Impacts and Risks.* Geological Survey of Finland, pp. 51–58.

Vivona, R., E. Presosi, G. Giuliano, D. Mastroianni, F. Falconi & A. Made. (2004) Geochemical characterization of a volcanic-sedimentary aquifer in Central Italy. In: R.B. Wanty & I. Seal (Eds), Proc. *11th Int. Symp. Water-Rock Interaction* (WRI–11), pp. 513–517.

Von Brömssen, M., M. Jakariya, P. Bhattacharya, et al. (2006) Targeting low-arsenic aquifers in groundwater of Matlab Upazila, southeastern Bangladesh. *Science of the Total Environment* 379(2–3), 121–132.

Von Ehrenstein, O.S., D.N.G. Mazumder, Y. Yuan, et al. (2005) Decrements in lung function related to arsenic in drinking water in West Bengal, India. *American Journal of Epidemiology* 162(6), 533–541

Von Ehrenstein, O.S., D.N. Guha Mazumder, M. Hira-Smith, et al. (2006) Pregnancy outcomes, infant mortality, and arsenic in drinking water in West Bengal, India. *American Journal of Epidemiology* 163, 662–669.

Voronov, A.N. (2000) Some features of mineral waters in Russia. *Environmental Geology* 39(5), 477–481.

Vuki, M., J. Limtiaco, T. Aube, J. Emmanuel, G. Denton & R. Wood. (2006) Arsenic speciation study in some spring waters of Guam, Western Pacific Ocean. *Science of the Total Environment* 379(2–3), 176–179.

Walker, M., W.D. Shaw & M. Benson. (2006) Arsenic consumption and health risk perceptions in a rural western U.S. Area. *Journal of the American Water Resources Association* 42, 1363–1370.

Wang, G.Q., Y.Z. Hang, B.Y. Xiao, X.C. Qian, H. Yao, Y. Hu & Y.L. Gu. (1997) Toxicity from water containing arsenic and fluoride in Xinjiang. *Fluoride* 80(2), 81–84.

Wang, S. & C.N. Mulligan. (2006) Occurrence of arsenic contamination in Canada: Sources, behavior and distribution. *Science of the Total Environment* 366(2–3), 701–721

Wang, W., L. Yang, S. Hou, S. Tan & H. Li. (2001) Prevention of endemic arsenism with selenium. *Current Science* 81, 1215–1217.

Warner K. L. (2001) Arsenic in glacial drift aquifers and the implications for drinking water – Lower Illinois River Basin. *Ground Water* 39(3), 433–442.

Warner, K.L., A. Martin Jr. & T.L. Arnold. (2003) *Arsenic in Illinois Ground Water Community and Private Supplies.* Retford, VA: U.S. Geological Survey Water-Resources Investigations Report 03–4103.

Warren, C., W.G. Burgess & M.G. Garcia. (2002) Arsenic and fluoride in quaternary loess and alluvial aquifers at Los Pereyras, Tucumán, Argentina. In: Bocanegra, E., Martinez, D. & Massone, H. (Eds) *Groundwater and Human Development.* Proceedings of the XXXII IAH and VI ALHSUD Congress, Mar del Plata, Argentina, pp. 722–730.

Warren, C., W.G. Burgess & M.G. Garcia. (2005) Hydrochemical associations and depth profiles of arsenic and fluoride in Quaternary loess aquifers of northern Argentina. *Mineral Magazine* 69, 877–886.

Warren, G.P., B.J. Alloway, N.W. Lepp, B. Singh, F.J.M. Bochereau & C. Penny. (2003) Field trials to assess the uptake of arsenic by vegetables from contaminated soils and soil remediation with iron oxides. *Science of the Total Environment* 311(1–3), 19–33.

Wasserman, G.A., X. Liu, F. Parves, et al. (2004) Water arsenic exposure and children's intellectual function in Araihazar, Bangladesh. *Environmental Health Perspectives* 112(13), 1329–1333.

Wasserman, G.A., X. Liu, F. Parvez, et al. (2006) Water manganese exposure and children's intellectual function in Araihazar, Bangladesh. *Environmental Health Perspectives* 114, 124–129.

Watanabe, C., A. Kawata, N. Sudo, M. Sekiyama, T. Inaoka, M. Bae & R. Ohtsuka. (2004) Water intake in an Asian population living in arsenic-contaminated area. *Toxicology and Applied Pharmacology* 198(3), 272.

Webster, J.G. (1999) The source of arsenic (and other elements) in the Marbel–Matingao river catchment, Mindanao, Philippines. *Geothermics* 28(1), 95–111.

Webster, J.G. & D.K. Nordstrom. (2003) Geothermal arsenic. In: Welch, A.H. & Stollenwerk, K.G. (Eds) *Arsenic in Groundwater: Geochemistry and Occurrence.* New York: Springer-Verlag, pp. 101–126.

Webster, R.C., H.I. Maibach, L. Sedik, J. Melendres & M. Wade. (1993) In vitro and in vivo percuataneous absorption and skin decontamination of arsenic from water and soil. *Fundamental Applied Toxicology* 20, 336–340.

Wei, J., J. Yang & M. Zhao. (2005) Analysis of drinking – water type endemic arsenism in Zhengzhou. *Chinese Journal of Controlling Endemic Diseases* 20(2), 99–101 [in Chinese].

Wei, C.Y., X. Sun, C. Wang & W.Y. Wang. (2006) Factors influencing arsenic accumulation by *Pteris vittata*: a comparative field study at two sites. *Environmental Pollution* 141(3), 488–493.

Weinberg, A. (1972) Science and trans-science. *Minerva* 10, 209–222.

Welch, A.H. & M.S. Lico. (1998) Factors controlling As and U in shallow ground water, southern Carson Desert, Nevada. *Applied Geochemistry* 13(4), 521–539.

Welch, A.H., M.S. Lico & J.L. Hughes. (1988) Arsenic in ground water of the western United States. *Ground Water* 26(3), 33–347.

Welch A.H., D.B. Westjohn, D.R. Helsel & R.B. Wanty. (2000) Arsenic in groundwater of the United States: occurrence and geochemistry. *Ground Water* 38, 589–604.

Westerhoff, P., M. De Haan, A. Martindale, M. Badruzzaman. (2006) Arsenic Adsorptive Media Technology Selection Strategies. *Water Quality Research Journal, Canada* 41(2), 171–184.

Whanger, P.D., J.C. Stoner & P.H. Weswig. (1977) Arsenic levels in Oregon waters. *Environmental Health Perspectives* 19, 139–144.

Whittemore, D.O. & D. Langmuir. (1975) The solubility of ferric oxyhydroxides in natural waters. *Ground Water* 13(4), 360–365.

WHO. (1993) *Environmental Health Criteria 18: Arsenic.* Geneva: World Health Organization.

WHO. (2001) *Environmental Health Criteria 224. Arsenic and Arsenic Compounds,* 2nd edn. Geneva: World Health Organization.

Wickramasinghe, S.R., B. Han, J. Zimbron, Z. Shen & M.N. Karim. (2004) Arsenic removal by coagulation and filtration: Comparison of groundwaters from the United States and Bangladesh. *Desalination* **169**(3), 231–244

Wilkie, J.A. & J.G. Hering. (1996) Adsorption of arsenic onto hydrous ferric oxide: effects of adsorbate/adsorbent ratios and co-occurring solutes. *Colloids and Surfaces, Part A* **107**(20), 97–110.

Wilkinson, S. (2005) *A hydrogeological study of the Rarangi area, Marlborough (New Zealand).* Unpublished MSc thesis, University of Canterbury (NZ).

Williams, M. (2001) Arsenic in mine waters: an international study. *Environmental Geology* **40**(32), 267–278.

Williams, M., F. Fordyce, A. Paijitprapapon & P. Charoenchaisri. (1996) Arsenic contamination in surface drainage and groundwater in part of the southeast Asian tin belt, Nakhon Si Thammarat Province, southern Thailand. *Environmental Geology* **27**(1), 16–33.

Williams, P. (2003) *Investigating Links Between Minerals in Rice Grain and Straighthead.* Final Report. Leeton, NSW: Ricegrowers' Cooperative Ltd.

Williams, P.N., A.H. Price, A. Raab, S.A. Hossain, J. Feldmann & A.A. Meharg. (2005) Variation in arsenic speciation and concentration in paddy rice related to dietary exposure. *Environmental Science and Technology* **39**(15), 5531–40.

Williams, P.N., M.R. Islam, E.E. Adomako, A. Raab, S.A. Hossain, Y.G. Zhu, J. Feldmann & A.A. Meharg. (2006) Increase in rice grain arsenic for regions of Bangladesh irrigating paddies with elevated arsenic in groundwaters. *Environmental Science and Technology* **40**(16), 4903–4908

Williams, P.N., A. Raab, J. Feldmann & A.A. Meharg. (2007) Market basket survey shows elevated levels of as in South Central U.S. processed rice compared to California: consequences for human dietary exposure. *Environmental Science and Technology* **41**(7), 2178–2183.

Wilson, S.D., W.R. Kelly, T.R. Holm & J.L. Talbott. (2004) *Arsenic Removal in Water Treatment Facilities: Survey of Geochemical Factors and Pilot Plant Experiments.* Illiinois Waste Management and Research Center, 79 pp.

Wolthers M., L. Charlet, C.H. van der Weijden, P.R. van der Linde & D. Rickard. (2005) Arsenic mobility in the ambient sulfidic environment: Sorption of arsenic(V) and arsenic(III) onto disordered mackinawite. *Geochimica Cosmochimica Acta* **69**(14), 3483–3492.

Woolson, E.A. & A.R. Isensee. (1981) Soil residue accumulation from three applied arsenic sources. *Weed Science* **29**, 17–22.

World Bank. (2005) *Towards a More Effective Operational Response: Arsenic Contamination of Groundwater in South and East Asian Countries. Vol. 1: Policy Report; Vol. 2: Technical Report.*

WSP. (2003) *Willingness to Pay for Arsenic-free, Safe Drinking Water in Bangladesh.* Water and Sanitation Program, World Bank and BRAC.

Wu, M.M., T.L. Kuo, Y.H. Hwang & C.J. Chen. (1989) Dose–response relation between arsenic concentration in well water and mortality from cancers and vascular diseases. *American Journal of Epidemiology* **130**, 1123–1132.

Wyatt, C.J., C. Fimbres, L. Romo, R. O. Méndez & M. Grijalva. (1998) Incidence of heavy metal contamination in water supplies in northern Mexico. *Environmental Research* **76**(2), 114–119.

Wyllie, J. (1937) An investigation of the source of arsenic in a well water. *Canadian Journal of Public Health* **28**, 128.

Wynne, B. (1980) Technology, risk and participation: on the social treatment of uncertainty. In: Conrad, J. (Ed.) *Society, Technology and Risk*. London: Academic Press, pp. 83–107.

Wynne, B. (1994) Scientific knowledge and the global environment. In: Redclift, M. & Benton, T. (Eds) *Social Theory and the Global Environment*. London: Routledge, pp. 169–189.

Xia, Y. & J. Liu. (2004) An overview on chronic arsenism via drinking water in PR China. *Toxicology* **198**(1–3), 25–29.

Yan, W., R.H. Dilday, T.H. Tai, et al. (2005) Differential response of rice germplasm to straighthead disease by arsenic. *Crop Science* **45**, 1223–1228.

Yanez, J., H. Mansilla, V. Fierro, et al. (2006) Arsenic exposure in rural population from Atacama Desert, Chile: characterization of arsenic species in water, urine, hair and nails. In: Bundschuh, J., Armienta, M.A., Bhattacharya, P., Matschullat, J., Birkle, P. & Rodriguez, R. (Eds) *Natural Arsenic in Groundwaters of Latin America*. Freiberg: Bergakademie, Abstract Volume.

Yang, C-Y. (2004) Reduction in kidney cancer mortality following installation of a tap water supply system in an arsenic-endemic area of Taiwan. *Archives of Environmental Health* **484**, 484–489.

Yang, L., P.J. Peterson, W.P. Williams, et al. (2002) The relationship between exposure to arsenic concentrations in drinking water and the development of skin lesions in farmers from inner Mongolia, China. *Environmental Geochemistry and Health* **24**(4), 293–303.

Yang, S., H-S. Jung & C. Li. (2004) Two unique weathering regimes in the Changjiang and Huanghe drainage basins: geochemical evidence from river sediments. *Sedimentary Geology* **164**(1–2), 219–34.

Yen, F.S., C.N. Long & T.H. Lu. (1980) An environmental model of high arsenic concentration in the groundwater aquifer of Taiwan. *Journal of Taiwan Environmental Sanitation* **12**(1), 66–80 [in Chinese].

Yu, G., D. Sun & Y. Zheng. (2007) Health effects of exposure to natural arsenic in groundwater and coal in China: an overview of occurrence. *Environmental Health Perspectives* **115**, 636–642

Yu, W.H., C.M. Harvey & C.F. Harvey. (2003) Arsenic in groundwater in Bangladesh: a geostatistical and epidemiology framework for evaluating health effects and potential remedies. *Water Resources Research* **39**(6), 17.

Yuan, Y., G. Marshall, C. Ferreccio, et al. (2007) Acute myocardial infarction mortality in comparison with lung and bladder cancer mortality in arsenic-exposed Region II in Chile from 1950 to 2000. *American Journal of Epidemiology* **166**, 1381–1391.

Zamfirescu, F., A. Danchiv, M. Bretotean & S. Wagstaff. (1999) Impact of intense urban abstraction on the regional aquifer beneath Bucharest, Romania. In: P.J. Chilton (Ed.). *Groundwater in the urban environment*. Balkema, Rotterdam.

Zarate, M.A. (2003) Loess of southern South America. *Quaternaty Science Reviews* **22**, 1987–2006.

Zhang, H. (2004) Heavy-metal pollution and arseniasis in Hetao region, China. *Ambio* **33**(3), 138–140.

Zhang, H., D. Ma & X. Hu. (2002) Arsenic pollution in groundwater from Hetao Area, China. *Environmental Geology* 41(6), 638–643.

Zheng, Y. (2007) The heterogeneity of arsenic in the crust: a linkage to occurrence in groundwater. *Quaternary Sciences* 27(1), 6–19.

Zheng, Y., M. Stute, A. van Geen, et al. (2004) Redox control of arsenic mobilization in Bangladesh groundwater. *Applied Geochemistry* 19(2), 201–214.

Zheng, Y., A van Geen, M. Stute, et al. (2005) Geochemical and hydrogeological contrasts between shallow and deeper aquifers in two villages of Araihazar, Bangladesh: Implications for deeper aquifers as drinking water sources. *Geochimica Cosmochimica Acta* 69, 5203–5218.

Zhenming, L., L. Zhongjie & Z. Lehong. (2000) An investigation in endemic arsenic disease in Jilin Province. *Chinese Journal of Controlling Endemic Diseases* 15(2), 77–79 [in Chinese].

Zhou, J., W. Zhu & X. Huang. (2004a) A survey of endemic arsenasis in Zhejiang Province. *Zhejiang Preventative Medicine* 16(7), 1–2 [in Chinese].

Zhou, J., X. Huang & W. Zhu. (2004b) Investigation and study of endemic arsenism in Tong Xiang City. *Chinese Journal of Controlling Endemic Disease* 19, 1 [in Chinese].

Zierold, K.M., L. Knobeloch & H. Anderson. (2004) Prevalence of chronic diseases in adults exposed to arsenic-contaminated drinking water. *American Journal of Public Health* 94(11), 1936–1937.

Zobrist, J., P.R. Dowdle, J.A. Davis & R.S. Oremland. (2000) Mobilization of arsenite by dissimilatory reduction of adsorbed arsenate. *Environmental Science and Technology* 34(22), 4747–4753.

Index

Note: Page numbers in *Italics* refer to figures and those in **bold** refer to tables.